Handbook of Experimental Pharmacology

Continuation of Handbuch der experimentellen Pharmakologie

Vol. 78

The Tetracyclines

Contributors

R. K. Blackwood · J. H. Boothe · I. Chopra · B. A. Cunha
J. J. Goodman · R. H. Gustafson · J. J. Hlavka · Z. Hošťálek
J. S. Kiser · W. Rogalski · Z. Vaněk

Editors

J. J. Hlavka and J. H. Boothe

Springer-Verlag Berlin Heidelberg New York Tokyo

J. J. Hlavka
American Cyanamid Company,
Medical Research Division, Lederle Laboratories,
Pearl River, NY 10987, USA

J. H. Boothe
418 E. Longport, P.O. Box 1004,
Ocean Gate, NJ 08740, USA

With 77 Figures

Library of Congress Cataloging in Publication Data. Main entry under title: The Tetracyclines. (Handbook of experimental pharmacology; vol. 78) Includes index. 1. Tetracyclines. I. Blackwood, R. K. II. Hlavka, J. J. (Joseph J.), 1927– . III. Boothe, J. H. (James H.), 1916– . IV. Series: Handbook of experimental pharmacology; v. 78). QP905.H3 vol. 78 615'.1 s [615'.329] 85–2793 [RM666.T33]

ISBN-13: 978-3-642-70306-5 e-ISBN-13: 978-3-642-70304-1

DOI: 10.1007/978-3-642-70304-1

Softcover reprint of the hardcover 1st edition 1985

2122/3130-543210

List of Contributors

R. K. Blackwood, Medical Research Laboratories, Central Research, Pfizer Inc., Groton, CT 06340, USA

J. H. Boothe, 418 E. Longport, P.O. Box 1004, Ocean Gate, NJ 08740, USA

I. Chopra, Department of Microbiology, University of Bristol, The Medical School, University Walk, Bristol BS8 1TD, Great Britain

B. A. Cunha, Chief, Infectious Disease Division, Department of Medicine, Nassau Hospital, 259 First Street, Mineola, NY 11501, USA

J. J. Goodman, Medical Research Division, American Cyanamid Company, Lederle Laboratories, Pearl River, NY 10965, USA

R. H. Gustafson, American Cyanamid Company, Agricultural Research Division, P.O. Box 400, Princeton, NJ 08540, USA

J. J. Hlavka, American Cyanamid Company, Medical Research Division, Lederle Laboratories, Pearl River, NY 10987, USA

Z. Hošťálek, Czechoslovak Academy of Sciences, Institute of Microbiology, Vídeňská 1083, CS-14220 Praha 4-Krč

J. S. Kiser, 930 North Florida Ave, De Land, FL 32720, USA

W. Rogalski, E. Merck, Pharmaceutical Research, Frankfurter Str. 250, D-6100 Darmstadt 1

Z. D. Vaněk, Czechoslovak Academy of Sciences, Institute of Microbiology, Vídeňská 1083, CS-14220 Praha 4-Krč

Preface

The history of antibiotics may well have begun with the ancient Sudanese-Nubian civilization (see Chapter 1, "Historical Introduction"), but this volume reflects a more contemporary appraisal of the antibiotic era. We have compiled a comprehensive review of the tetracyclines which includes all the major subdivisions of these chemically important and clinically useful antibiotics.

There can be little doubt about the contribution of antibiotics to both the increase in human life span and the alleviation of much human suffering. The tetracyclines are still playing an important role in these areas and will continue to do so in the foreseeable future.

We hope this volume will be an important contribution to a better understanding of the chemistry, biochemistry, and medical aspects of tetracycline antibiotics.

We are indebted to the individual authors who have given so much of their time and effort in the preparation of the chapters.

Pearl River, NY
Ocean Gate, NJ

Joseph J. Hlavka
James H. Boothe

Contents

E. Regulation of the Biosynthesis of Tetracyclines 159

CHAPTER 5

Chemical Modification of the Tetracyclines. W. ROGALSKI
With 46 Figures

CHAPTER 6

Mode of Action of the Tetracyclines and the Nature of Bacterial Resistance to Them

I. CHOPRA. With 27 Figures

CHAPTER 7

Clinical Uses of the Tetracyclines. B. A. CUNHA

CHAPTER 8

Nonmedical Uses of the Tetracyclines. R. H. GUSTAFSON and J. S. KISER

CHAPTER 1

Historical Introduction

J. H. BOOTHE and J. J. HLAVKA

The tetracyclines have been an important component in the treatment of bacterial infections since their discovery in 1948. During this time the literature relating to these antibiotics has become quite voluminous, complex, and scattered among publications in many different scientific disciplines and languages. Numerous reviews of specific areas have been written in the past, such as the recent comprehensive review by MITSCHER (1978), but the present work is, to our knowledge, the first attempt to combine reviews of all the major subdivisions from chemistry to clinical applications of the tetracyclines in one volume. It should be understood, however, that no review could (or should) contain every literature reference to the subject being reviewed, but rather that important and pertinent literature be selected to illustrate the various chapters.

The history of antibiotics began with the often-told events related to the observations of penicillin activity by Fleming in 1928, the rediscovery and purification by Florey and Chain in 1938, and the large-scale development and clinical use of penicillin during World War II. By 1946–1947, the problems related to penicillin production had essentially been solved. The material was readily available at a reasonable price, and in fact the world's needs could be satisfied by a few large efficient pharmaceutical producers. Stimulated by the tremendous successes of penicillin, many of the drug companies and academic institutions now began to search for new antibiotics by screening soil samples for antibiotic-producing microorganisms. Such a screening program was established at Lederle Laboratories and surprisingly quickly the producer of what became known as chlortetracycline or Aureomycin was discovered (DUGGAR 1948). In retrospect, the early discovery of the penicillin and the tetracycline families of antibiotics seems especially fortuitous since large screening programs in the succeeding 30–40 years have discovered relatively few, new and useful families of antibiotics even though about 6,000 antibiotics have now been described in the literature.

Chlortetracycline was introduced to the medical profession in 1948 and was enthusiastically accepted on the basis of its merits. It first of all inhibited a much wider spectrum of microorganisms than the then available penicillins, covering not only the gram-positive organisms but many of the gram-negative ones as well. Secondly, it was orally active, being very well absorbed from the stomach and upper small intestine. The second member of the family, oxytetracycline, was discovered independently by the Charles Pfizer Company and introduced in 1950 (FINDLAY et al. 1950). In 1953, the nomenclature parent of the series, tetracycline, was discovered (BOOTHE et al. 1953; CONOVER et al. 1953) and introduced, and rather quickly became the favorite of the medical profession. Tetracycline was discovered almost simultaneously as a product of reductive dechlorination of chlortetracycline and as a fermentation product of a *Streptomyces* species (MINIERI et al. 1953, 1954). The study of mutant strains of *Streptomyces*, both natural and induced, undertaken in attempts to improve fermentation yields, provided the next medically useful tetracycline, 6-demethylchlortetracycline (McCORMICK et al. 1957). This compound provided clinically useful antibiotic blood levels for longer periods, thus permitting the use of lower dose levels to produce the same therapeutic effect.

The remaining medically useful members of the tetracycline family, rondomycin (BLACKWOOD et al. 1963), doxycycline (STEPHENS et al. 1963), and minocycline (MARTELL and BOOTHE 1967) were all the results of lengthy programs of chemical modification of members of the naturally occurring tetracyclines. These semisynthetic tetracyclines will be reviewed in some detail later in this book, but briefly these compounds offer improved therapeutic efficacy in the areas of potency, serum half-life, and, in some cases, broadened spectrum of activity.

Having reviewed the relatively brief, 50-year history of antibiotics in medicine, and the even shorter history of the tetracyclines, it should be noted that these compounds probably played a role in ancient history that has not yet been fully appreciated or studied. In 1980, a group of anthropologists from the University of Massachusetts observed fluorescent areas in bones obtained from an ancient (350 A.D.) Sudanese-Nubian civilization. These fluorescent areas were identical both as to location in the bone and fluorescent characteristics to modern bone from patients treated with tetracycline antibiotics (BASSETT et al. 1980). This observation has been at least partially confirmed by fluorescence spectrum measurements and by microbiological inhibition studies of the old bone (BOOTHE 1984). The deposition of tetracycline antibiotics in developing bones and teeth as a very stable calcium chelate complex was observed early in biological studies. In fact, it is the basis for the recommendation that children below the age of 8 years should not be treated with tetracyclines because of occasional teeth staining.

If we assume that at least some ancient civilizations were exposed to tetracycline antibiotics (and perhaps to other antibiotics which were less stable and thus decomposed in the intervening years) the question arises as to the source. The most likely answer seems to be that they were produced during the growth of an antibiotic-producing organism either in stored grain or in some fermented liquid such as a beer.

It may be instructive to make future determinations as to which competing civilizations were exposed to these antibiotics, for example, the Greeks or the Persians, the Romans or the Carthaginians, the Philistines or the Israelites.

The scientific and medical history of the tetracycline antibiotics seems to have been paralleled by a long and complicated series of legal entanglements. It often seemed that the legal minds were as numerous and as active as the scientific ones. Some of the more prominent of these legal affairs are briefly described: (1) In the late 1950s a number of cultures of tetracycline-producing streptomycetes, along with much technical information, were stolen from the Lederle Laboratories by a few employees and sold to some foreign producers. The solving of the case and the prosecution of the leader is described in some detail in *The Million Dollar Bugs* (PEARSON 1969), which makes a lively detective yarn. (2) Congressional hearings on the questions of pricing and price fixing were held by various committees over a number of years beginning in 1959 with those held by the late Senator Estes Kefauver. (3) The Federal Trade Commission held hearings and proceedings at various times from 1958 to 1968 which resulted in an order to allow open licensing of tetracycline. (4) Criminal proceedings involving conspiracy to fix prices were brought in 1961 by the US Department of Justice against the five companies who made and sold tetracycline antibiotics. The companies were first convicted of price fixing, but the US Court of Appeals later reversed the conviction, and the reversal was affirmed by the US Supreme Court. The case was remanded for a new trial, and on retrial the companies were found not guilty. (5) The original conviction for price fixing stimulated the filing of civil suits by large users of tetracycline to recover overpayments. One hundred and fifty-eight treble damage actions were filed, many of which were settled before the reversal of the conviction. After the price-fixing conviction was reversed, the civil suits were based mainly on the contention that the original patent on tetracycline had been obtained fraudulently by withholding information from the patent examiner. The most recent and final judicial decision has affirmed the validity of the 1955 tetracycline patent and the last legal action against the companies was dropped in 1982.

References

Bassett EJ, Keith MS, Armelagos GJ, Martin DL, Villanueva AR (1980) Tetracycline labeled human bone from ancient Sudanese Nubia (A.D. 350). Science 209:1532

Blackwood RK, Beereboom JJ, Rennhard HH, Schach von Wittenau M, Stephens CR (1963) 6-Methylenetetracyclines. III. Preparation and properties. J Am Chem Soc 85:3943

Boothe JH, Morton J, Petisi JP, Wilkinson RG, Williams JH (1953) Tetracycline. J Am Chem Soc 75:4621

Boothe JH (to be published) Tetracycline antibiotics in an ancient civilization. Science

Conover LH, Moreland WT, English AR, Stephens CR, Pilgrim FJ (1953) Terramycin. XI. Tetracycline. J Am Chem Soc 75:4622

Duggar BM (1948) Aureomycin. Ann NY Acad Sci 51:177

Findlay AC, Hobby GL, Pan SY, Regna JB, Routien DB, Seeley DB, Shull GM, Sobin BA, Solomens IA, Vinson JW, Kane JH (1950) Terramycin, a new antibiotic. Science 111:85

Martell MJ, Boothe JH (1967) The 6-deoxytetracyclines. VII. Alkylated aminotetracyclines possessing unique antibacterial activity. J Med Chem 10:44

McCormick JRD, Sjolander NO, Hirsch U, Jensen ER, Doerschuk AP (1957) A new family of antibiotics: The demethyltetracyclines. J Am Chem Soc 79:4561

Minieri PP, Firman MC, Mistretta AG, Abbey A, Bricker CE, Rigler NE, Sokol H (1953–1954) A new broad spectrum antibiotic product of the tetracycline group. Antibiotics Annual. Proc Symposium Antibiotics, Washington DC, pp 81–87

Mitscher LA (1978) The chemistry of the tetracycline antibiotics. In: Medicinal research, vol 9. Dekker, New York

Pearson M (1969) The million dollar bugs. Putnam, New York

Stephens CR, Beereboom JJ, Rennhard HH, Gordon PN, Murai K, Blackwood RK, Schach von Wittenau M (1963) 6-Deoxytetracyclines. IV. Preparation C-6 stereochemistry, and reactions. J Am Chem Soc 85:2643

CHAPTER 2

Fermentation and Mutational Development of the Tetracyclines

J. J. GOODMAN

A. Introduction

The first of the tetracycline family of antibiotics, chlortetracycline (CTC), was introduced over 3 decades ago (DUGGAR 1948) and in the following years, with the introduction of new members of the family, the tetracyclines have retained their importance in both human therapy and animal feed use. According to reports of the US Tariff Commission, annual production is in the order of 11,000–13,000 tonnes. Numerous reviews dealing with the pathways of biosynthesis and the genetics and biochemistry of the producing organisms have appeared and these will be cited in the appropriate sections. The production aspects of the fermentation and the factors leading to higher yields have been dealt with less frequently and this is understandable in view of the proprietary nature of much of the information. An excellent review by DI MARCO and PENNELLA appeared in 1959 (DI MARCO and PENNELLA 1959) and the most recent general review is by HOSTALEK et al. (1979). A great deal of the pertinent information is to be found in the patent literature, where, again for obvious reasons, only minimal disclosures are often made. A compendium giving excerpts from the United States patent literature appeared in 1968 (EVANS 1968). This review will attempt to deal with the fermentation and mutational development of the tetracyclines from the practical perspective of increasing fermentation potencies. The large number of enzymes and individual steps involved in biosynthesis and the large number of possible compounds on the pathway to the final products (see HOSTALEK et al. 1974 for a review) can all have a potential effect on ultimate yield. As products of fermentation the tetracyclines are "mature" products. If a recent report (BASSETT et al. 1980) on their detection in ancient bones holds up, their existence predates the antibiotic era by at least 1,400 years! In the modern antibiotic era as products mature, improved production strains come along more slowly and useful media combinations are more likely already to have been tested. Maintenance of high yields becomes increasingly a matter of constant attention to small details rather than through some dramatic change. As more sophisticated production technologies get locked in place it becomes more difficult to introduce changes. The gap between tank results and shaken flask results becomes wider though one may hope that the latter will still be predictive of the potential of a new strain or medium ingredient.

This review will include both older as well as the more recent literature citations. Where no specific organism is stated all reference to oxytetracycline (OTC) production will be by *Streptomyces rimosus*, and similarly unless otherwise stated in the text references to production of any of the other tetracyclines will be by

S. aureofaciens. Citations will all be from the published literature. In some instances the citation will refer to Chemical Abstracts rather than to the original publication, which was not available. In such cases, however, the abstract was judged to be sufficiently complete to be used in the context of the particular discussion.

B. The Producing Microorganisms

I. Morphology and Ultrastructure

When grown on agar media of diverse composition, the tetracycline producers display wide variations in colonial morphology. The morphology in submerged culture exhibits less variability, but in both *S. aureofaciens* and *S. rimosus* differences between high and low producing variants can be distinguished and differences between favorable and infavorable production conditions are reflected in the morphology of the submerged mycelium.

Studies by a number of investigators (Van Dyck and De Somer 1952; Biffi et al. 1954; Boretti et al. 1955; Scotti and Zocchi 1955; Di Marco 1956) all confirm the two-phase nature of the submerged mycelial growth. These phases may be further subdivided into five to six stages based not only on the morphology but also on the biochemical and productive activity of the mycelium (Doskocil et al. 1958, 1959). The exact timing of the transitions varies with strains and with the medium used. The initial hyphae are thick and branched, heavily basophilic, and rapidly growing. They are characterized by an abundant synthesis of nucleic acids. These hyphae in turn give way to the thinner more lightly staining hyphae characteristic of the productive phase, exhibiting no protein or RNA synthesis and having a much lower growth rate. During the rapid early growth stage, which may last for the first 10–12 h, phosphate is rapidly utilized and its exhaustion triggers the beginning of the productive stage.

Addition of phosphate to media otherwise favorable to antibiotic production causes a change in the normal sequences of mycelial morphology that accompanies the unfavorable effect on antibiotic production (Boretti et al. 1955; Prokofieva-Belgovskaya and Popova 1959). There is an increase in the number of thick hyphae; they remain basophilic and do not differentiate into the thinner productive form. There is an increase in the ratio of nuclear to cytoplasmic elements in the mycelium which also becomes rich in the so-called volutin granules, polyphosphates, in both *S. aureofaciens* and *S. rimosus* (Prokofieva-Belgovskaya and Kats 1960). Both DNA and RNA are detectable in the mycelium at all stages of development but DNA is more difficult to detect in the early stages due to the masking effect of unused medium ingredients (Guberniev et al. 1960).

Some differences between *S. aureofaciens* and *S. rimosus* can be distinguished. *S. rimosus* consistently exhibits a fragmentation phase following the first growth of the primary mycelium (Doskocil et al. 1958). This is of particular importance from the standpoint of inoculum since it serves to increase greatly the number of growth centers available for starting subsequent fermentation cycles. Tresner et al. (1967) noted distinctive thickened arthrospore entomoid-like structures characteristic of *S. aureofaciens* grown in submerged culture in broths containing 2%–4% peptone. Such structures were only sparingly produced, if at all, in other media.

BEKHTEREVA and KOLESNIKOVA (1961) subjected an aging culture of *S. aureofaciens*, whose mycelium had already lost its basophilic property and which contained large volutin granules, to continuous culture. Within 27 h there was a resurgence of basophilic hyphae with homogeneous cytoplasm characteristic of young nonproducing hyphae. This condition was maintained for 5 days, during which little CTC was produced. ZASLAVSKAYA et al. (1977) studied a nonproducing proactinomycete-like variant and a producing culture of *S. aureofaciens* without and with the controlled periodic addition of nutrients to prolong the biosynthetically active phase. Without nutrient addition the producing culture exhibited widespread hyphal fragmentation and thickening of cell walls characteristic of the final stages of culture growth. With nutrient addition this stage was delayed and viable cells persisted for a longer period. The inactive mutant exhibits very early thickening of cell walls and fragmentation of hyphae compared with the producing strain.

It has been known for some time that the antibiotic itself is associated with insoluble precipitates formed in the medium as growth and synthesis progress (NIEDERCORN 1952). The amount of antibiotic free in the medium depends upon the solubility of the Ca^{2+} or Mg^{2+} complexes of the antibiotic at the pH of the fermentation broth. ZELINKOVA et al. (1976b) found 10% of the CTC to be excreted into the medium with the remainder bound up in the mycelium. This ratio of course depends upon the potency of the particular broth. ROSOVA and ZELINKA (1968) found that at all stages of the fermentation the CTC present was associated with insoluble cellular material. It is concentrated in the sediment after centrifugation of a mycelial homogenate at 30,000 × g. KURYLOWICZ and MALINOWSKY (1970, 1971, 1972a, b) examined the surface structure and the ultrastructure of both high and low, 4,000 and 100 µg/ml, tetracycline (TC) producers by electron microscopy. In the high-producing variant, bubble-like substructures originating from the external cell layers of the mycelium begin to form at about 48 h. These substructures increase in number and size, reaching dimensions of 30–60 nm. They were shown to contain 70% of the total antibiotic and to disintegrate and release the antibiotic on treatment with oxalic acid without damage to the remaining mycelium. The low-yielding strain has few of these substructures associated with it. Sections through the mycelium of the high-yielding variant show internal double-walled tubular structures, mesosomes, and vacuoles present to a high degree. These internal structures appear to be associated with the secretion of the antibiotic toward the outer layers of the cellular membrane, where it is excreted in association with the bubble-like external substructures. These phenomena were also found in an intermediate degree in a 6-demethylchlortetracycline (DMCTC)-producing strain of intermediate potency – 1,000 µg/ml. Lipids also appear to participate in the transport of antibiotic through the membranous structures. Analysis of lyophilized mycelium of both low- and high-producing variants show that over 90% of the cellular lipids are in the membranous structures (KURYLOWICZ and MALINOWSKI 1972b). In the high producers the ratio of saturated to unsaturated fatty acids in the mycelial lipids is 1.26–1.39 and in the lower producers it is 0.86–0.89 and these ratios remain constant with time. WILLIAMS et al. (1977) and KURYLOWICZ (1977) find similar globular structures present in a number of antibiotic-producing actinomycetes, *S. noursei*, *S. erythreus*, and *S. vinaceus*; but interestingly *S. rimosus* was not reported on. LUDVIK et al. (1971, 1973), on examining *S. aureofaciens* by transmission and scanning electron microscopy, have in general confirmed the previous observations and the differences to be found in high- and low-yielding variants. ZASLAVSKAYA et al. (1977) also confirm to a large degree the existence of the globular structures in *S. aureofaciens* and their absence in a nonproducing proactinomycete-like variant.

In all of these more recent electron microscopic observations, as well as the earlier ones using light microscopy, the substructures seen and the morphological phases of the developmental cycles are associated with antibiotic production. This is especially true when comparing high- and low-yielding variants, but which is cause and which is effect? The sequence of changes observable in batch culture does not occur under the conditions of continuous culture, where at any given time the concentration of antibiotic is much lower. Poor producers or good producers grown under conditions unfavorable to antibiotic production do not go through the sequences characteristic of good antibiotic production.

It is interesting to speculate whether mycelial monitoring might be used to keep a fermentation "on track." Such monitoring might well reveal changes ahead of other parameters being measured and allow earlier corrective action to be taken. LAZNIKOVA and DMITRIEVA (1973) found that the structure of 72-h mycelium as revealed by sucrose density gradient centrifugation could be used to draw conclusions on the course of the fermentation.

II. Mutation and Strain Selection

The genetics of antibiotic producers and production has been extensively dealt with in a number of reviews. Among those which deal in part with the tetracyclines are the following: ALIKHANIAN (1962, 1979), ALIKHANIAN and DANILENKO (1979), CALLAM (1970), DEMAIN (1973), ELANDER (1966, 1976), ELANDER et al. (1977), HOPWOOD (1974, 1976, 1978), HOPWOOD and MERRICK (1977), HOPWOOD and CHATER (1980), QUEENER (1976), and QUEENER et al. (1978). Among reviews dealing specifically with the genetics of tetracycline producers and production may be mentioned the following: ALIKHANIAN et al. (1959), BLUMAUROVA et al. (1971, 1972), HOSTALEK et al. (1971, 1974), and VANEK et al. (1971, 1973). In the case of the tetracyclines, the mutational approach to yield improvement has been the most productive, and a number of papers dealing specifically with the relative effectiveness of a variety of mutational agents may be cited: MRACEK et al. (1969), BLUMAUEROVA et al. (1971, 1973), and JARAI (1962). In addition to yield improvement, the induction of mutants has several other goals which are not mutually exclusive: (1) to provide new, modified antibiotics, (2) to provide blocked mutants which can be used to elucidate biosynthetic pathways or to provide intermediates for synthetic work, and (3) to provide suitable nutrition and resistance markers to be used for genetic analysis.

Use of mutation as a tool for yield improvement is more likely to be immediately productive during the early years of development of an antibiotic than at a later date, where a more "mature" antibiotic calls for a more sophisticated approach. In the very initial stages, natural selection without mutation treatments can lead to improved variants. From its first discovery it was evident that *S. aureofaciens* as found in nature is a highly variable species (BACKUS et al. 1954; DUGGAR et al. 1954). *Streptomyces rimosus* is also a variable species. NYIRI (1961) studied three different strains and their natural and mutagen-induced variants for growth, and morphological, physiological, and biochemical properties on a number of media and concluded that there were only a few properties which would serve as being unequivocally characteristic of the species. The best of these were colony form and shape of sporangia and spores. RUDAYA and SOLOVEVA (1960) subjected four diverse strains of *S. rimosus* to a variety of cultivation conditions of pH, temperature, media, etc. and found that a single strain could give rise to diverse variants but also that identical variants could arise from different strains. They emphasized the importance of this natural variability to taxonomy. If to the natural variability is added the variability induced by mutagens the consequences for species designation are great indeed. The formation of a specific product is not a reliable criterion; for instance, PREOBRAZHENSKAYA et al. (1961) described a newly isolated strain which produced OTC but was taxonomically *Actinomyces* (*Streptomyces*) *aureofaciens* and was given the varietal designation *oxytetracyclini* var. nov. PETTY (1961) has addressed himself to the problem of species designation in the tetracycline producers, and the legal patent implications were discussed by WHITTENBURG (1970). The recent adoption of an approved list of bacterial names by the International Committee on Systematic Bacteriology (SKERMAN et al. 1980) should serve to reduce the problem of proliferation of species names.

The mutation treatments used for the tetracyclines differ little from those described by FANTINI (1975) for use with newly isolated antibiotic producers synthesizing low levels of an antibiotic. It is the selection process after mutational treatment that requires the skill born of experience. It requires a knowledge of the inherent variability of the organism and a keen eye for recognizing small and perhaps unique morphological or color variations which lead to variants with higher productivity or greater stability or indeed to variants producing new tetracyclines. In the latter case the ready availability of a variety of assay methods can play an important role when discrepancies in results may be indicative of the presence of new entities.

The discovery of a 5a-(11a)-dehydro CTC producer (MCCORMICK et al. 1958a; GROWICH and MILLER 1961) was the result of a simultaneous program in which inactive mutants were not discarded but were screened as well in a blocked mutant program. The product was important as a key intermediate in several potential alternative routes to an active tetracycline, but of ultimate greater importance was the role of the producing strain S-1308, as the starting point for a series of investigations by MCCORMICK and co-workers leading to the elucidation of the pathways of tetracycline biosynthesis. This work has been reviewed in a number of papers by MCCORMICK (1966, 1967, 1968).

The original strains carrying a block in C6 methylation (MCCORMICK et al. 1957a, 1959b) produced CTC and TC along with the demethylated analogues. They were also characterized by a reddish purple pigment in the colony itself on agar and in liquid culture. This characteristic was then used in future selection work. It enabled GROWICH (1971a) to select strains which no longer made any CTC or TC but only the 6-demethylated analogues and even strains making exclusively DMTC. Color differences exhibited in liquid culture could be characterized and quantitated by means of reflectance curves. A similar application of color observation and reflectance curves enabled GROWICH and DEDUCK (1963) to recognize strains producing exclusively TC. Similar attention to color variation has enabled others (HSU et al. 1974; CHENG and LI 1975; CHENG et al. 1975) also to select for 6-demethylating strains of *S. aureofaciens* after mutation treatments. This can be done without any knowledge of how or where the block in C6 methylation occurs.

Sulfonamides were found (GOODMAN and MATRISHIN 1961; PERLMAN et al. 1961) to cause normal CTC/TC procedures to synthesize the demethylated analogues. This observation was then used by ZAITSEVA and MINDLIN (1965) to isolate mutants with increasing resistance to sulfonamides which synthesized 2%–16% of the total antibiotic as the demethylated analogues even in the absence of sulfonamide addition. These mutants were deficient for, and could be reversed by the addition of, *p*-aminobenzoic (PABA) acid. None of the American Cyanamid Company strains show such a deficiency for PABA.

A patent granted to CHINOIN (1963) disclosed the use of both sulfonamide- and aminopterin- or amethopterin-(NEIDLEMAN 1962; NEIDLEMAN et al. 1963a) containing agars to select recombinant colonies of *S. aureofaciens* capable of synthesizing a small amount of 6-demethylated analogues. These recombinant strains were capable of very high levels of DMCTC production on the addition of sulfonamides to the medium. Similar methodology was used (JARAI 1969) to isolate strains with cobalamin-dependent 6-methylation blocks.

Many antibiotic producers are known to be susceptible to their own antibiotic at some stage of the fermentation process (VINING 1979). Even before the biochemical basis for such sensitivity in the tetracycline producers was known, investigators were incorporating antibiotic in the selection procedures to isolate strains which would be higher producers by virtue of a greater resistance to their own antibiotic. The earliest use of this approach was by KATAGIRI (1954), who on plating *S. aureofaciens* spores on CTC-containing agar, obtained a strain with a fourfold increase in activity over the starting culture. The method has continued to be used. VESELOVA and KOMAROVA (1968) eliminated low-producing *S. rimosus* variants by plating spore suspensions on agar containing 3,000–5,000 μg/ml OTC. Twelve out of 169 such resistant selections were more productive. VESELOVA (1969) used 1,000–1,500 μg/ml CTC to selectively choose higher-producing *S. aureofaciens* variants. PALECKOVA et al. (1969) used 1,200 μg/ml CTC in the agar to select a higher-producing TC strain. ARDELEAN et al. (1972) selected higher-producing *S. aureofaciens* cultures in the presence of increasing amounts of CTC up to 1,500 μg/ml. RYABUSHKO (1972, 1976) found brown pigmented TC producers to be higher producers and less sensitive to added TC than were non-pigmented nonproducers. He suggested that the pigment plays a role in sensitivity to the antibiotic through its effect on the cell membrane. The combined use of mutagens and antibiotics is more effective for the selection of higher-producing

S. aureofaciens and *S. rimosus* cultures than is the use of a mutagen alone (VESELOVA 1969, 1978).

Very low levels, 1 μg/ml, of OTC, CTC, or TC were found by NYIRI (1962) to induce the production of OTC by nonproducing strains of *S. rimosus*. Higher levels of added OTC inhibited development of the young hyphae but these became more resistant once OTC production began. A pseudoantagonism could be demonstrated on agar between producing and nonproducing strains. Added OTC inhibits the oxidation of maltose by young (first-generation) hyphae of both producing and nonproducing strains. Older hyphae (second generation) are more resistant to the added OTC and the inactive strains respond by initiating OTC synthesis (NYIRI et al. 1963). MIKULIK et al. (1971 a–c) found a relationship between CTC production and the protein-synthesizing system of *S. aureofaciens*. Addition of 500 μg/ml CTC to a 4-h-old culture completely inhibits TC production but decreases protein synthesis by only 37%. Adding the same level of TC to a 16-h-old producing culture has no such effect. The addition of 500 μg/ml TC to a 4-h-old nonproducing culture completely inhibits protein synthesis. The ribosomes of TC-producing strains are more resistant to added TC than are those of nonproducers or of bacteria sensitive to TC.

Plasmids are also associated with losses in productivity and losses in resistance to tetracyclines by the producing organism. JARAI (1962) found that acridine orange had no effect on causing loss of productivity in *S. aureofaciens* and in fact had a slight mutagenic effect. ZELINKOVA et al. (1976a) found growth and CTC formation to be inhibited by acridine orange in a dose-dependent manner, with antibiotic synthesis completely inhibited by 20 μg/ml. This would at least suggest plasmid involvement. In *S. rimosus* plasmids also appear to be involved in OTC synthesis. BORONIN and SADOVNIKOVA (1972) found strain LST-118 to give rise spontaneously to OTC-sensitive mutants and to do so even more after acridine orange treatment. BORISOGLEBSKAYA et al. (1979) found a high degree of reversion to OTC sensitivity after acridine orange and UV treatment and a plasmid present in the original culture was absent after treatment. Most genes for OTC production are, however, chromosomal (BORONIN and MINDLIN 1971).

Thus, several mechanisms – the protective effect of pigments on permeability; the sensitivity of ribosomes; plasmids; and the "compartmentalization" of antibiotic in vesicles as described earlier – may all, together or separately, play a role in the selection for increased yield in the presence of antibiotic. Since often these latter observations are carried out retrospectively on producing and nonproducing strains obtained by other means, it is difficult to distinguish cause and consequence. It is obviously easier to find improved strains almost empirically than it is to carry out studies on ribosomal sensitivity or to examine the ultrastructure of many strains by electron microscopy. While not easily used as a predictive tool, such studies, however, are invaluable to an understanding of the underlying mechanisms involved.

Strain selection using resistance to high levels of tetracyclines as a selective agent may have little relevance to actual production conditions where the level of free antibiotic is only a small fraction of the total antibiotic content of the fermentation broth. Other properties can also be selected for as, for example, cultures capable of higher yields in surface culture (KVASHNINA 1966) or strains adapted to richer media (FEDOROVA et al. 1971).

More directed genetic approaches to strain improvement have also been made. DULANEY and DULANEY (1967) bypassed the regulatory mechanisms limiting CTC production by selecting for prototrophic revertants of induced auxotrophs of *S. viridifaciens* and obtained some higher-yielding cultures. Recombination of mutants bearing suitable resistance or nutritional markers has also been reported. ALIKHANIAN and BORISOVA (1961) using *S. aureofaciens* recombined arginine auxotrophs (which formed the bulk of the mutant population) with histidine or isoleucine-valine auxotrophs. The prototrophs obtained all exceeded the auxotrophic parents and some even exceeded the original strains in productivity. JARAI (1961 a) reported similar increases in CTC productivity in prototrophic recombinants of *S. aureofaciens*. The increased productivity was more frequent when the recombining auxotrophs were descendent from separate original lines.

Recombinations in *S. rimosus* were reported by ALIKHANIAN and MINDLIN (1957 a, b), who found the prototrophic recombinants to exceed the auxotrophic combining strains and even the original lines in OTC production. MINDLIN et al. (1961 b) found one such hybrid in *S. rimosus* which exceeded the original prototrophic parent by 10%–15%. This improved yield was attained in shaken flasks and in tanks where in addition the hybrid had the desirable property of lower foam formation. Levels of 4,900 μg/ml OTC were reported, which is a reasonably respectable titre. Another practical example already discussed is the recombination by investigators at CHINOIN (CHINOIN GYOGYSZER 1963) of methionine auxotrophs to yield a strain highly responsive to production of demethylated tetracyclines when using sulfonamides.

POLSINELLI and BERETTA (1966) successfully obtained crosses between auxotrophs of *S. aureofaciens* and *S. rimosus*, most of which resembled the *S. rimosus* parent. No data on the antibiotic capabilities were reported. BLUMAUEROVA (1971) reported similar interspecific hybrids. Despite such instances of success, FANTINI and WALLO (1967) in their study of recombination in *S. aureofaciens* were not overly encouraged by the results insofar as having a direct application to yield improvement, especially when compared with programs of induced mutation and selection. HOPWOOD (1974) has pointed out that the strategies of mutation and recombination are complementary in strain improvement programs, the first being a divergent, the second being a convergent process. The newer techniques of protoplast fusion should greatly increase the recombinant frequencies but no reports of yield improvement in the tetracyclines using this technology have yet come to our attention.

Transformations in tetracycline producers have also been reported. *S. aureofaciens* auxotrophs were transformed by purified DNA from prototrophic *S. aureofaciens* strains and from *S. griseus* but not with *S. rimosus* as the donor (JARAI 1961). Transformation of nonproducing *S. rimosus* was achieved using DNA from producing strains (MATSELYUKH 1964). BISWAS and SEN (1971), testing a number of tetracycline producers as donors and antibiotically inactive strains as recipients, found the only successful combination to be *S. aureofaciens* prototrophic DNA which transformed an inactive *S. viridifaciens*.

III. Cosynthesis

This term was coined by McCormick et al. (1960) to describe the cooperative biosynthesis of active antibiotics by the joint cultivation of pairs of inactive mutant strains. The process is to be distinguished from simple cross-feeding to overcome nutritional deficiencies since both of the cosynthetic partners grow very well by themselves. The simple case of cross-feeding has also been described for the tetracyclines. Shen and Shan (1957) jointly cultivated a strain which produced poorly on sucrose with a nonproducing strain which was an active invertase secretor to achieve a CTC production level which was normal for cultivation on glucose. No fusions were observed and no new strains were isolated from the mixture. McCormick et al. (1960) found that filtrates of a non-tetracycline-producing strain when added to S-1308 which produced 5a-(11a)-dehydro CTC caused the latter to synthesize CTC instead. The factor involved was called cosynthetic factor 1 (CF-1), which, when added to S-1308, has the same effect as filtrates. CF-1 has an extremely high catalytic activity, 1 μg being sufficient to stimulate formation of 50,000 μg CTC (Miller et al. 1960a). CF-1 is produced by a number of species which synthesize tetracyclines, as well as by species such as *S. griseus*, *S. albus*, and *S. alboniger* which do not synthesize tetracyclines; but *S. aureofaciens* is the richest source. Had sufficiently active 5a-(11a)-dehydro CTC been made available through yield improvement, the catalytic activity of CF-1 would have made this an attractive route to CTC. In addition, 5a-(11a)-dehydro CTC is itself convertible by catalytic reduction (McCormick et al. 1958a; Miller 1961b) and biological reduction (McCormick et al. 1957b, 1958b) to active tetracyclines. In the case of catalytic reduction, however, both active TC and inactive 5a-epi TC are produced and in the case of the biological reduction only 20%–40% reduction to CTC was achieved. McCormick et al. (1961c) described numerous cosynthetic pairs derived from CTC-, TC-, DMCTC-, and OCT-producing cultures where one or both partners were nonproducing and on mixing after an initial 48-h growth period produced in some instances >4,000 μg/ml of an active tetracycline. Martin et al. (1966) prepared 5-hydroxy-7 CTC by addition of 5a-(11a)-dehydro CTC to washed cells of *S. rimosus*.

It is interesting to note that not all 5a-(11a)-dehydro CTC producers are responsive to CF-1. Growich (1971c) described strains which, unlike the original S-1308, are completely blocked, making no detectable CTC and responding neither to added CF-1 nor to riboflavin.

Cosynthetic processes analogous to those found in *S. aureofaciens* have been described in *S. rimosus*. Alikhanian et al. (1961) found two groups of nonproducers characterized in one case by white aerial mycelium and in the second case by gray aerial mycelium with a dark brown pigment secreted into the medium. Conjoint cultivation of these two types led to the production of OTC. The culture fluid of the "white" mutants produced a substance "X" which caused the "dark" mutants to produce OTC. The reverse situation did not hold. The two types of mutants could be crossed to yield recombinants capable of OTC production (Mindlin et al. 1961a). The X factor from the white mutants has been isolated and found to be coenzyme-like (Orlova et al. 1961). The factors affecting its maximum production differ to some extent, less phosphate for instance is required, from those for maximum OTC production. The substance isolated from the dark mutants resembles OTC but has no bioactivity (ZAITSEVA and ORLOVA 1962). As in the case of CF-1 the X factor for *S. rimosus* is produced by nontetracycline producers as well. Almost all of 27 actinomycetes tested by ORLOVA et al. (1964) were found to produce it, but none of the fungi, bacteria, or yeasts tested did so.

Cosynthesis has been detected between pairs of inactive *S. rimosus* mutants and between pairs of inactive *S. aureofaciens* mutants using an agar method (DELIC et al. 1969). Interspecific cosynthesis was also detected. The method has the advantage of rapid detection and discrimination between donor and recipient strains.

C. The Fermentation Process

I. Inoculum

While almost every paper and patent dealing with the fermentation of various tetracyclines cites the conditions for the inoculum stages used, there are surprisingly few published references dealing with the effect of inoculum per se on the subsequent fermentation of the antibiotic.

Well-sporulated cultures are often maintained and used as such for initiating the inoculum sequence though this is not a necessity for optimum yield since nonsporulating cultures may at times be better producers (VAN DYCK and DE SOMER 1952; NIEDZWIECKA-TRZASKOWSKA and SZTENCEL 1958). Spores of *S. aureofaciens* can be used directly to inoculate surface fermentations of cracked grains or bran (NOVOTNY and HEROLD 1960), and they have also been used in synthetic media studies to avoid carryover of nutrients but when this is done poorer yields are obtained than when using vigorously grown vegetative inoculum (MCCORMICK et al. 1959a). The more usual procedure is to use spores to start the buildup of a series of vegetative stages, using progressively larger vessels, the last of which is used to inoculate the production fermentor. While excess inorganic phosphate in the production stage is inhibitory to growth, its presence in the agar media in the prior stages may be an advantage in inducing well-sporulated growth without any adverse effect on subsequent fermentation (ORLOVA 1971).

The vegetative inoculum medium should allow for a rapid and abundant growth of the organism. MAKAREVICH and LAZNIKOVA (1970) found that increasing the levels of corn flour, NH_4NO_3, and $CaCO_3$ in the inoculum medium led to higher rates of carbohydrate and nitrogen consumption in the inoculum and to an increase in subsequent CTC synthesis by 25%. Similar effects were obtained with inoculum media enriched in amino acids (LAZNIKOVA and MAKAREVICH 1971).

Despite the sequence of stages exhibited by *S. rimosus* in submerged cultivation, ORLOVA and PROKOFIEVA-BELGOVSKAYA (1961) found that the amount rather than the age of inoculum exerted a greater effect on subsequent growth rate and OTC production. *Streptomyces rimosus* tends to form spores in submerged culture often within the first 24 h (ORLOVA and VERKHOVTSEVA 1957). In some cases up to 10^8–10^{10} spores/ml were formed (HORVATH et al. 1958c). This characteristic is significant for inoculum buildup.

Streptomyces aureofaciens does not form spores in submerged culture. MAKAREVICH and LAZNIKOVA (1961b) suggested very young inoculum of *S. aureofaciens* should be used for best results. Inoculum "quality" is difficult to predict. SHEN et al. (1955) studied five different inoculum media and despite the low potencies obtained were able to demonstrate marked differences in the subsequent fermentations in CTC accumulation, carbohydrate use, and lactic and volatile fatty acid accumulation while no significant effect was noted on the growth of *S. aureofaciens* in either the inoculum or production stage.

The schedule in a busy operating situation often does not allow the luxury of variable inoculum ages or excessive or laborious measurements of inoculum quality and decisions as to readiness must be based on experience. LAZNIKOVA and DMITRIEVA (1973) and LAZNIKOVA (1973) found that the behavior of the mycelium on centrifugation in a sucrose density gradient was a measure of its quality. Such procedures, while perhaps useful for retrospective evaluations of inoculum, would appear to be too sophisticated and unnecessary for routine use where a simple settling measurement in a graduated cylinder is often sufficient. In a stirred inoculum tank, conditions which delay growth and decrease consumption of carbon and nitrogen, such as poor aeration, adversely affect the capacity of *S. rimosus* for OTC synthesis in the subsequent stage (OBLOZHKO et al. 1974).

It is important to consider at all times a possible carry-over effect. High levels of inorganic phosphate in the inoculum medium have no adverse effect on growth and in fact result in better inoculum growth but can also result in a significantly high amount of inorganic phosphate transferred into the fermentation stage. This could have a depressing effect on subsequent tetracycline biosynthesis. Similarly, the carry-over of significant amounts of free antibiotic with the inoculum could have a depressing effect on subsequent biosynthesis. GOODMAN et al. (1955) found the tetracycline-producing microorganisms to be sensitive to a level of 10–50 μg/ml of added antibiotic. The production of TC by CTC-producing strains using halide denial can be compromised by carry-over of sufficient chloride with the inoculum to allow excessive levels of CTC to be synthesized. This is avoided by reduction of chloride levels in the inoculum as well. In the production of TC by means of chlorination inhibitors these can be added to both the inoculum and fermentation media (MAKAREVICH and LAZNIKOVA 1969). Their inherent toxicity, however, does not make this an attractive alternative to use in the inoculum stages.

Inoculum production for the tetracyclines has been investigated under continuous or semicontinuous conditions (BOSNJAK and KAPETANOVIC 1971). *S. aureofaciens* inoculum for either CTC or TC production has been continuously transferred 15–20 times after an initial 24- to 30-h growth period (KRUSSER et al. 1963). It was kept productive provided that the intervals between successive transfers into fresh inoculum were shortened to 13–18 h and less inoculum was used for inoculation of the production stage when using inoculum from later transfers in the continuous inoculum cycle. Similar results were reported by DRAZHNER et al. (1969) using off-takes from production fermentors as seed. In continuous production of CTC, SLEZAK and SIKYTA (1964) and SHU (1966) found a loss of productivity due to degeneration of the culture in part through the gradual overgrowth of nonproductive variants. These were either introduced with the inoculum or generated by mutations during the operation. Continuous production of inoculum is likely to be subject to the same danger and it would appear to be prudent to make certain that the starting point for continuous fermentation, the inoculum stage, be run in a batch mode to insure as low a burden of initial "off types" as possible.

II. Contamination

Despite the fact that they are broad-spectrum antibiotics, the tetracyclines, in common with all fermentations, are subject to bacterial contamination. The extent of economic loss due to such contamination may not always be easy to estimate. In cases of complete failure a "price tag" can be assigned. Less severe contamination may occur which has no apparent effect on yield. There are also instances where the decrease in yield is only moderately severe and from which the product might normally by salvageable, but processing difficulties beyond the fermentation stage such as clogged filters, etc. make such salvage impractical. HEROLD and NECASEK (1959) have dealt with the problems of microbial contamination of fermentation processes in general. Among these problems which apply to the tetracyclines as well are the specific properties of the production culture, the type of nutrient medium, and the raw materials used in its preparation and the technology of the process itself. In our experience the DMCTC fermentation has a higher incidence of contamination than does the CTC process despite the fact that the two antibiotics are closely related and are produced in the same equipment. The answer lies in part in the somewhat less vigorous growth pattern of the DMCTC mutant. Of greater significance is the medium which contains cottonseed flour, making it more difficult to sterilize and more subject to buildup of particulate matter than is the corn-steep-liquor-based medium used in CTC. Taking the tetracyclines produced at American Cyanamid Company as a whole it is estimated that in a comparison of contaminated batches with uncontaminated batches the loss in yield is in the order of 10%. It is of obvious importance to maintain the incidence of contamination as low as possible.

KOSHEL et al. (1971 b) found six species of bacteria most frequently occurring in contamination of the tetracyclines. In order of importance these were: *Bacillus, Bacterium, Pseudomonas, Micrococcus, Lactobacterium*, and *Sarcina* species, with the first four being the ones least sensitive to CTC and responsible for 90% of the contaminations found. WELWARD and HALAMA (1978) found the eight most frequent contaminations to be: *Aerobacter aerogenes, Alcaligenes faecalis, Escherichia coli, Micrococcus ovalis, Pseudomonas aeruginosa, Bacillus subtilis, Proteus vulgaris*, and *Streptococcus lactis*. Pathogenic bacteria have no significant effect on the biosynthesis of CTC. GREZIN et al. (1964) added *Bacillus anthracis, Salmonella breslau,* and other pathogens along with the inoculum into a CTC fermentation and found that all except *Salmonella breslau* decreased in virulence.

The presence of a broad-spectrum antibiotic is thus not always sufficient insurance against contamination particularly if this were to occur before sufficient tetracycline were present. While the addition of 300 μg/ml OTC was found by

HREBENDA et al. (1969) to be sufficient to "sterilize" media used for OTC and TC fermentations, this amount approaches, if not exceeds, the self-inhibitory levels for these antibiotics (GOODMAN et al. 1955; MIKULIK et al. 1971 c; NYIRI et al. 1963). Somewhat lower levels of antibiotic are introduced into the fermentation with the inoculum itself and this appears to be the basis of the protection afforded in CTC fermentations which have been run without maintenance of aseptic conditions. BELIK et al. (1958) were able to run the CTC fermentation in a nonaseptic manner for an uninterrupted period of 1.5 years. They used wooden tanks of 2,000-liter capacity and relied solely upon a 40-min boiling of the medium, which contained such highly contaminating materials as soy flour, corn-steep liquor, and molasses. They also relied on the carry-over of CTC in the inoculum, which was grown with the maintenance of normal aseptic conditions. ZELINKA and HUDEC (1962) found that fermentations carried out in such wooden containers showed the same metabolism in respect to sugar, total nitrogen, and amino nitrogen as did similar nonaseptic fermentations run in aluminum tanks of 50,000-liter size. It will be noted that tanks of 2,000-liter size are no longer a "cottage industry." The carry-over of CTC with the inoculum amounts to 10–20 μg/ml in the starting fermentation. This amount in shake flask fermentations was found to protect against deliberate contamination by soil or river water or by artificial contamination by pure cultures of microorganisms. Production of CTC was lowered by 40% only by two strains of *Torulopsis utilis* (HEROLD and NECASEK 1959).

A combination of antibiotic carry-over plus other antimicrobial agents along with a short thermal sterilization were found by WELWARD and HALAMA (1978) to protect against a mixture of the eight most common contaminants added before the treatment. Of the various chemical agents tested, formaldehyde at 0.01% and nitrofurazone at 20 μg/ml did not protect by themselves but when used in conjunction with a sterilization of 5 min at 120 °C afforded complete protection. A combination of formaldehyde added before and nitrofurazone after the short heat sterilization gave the best results. Yields of CTC were actually higher by up to 10% than those achieved with a control sterilization period of 30 min. Whether protection would occur against massive contamination introduced after rather than before the treatment is not stated.

The short sterilization period of 5 min apparently prevented some thermal degradation of the medium compared with the normal 30-min treatment. HREBENDA et al. (1969) found reduced potency in the OTC and TC fermentations and impaired carbohydrate and amino nitrogen uptake when media were sterilized at 130 °C for 3–6 h compared with 120 °C for 1 h. It is not unreasonable then that a short heat treatment of 5 min if combined with an antimicrobial agent might perform better than a normal 30-min sterilization. The use of formaldehyde for such a purpose is now prohibited in the United States. KOSHEL et al. (1971 a) successfully used cetylpyridinium chloride as an antiseptic against cocci and species of *Pseudomonas* and *Bacterium* in CTC production. The amount used was 0.0005%–0.005%, depending upon the severity of infection.

Contamination can also be a problem in the production of feed-grade CTC by the surface growth method. NOVOTNY and HEROLD (1960) found that a layer of dry sterile wheat flour dusted over the inoculated substrate, which consisted of ground moistened wheat in trays, would protect against contamination in an incubation tunnel for 6 days.

III. Complex Media

The wide variety of media that have been used in the fermentation of the various tetracyclines is most obviously evident in even a casual perusal of the patent literature. While it is not the intention to present here a complete "recipe book" of all of the variations that have been reported it may still be useful to list some of the fermentation media which have been used. Table 1 is a sampler taken only from the patent literature.

Common to all these media is a carbohydrate or glyceride oil serving as the source of energy and ultimately as the source of the basic structural elements for antibiotic formation and a protein with or without supplemental inorganic nitrogen serving as the source of nitrogen. Mineral salts may be added or may be present in sufficient quantity in the other raw materials. Calcium carbonate serves as a buffer against excessive acidity and also to bind the antibiotic in an insoluble form (NIEDERCORN 1952). In the case of CTC, chloride must be provided or in the case of the TC fermentation special provision must be made under certain circumstances to exclude it. Special additives such as chlorination or methylation inhibitors or copper ion will be dealt with separately.

Table 1. A sampler of fermentation media taken from the patent literature

Medium		Reference
1. Corn steep liquor	20 g/liter	NIEDERCORN (1952)
$(NH_4)_2SO_4$	2 g/liter	
Sucrose	30 g/liter	
$CaCO_3$	3 g/liter	
2. Cottonseed flour	45 g/liter	GOODMAN (1964b)
Starch	45 g/liter	
Brewer's yeast	1.5 g/liter	
$CaCO_3$	10.5 g/liter	
NH_4Cl	1.5 g/liter	
$CuSO_4 \cdot 5H_2O$	50 mg/liter	
3. Corn steep liquor	25 g/liter	GOODMAN (1959)
Starch	47 g/liter	
Corn flour	14.5 g/liter	
Cottonseed flour	5 g/liter	
$(NH_4)_2SO_4$	5.6 g/liter	
$CaCO_3$	9 g/liter	
NH_4Cl	1.7 g/liter	
$MnSO_4$ (technical)	80 mg/liter	
$CoCl_2 \cdot 6H_2O$	5 mg/liter	
Lard oil	2% v/v	
4. Corn steep liquor (resin dehalogenated)	30 g/liter	SZUMSKI (1959a)
Low chloride starch	55 g/liter	
Cottonseed flour	5 g/liter	
$(NH_4)_2SO_4$	5 g/liter	

Table 1 (continued)

Medium		Reference
$CaCO_3$	7 g/liter	
$MnSO_4 \cdot 4H_2O$	50 mg/liter	
H_3PO_4 (85%)	200 mg/liter	
Lard oil	2% v/v	
5. Corn steep liquor	30 g/liter	PETTY (1955)
Sucrose	30 g/liter	
$CaCO_3$	9 g/liter	
$(NH_4)_2SO_4$	3.3 g/liter	
NH_4Cl	1 g/liter	
$MgCl_2 \cdot 6H_2O$	2 g/liter	
$FeSO_4 \cdot 2H_2O$	41 mg/liter	
$MnSO_4 \cdot 4H_2O$	50 mg/liter	
$ZnSO_4 \cdot 7H_2O$	100 mg/liter	
$CoCl_2 \cdot 6H_2O$	5 mg/liter	
Lard oil with or without octadecanol or silicone oil for antifoam		
6. Corn steep liquor	6 g/liter	CHINOIN (1962)
Starch	25 g/liter	
$(NH_4)_2SO_4$	5 g/liter	
KNO_3	2 g/liter	
$CaCO_3$	4 g/liter	
Palm oil	0.2% v/v	
7. Soybean oil meal	50 g/liter	PERLMAN (1962)
Glucose	50 g/liter	
$CaCO_3$	5 g/liter	
8. Soybean oil meal	40 g/liter	CULIK et al. (1969a)
Sucrose	50 g/liter	
$CaCO_3$	6.3 g/liter	
$(NH_4)_2SO_4$	6.3 g/liter	
Molasses	2.5 g/liter	
Corn steep liquor (solids)	3.0 g/liter	
Benzyl thiocyanate	0.054 mg/liter	
Soybean oil	2% v/v	
9. Soybean oil meal	30 g/liter	STOUDT and TAUSIG (1963)
Distiller's solubles	7.5 g/liter	
NaCl	2.5 g/liter	
Glucose	20 g/liter	
$CaCO_3$	10 g/liter	
10. Filtrate[a] of *Zea mays* plus:		ZANNINI et al. (1968a)
NH_4Cl	4 g/liter	
Starch	55 g/liter	
Soybean oil meal	10 g/liter	
$SrCO_3$	8 g/liter	
11. Dextrin	120 g/liter	BONNAT and CHAUSSIER (1968)
Soyflour	25 g/liter	
Cottonseed flour	15 g/liter	
$(NH_4)_2SO_4$	7.5 g/liter	
$CaCO_3$	12 g/liter	
Lard oil	3.3% v/v	
Silicone oil	1.7% v/v	
Mercapto benzothiazole	60 mg/liter	

Table 1 (continued)

Medium		Reference
12. Starch	20 g/liter	ARDELEAN (1971)
Soyflour	38 g/liter	
Corn steep liquor	2.5 g/liter	
Urea	1 g/liter	
Corn meal	10 g/liter	
Benzyl thiocyanate	4 mg/liter	
13. Peanut flour	20 g/liter	SZCZESNIAK et al. (1975)
Potato flour	20 g/liter	
Oat flour	20 g/liter	
Corn steep liquor	12.5 g/liter	
$CaCO_3$	4 g/liter	
NH_4Cl	2 g/liter	
NH_4NO_3	5 g/liter	
Animal fat	1% v/v	

[a] Acid or neutral hot water extract of corn

1. Carbohydrate Source

Protein and carbohydrate may be combined in a single raw material such as corn flour (LAB PRO-TER 1963 b). More usually the preferred carbohydrate is some form of starch which may be from a variety of sources. Starch-containing media favorable to OTC biosynthesis result in virtually no pyruvic, lactic, or volatile acids compared with their formation in glucose medium less favorable to OTC production (BRYZGALOVA and ORLOVA 1975).

Corn is the usual source of starch but potato, raw or boiled (YAKIMOV and NESHATEVA 1961), potato flour (SZCZESNIAK et al. 1975), or spent potato washings (FREMEL et al. 1963) have also been used. Also used have been yams (LAB SAILLY 1974), millet (*Panicium miliaceum*) flour (SMEKAL and ZAJICEK 1976), barley flour (SZUMSKI 1961), oat flour (SZCZESNIAK 1975), and wheat flour (FREMEL et al. 1963).

Starch may cause viscosity problems in large-scale fermentations. Modified starches, the so-called fluidity starches and dextrins, are commercially available in a range of viscosities. Such fluidity starches allowed GOODMAN (1954) to prepare media in concentrated form in available equipment. Alternatively the starchy substrate may be hydrolyzed by amylase (BAEV et al. 1980) or be first subjected to the action of amylase-producing organisms such as *Aspergillus oryzae* (NITELEA et al. 1968). *S. aureofaciens* is itself a strong amylase producer (KOAZE et al. 1974; HOSTINOVA et al. 1979) and has been used as a preliminary hydrolyzing agent prior to medium sterilization (ANKERFARM 1971). VECHER et al. (1969) found the amylase activity of *S. aureofaciens* grown on a starch-containing medium to be maximum at 5 h. Amylase is, however, present and diffuses from the cells into the culture fluid throughout the fermentation (CHALENKO and MALTSEV 1971). Starches tend to present a more slowly available source of carbohydrate that is to a degree self-regulating since excessive glucose accumulation depresses the amylolytic activity of *S. aureofaciens* (VECHER et al. 1969).

The ability of starchy substrates to support increased production of antibiotic may depend on particle size. MAKAREVICH et al. (1969) find that more finely screened or ground corn meal results in increased yields. Ground cereal grains are the sole nutrient in the surface production of feed-grade antibiotics where the hydrolysis of the starchy substrate is accomplished by the producing culture. NOVOTNY and HEROLD (1960) achieved yields of 2,000 μg/g CTC using ground wheat and PIVNYAK (1962) achieved 18,000 μg/g OTC using coarse barley flour.

While starch in some form is the usual preferred carbohydrate, special conditions of availability may dictate the choice of carbohydrate. ABOU-ZEID and ABOU-EL-ATTA (1973) and ABOU-ZEID et al. (1979) found local (Egyptian) molasses to be a suitable replacement for starch in CTC and OTC production. Other carbohydrates have been reported to be optimum for CTC production. Thus HOSTALEK et al. (1959), MOSTAFA et al. (1972), and ROKOS and PROCHAZKA (1962) report sucrose as an optimium carbohydrate. NESHATAEVA et al. (1963) report glycerol, maltose, and glucose to be optimum und ROKOS and PROCHAZKA (1962) report fructose to be suitable, though in our experience and in others' (HOSLALEK et al. 1959) it is a poor carbohydrate source. The differences observed are almost certainly a matter of strain differences and in most reports starch appears to be the carbohydrate of choice.

The productive period of the fermentation can be prolonged by the addition of carbohydrate during the run. ADAMOVIC et al. (1969) found that addition of starch and maltose during the fermentation improved OTC yields but the addition of hydrolyzed starch or glucose depressed yields. ORLOVA and PUSHKINA (1972) found that addition of both carbon and nitrogen in small doses after their initial exhaustion during the phase of intensive OTC biosynthesis led to higher productivity for a longer period. MAKAREVICH et al. (1978) found increased TC production (240%) by initial enrichment of the corn flour level from 50 to 80 g/liter. *S. aureofaciens* cells became adapted to such enriched media and produced lower yields when taken from an enriched medium and put into a medium of lower carbohydrate content.

2. Triglyceride Oils

Animal and vegetable oils, the second major carbon source in tetracycline fermentation media, have long been used both as antifoams with or without additives such as octadecanol (PETTY 1955) and as major nutrients (SZUMSKI 1957). They are particularly effective in the CTC fermentation when used in conjunction with starch (GOODMAN 1957) or with casein (SZUMSKI 1967). As high as 14-fold increases in CTC yields were cited by BORISOV and GORBASH (1963) with 0.1%–0.5% sunflower or spermaceti oil added to the medium. Animal or vegetable oils have also been used in OTC production (MANCY-COURTILLET et al. 1959). If added incrementally over a period of 72 h, peanut oil could substitute for sucrose in OTC production (BORENSZTAJN and WOLF 1955). ENGELBRECHT and MACH (1967) found vegetable oils and fatty acids both to the better than glucose for OTC production. ORLOVA (1961) found that while oils could replace starch for OTC production the yields obtained varied with the type of oil used, ranging from 47% of the starch control when using the saturated coconut oil to 115% when using olive oil, with most others being in the 90% range of the starch control. Regardless of the amount added only 40%–60% of the oil was utilized and the unsaturated fatty acids were preferentially used as determined by the change in iodine number. The optimum phosphorus concentration is higher for oil-based than for starch-based media.

The degree of saturation of the fatty acids in the oil significantly affects its quality and suitability for use in media. The ability of *S. aureofaciens* to oxidize oleate is distinct from its ability to use it as a substrate for growth. HIRSCH and WALLACE (1951) found that *S. aureofaciens* washed cells would oxidize 0.028% oleate but that such an amount added to their complete medium partially inhibited growth.

Improper storage of oils leads to increases in free fatty acids and peroxides affecting their quality both as an antifoam and as a nutrient. LAZNIKOVA and MAKAREVICH (1969) found a 16% decrease in TC production after a 1-month storage of sperm oil, where the peroxide value increased from 0.07 to 3.8. Further storage led to more drastic yield decreases. Oils of acid numbers <0.7 and peroxide numbers of <0.1 were suitable for TC production. Higher fatty acids and their esters are poor antifoaming agents and severely reduce production of CTC (IVANOV and BLIZNAKOVA 1971).

The sensitivity of the OTC fermentation to iron is affected by the degree of unsaturation of the oils used in the medium (HORVATH et al. 1958a, b). The simultaneous presence of iron and unsaturated oil leads to the catalytic production of peroxides and a drop in OTC production. With palm oil up to 200 μg/ml Fe^{2+} was tolerated while with sunflower oil even 20–40 μg/ml Fe^{2+} led to a decrease in yield.

Oils used in production of tetracyclines are usually protected against deterioration by the addition of antioxidants. SZUMSKI (1957) found that 0.05%–0.5% antioxidant (Tenox II Eastman Chemical) prevented deterioration of the oil as a nutrient in CTC production. Its use even with fresh unstored oil led to better CTC yields. RAKYTA et al. (1980) reported similar results and suggested that during the fermentation *S. aureofaciens* oxidizes the oil to form peroxides, aldehydes, and carboxylic acids and that this is prevented by the addition of an antioxidant.

Consistent with economic consideration, it is desirable to use the highest quality oils available since antioxidants do not compensate for poor quality oil. Lard oils, for instance, are available in a number of grades and these have a significant affect on yields. Pure, chemically defined triglycerides have been used particularly in synthetic media work. ZYGMUNT (1964) used gylcerol dioleate in OTC synthetic media and MCCORMICK et al. (1959a) used glycerol trioleate in CTC synthetic media. BISHOP (1970) used oleyl alcohol in place of normally used triglycerides in both CTC and OTC fermentation. This material does not oxidize and does not interfere with subsequent isolation procedures through formation of calcium soaps.

One further potential source of carbon may be CO_2. MILLER et al. (1956) found no incorporation of carbon-labeled carbonate in *S. aureofaciens*, but PLAKUNOVA (1969) reported heterotrophic fixation of CO_2 at a rate of 10%–20% in *S. aureofaciens* and 30%–45% in *S. rimosus*. The rate of fixation varied inversely with the age of the culture. The major fixation products were aspartic and glutamic acids which were then used by the growing cultures. In *S. aureofaciens* 5%–7% of the total fixed carbon was incorporated into CTC.

3. Nitrogen Sources

A wide variety of organic nitrogen sources have been used for production of the tetracyclines – corn steep liquor (CSL), cottonseed meal or flour, soybean meal or flour, peanut flour, distillers solubles, and yeast have been widely reported. Combined carbon and nitrogen sources such as corn flour, and cracked cereal grains in the surface method of fermentation have already been mentioned. Other reported organic nitrogen sources have been malt extracts (LEPETIT 1958 b) or malt sprouts used alone or substituting for part of the CSL (FERTMAN 1965; GIRS et al. 1980). Deproteinized potato juice concentrate (VECHER et al. 1978) and waste mycelium from penicillin fermentations (QUADEER 1970) have been used in the CTC fermentation. Waste sludge from L-lysine production by *Micrococcus glutamicus* in combination with peanut meal or acid hydrolyzed peanut meal has been used for both CTC and TC production (WELWARD et al. 1975, 1976 b). The residual lysine content of such sludge makes it a particularly valuable ingredient, ZILBERMAN et al. (1978) finding up to 30% improvement in TC yields by supplementing corn steep with lysine. Blood meal has been used for TC production (KRUPENSKI et al. 1978) and lucern flour has been used for OTC production (ZANNINI et al. 1968 b).

The availability of CSL as an inexpensive source of inorganic nitrogen and essential minerals has resulted in its widespread use but it is not without its disadvantages. It is above all a highly variable material being itself the product of a lactic fermentation of the steeping water used in the first stages of corn starch manufacture. Manufacturers analyses in the author's experience are no reliable guide as to the suitability of any given lot for tetracycline production. The quality of any given lot is in largest part a reflection of its inorganic phosphate content (ORLOVA and VERKHOTSEVA 1959), to which, when present to excess, the tetracyclines are particularly sensitive. An examination of some patents (MILLER and MCCORMICK 1960; GROWICH and DEDUCK 1963) will show the CSL content of media to be given as a range. This reflects the fact that each lot of CSL has its optimum usage level which strikes a balance between the optimum phosphate level and the optimum levels of other essential ingredients in the particular lot being used. Organic phosphate present as phytates has no adverse effect. They can be removed by boiling the steep under alkaline conditions and removing the precipitate. Such treatment does not harm the CSL for CTC production and such treatment of CSL has been found (PASKOVA and SMOLEK 1967) to give higher OTC yields. The process of dehalogenating CSL with ion exchange resins for use in TC production removes both phytates and inorganic phosphorus and the latter must then be added back to the medium. Such treated CSLs with chloride also added are often better for CTC production than is the original CSL (J. J. GOODMAN 1954, unpublished results). The improved yield, however, does not justify the expense of the treatment since on a commercial scale CSL lots can easily be pretested for suitability and optimum use levels.

The inorganic phosphate content of CSL is an indicator of its quality for OTC production as well. ORLOVA and VERKHOTSEVA (1959) found that CSLs freed of inorganic phosphate could then be used to supplement normal CSL medium resulting in stimulation of OTC synthesis in some cases. Total phosphorus, nitrogenous substances, and lactic acid were not sufficiently reliable to be used as indicators of quality of CSL for OTC production. Addition of amino acids to the medium did not affect OTC production (VERKHOTSEVA and ORLOVA 1960).

SZUMSKI (1959b) found CSLs with an oxidation-reduction potential more positive than −170 mV tended to result in higher yields of both CTC and OTC. This was based on retrospective measurements of a large number of corn steeps used in production of CTC. Consideration of availability, however, made it frequently necessary to use CSL lots outside of the preferred range of oxidation-reduction potential.

Since CSLs are variable in phosphate the use of oilseed meals and cakes as partial or even major substitutes for corn steep has often resulted in an improved yield (MAKAREVICH and LAZNIKOVA 1961a). VAN DYCK and DE SOMER (1952) were among the first to develop a medium with peanut meals as the major and CSL as a minor organic nitrogen source. They found, however, that peanut meals also differed from lot to lot in respect to CTC production and that, further, different *S. aureofaciens* strains responded differently to batches of peanut meal. Soybean meals and flours though perhaps less variable are commercially available in a wide range of particle size, protein contents, and solubility of the protein fractions; and such factors must be taken into consideration for use in media. In our own laboratories we have not found isolated soy proteins to be suitable for antibiotic production by *S. aureofaciens*.

Cottonseed flour is used as the major protein in the production of the 6-demethyl tetracyclines. It may be noted that the early disclosure (McCORMICK et al. 1959b) featured the use of CSL media typical for CTC. Later patents, however (SZUMSKI 1961; GOODMAN 1964b), featured the use of cottonseed meal or flour. This development is an illustration of the interaction of strain and media development. At an early stage of development CSL and cottonseed flour media gave approximately equal yields of DMCTC, but given the known variability of CSL the choice was made to proceed with cottonseed flour media. Further strain development was carried out on such media and a point was reached where production strains no longer did well on the original CSL media. Such an experience is probably not unique and it emphasizes the variation in results to be expected among investigators when the producing organisms start from a different genetic base and proceed along a different selective path.

Free amino acids in CSL or in the proteolysis products of proteinaceous ingredients are the ultimate source of organic nitrogen. Both the amine nitrogen and the carbon skeleton of the amino acids are assimilated by *S. aureofaciens* (LAZNIKOVA and MAKAREVICH 1971). During the initial stages of growth, free amino acids in CSL medium decrease and appear in the mycelium of *S. aureofaciens* after which the amino acid content of the mycelium decreases and that of the medium increases, but the proportions of glutamic, arginine, lysine, valine, leucine, glycine, and aspartic acids in the mycelium differ from those in the original corn steep (TER-KARPETYAN and AVAKYAN 1963). HOFMAN (1961) found two maxima of amino acid concentration in soyflour and CSL media used for CTC production. The first was due to hydrolysis of proteins and peptides and was reached in 12–13 h. The content of amino acids became constant over the next 30–60 h and a second maximum was reached at 72 h. Mycelial amino acid proportions did not change with time but medium amino acids changed both in concentration and kinds with time.

Amino acids have been used to supplement media in an attempt to counteract normal fluctuations found in complex nitrogen sources. ZELINKA et al. (1962) added 32 individual amino acids and related substances at up to 2 g/liter to a soyflour-corn steep medium. Valine, hydroxyproline, tyrosine, cadaverine, and glucosamine stimulated yields by up to 30% while distinct inhibition was observed with norleucine, cystine, cysteine, alanine, methionine, and valine. Cadaverine stimulates CTC biosynthesis only if added at the beginning of the fermentation (ZELINKA 1968). As already noted, ZILBERMAN (1978) finds lysine supplementation of corn steep results in higher CTC yields.

Inhibitors of aromatic acid biosynthesis, *N*-methyl anthranilic and 3-hydroxybenzoic acids and benzyl thiocyanate, were found by SHAPOSHNIKOV and PLAKUNOVA (1964a, b) to stimulate CTC synthesis. This stimulation is not likely due to any overlap in the pathways of CTC and aromatic amino acid biosynthesis.

4. Carbon/Nitrogen Ratios

Absolute levels may be of less importance than is the ratio of carbon to nitrogen in the medium. This ratio will, of course, be altered during the course of the fermentation. LUBA et al. (1968) found an initial C/N ratio of 25 to give the best TC yield and maintained this ratio through the fermentation by the addition of dextrin. Reduction of the C/N ratio to 10 or an increase to 40 resulted in a decrease to 74% and 66% of normal yields respectively. Thus nitrogen shortage decreases yield more severely than does carbon shortage. The C/N ratio can affect the utilization of carbohydrate. CHANG (1961) found sucrose to be utilized by *S. aureofaciens* at C/N ratios of 10 and 50 but not at C/N ratios of 1 or 0.5.

MAKAREVICH et al. (1976) found that maintaining NH_4 nitrogen levels at a constant 10–20 mg/ml along with phosphate at 10–20 µg/ml resulted in a five fold increase in TC. ORLOVA and PUSHKINA (1972) found repeated small additions of carbon and nitrogen sources during the intensive stage of OTC synthesis prolonged the active production phase. The same was true of TC (ORLOVA et al. 1978) where the added NH_4OH is used both as a nutrient and for pH control. Addition of only two-thirds of the total $(NH_4)_2SO_4$ at zero hour and one-third as a sterile solution at 60–80 h into the fermentation led to higher OTC yields (PIERREL SpA 1964). Addition of urea at 48 and 96 h led to increases in CTC yields (SZUMSKI 1964).

5. Inorganic Ingredients

Inorganic nitrogen for *S. aureofaciens* is usually supplied as an ammonium salt. *Streptomyces rimosus* will use both ammonium and nitrate nitrogen. Calcium and magnesium are the other major inorganic substances added. All of the remaining requirements, particularly phosphate, are satisfied by the use of complex ingredients such as CSL or soy and cottonseed flours.

a) Phosphate

Phosphate has an important influence on the production of many antibiotics (MARTIN 1977), and the extreme sensitivity of the tetracycline fermentations to phosphate has been known for many years (BIFFI et al. 1954). The subject has been most recently reviewed by HOSTALEK et al. (1979). The influence of excessive phosphate is exerted on a morphologic level for both *S. aureofaciens* (BORETTI et al. 1955; DOSKOCIL et al. 1959; PROKOFIEVA-BELGOVSKAYA and POPOVA 1959) and *S. rimosus* (Doskocil et al. 1958). The changes in the mycelium include an increase in the nuclear substance to cytoplasm ratio, an increase in the phosphorus-containing elements, thicker hyphae, accelerated growth, and a decreased capacity for antibiotic synthesis. There is an increased accumulation of organic acids, mainly pyruvic, in the medium (BORETTI et al. 1956; BARANOVA and EGOROV 1963; SHEN and CHEN 1959; SHEN and CHANG 1960) and an inhibition of the enzymes of the pentose pathway in favor of those of the glycolytic pathway. This was recently reviewed by VANEK et al. (1978). An increase in phosphate depresses the level of anhydro-tetracycline oxygenase, the penultimate enzyme involved in the biosynthetic pathway, to one-third of its normal activity (BEHAL et al. 1979).

The amount of phosphate which is excessive has been variously stated as 35–55 mg/liter by MAKAREVICH and LAZNIKOVA (1959), as 80 mg/liter by ABOU-ZEID and YOUSEF (1971), and, if maintained at a constant level, as 15–20 mg/liter by TARASOVA et al. (1976). Phosphate is more inhibitory if added during the period of intensive mycelial growth than if added after growth has slowed (BELOUSOVA and POPOVA 1961 b). It is more inhibitory with a readily utilized carbohydrate such as starch or glucose than with a poorly utilized carbohydrate such as sucrose (SHEN and CHEN 1959). The more enriched the medium the less sensitive it is to inorganic phosphate (MAKAREVICH and LAZNIKOVA 1961 b), and synthetic media are also less sensitive to phosphate than are complex media (GUBERNIEV et al. 1954). The tolerance to phosphate is also a function of the specific strain used (MINDLIN et al. 1961 b). The maximum growth rate and amount of mycelium production by *S. aureofaciens* is achieved at phosphate levels two to four times higher than that required for optimum TC synthesis (MAKAREVICH et al. 1975), and maximum production of other unrelated metabolites such as the antifungal antibiotic and vitamin B_{12} by *S. aureofaciens* are achieved at phosphate levels of four and eight times higher than those required for CTC synthesis (ABOU-ZEID and YOUSEF 1971).

b) Calcium

Calcium per se in any major amount is not required for the synthesis of tetracyclines; yet it along with magnesium plays an important role in the fermentation medium. Calcium carbonate provides a convenient pH control mechanism and the formation of insoluble Ca^{2+} and Mg^{2+} tetracycline salts serve to reduce the level of free antibiotic in the fermentation broth to below autotoxic levels (NIEDERCORN 1952).

Calcium carbonates are highly variable in the degree of pH control they provide. Chemically precipitated carbonates generally buffer at a higher pH than do mineral carbonates. Mineral carbonates also differ in the amounts of calcite and aragonite present which in turn affect dissolution rates. WELWARD et al. (1976a) outlined the criteria for evaluating the suitability of various calcium carbonates for CTC production and found a particular microfine ground mineral carbonate to give up to 20% greater yield than did six other samples tested. Strontium carbonate has also been used for buffering the fermentation medium (ZANNINI et al. 1968a). Magnesium and aluminum carbonates are much less useful compared with calcium carbonate (J.J. GOODMAN 1960, unpublished results). PLAKUNOVA (1961) suggested the use of calculated amounts of ion exchange resins as buffering agents in the CTC fermentation.

c) Other Elements

Contradictory observations may be found in the literature on the effect of a number of metals on yields. SHEN (1962) found iron to be inhibitory to CTC production as did PETTKO et al. (1956), who recommended the use of aluminum rather than iron fermentors. MESHKOV et al. (1973) on the other hand found iron to increase CTC production and aluminum to inhibit it. MAJCHRZAK and MAJCHRZAK (1965) found OTC yield to depend on iron with an optimum level of 14–15 mg/liter. Iron toxicity in OTC media is related to the unsaturatedness of the oil used as has already been discussed. In such media methylene blue can protect against iron toxicity and conversely iron can protect against the toxic effect of methylene blue (HORVATH et al. 1959).

UZKURENAS (1969) found zinc and manganese to increase CTC yields and copper to depress yields. Copper is involved in halogenations by *S. aureofaciens* through a copper-containing oxidase (GOODMAN 1959a). In normal CTC and DMCTC fermentations the proportion of nonhalogenated analogues which are difficult to remove by normal refining procedures may be reduced to acceptable levels by the addition of 100 mg/liter $CuSO_4 \cdot 5H_2O$ to the medium (GOODMAN 1962b). Among a number of unrelated materials causing the 5a-(11a)-dehydro CTC producing culture, S1308, to shift to CTC production are a number of copper-chelating oximes the most active of which is 1,-2-naphthoquinone-1-oxime (MILLER et al. 1961).

IV. Synthetic Media

Though yields of tetracyclines using complex media have invariably been superior to those using synthetic defined media, the latter are invaluable in determining basic nutritional requirements for antibiotic production and often also for the elucidation of biosynthetic pathways. PETTY and MATRISHIN (1950) devised a medium based on an analysis of corn steep liquor to study chloride utilization by *S. aureofaciens* as various levels of KCl were added. The medium consisted of the following:

Sucrose	30 g/liter	$MnSO_4 \cdot 7H_2O$	25 mg/liter
$CaCO_3$	5 g/liter	$CuSO_4 \cdot 5H_2O$	5 mg/liter
$(NH_4)_2SO_4$	1 g/liter	Co acetate	5 mg/liter
Mg lactate	5 g/liter	DL-Alanine	450 mg/liter
$NH_4H_2PO_4$	1 g/liter	L-Arginine	550 mg/liter
$MgHPO_4$	1 g/liter	DL-Methionine	200 mg/liter
K lactate	3 ml/liter	D-Glutamic acid	260 mg/liter
$FeSO_4 \cdot 7H_2O$	60 mg/liter	L-Histidine	200 mg/liter
$ZnSO_4 \cdot 7H_2O$	33 mg/liter	DL-β-Asparagine	200 mg/liter

While all six amino acids were required to initiate mycelial growth and CTC production from spore inoculum, mycelial growth once established could then be used as inoculum into a medium in which only a single amino acid, glycine, was sufficient for the production of CTC (PETTY et al. 1953).

MILLER et al. (1956) and MCCORMICK et al. (1959a) found that a medium containing glycerol as the only carbon source and ammonium salts as the only nitrogen source would support up to 500 µg/ml CTC using washed inoculum grown in a CSL-containing medium and up to 240 µg/ml CTC using spore inoculum. The inorganic salts consisted of:

$CaCO_3$	9 g/liter	H_3PO_4	0.4 g/liter
$(NH_4)_2SO_4$	5 g/liter	$FeSO_4 \cdot 7H_2O$	60 mg/liter
NH_4Cl	1 g/liter	$ZnSO_4 \cdot 7H_2O$	50 mg/liter
$MgCl_2 \cdot 6H_2O$	2 g/liter	$MnSO_4 \cdot 4H_2O$	50 mg/liter
KCl	1.3 g/liter	$CoCl_2 \cdot 6H_2O$	5 mg/liter

When supplemented with carbohydrate at 55 g/liter, and 0.8 g/liter each of L-histidine and L-methionine and a lipid source – lard oil or glycerol trioleate – at 20 ml/liter, the medium was capable of producing up to 4,000 µg/ml CTC using washed inoculum previously grown in a complex medium and 2,000 µg/ml CTC using inoculum previously grown in a defined medium.

A synthetic medium (J. J. GOODMAN 1962, unpublished) useful for the production of DMCTC consists of:

Dextrin	50 g/liter	K_2HPO_4	0.65 g/liter
$CaCO_3$	10 g/liter	$ZnSO_4 \cdot 7H_2O$	100 mg/liter
NH_4 tartarate	3 g/liter	$FeSO_4 \cdot 5H_2O$	50 mg/liter
$(NH_4)_2SO_4$	3 g/liter	$MnSO_4 \cdot 4H_2O$	50 mg/liter
L-Proline	2 g/liter	$CuSO_4 \cdot 5H_2O$	50 mg/liter
$MgCl_2 \cdot 6H_2O$	2 g/liter	Triglyceride oil	2% v/v

Other synthetic media formulations for CTC production have been disclosed. LAVATE (1960) using a starch salts medium found 1 g/liter tyrosine to be the best of a number of amino acids tested and phenylalanine to be almost as useful. SHULO and ZELINKA (1970) published a sucrose-salt medium containing glycine, phenylalanine, and tyrosine as organic nitrogen sources. In this medium, biotin (0.5 µg/ml) resulted in an increase in mycelial RNA, phosphorus, and biotin. CTC production was decreased, an effect reversed by benzyl thiocyanate, leading to the suggestion that benzyl thiocyanate affects carbohydrate metabolism through an inhibition of biotin synthesis. SEKIZAWA (1960) found L-lysine to be the best nitrogen source and biotin to be stimulatory to CTC production, as was shikimate, pantothenate, dimethylthetin, and vitamin B_{12}.

DARKEN et al. (1960) developed synthetic chloride-free media based on citric acid, sucrose, and mineral salts for production of TC. A simultaneous mutation and strain selection program resulted in a strain requiring ammonium nitrogen for optimum TC production. Yields of 2,000 μg/ml were achieved with no organic nitrogen present. Interestingly the strains used by DARKEN et al. (1960) were not suited for optimum yields in the media of MCCORMICK et al. (1959a) and the reverse was also true (J.J. GOODMAN 1960, unpublished results). MOLINARI (1964) also found no other nitrogen source superior to ammonium salts for TC production in synthetic medium and Mn^{2+}, Co^{2+}, K^{2+}, and SO_4^{2-} to be essential as well. Both inorganic and organic phosphorus could be used. Discrepancies in results between investigators are most probably due to differences in strains and inoculum procedures.

Growth and biosynthetic requirements are separable by the use of washed resting cell techniques. DESHPANDE (1965) resuspended cells of *S. aureofaciens* in nitrogen-free salt solution and obtained CTC synthesis with a number of mono- and disaccharides the best of which were fructose and dextrin, with starch being a poor carbohydrate source probably because of a lack of amylase secretion.

Washed resting cell systems respond to excess phosphate and to benzyl thiocyanate in the same way that growing systems do (DESHPANDE 1968). Pyruvic, malonic, and lactic acids stimulated while acetic and propionic acids inhibited CTC synthesis (DESHPANDE 1967). Aromatic amino acids, particularly L-tyrosine, stimulated CTC synthesis (MALADKAR and DESHPANDE 1978).

Synthetic media for OTC production have also been described. One of these (SHAPOSHNIKOV et al. 1958), widely used by Soviet investigators, consists of:

Starch	30 g/liter	K_2HPO_4	0.3 g/liter
Glucose	2 g/liter	$MgSO_4 \cdot 7H_2O$	0.1 g/liter
$(NH_4)_2SO_4$	1 g/liter	$FeSO_4 \cdot 7H_2O$	10 mg/liter
NH_3	1 g/liter	$ZnSO_4 \cdot 7H_2O$	18 mg/liter
Succinic acid	1.6 g/liter	$MnCl_2$	8 mg/liter

This medium was capable of yielding 1,500–1,900 μg/ml OTC in 4–5 days. With an enrichment in the levels of starch and $(NH_4)_2SO_4$, up to 3,800 μg/ml OTC was obtained (ORLOVA and ZAITSEVA 1960) and eventually yields as high as 5,000 μg/ml were reported (LISTVINOVA et al. 1968). The developmental sequences and the responses to phosphate seen with this medium are the same as those observed in complex media (ORLOVA and ZAITSEVA 1960).

HORVATH et al. (1958c) achieved 25%–30% of OTC yields obtainable in complex media using a medium consisting of:

Starch	15 g/liter	KH_2PO_4	130 mg/liter
Glycine	5 g/liter	$Co(NO_3)_2$	5 mg/liter
NaCl	3 g/liter	Tween 80	0.02 ml/liter

For use in tanks the carbohydrate was reduced to 10 g/liter and 4 g/liter palm oil was used in place of Tween 80. In this latter medium the optimum phosphate level was found to be twice that of the optimum shake flask level. Comparing several *S. rimosus* strains on this medium, GADO et al. (1961) found one strain which yielded better in synthetic than in complex medium and also found that the optimum phosphate level varied with strain, the better procedures requiring a higher phosphate level. The series of strains used in these investigations apparently do not utilize inorganic nitrogen well. Amino acids other than glycine, such as glutamic, aspartic, histidine, citrulline, arginine, and lysine used at equivalent amino nitrogen levels gave equal yields (GADO and HORVATH 1962).

Response to serine is particularly indicative of productivity of various strains. Serine was found by PARADA (1981) to inhibit OTC production by *S. rimosus* and CTC production by *S. aureofaciens* in complex media without significant effect on growth. In minimal medium, growth of both species was inhibited by serine and this was reversed by glycine and methionine. Amino acids which in synthetic media supported only poor OTC production were found by GADO and HORVATH (1963) to be potentiated by the addition of adenine and guanine but not by uracil, cytosine, or thymine. Amino acids which allowed no initiation of growth – valine, isoleucine, leucine, and oxyproline – did so on supplementation with the purines.

ZYGMUNT (1961), using washed *S. rimosus* inoculum growth in complex media, devised a synthetic medium where glucose and glycerol supported the best antibiotic yields and aspartic, proline, threonine, and β-alanine were the best among the amino acids tested for both growth and OTC production, while the other amino acids supported only growth but no OTC production. Such amino acids – alanine, glycine, and methionine – did support OTC synthesis when used as the *N*-acetyl derivatives (ZYGMUNT 1963). A subsequent medium published by ZYGMUNT (1964) very similar to the one devised by MCCORMICK (1959 a) for CTC but with no amino acids included gave OTC yields of 500–600 μg/ml.

Washed cell studies with *S. rimosus* were carried out by MAMANOVA and ORLOVA (1979), who found that the requirements of carbohydrate and $(NH_4)_2SO_4$ for maximum growth were twice as great as those for maximum OTC synthesis. Optimum phosphate levels were the same for both growth and OTC synthesis.

V. Stimulators and Inhibitors

In the absence of detailed knowledge of biosynthesis pathways, numerous compounds, particularly aromatic compounds, suggest themselves as potential precursors of tetracycline biosynthesis. A large number of these have been reported to cause increased antibiotic production. Such reports have not always been confirmed and such stimulation that has been observed is usually found with less productive strains (VANEK 1958; SHAPOSHNIKOV and PLAKUNOVA 1964 b). It is evident that the effects are not due to any direct incorporation into the antibiotic molecule. Among the compounds reported stimulatory to CTC production are: quinic and shikimik acids and their 5-dehydro derivatives (GOUREVITCH and LEIN 1955); ammonium benzoate, *p*-hydroxybenzoic acid, *p*-aminobenzoic acid, catechol, *p*-chlorophenoxyacetic acid, gallic acid, hippuric acid, β-indolylacetic acid, β-naphthol, α-naphthylamine, α-naphthylacetic acid, phenylacetic acid, and phlorglucinol (VANEK 1958); *p*-dimethylaminobenzaldehyde and *n*-methylanthranilic acid

(EGOROV and BARANOVA 1959; SHAPOSHNIKOV and PLAKINOVA 1964b); and diphenylamine, diphenylformamide, and α-naphthol (ABOU ZEID and YOUSEF 1972).

As stimulatory to OTC production may be listed indole butyric and indole acetic acids (SMOLEK et al. 1961; TOKADI 1962) and β-naphthoxyacetic and indole acetic acids and rutin (TOKADI 1962).

Lactic acid, a major ingredient of CSL, was reported (ORLOVA 1959) to stimulate OTC synthesis though addition of lactic acid to corn steep liquors low in this ingredient does not improve them. Poor-producing strains lack the ability to utilize lactic acid well (BRYZGALOVA and ORLOVA 1975). A specific *S. aureofaciens* mutant increased its CTC productive capacity from 5,900 μg/ml to 8,600 μg/ml on addition of 2 mg/ml thiamine mononitrate (MARINI 1972). Cadaverine (0.1%) added initially stimulated CTC formation but when added at 24 or 48 h inhibited antibiotic synthesis (ZELINKA 1968; ZELINKA and BIELY 1967). Cadaverine acts as a stabilizer of ribosomes of the producing organism in the presence of CTC. Saponin and *Claviceps* alkaloids also act as stabilizers and promote OTC formation (BOSTAN et al. 1979). Kinetin at 3 μg/ml increased TC production by 39% in a medium containing indole acetic acid (PRAVE and HUBER 1967). Polymers and coating made from them have been reported to increase TC production (KESTEL'MAN and VIL'NINA 1971).

Materials which specifically inhibit antibiotic production but not growth are propylalcohol (LISTVINOVA and GRYZANOVA 1969) bromethynol blue, methylene blue, and bromecresol green (ZYGMUNT 1962) for OTC and acridine orange (ZELINKOVA et al. 1976a) for CTC.

Benzyl thiocyanate deserves special mention because its mechanism of action is firmly established. It is widely used and effective not only with low-producing but also with high-producing strains. Added at the beginning or during the first 10 h it stimulates CTC production (PECAK et al. 1958). The optimum concentration for a high-producing strain was found to be 0.5–1.0 μg/ml and for a low-producing strain 3.0 μg/ml, resulting in a 40% and 78% increase in CTC production respectively. In tanks the optimum level of use is 2.0 μg/ml. The stimulation of CTC biosynthesis is more pronounced in media containing readily assimilable than in those containing poorly assimilated carbohydrates (HOSTALEK et al. 1958). In contrast to phosphate, benzyl thiocyanate decreases the rate of carbohydrate utilization. The relationships between carbohydrate metabolism and the biosynthesis of CTC as influenced by benzyl thiocyanate were described in a series of papers by HOSTALEK (1964a, b, c). Oxidation of sucrose but not endogenous respiration is inhibited by $6 \times 10^{-4} M$ concentration. At higher levels endogenous respiration is blocked and the block can be removed by washing. Oxidation of only the sugar which had served as the source of carbon but not other sugars is blocked. The inhibitory effect of interrupted aeration is reduced by benzyl thiocyanate. CTC production by washed resting cells is also increased by benzyl thiocyanate (DESHPANDE 1968). SHULO and ZELINKA (1970) found a reversal of the negative effect of biotin on CTC accumulation by benzyl thiocyanate. A reversal of the toxic effect of chlorination inhibitors can also be obtained by their combined use with benzyl thiocyanate (CULIK and HEROLD 1966; CULIK et al. 1969b).

NITESCU et al. (1962) found that OTC production as well as CTC production was stimulated by benzyl thiocyanate with increases of up to 85% in laboratory fermentations and 45%–60% in tanks.

It is of interest to note that though the use of benzyl thiocyanate is widespread and is obviously of benefit, none of the various production strains available to this author have responded to its addition.

VI. Directed Fermentations

The original reports on the production of TC by catalytic reduction of CTC (BOOTH et al. 1953; CONOVER et al. 1953) were soon followed by reports on the biosynthesis of TC (BOHONOS et al. 1953–1954; MINIERI et al. 1953–1954). These processes involved chloride denial by the use of synthetic media (DARKEN et al. 1960; MINIERI et al. 1953–1954) or the use of complex media ingredients naturally low in chloride such as cereal extract (ROLLAND and SENSI 1955) or cottonseed flour (HATCH et al. 1956; MCGHEE and MEGNA 1957). Other methods used silver or mercury to precipitate chloride from soluble media ingredients such as corn steep liquor (AMERICAN CYANAMID COMPANY 1957; CHERTOW 1961), dialysis to free insoluble ingredients, such as soy flour and peanut flour, from chloride ion (LEPETIT SpA (1958 a), and the use of ion exchange resins to free corn steep liquor of chloride (MINIERI et al. 1956, 1958).

1. Inhibition of Chlorination

Using chlorination inhibitors rather than chloride denial to promote TC formation allows the use of media without regard to their chloride content. GOUREVITCH et al. (1955) found bromide ion competitively inhibited chloride uptake, the extent of which depended on the Br/Cl ratio rather than on the absolute amount of halide. SEKIZAWA also found bromide inhibition of chloride uptake (1955) and in searching for a total inhibition of the residual amount of chlorination also found a number of mercapto type inhibitors whose actions will be discussed below. ARISHIMA et al. (1956) found bromide inhibition to be independent of the Br/Cl ratio, increasing with increasing bromide concentration. Certain mutants of *S. aureofaciens* will synthesize bromotetracycline if provided with bromide in place of chloride (SENSI et al. 1955; DOERSCHUK et al. 1956, 1959). Iodide (LEIN and GOUREVITCH 1956; KOLLAR and JARAI 1960 a) and fluoride (KOLLAR and JARAI 1960 a) have also been reported to inhibit chlorination. In our laboratories, we have not been able to confirm the effect of iodide and have found in some cases that fluoride actually increases the proportion of CTC to TC (SZUMSKI 1959 a). In *S. rimosus* addition of fluoride increases OTC production (GOODMAN 1959).

The discrepancies may perhaps be explained on the basis of types of mutants (DOERSCHUK et al. 1956, 1959), which differ in their halide metabolism and can broadly be distinguished as scavengers and nonscavengers. The differences between the two classes which incorporate the results of other investigators with our own are shown in Table 2.

Table 2. Classes of *S. aureofaciens* mutants and their response to halides

	Scavengers	Nonscavengers
Chloride	1. Rate of chlorination is dependent on chloride ion concentration 2. Maximum rate of chlorination assumed immediately after chloride addition to a halide-free medium	1. Rate of chlorination is independent of chloride ion concentration 2. Maximum rate of chlorination assumed gradually after chloride addition to a halide-free medium
Bromide	1. Used for BTC synthesis 2. Does not inhibit chlorination	1. Not used for BTC synthesis 2. Inhibits chlorination, reversible by Cl^-
Iodide	Does not inhibit chlorination	Inhibits chlorination
Fluoride	Increases chlorination	Inhibits chlorination
Thiocyanate	Inhibits chlorination, not reversible by Cl^-	Inhibits chlorination, slightly reversible by Cl^-

Given excess chloride, scavenging strains are able to synthesize 90%–93% of the total tetracyclines as CTC (DOERSCHUK et al. 1956, 1959). Nonscavenging strains exhibit gradations in chlorinating capacity ranging from those able to synthesize 75% (DOERSCHUK et al. 1956, 1959) to others synthesizing 20% (KOTIUSZKO et al. 1958) of the total tetracycline capacity as CTC. At the other end of the spectrum are the strains which have a complete block in their halide metabolism and completely ignore chloride. KOLLAR and JARAI (1960a) claimed to have obtained such strains by undisclosed mutagenic treatments and such strains were completely described by GROWICH and DEDUCK (1963).

Both DOERSHUK et al. (1956, 1959) and LEIN and GOUREVITCH (1956) found thiocyanate to inhibit chlorination. Though originally it was tested because it is a halogenoid, its known effect as an antithyroid agent led to the examination of other antithyroid compounds. SEKIZAWA (1955, 1956a, 1956b) found out of 18 such compounds tested that 2-thiouracil, thiourea, 2-mercaptobenzothiazole, and α-mercapto-*N*-2-naphthyl acetamide were effective chlorination inhibitors. GOODMAN et al. (1959) found 2,5-dimercapto-1,3,4-thiadiazole, 2-phenyl-5-mercapto-1,3,4-oxadiazole, and 2-(2-furyl)-5-mercapto oxadiazole to be particularly effective with as little as 5–10 mg/liter resulting in the production of over 95% TC. LEIN et al. (1959) added 2-benzoxazolethiol and 2-mercaptobenzimidazole to the list of active compounds. Highly active compounds all contain the structural feature:

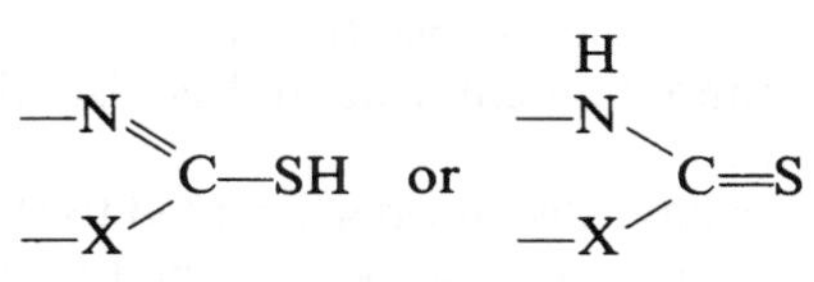

where X=N, S, or 0.

A number of patents have been issued on the use of such compounds as chlorination inhibitors for TC fermentation (GOODMAN and YOUNG 1960 a, b; TANNER 1960; ARISHIMA and SEKIZAWA 1960, 1962; GOODMAN 1962 a).

The action of the mercapto-type inhibitors is characterized by the following features:

1. They are equally active against both scavenging and nonscavenging CTC strains.
2. They are not reversible by excess chloride.
3. They are effective immediately on addition to the system.
4. They are reversible by Cu^{2+} and Ag^{2+}.

A number of such inhibitors, as is also bromide, are reversible by chloropropanediol (SEKIZAWA 1960; JARAI 1964). This led to the proposal (SEKIZAWA 1960) that chloropropanediol was incorporated into the biosynthetic pathway at some point before the chlorination step. GOODMAN et al. (1963) offered strong evidence that the reversal is due to the alkylation of the inhibitor by chloropropanediol. Inhibitors without a free SH group such as dibromothiazole are not reversed. In chloride-free media chloropropanediol can serve as an efficient source of chloride ion, which explains its reversing effect on bromide.

Halogenated pyrimidines also are chlorination inhibitors. CULIK et al. (1969 a) found that their effect is potentiated by benzyl thiocyanate. GOODMAN and MATRISHIN (1968) found 2,4-dichloro-5-methylpyrimidine to be the most effective among 30 such compounds tested and for their strains bromide was found to be a potentiating agent. Their mechanism of action is unknown. They are not reversed by Cu^{2+} or chloropropanediol as are the mercapto type of inhibitors.

A final group of chlorination inhibitors are 1,1,3-tricyano-2-amino-1-propene, a known antithyroid agent, and a number of other nitrile and cyano compounds (GOODMAN and MATRISHIN 1973). As a group, these are the least effective of those so far noted. They are strongly potentiated by bromide. They are slightly reversed by Cu^{2+} and more strongly reversed by *p*-aminopropiophenone and methylene blue, the latter requiring addition after 48 h of growth to prevent its own toxicity. Both of these last two reversing agents are known antidotes to cyanide poisoning.

All of the organic chlorination inhibitors cause a reduction in total antibiotic yield in the CTC/TC-producing strains. The more effective the compound as a chlorination inhibitor the greater is the toxicity and the narrower the range of concentrations at which it can be used effectively. These inhibitors are also effective with the nonmethylating DMCTC-producing strains, causing them to synthesize DMTC but at an even greater sacrifice in total potency than is the case with CTC/TC production. This loss is accompanied – but not to the same extent as the loss – by an increase in the purple pigment characteristic of nonmethylating strains (MCCORMICK et al. 1959 b; MCCORMICK and GARDNER 1963). This increased pigment production is not a specific effect due to the inhibitors because it is noted as well on withholding chloride and is also characteristically high in DMTC-producing strains.

All of the inhibitors we have discussed are added to the medium as chemically defined entities. Similar results can also be obtained using less "defined" inhibitors. For instance, CULIK et al. (1962) react bromine with one of the medium ingredients such as soyflour or with a mixture of unsaturated fats to form nontoxic organic compounds containing covalently bound bromine which, on use in the medium, then function as chlorination inhibitors. Natural substances such as rapeseed meal or mustard seed meal at a level of 5 g/liter in the medium have resulted in a shift to a 95/5 TC/CTC ratio from the normal 35/65 TC/CTC ratio produced by the nonscavenging mutant used (CULIK and HEROLD 1966). Rapeseed and many other seeds of *Brassica* and related species are known to contain natural antithyroid substances (SELENKOW and COLLACO 1961; GREER 1956; BELL 1956).

Somewhat more surprising is the claim that oat products (Institut Antibiotykow 1961) act in a similar way, causing only TC to be produced at a 3,000- to 4,000-µg/ml level in a medium containing chloride, while without the oat flour both CTC and TC are produced. We have noted no such effect in extensive experience using cereal flours such as corn, wheat, barley, and oat flours nor have such reports appeared in the literature when using flours from rice or sorghum millet.

At times it may be desirable to direct the fermentation toward the chlorinated rather than the nonchlorinated product. A particular example is the DMCTC fermentation, where before improved strains were developed the nonchlorinated DMTC exceeded specified limits. In this case and also in the CTC fermentation the addition of 50–100 mg/liter $CuSO_4 \cdot 5H_2O$ to the medium increased the ratio of the halogenated to nonhalogenated antibiotic (GOODMAN 1962b). The same effect was observed on adding 1 mg/liter 5-fluorouracil or 0.5 g/liter D-methionine (GOODMAN 1964b). A similar effect was noted in the CTC fermentation with 4 mg/liter *p*-dimethylaminobenzaldehyde (WELWARD and HALAMA 1974).

Deviations from optimal conditions tend to increase the minor component level. Thus an improper corn steep level or improper aeration conditions increase the TC content in the CTC fermentation or the CTC content in a TC fermentation (LAZNIKOVA and MAKAREVICH 1963). This may also explain in part the observations of PETTY (1968), who found that higher growth temperatures favored TC production in five diverse strains of *S. aureofaciens*. In some cases TC was made almost exclusively but at a sharply reduced total yield.

In *S. rimosus* TC has been noted as a minor component by PERLMAN et al. (1960) and by ZYGMUNT (1962). There appears to be no report, however, of a directed fermentation toward increased TC production at the expense of the normal OTC production.

2. Inhibition of Methylation

Inhibition of methylation at C6 of the tetracycline nucleus in strains which normally make only CTC and TC has also been accomplished but since methylation is a more fundamental and widespread reaction yield losses are significantly greater than for the inhibition of chlorination. At the time this work was undertaken in our laboratories, the yields achieved by CTC-producing strains were so much superior to those of the DMCTC producers that continued efforts were justified in the search for a reasonably successful inhibition route.

The source of the C6 methyl group being methionine (MILLER et al. 1956), methionine analogues were the first to be tested. Addition of 400 μg/ml DL-ethionine to a normal CTC producer led to the production of DMCTC in the amount of about 7% of the total tetracyclines. Only the L-isomer was active GOODMAN and MILLER 1962). Other workers have essentially confirmed these results. NEIDLEMAN et al. (1963 a) found both D- and L-isomers to be active and to be reversed by methionine, methionine sulfoxide, methoxinine, glycine, serine, threonine, homocysteine, cyanocobalamin, and Co^{2+}. Using an auxotrophic mutant of *S. viridifaciens* blocked between cystathionine and homocysteine in the methionine pathway, HENDLIN et al. (1962) found that the small amount of DMCTC normally produced could be shifted toward higher DMCTC production by the addition of ethionine or back to CTC by the addition of methionine.

Adding ethionine to *S. rimosus* leads to different results. ZYGMUNT (1962) found a reduction in OTC synthesis which was readily reversed by methionine. However, DULANEY et al. (1962), again using methionine auxotrophs, found ethionine to inhibit methylation not at C6 but rather at C4, leading to small amounts of *N*-methylethyl OTC. *N*-Demethyl precursors of anhydrotetracyclines were found by MILLER et al. (1964) on adding ethionine to selected *S. aureofaciens* mutants.

Other methionine analogues and antagonists have also led to the production of small amounts of DMCTC. These substances include D-methionine (GOODMAN and MILLER 1962); D-methionine ethyl ester (GOODMAN 1964 a); and the *S*-2-hydroxy-ethyl, *S*-2-chloroethyl, and *S*-ethyl derivatives of homocysteine (NEIDLEMAN et al. 1963 b). In none of these cases was DMCTC the major product.

Interference with the folic-acid-dependent 1-carbon transfer system has also led to the production of DMCTC by CTC-producing strains. Thus NEIDLEMAN et al. (1963 a) found aminopterin (4-amino folic acid) to be active and reversible by methionine but not by PABA, folic acid, or cyanocobalamin.

A shift toward DMCTC as the major product was most successfully achieved through the use of a number of sulfonamides to interfere with the 1-carbon transfer system. Both PERLMAN et al. (1961) and the author (GOODMAN and MATRISHIN 1961, 1962) have reported that up to 65% of DMCTC is synthesized by CTC-producing strains on adding 50–100 μg/ml of sulfapyridines, sulfadiazines, sulfapyridazines, and sulfatriazines with methyl, thiomethyl, methoxy, or chlorine substituents on the heterocyclic nitrogen moiety. Other sulfonamides active at higher levels include sulfanilamide, sulfacetamide, sulfaguanidine, and sulfathiazole. Typical results obtainable with sulfadiazine are illustrated in Table 3, where it will be seen that a 67% level of DMCTC can be achieved but only with an unacceptable loss in total yield.

In cases where DMCTC is produced both growth and potency are sharply reduced, but not all sulfonamides causing growth reduction result in DMCTC production. The action of sulfonamides is reversible by PABA and folic or folinic acids; and to a lesser extent by thymine, adenine, and methionine. In all cases production of DMCTC was accompanied by the production of the reddish-brown to violet pigment characteristic of demethylating strains. Attempts to cause the synthesis of DMCTC without at the same time causing an adverse effect on the producing organism by using a strain made resistant to up to 500 μg/ml sulfa-

Table 3. Effect of sulfadiazine on the synthesis of CTC and DMCTC by *S. aureofaciens*

Sulfadiazine (μg/ml)	CTC (μg/ml)	6-DMTC (μg/ml)	% DMCTC (μg/ml)	% Yield reduction
0	7,350	0	0	0
10	6,175	0	0	16
30	3,920	Trace	Trace	46
50	565	260	34	89
70	170	340	67	93

diazine were without effect. Also adding the drug 16 h into the fermentation allowed the final amount of growth to approach control levels but again with no DMCTC synthesis (GOODMAN and MILLER 1962).

The problem of yield loss was solved to some degree by workers at CHINOIN (1963) by using a prototrophic recombinant of two methionine auxotrophs which synthesized 4% of its total tetracyclines as DMCTC. Adding 4 g/liter sulfaguanidine to this strain in gradually increasing doses at 3-h intervals after inoculation resulted in a final DMCTC level of 77% with no loss and even with some increase in overall yield over the control without added sulfaguanidine.

Using a similarly derived strain normally synthesizing 45% DMCTC, JARAI (1969) found a cobalamin rather than a folic-dependent methylation. Addition of cobinamides but not Co^{2+} within the first 16 h of fermentation caused a shift to complete CTC production. Addition of a vitamin B_{12} antagonist, α-5,6-dimethylbenzimidazolecobamic acid-a,b,c,d,g-pentaamide-cyanide (DCAPA), caused a shift to a 60%–85% DMCTC level but with a loss of up to 75% of total tetracyclines produced. None of the methylation inhibitors discussed are as efficient in causing a shift to DMCTC production as are chlorination inhibitors in causing a shift to TC production. Mutant strains completely lacking 6-methylating capacity are the preferred route to the demethyltetracyclines.

Two other instances of directed fermentation in the tetracyclines may be noted. ORLOVA (1968) found L-glutamine or L-asparagine added at 24 h to a 2-acetyl-2-decarboxamido OTC synthesizing *S. rimosus* culture turned the process in the direction of OTC formation. Previously synthesized 2-acetyldecarboxamido OTC was not converted. Glutamine and aspartic acids, urea, and ammonium salts had a similar effect. *Streptomyces aureofaciens* strain S1308 produces 7-chloro-5a(11a)-dehydrotetracycline in amounts of 2,500–4,000 μg/ml in a medium lacking or low in riboflavin and up to 8,000–10,000 μg/ml in media containing 0.1–2.0 μg/ml riboflavin (GROWICH and MILLER 1961). However, larger amounts of riboflavin (up to 5 μg/ml) direct the process toward the formation of CTC (MILLER et al. 1961). A number of other materials, particularly glycerol, sorbitol, and barbaloin and a number of oximes such as 1,2-naphthoquinone-1-oxime, 2-butanone oxime, and furil dioxime, have a similar effect but at a lower specific activity than riboflavin. Cosynthetic factor 1 (MILLER et al. 1960; MCCORMICK et al. 1961 b) isolated from several strains forming cosynthetic pairs with S-1308 acts in the same manner and being a pteridin or flavin could be related in its catalytic mode of action to riboflavin[1]. The mode of action of the other alcohols and oximes is not known.

D. Fermentation Technology

A detailed discussion of the biochemical engineering aspects of tetracycline production is beyond the scope of this review; however, some mention of a few topics properly belong here. While feed-grade tetracyclines have been produced to a small extent in surface culture, the bulk of production is carried out in submerged culture in aerated tanks, where improved strains and media must ultimately perform. Changes in technology are introduced more slowly compared with strain or media improvements because of the constraints fixed by original fermentor designs and the large capital costs involved in changing them. There is, understandably, less information published on the technology of the tetracycline fermentations than there is on other areas of the subject. The translation from laboratory shake flask through small fermentors to large-scale equipment is largely a problem of oxygen supply, and this is what the literature is mostly concerned with.

I. Aeration

Oxygen must certainly be considered an important medium ingredient, the availability of which is severely limited by its low solubility in water. It is usually introduced into the fermentor by means of a sterile air supply. It is the task of the fermentation engineer to insure an adequate supply of dissolved oxygen at all times. The tetracycline producers are quite sensitive to reduction in adequate air supply. HRIBALOVA and STARKA (1959) found the mycelium from continuously aerated *S. aureofaciens* to differ in its response to inhibitors of glycolysis and the hexose monophosphate shunt from that of the mycelium subjected to interrupted aeration. HOSTALEK et al. (1958) found interruptions of aeration of *S. aureofaciens* between the 6th and 12th h of growth severely depressed yields of CTC. A single 10-min pause resulted in a 50% yield reduction while six 10-min pauses during that critical period resulted in a greater than 75% yield reduction. Pauses in aeration outside of the critical period had a much less drastic effect. Benzyl thiocyanate addition antagonized the effects of interrupted aeration which were exerted through an interaction with carbohydrate metabolism. The extreme sensitivity to interrupted aeration during the early stages may be confined to certain strain lines of *S. aureofaciens* since, with the production strains available to him, this author has not been able to duplicate the effects of interrupted aeration in the early hours of the fermentation.

MATELOVA (1964) found that for any of a series of variables such as medium, flask size, media volumes, shaker speeds, or the number and rpm of agitators in a stirred vessel, the maximum total productivity varied. In any combination, however, on keeping all but one of the variables constant, the highest yield was always obtained at an oxygen transfer rate of 0.59 ml O_2/ml per hour.

---

1 Since the preparation of this manuscript, cosynthetic factor 1 has been identified as 7,8-didemethyl-8-hydroxy-5-deazariboflavin (MCCORMICK and MORTON 1982)

GRINYUK and BRINBERG (1960) found that as medium concentration was increased, higher yields of CTC were obtained but the solubility of oxygen in the medium decreased while the oxygen requirement of the culture remained the same, thus limiting the biosynthetic process. At lower levels of aeration BELOUSOVA and POPOVA (1961 a) and CHERKASOVA et al. (1978) found an increase in the pyruvic and acetic acid in the medium and a decrease in TC production similar to the effect of excess phosphate. OBLOZHKO et al. (1977) found that as medium richness was increased twofold there was also a twofold increase in mycelium but only a 54% increase in OTC formation limited by a decrease in the dissolved oxygen level. A lack of dissolved oxygen in the OTC fermentation also leads to an accumulation of organic acids in the medium (OBLOZHKO and ORLOVA 1975). JENSEN et al. (1966) were able to duplicate patterns of oxygen utilization, CTC accumulation, and mycelial accumulation in tank-to-tank, flask-to-flask, or flask-to-tanks runs using oxygen utilization as a scale-up parameter with very little discrepancy between runs. Variable agitator speed was used to duplicate the oxygen utilizations from one vessel to the other.

The optima for oxygen have been expressed in a variety of ways – as dissolved oxygen levels, as oxygen uptake rates in milligrams or milliliters, or simply as volumes of air supplied per volume of medium per minute, making translation for the nonengineer difficult. There is general agreement, however, that critical levels do exist. Excessive oxygen has also been reported to result in decreased CTC yields due to a destruction of cellular metabolites (PLAKUNOVA and KISELEVA 1965; PLAKUNOVA 1967).

The CO_2 level in the medium is also affected by the amount swept out through aeration. Optimal CO_2 concentrations for TC fermentation have been reported as 2–8 ml CO_2/100 ml medium (SHERSTOBITOVA et al. 1976). A level greater than 15 ml/100 ml decreases the rate of respiration of various tetracycline producers (NIKITINA et al. 1974). CHAGIN and BIRYUKOV (1980) found that changes in CO_2 concentration paralleled changes in TC production by *S. aureofaciens*. Slowing the aeration rate increased the CO_2 concentration in the medium and increased antibiotic formation by 25%–30%.

The general trend has been to increase oxygen supply as the concentration of media has increased and as more productive strains have been developed. Air entering the fermentor has been enriched with oxygen. PLICHON et al. (1976) found that air enriched to 40% oxygen gave a 50% increase in OTC yield and a 20% increase in mycelial growth. Air enriched to 60% oxygen gave no further increases in yield. GOUGES (1978) added air with or without supplemental pure oxygen to keep the dissolved oxygen level at 0.3 ppm in the OTC fermentation with *S. varsoviensis*. Other such "programmed" aeration patterns have been described. BAEV et al. (1980) maintained an aeration rate of 0.5 vvm until the last 20–30 h of an *S. rimosus* fermentation, when the rate was increased to 0.6 vvm, achieving a yield of 18,500 μg/ml OTC after 160 h. SHTOFFER et al. (1973) chose an aeration and agitation schedule for OTC production based on maintaining a maximal rate of oxygen consumption by the culture. A stepwise alteration of the pattern during the course of the fermentation resulted in a substantial decrease in power consumption. Agitation rate was the parameter most often varied, with early and late stages of the fermentation being able to use less agitation. Air supply had a smaller effect on oxygen consumption than did agitation though either could be varied based on economics, foam production, or CO_2 concentration. Oxygen consumption was measured by off-gas analysis.

Excessive aeration and agitation, which may be harmful and are certainly wasteful, have an effect also on foam production in submerged fermentations. In the tetracyclines this foam is most often controlled by the triglyceride oils which are added both as nutrients and natural antifoams. Their antifoam properties may, however, be enhanced by the addition of supplementary substances such as octadecanol added at the rate of 1% to the lard oil (PETTY 1955) or the sludge from rice bran oil at 0.5–10% (SZUMSKI 1960) or by the addition of 0.01%–0.2% of water-soluble antifoams such as Pluronic L61 or L81 to the medium (PHILLIPS 1964).

II. Temperature

The tetracyclines are usually fermented at moderate temperatures of 24°–28 °C. A fermentation capable of running at a higher temperature would be a definite advantage because of lower cooling water requirements. Some higher temperature fermentations have been described. In the OTC fermentation PIVNYAK (1963) found that at an air temperature of 27°–28 °C the medium temperature in the flasks is 30°–31 °C but that raising the flask temperature slightly to 31°–32.5 °C slightly accelerated the rate of biosynthesis of OTC but was without effect on the ultimate potency or length of the fermentation. However, in the surface culture method for OTC, PIVNYAK (1962) found an advantage in running the fermentation at temperatures as high as 36 °C. A patent was granted to LAB PRO-TER (1963 b) in which the OTC fermentation using *S. ticinensis* yielded 4,950 mg/ml running at 36 °C after 70 h. A patent for TC production by *S. aureofaciens* var *mediolanum* also granted to LAB PRO-TER (1963 a) described a slightly more accelerated production at 38 °C but an ultimately higher yield when carried out at 35 °C.

E. Concluding Remarks

This review has attempted to illustrate how developments in strains and media in particular have resulted in increased yields in the fermentation of tetracyclines. Though much of media development and much of strain selection is a matter of trial and error, still some rationales do exist. While media cost is not a significant factor in the case of a newly discovered antibiotic, in the case of mature antibiotics such as the tetracyclines produced in large volumes it may be quite significant. Variability of raw materials must be considered, a uniform material obviously being more desirable. Given the present-day uncertainties of supply it is also desirable to have alternative media formulations available.

The selection of improved strains has in most instances not used a directed genetic approach but has been a matter of mutation and selection. The newer genetic approaches continue to hold out a promise that has not yet been fulfilled.

We have discussed several processes which were supplanted as new fermentation improvements were introduced. These old processes were included because they were part of a developmental continuum. It is interesting to note that in our experience, though TC processes through halide denial and chlorination inhibitors were available by mid-1955 and pure TC-producing strains were available by 1962 (GROWICH and DEDUCK 1963), it was not until 1966 that direct fermentation supplanted the reduction process as a source of TC. This is a tribute to the ongoing process improvements in CTC fermentation yields which made it possible for the reduction process to be competitive for such a long period.

Strain development and media development programs usually go on simultaneously and it is useful to assess if possible the individual effect such programs have had on improvements in yield. This can be done as a retrospective exercise without regard to any advances simultaneously being made in the strictly engineering aspect of the fermentation. A "library" of strains is usually maintained and the media are simple to duplicate. Four such CTC-producing strains of increasingly higher yield potential and four media qualitatively similar but of generally increasing concentration all of which, strains and media, had been introduced into production-scale operations over a 25-year period were run together in a single experiment by the author. The results are shown in Table 4, which, for the purposes of illustration, normalizes the potencies obtained with the earliest strain and earliest medium at a value of 100.

Table 4. Combined effect of strains and media on increasing yields in CTC production

Strains of increasing potency	Media of increasing concentration			
	1	2	3	4
A	100	316	466	443
B	154	363	635	762
C	188	378	680	830
D	155	405	800	1,050

It is evident that any strain, even an early one, responds to media improvements introduced at a much later date and that for any given medium all strains could be ranked in about the same order. The maximum improvements are achieved when both improved strains and media are used together.

The above experiment does not assess the effect of engineering advances on yield increases. A somewhat similar assessment for a typical antibiotic based on historical data was released by Bristol Laboratories and published in the *Second Edition of Biochemical Engineering* (AIBA et al. 1973, pp 218–219). In this case the improvement that can be ascribed to strain and medium improvement account for roughly 30% each while engineering advances are responsible for 40% of the yield improvement over a 14-year period. Roughly the same values could reasonably be expected to hold for the tetracyclines.

References

Abou-Zeid A, Abou-El-Atta (1973) Utilization of Egyptian raw materials in production of tetracyclines by *Streptomyces aureofaciens*. Chem Abstr 78:14446

Abou-Zeid A, Yousef AE (1971) Influence of phosphorous on the fermentation production of chlortetracycline (CTC), cobalamin (vitamin B_{12}) and antifungal antibiotic AYF by *Streptomyces aureofaciens*. Pak J Sci Ind Res 14:244–246

Abou-Zeid A, Yousef AE (1972) Influence of some organic compounds on the production of chlortetracycline, vitamin B_{12}, and antiyeast factor (AYF) by *Streptomyces aureofaciens*. Indian J Appl Chem 35:26–29

Abou-Zeid A, El-Dewany AI, Eissa AEI, Fouad M, Yessein M (1979) Production of oxytetracycline, by *Streptomyces rimosus* 12907, as an animal feed supplement. Chem Abstr 91:106534

Adamovic V, Bosnjak J, Vebel D (1969) Effect of different sources of carbon on the biosynthesis of oxytetracycline. Chem Abstr 70:95406

Aiba S, Humphrey AE, Millis NF (1973) Biochemical engineering, 2nd edn. Academic, New York

Alikhanian SI (1962) Induced mutagenesis in the selection of microorganisms. Adv Appl Microbiol 4:1–50

Alikhanian SI (1979) Achievements of genetic engineering and their practical application. Biol Zbl 98:513–526

Alikhanian SI, Borisova LN (1961) Recombination in *Actinomyces aureofaciens*. J Gen Microbiol 26:19–28

Alikhanian SI, Danilenko VN (1979) Sources and perspectives in the studies of genetic control of antibiotic synthesis in Actinomycetes. Hindustan Antib Bull 24:125–132

Alikhanian SI, Mindlin SZ (1957a) Development of biochemical mutants of *Streptomyces rimosus* for derivation of hybrid forms. Dokl Akad Nauk SSSR 114:1113–1115

Alikhanian SI, Mindlin SZ (1957b) Recombinations in *Streptomyces rimosus*. Nature 180–1208–1209

Alikhanian SI, Mindlin SZ, Goldat SV, Vladimizov AV (1959) Genetics of organisms producing tetracyclines. Ann NY Acad Sci 82:914–949

Alikhanian SI, Orlova NV, Mindlin SZ, Zaitseva ZM (1961) Genetic control of oxytetracycline biosynthesis. Nature 189:939–940

American Cyanamid Company (1957) Tetracycline. British Patent 773,453

Ankerfarm SpA (1971) Enzymatic hydrolysis of carbohydrate-rich fermentation media for producing tetracycline-group antibiotics. French Patent 1,603,121

Ardelean V, Alupei G, Jaluba M (1972) Biosynthesis of aureocycline by *Streptomyces aureofaciens*. German Patent 2,033,447

Arishima M, Sekizawa Y (1960) Method for preparing tetracycline. US Patent 2,949,406

Arishima M, Sekizawa Y (1962) Method for preparing tetracycline. US Patent 3,019,173

Arishima M, Sekizawa Y, Sakamoto J, Miwa K, Okada E (1956) Tetracycline fermentation. Bull Ag Chem Soc Japan 30:407–409

Backus EJ, Duggar BM, Campbell TH (1954) Variation in *Streptomyces aureofaciens*. Ann NY Acad Sci 60:86–101

Baev V, Manafova N, Baeva Z, Again I, Georgieva-Borisova L, Kostova R, Patsadzhi A, Rutkova E, Kostova T, Strashilov T (1980) Improvement of oxytetracycline production. Chem Abstr 93:148039

Baghlaf AO, Abou-Zeid AA, El-Diwamy AI, Eissa AI (1980) Production of oxytetracycline by *Streptomyces rimosus* 12907 as an animal feed supplement. Chem Abstr 92:162097

Baranova IP, Egorov NS (1963) Pyruvic acid metabolism and biosynthesis by *Actinomyces aureofaciens*. Mikrobiologiia 32:209–215

Bassett EJ, Kieth MS, Armelagos GJ, Martin DA, Villanueva AR (1980) Tetracycline labeled human bone from ancient Sudanese Nubia. Science 209:1532–1534

Behal V, Hostalek Z, Vanek Z (1979) Anhydrotetracycline oxygenase activity and biosynthesis of tetracyclines in *Streptomyces aureofaciens*. Biotechnol Lett 1:177–182

Bekhtereva MN, Kolesnikova IG (1961) Morphological peculiarities of *Actinomyces lavendulae* and *Actinomyces aureofaciens* long cultivated in a streaming medium. Mikrobiologiia 30:402–408

Belik E, Herold M, Hudec M, Misecka J, Zelinka J (1958) New methods for biosynthetic manufacture of antibiotics. I. Manufacture of technical chlortetracycline. Chemicke Zvesti 12:122–127

Bell DJ (1956) 2-Mercapto-Δ^2-1:3 oxazolines (2-thio-1:3-oxazolidines) as anti-thyroid substances from vegetable sources. Annual reports on the progress of chemistry. Chem Soc 52:291–295

Belousova II, Popova LA (1961 a) The formation of organic acids in biosynthesis of tetracycline under varied conditions of fermentation. Antibiotiki 6:115–118

Belousova II, Popova LA (1961 b) Effect of mineral phosphorus on biosynthesis of tetracycline and composition of the phosphorus fractions of *Streptomyces aureofaciens* in relation to the cultivation conditions and growth of mycelium. Antibiotiki 6:302–307

Biffi G, Boretti G, DiMarco A, Pennella P (1954) Metabolic behavior and chlortetracycline production of *Streptomyces aureofaciens* in liquid culture. Appl Microbiol 2:288–293

Bishop H (1970) Fermentative biosynthesis of tetracycline antibiotics. US Patent 3,516,909

Biswas GD, Sen SP (1971) Transformation in *Streptomyces* with respect to antibiotic production. J Appl Bacteriol 34:287–293

Blumauerova M (1971) Contribution to the study of genetic recombination in tetracycline-producing streptomycetes. Folia Microbiol 16:504

Blumauerova M, Ismail AA, Hostalek Z, Vanek Z (1971) Mutation studies in *Streptomyces aureofaciens*. Radiation and radioisotopes for industrial microorganisms. Int Atomic Energy Agency, Symp Vienna, pp 157–166

Blumauerova M, Hostalek Z, Vanek Z (1972) Biosynthesis of tetracyclines: problems and perspectives of genetic analysis. Proc IV Int Ferm Symp. Terui G (ed) Fermentation technology today, pp 223–232

Blumauerova M, Hostalek Z, Vanek Z (1973) Mutagenesis by UV-irradiation and *N*-methyl-*N*-nitrosoguanidine in *Streptomyces aureofaciens*. Studia Biophysica (Berlin) 36/37:311–318

Bohonos N, Dornbush AC, Feldman LI, Martin JH, Pelcak E, Williams JH (1953–1954) *In vitro* studies with chlortetracycline oxytetracycline and tetracycline. Antibiot Annu: 49–55

Bonnat R, Chaussier M (1968) Tetracycline preparation procedure. French Patent 1,580,921

Booth JH, Morton J, Petisi JP, Wikinson RG, Williams JH (1953) Tetracycline. J Am Chem Soc 75:4621

Borensztajn D, Wolf J (1955) Laboratory and pilot-plant production of oxytetracycline. Chem Abstr 49:11781

Boretti G, DiMarco A, Scotti T, Zocchi P (1955) Morphologic and biochemical variations in *Streptomyces aureofaciens* in relation to the production of chlortetracycline. G Microbiol 1:97–105

Boretti G, DiMarco A, Julita P, Raggi F, Bardi U (1956) Presenza degli enzimi della via esosomonofosfato ossidativa nello *Streptomyces aureofaciens*. G Microbiol 5:406–416

Borisoglebskaya AN, Perebityuk AN, Boronin M (1979) Study of the resistance of *Actinomyces rimosus* to oxytetracycline. Antibiotiki 24:883–888

Borisov VP, Gorbash AA (1963) Vegetable oil for the production of biomycin. Chem Abstr 58:14655

Boronin AM, Mindlin SZ (1971) Genetic analysis of *Actinomyces rimosus* mutants with impaired synthesis of oxytetracycline. Genetika (Moskva) 7:125–131

Boronin AM, Sadovnikova G (1972) Use of acridine dyes to eliminate oxytetracycline resistance in *Streptomyces rimosus*. Genetika (Moskva) 8:174–176

Bosnjak M, Kapetanovic E (1971) Pilot-plant semicontinuous cultivation of oxytetracycline inoculum. Chem Abstr 75:18546

Bostan R, Toma M, Rugina V, Mihalache A, Ciocan R (1979) Biosynthesis of 5-hydroxytetracycline. Chem Abstr 91:191360.

Bryzgalova TE, Orlova NV (1975) Organic acid production by an active strain of *Actinomyces rimosus* and an inactive mutant in oxytetracycline biosynthesis. Antibiotiki 20:11–15

Callam CT (1970) Improvement of micro-organism by mutation, hybridization and selection. In: Norris RJ, Ribbons DW (eds) Methods in microbiology. Academic, New York, pp 435–459

Chagin BA, Biryukov VV (1980) Automatic monitoring of the partial pressure of dissolved carbon dioxide in tetracycline biosynthesis. Chem Abstr 93:184219

Chalenko NV Malt'tsev PM (1971) Amylolytic activity of *Actinomyces aureofaciens*. Chem Abstr 74:139543

Chang SL (1961) The effects of sugars and nitrogenous compounds upon the metabolism of *Streptomyces aureofaciens*. Sci Sin 10:349–360

Cheng HF, Li HL (1975) Selection for producer of demethylchlortetracycline I. Selection of demethylchlortetracycline producing strain of *Streptomyces aureofaciens*. Chem Abstr 82:168786

Cheng HF, Liu JL, Chou SY (1975) Selection for producer of demethylchlortetracycline II. Selection of *Streptomyces aureofaciens* 635 and its characters. Chem Abstr 83:112279

Cherkasova GN, Sherstobitova TS, Orekhova VM (1978) Study of aeration conditions during tetracycline biosynthesis. Role of organic acids. Chem Abstr 88:87589

Chertow B (1961) Process for the production of tetracycline by fermentation. US Patent 2,970,946

Chinoin Gyogyszer (1962) Mutant of *Streptomyces aureofaciens* which produces tetracycline. German Patent 1,128,599

Chinoin Gyogyszer (1963) Demethyltetracycline from selected *Streptomyces* strains. French Patent 1,414,222

Conover LH, Moreland WT, English AR, Stephens CR, Pilgrim FJ (1953) Terramycin XI. Tetracycline. J Am Chem Soc 4622–4623

Culik K, Herold M (1966) The inhibition of chlorination in the biosynthesis of tetracycline by agents from diverse natural substances. In: Herold M, Gabriel Z (eds) Antibiotics. Advances in research production and clinical use. Butterworth's, London, pp 580–581

Culik K, Herold M, Palkoska J, Belik E, Dasek J (1962) Method of producing tetracycline. US Patent 3,037,917

Culik K, Herold M, Palkoska J, Sikyta B (1967) Manufacturing tetracycline. Chem Abstr 66:104024

Culik K, Palkoska J, Vondracek M, Skoda J, Herold M (1969 a) Fermentation process for the production of tetracycline. US Patent 3,429,780

Culik K, Herold M, Palkoska J, Sikyta B, Slezak J (1969 b) Production of tetracycline by *Streptomyces aureofaciens* in synthetic media. Appl Microbiol 8:46–51

Darken MA, Berenson H, Shirk RJ, Sjolander NO (1960) Production of tetracycline by *Streptomyces aureofaciens* in synthetic media. Appl Microbiol 8:46–51

Delic V, Pigac J, Sermonti G (1969) Detection and study of cosynthesis of tetracycline antibiotics by an agar method. J Gen Microbiol 55:103–108

Demain AL (1973) Mutation and production of secondary metabolites. Adv Appl Microbiol 16:177–202

Deshpande VN (1965) Biosynthesis of chlortetracycline by washed resting cells of *Streptomyces aureofaciens*. Hindustan Antibiot Bull 8:64–66

Deshpande VN (1967) Biosynthesis of chlortetracycline. Effect of organic acids on the biosynthesis of chlortetracycline by washed resting cells of *Streptomyces aureofaciens*. Indian J Biochem [Suppl] 4:19

Deshpande VN (1968) Biosynthesis of chlortetracycline. II. Carbohydrate metabolism by resting cells of *Streptomyces aureofaciens* in relation to the biosynthesis of chlortetracycline. Hindustan Antibiot Bull 11:106–112

DiMarco A (1956) Metabolism of *Streptomyces aureofaciens* and biosynthesis of chlortetracycline. G Microbiol 2:285–301

DiMarco A, Pennella P (1959) The fermentation of the tetracyclines. Prog Ind Microbiol 1:47–91

Doerschuk AP, McCormick JRD, Goodman JJ, Szumski SA, Growich JA, Miller PA, Bitler BA, Jensen ER, Petty MA, Phelps AS (1956) The halide metabolism of *Streptomyces aureofaciens* mutants. The biosynthesis of 7-chloro,7-chloro^{36}- and 7-bromotetracyline and tetracycline. J Am Chem Soc 78:1508–1509

Doerschuk AP, McCormick JRD, Goodman JJ, Szumski SA, Growich JA, Miller PA, Bitler BA, Jensen ER, Martrishin M, Petty MA, Phelps AS (1959) Biosynthesis of tetracyclines. I. The halide metabolism of *Streptomyces aureofaciens* mutants. The preparation and characterization of tetracycline, 7-chloro^{36}-tetracycline and 7-bromotetracycline. J Am Chem Soc 81:3069–3075

Doskocil J, Sikyta B, Kasparova J, Doskocilova D, Zajicek J (1958) Development of the culture of *Streptomyces rimosus* in submerged fermentation. J Gen Microbiol 18:302–314

Doskocil J, Hostalek Z, Kasparova J. Zajicek J, Herold M (1959) Development of *Streptomyces aureofaciens* in submerged culture. J Biochem Microbiol Technol Eng 1:261–271

Drazhner TM, Ashkinuzi ZK, Grigor'eva GP (1969) Use of offtakes of a cultural liquid as seed. Chem Abstr 70:86219

Dulaney EL, Dulaney DD (1967) Mutant populations of *Streptomyces viridifaciens*. Trans NY Acad Sci Ser II 29:782–799

Dulaney EL, Putter I, Drescher D, Chaiet L, Miller WJ, Wolf FJ, Hendlin D (1962) Transethylation in antibiotic biosynthesis I. An ethyl homolog of oxytetracycline. Biochem Biophys Acta 60:447–449

Duggar BM (1948) Aureomycin: a product of the continuing search for new antibiotics. Ann NY Acad Sci 51:171–181

Duggar BM, Backus EJ, Campbell TH (1954) Types of variation in actinomycetes. Ann NY Acid Sci 60:71–86

Egorov NS, Baranova IP (1959) Effect of *p*-dimethylaminobenzaldehyde on formation of chlortetracycline. Antibiotiki 4:35–40

Elander RP (1966) Two decades of strain development in antibiotic-producing microorganisms. Dev Ind Microbiol 7:61–73

Elander RP (1976) Mutation to increased product formation in antibiotic-producing microorganism. Microbiology (ASM) 1976:517–521

Elander RP, Chang LT, Vaughan RW (1977) Genetics of industrial microorganisms. In: Perlman D (ed) Annual reports on fermentation processes, vol 1. Academic, New York, pp 1–40

Engelbrecht H, Mach H (1967) Physiological investigations of the interrelationships between fat metabolism and hydroxytetracycline biosynthesis in *Actinomyces rimosus*. Mikrobiologiia 36:976–987

Evans RC (ed) (1968) The technology of the tetracyclines. Quandrangle, New York

Fantini AA (1975) Strain development. Methods Enzymol 43:24–41

Fantini AA, Wallo KG (1967) *Streptomyces* genetics and industrial microbiology. Trans NY Acad Sci II. 29:800–809

Fedorova NY, Pisarchuk EN, Fedorenko IN (1971) Reaction of strain LBS-2201, a biomycin producer, to the enrichment and impoverishment of a culture medium. Chem Abstr 75:18553

Fertman GI (1965) Malt sprouts in the production of biomycin. Chem Abstr 62:4571

Fremel VB, Losyakova LS, Ustinnikova YI (1963) Flour and spent wash in the production of Terramycin. Chem Abstr 58:8383

Gado I, Horvath J (1962) Oxytetracycline production in different amino acid containing media. Acta Microbiol Acad Sci Hung 9:1–9

Gado I, Horvath J (1963) The influence of purine bases upon the growth of *Streptomyces rimosus*. Arch Mikrobiol 46:305–307

Gado I, Szentirmai A, Steczek K, Horvath J (1961) Metabolic studies with *Streptomyces rimosus*. Acta Microbiol Acad Sci Hung 8:291–302

Girs VT, Fertman GI, Malamud IK (1980) Malt sprouts as a stimulant in feed biomycin production. Chem Abstr 92:74299

Goodman JJ (1954) Process for production of chlortetracycline. Canada Patent 499,649

Goodman JJ (1957) *Streptomyces aureofaciens* fermentation process. US Patent 2,911,339
Goodman JJ (1959) Fermentation of oxytetracycline by *Streptomyces rimosus*. US Patent 2,871,166
Goodman JJ (1962a) Fermentation of tetracycline. US Patent 3,037,916
Goodman JJ (1962b) Fermentation of chlortetracycline and tetracycline. US Patent 3,050,446
Goodman JJ (1964a) Process of preparing 6-demethyltetracyclines. US Patent 3,137,328
Goodman JJ (1964b) Production of chlortetracycline and demethylchlortetracycline. US Patent 3,145,154
Goodman JJ, Martishin M (1961) Effect of sulfadiazine on the synthesis of demethylchlortetracycline by *Streptomyces aureofaciens*. J Bacteriol 82:615
Goodman JJ, Matrishin M (1962) Production of 7-chloro-6-demethyl-tetracycline. US Patent 3,019,172
Goodman JJ, Matrishin M (1964) Effect of norleucine on the synthesis of demethylchlortetracycline by *Streptomyces aureofaciens*. Nature 201:190
Goodman JJ, Matrishin M (1968) Chlorination inhibitors in *Streptomyces aureofaciens*. Nature 219:291–292
Goodman JJ, Matrishin M (1973) Inhibition of chlorination in *Streptomyces aureofaciens* by nitriles and related compounds. Antimicrob Agents Chemother 3:138–140
Goodman JJ, Miller PA (1962) The effect of antimetabolites on the biosynthesis of tetracyclines. Biotech Bioeng 4:391–402
Goodman JJ, Young RW (1960a) Chlorination inhibitors in chlortetracycline-tetracycline fermentations. US Patent 2,923,667
Goodman JJ, Young RW (1960b) Chlorination inhibitors in chlortetracycline-tetracycline fermentations. US Patent 2,923,668
Goodman JJ, Matrishin M, Backus EJ (1955) The effect of anhydrochlortetracycline on the growth of actinomycetes. J Bacteriol 69:70–72
Goodman JJ, Matrishin M, Young RW, McCormick JRD (1959) Inhibition of the incorporation of chloride into the tetracycline molecule. J Bacteriol 78:492–499
Goodman JJ, Matrishin M, McCormick JRD (1963) Reversal of chlorination inhibitors in *Streptomyces aureofaciens*. Nature 198:1903–1904
Gouges Y (1978) Antibiotics of the tetracycline group. German Patent 2,823,469
Gourevitch A, Lein J (1955) Production of tetracyclines and substituted tetracyclines. US Patent 2,712,517
Gourevitch A, Misiek M, Lein J (1955) Competitive inhibition by bromide of incorporation of chloride into the tetracycline molecule. Antibiot Chemother 5:448–452
Greer MA (1956) Isolation from rutabaga seed of progoitrin, the precursor of the naturally occurring antithyroid compound goitrin (L-5 vinyl-2-thiooxazolidone). J Am Chem Soc 78:1260–1261
Grezin VF, Kovalev VF, Nechaev GE (1964) Biosynthesis of chlortetracycline in the presence of pathogenic bacteria. Chem Abstr 60:4886
Grinyuk TI, Brinberg SL (1960) Interrelation between medium composition and conditions of aeration in the biosynthesis of antibiotics. Antibiotiki 5:24–27
Growich JA (1971a) 7-Chloro-6-demethyl-tetracycline fermentation. US Patent 3,616,239
Growich JA (1971b) 7-Chloro-6-demethyl-tetracycline fermentation. US Patent 3,616,240
Growich JA (1971c) Process for the production of 7-chloro-5a,11a-dehydro-tetracycline. US Patent 3,616,241
Growich JA, Deduck N (1963) Tetracycline fermentation. US Patent 3,092,556 (Reissue 25,840, 1965)
Growich JA, Miller PA (1961) New tetracyclines produced by *Streptomyces aureofaciens*. US Patent 3,007,965
Guberniev MA, Torbochkina LI, Kats LN (1954) Polyphosphates of *Actinomyces aureofaciens*. Antibiotiki 4:24–30

Guberniev MA, Ugelova NA, Kats LN (1960) Desoxyribonucleic acid in the mycelium of *Streptomyces aureofaciens* strain LS-12 under conditions of submerged cultivation. Mikrobiologiia 29:512–515

Hatch AB, Hunt GA, Lein J (1956) Tetracycline production using cottonseed endosperm flour. US Patent 2,763,591

Hendlin D, Dulaney EL, Drescher D, Cook T, Chaiet L (1962) Methionine dependence and the biosynthesis of 6-demethylchlortetracycline. Biochim Biophys Acta 58:635–636

Herold M, Necasek J (1959) Protected fermentations. Adv Appl Microbiol 1:1–21

Herold M, Belik E, Doskocil J (1956) Biosynthesis of chlortetracycline without maintenance of aseptic conditions. G Microbiol 2:302–311

Hirsch HM, Wallace GI (1951) The octanoxidase system of *Streptomyces aureofaciens*. Rev Can Biol 10:191–214

Hofman J (1961) Metabolism of amino acids by *Streptomyces aureofaciens*. Folia Microbiol (Praha) 6:64–65

Hopwood DA (1974) The impact of genetics on the study of antibiotic-producing actinomycetes. Postepy Hig Med Dosw 28:427–439

Hopwood DA (1976) Genetics of antibiotic production in *Streptomyces*. Microbiology (ASM) 1976:558–562

Hopwood DA (1978) Extrachromosomally determined antibiotic production. Ann Rev Microbiol 32:373–392

Hopwood DA, Chater KF (1980) Fresh approaches to antibiotic production. Phil Trans R Soc Lond B 290:313–328

Hopwood DA, Merrick MJ (1977) Genetics of antibiotic production. Bacteriol Rev 41:595–635

Horvath I, Magyar K, Gado I, Szanto J, Vadkerty T (1958 a) Toxic effects of oil peroxides formed during fermentation. Chem Industry 1958:916–917

Horvath I, Magyar K, Gado I, Szanto J, Vadkerty I (1958 b) The influence of iron upon oxytetracycline production by *Streptomyces rimosus*. Acta Microbiol Acad Sci Hung 5:253–260

Horvath I, Gado I, Szentirmai A (1958 c) Production of oxytetracycline in synthetic media. Acta Microbiol Acad Sci Hung 5:317–327

Horvath I, Magyar K, Gado I (1959) The effect of methylene blue on the iron sensitivity of *Streptomyces rimosus* fermentations. Acta Microbiol Acad Sci Hung 6:47–50

Hostalek Z (1964 a) Relationship between the carbohydrate metabolism of *Streptomyces aureofaciens* and the biosynthesis of chlortetracycline I. The effect of interrupted aeration, inorganic phosphate and benzyl thiocyanate on chlortetracycline biosynthesis. Folia Microbiol (Praha) 9:78–88

Hostalek Z (1964 b) Relationship between the carbohydrate metabolism of *Streptomyces aureofaciens* and the biosynthesis of chlortetracycline II. The effect of benzyl thiocyanate on the respiration of washed mycelium of *Streptomyces aureofaciens*. Folia Microbiol (Praha) 9:89–95

Hostalek Z (1964 c) Relationship between the carbohydrate metabolism of *Streptomyces aureofaciens* and the biosynthesis of chlortetracycline III. The effect of benzyl thiocyanate on carbohydrate metabolism of *Streptomyces aureofaciens*. Folia Microbiol (Praha) 9:96–102

Hostalek Z, Herold M, Necasek J (1958) Die Beeinflußung der Chlortetracyclin Produktion durch Belüftungspausen, durch Orthophosphat und durch Benzylrhodanid. Naturwissenschaften 45:543–544

Hostalek Z, Herold M, Sikyta B, Necasek J (1959) Substitution of starch for saccharose in the nutrient medium during the biosynthesis of chlortetracycline. Antibiotiki 4:8–12

Hostalek Z, Blumauerova M, Cudlin J, Vanek Z (1971) Speculations on genetic loci controlling the biosynthesis of tetracyclines. Radiations and radioisotopes for industrial microorganisms. Int Atomic Agency Symp, Vienna, pp 189–198

Hostalek Z, Blumauerova M, Vanek Z (1974) Genetic problems of the biosynthesis of tetracycline antibiotics. In: Ghose TK (ed) Advances in biochemical engineering, vol 3. Springer, Berlin Heidelberg New York, pp 13–67

Hostalek Z, Blumauerova M, Vanek Z (1979) Tetracycline antibiotics. In: Rose AH (ed) Econ microbiol, vol 3. Secondary products of metabolism. Academic, New York, pp 293–354

Hostinova E, Bacova M, Polivka L, Gasperik J, Zelinka J (1979) Studies on amylases from *Streptomyces aureofaciens*. Biologia (Bratisl) 34:939–946

Hrebenda J, Luba J, Szewczak R, Ulikowski S (1969) Effect of conditions of medium sterilization upon carbohydrate and ammonium nitrogen uptake and biosynthesis of oxytetracycline and tetracycline. Chem Abstr 79:66763

Hribalova V, Starka J (1969) Relation between the respiratory activity and the biosynthesis of chlortetracycline by *Streptomyces aureofaciens*. Ann Inst Pasteur 96:120–124

Hsu CY, Yao TC, Li HL (1974) Selection of demethylchloretetracycline producing mutants from *Streptomyces aureofaciens* 38. Chem Abstr 81:165937

Institut Antybiotykow (1961) Tetracycline. French Patent 1,279,692

Ivanov SA, Bliznakova L (1971) Antifoaming effect of some individual organic alcohols, acids, or esters and their mixtures on the biosynthesis of biovit in submerged cultures of *Actinomyces aureofaciens (Streptomyces aureofaciens)* strain 2201. Antibiotiki 16:254–258

Jarai M (1961 a) Genetic recombination in *Streptomyces aureofaciens*. Acta Microbiol Acad Sci Hung 7:73–80

Jarai M (1961 b) Transformation in *Streptomyces*. Acta Microbiol Acad Sci Hung 7:81–87

Jarai M (1962) Action of mutagenic agents on auxotrophic strains of *Streptomyces*. Acta Microbiol Acad Sci Hung 9:273–284

Jarai M (1969) Biochemical studies on *Streptomyces aureofaciens*. V. The role of cobalamins and methionine in methylation reactions in tetracycline biosynthesis. Acta Microbiol Acad Sci Hung 16:85–96

Jarai M, Josza A, Kollar J (1964) Biochemical chlorination in *Streptomyces aureofaciens*. Nature 204:1307–1308

Jensen AL, Schultz JS, Shu P (1966) Scale-up of antibiotic fermentations by control of oxygen utilization. Biotechnol Bioeng 8:525–537

Katagiri K (1954) Study on the chlortetracyclines. Improvement of chlortetracycline-producing strains by several kinds of methods. J Antibiotics Ser A 7:45–52

Kestel'man VM, Vil'nina GL (1971) Influence of polymers on fermentative and other activities of microorganisms. Int Biodeterior Bull 7:99–103

Koaze Y, Nakajima J, Hidaka H, Niwa T, Adachi T, Yoshida K, Ito J, Nida T, Shomura T, Ueda M (1974) Production of new amylases by cultivation of *Streptomyces* and uses of these new amylases. US Patent 3,840,717

Kollar J, Jarai M (1960 a) Biochemical studies on *Streptomyces aureofaciens*. I. Studies on the chlorination mechanism. Acta Microbiol Acad Sci Hung 7:5–10

Kollar SJ, Jarai M (1960 b) Biochemical chlorination in *Streptomyces aureofaciens*. Nature 168:665

Koshel TN, Slyusarenko TP, Tkachenko EM (1971 a) Use of cetylpyridinium chloride in the production of food antibiotics. Chem Abstr 74:86344

Koshel TN, Dudnik DS, Slyusarenko TP (1971 b) Microorganisms affecting the production of fodder biomycin. Chem Abstr 75:62323

Kotiuszko D, Lubinsky O, Ruczaj Z, Ruszczynski J, Sobiewski W (1958) Production of tetracycline (Achromycin) by subsurface fermentation of *Streptomyces aureofaciens*. Med Dosw Mikrobiol 10:153–164

Krupenski A, Rusan M, Pop I, Rusan S, Burga V (1978) Tetracycline biosynthesis. Chem Abstr 89:40865

Krusser OV, Yakimov PA, Neshataeva E, Hao S, Loshkareva AE (1963) Vegetative proliferation of *Streptomyces aureofaciens* mycelium. Chem. Abstr 58:8383

Kurylowicz W (1977) The site of antibiotic accumulation in Streptomycetes and *Penicillium chrysogenum*. Chem Abstr 88:148857

Kurylowicz W, Malinowski K (1970) Electron microscopy of surface of two strains of *Streptomyces aureofaciens* during tetracycline biosynthesis. Acta Microbiol Polonica Ser B 2:223–228

Kurylowicz W, Malinowski K (1971) The ultrastructure of the mycelium of *Streptomyces aureofaciens* in the course of biosynthesis of tetracycline. Acta Microbiol Polonica Ser B 3:3–6

Kurylowicz W, Malinowski K (1972a) Ultrastructure of the mycelium of *Streptomyces aureofaciens* in the course of biosynthesis of tetracycline. Post Hig Med Dosw 26:563–569

Kurylowicz W, Malinowski K (1972b) Modification of mycelium ultrastructure in *Streptomyces aureofaciens* in the course of tetracycline biosynthesis. Mikrobiologiia 41:704–712

Kurylowicz W, Malinowski K, Kurzatkowski W (1971) Fatty acids of the mycelium of *Streptomyces aureofaciens* during tetracycline biosynthesis. Acta Microbiol Polonica Ser B 3:179–187

Kvashnina ES (1966) Natural selection of *Actinomyces rimosus* variants for surface fermentation. Antibiotiki 11:1004–1007

Lab Pro-Ter (1963a) Tetracycline. Belgian Patent 628,257

Lab Pro-Ter (1963b) Oxytetracycline by fermentation. Belgian Patent 632,332

Lab Sailly (1974) Tetracycline by the fermentation of hydrolyzed yams. French Patent 2,276,380

Lavate WV (1960) Chlortetracycline biosynthesis in synthetic medium. Hindustan Antibiot Bull 3:64–65

Laznikova TN (1973) Study of the effect of spore seed material quality on tetracycline accumulation level using the method of differential centrifugation in sucrose density gradient. Antibiotiki 18:887–890

Laznikova TN, Dmitrieva SV (1973) Effect of biosynthetic conditions on tetracycline accumulation and the characteristics of mycelium distribution in a sucrose density gradient during differential centrifugation. Antibiotiki 18:780–784

Laznikova TN, Makarevitch VG (1963) A study of tetracycline production conditions in the process of chlortetracycline biosynthesis. Antibiotiki 8:579–583

Laznikova TN, Makarevich VG (1969) Effect of whale oil and its quality on tetracycline biosynthesis. Antibiotiki 14:311–316

Laznikova TN, Makarevich VG (1970) Effect of hydrogenated fats on tetracycline biosynthesis. Chem Abstr 72:65362

Laznikova TN, Makarevich VG (1971) Effect of amino acids on the growth of *Actinomyces aureofaciens (Streptomyces aureofaciens)* and the biosynthesis of tetracycline. Antibiotiki 16:207–212

Lein J, Gourevitch A (1956) Production of tetracycline. US Patent 2,739,924

Lein J, Sawmiller LF, Cheney LC (1959) Chlorination inhibitors affecting the biosynthesis of tetracycline. Appl Microbiol 7:149–151

Lepetit SpA (1957) Brometetracycline. British Patent 772,149

Lepetit SpA (1958a) Production of tetracycline by fermentation. British Patent 790,953

Lepetit SpA (1958b) Tetracycline by fermentation. British Patent 799,051

Listvinova SN, Levitov MM, Kapustina NA (1968) A synthetic medium for studying antibiotic-producing actinomycetes. Antibiotiki 13:604–610

Listinova SN, Gryaznova NS (1969) Effect of propyl alcohol on oxytetracycline. Antibiotiki 14:808–813

Luba J, Szewczak R, Ulikowski S (1968) A study on the influence of the ratio C/N in the media on biosynthesis of tetracycline. Acta Poloniae Pharmaceutica 25:154–157

Ludvik J, Mikulik K, Vanek Z (1971) Fine structure of *Streptomyces aureofaciens* producing tetracycline. Folia Microbiol (Praha) 16:479–480

Ludvik J, Vorisek J, Behal V, Hostalek Z, Jurkech L (1973) Morphology of the submerged mycelium of *Streptomyces aureofaciens* in a scanning electron microscope. Folia Microbiol (Praha) 18:150–151 (abstract)

Majchrzak R, Majchrzak M (1965) The effect of iron on the yield of oxytetracycline. Chem Abstr 63:15503

Makarevich VG, Laznikova TN (1959) Significance of phosphorus for biosynthesis of chlortetracycline. Antibiotiki 4:46–49
Makarevich VG, Laznikova TN (1961 a) Media with different oilcakes as a source of organic nitrogen for the fermentation of chlortetracycline. Antibiotiki 6:308–311
Makarevich VG, Laznikova TN (1961 b) New media for the fermentation of chlortetracycline. Antibiotiki 6:994–998
Makarevich VG, Laznikova TN (1969) Decrease in chlortetracycline produced during the directed fermentation of tetracycline. Antibiotiki 14:695–698
Makarevich VG, Laznikova TN (1970) Effect of vegetative inoculum on tetracycline biosynthesis. Antibiotiki 15:972–977
Makarevich VG, Laznikova TN, Lyubishkin VT, Donetskaya TF (1969) Effect of cornmeal quality on tetracycline biosynthesis. Antibiotiki 14:977–981
Makarevich VG, Upiter GD, Slugina MD, Tarasova SS, Gravit NF (1975) Effect of orthophosphate on growth rate of *Actinomyces aureofaciens* and tetracycline biosynthesis by it. Antibiotiki 20:295–299
Makarevich VG, Slugina MD, Upiter GD, Zaslavskaya PL, Gerasimova TM (1976) Regulation of tetracycline biosynthesis by controlling the growth of the antibiotic-producing organism. Antibiotiki 21:205–210
Makarevich VG, Laznikova TN, Orlova NV, Gorskaya SV, Surikova EI, Dmitrieva SV, Gracheva IV, Brinberg SL (1978) Some methods for improving the biosynthesis of antibiotics. Chem Abstr 89:195353
Maladkar NK, Deshpande VN (1978) Effect of L-aromatic amino acids on the biosynthesis of chlortetracycline by washed resting cells of *Streptomyces aureofaciens*. Indian J Exp Biol 16:394–396
Mamonova EI, Orlova NV (1979) Methodological approaches to the development of methods for the controlled biosynthesis of antibiotics. Antibiotiki 24:574–581
Mancy-Courtillet D, Florent J, Ninet L, Preud'Homme J (1959) Oxytetracycline. French Patent 1,084,203
Marini F (1972) Stimulatory effect of thiamine on the biosynthesis of tetracycline in a mutant strain of *Streptomyces aureofaciens*. Ann Microbiol Enzimol 22:81–83
Martin JF (1977) Control of antibiotic synthesis by phosphate. Adv Biochem Eng 7:106–127
Martin JH, Mitscher LA, Miller PA, Shu P, Bohonos N (1966) 5-Hydroxy-7-chlortetracycline. I. Preparation, isolation and physiochemical properties. Antimicrob Agents Chemother, pp 563–567
Matelova V (1964) Investigations of conditions for production of penicillin and chlortetracycline in submerged fermentation. Biotechnol Bioeng 6:329–345
Matselyukh BP (1964) Transformation of antibiotic formation in *Actinomyces* by means of DNA. Chem Abstr 60:11086
McCormick JRD (1966) Biosynthesis of the tetracyclines. An integrated biosynthetic scheme. In: Herold M, Gabiel Z (eds) Antibiotics. Advances in research, production and clinical use. Proc congr antibiotics, Prague. Butterworth's, London, pp 556–574
McCormick JRD (1967) Tetracyclines. In: Gottlieb D, Shaw PD (eds) Antibiotics II. Biosynthesis. Springer, Berlin Heidelberg New York, pp 113–122
McCormick JRD (1968) Point blocked mutants and biogenesis of tetracyclines. In: Sermonti G, Alecevic M (eds) Genetics and breeding of Streptomycetes. Yugoslav Acad Sci and Arts, Zagreb, pp 163–176
McCormick JRD, Gardner WE (1963) Naphthacenequinones. US Patent 3,074,975
McCormick JRD, Morton CO (1982) Identity of cosynthetic factor I of Streptomyces aureofaciens and fragment FO from coenzyme F 240 of *Methanobacterium* species. J Am Chem Soc 104:4014
McCormick JRD, Sjolander NO, Hirsch U, Jensen ER, Doerschuk AP (1957 a) A new family of antibiotics: the demethyltetracyclines. J Am Chem Soc 79:4561–4563
McCormick JRD, Sjolander NO, Hirsch U (1957 b) Biological conversion of 5a(11a)-dehydrotetracycline to broad-spectrum antibiotics. US Patent 2,965,546
McCormick JRD, Miller PA, Growich JA, Sjolander NO, Doerschuk AP (1958 a) Two new tetracycline related compounds: 7-chloro-5a-(11a)-dehydrotetracycline and 5a-epi-tetracycline. A new route to tetracycline. J Am Chem Soc 80:5572

McCormick JRD, Sjolander NO, Miller PA, Hirsch U, Arnold NH, Doerschuk AP (1958 b) The biological reduction of 7-chloro-5a-(11a)-dehydrotetracycline by *Streptomyces aureofaciens*. J Am Chem Soc 80:6460

McCormick JRD, Sjolander NO, Johnson S, Doerschuk AP (1959 a) Biosynthesis of tetracyclines. II. Simple defined media for growth of *Streptomyces aureofaciens* and elaboration of 7-chlortetracycline. J Bacteriol 77:475–477

McCormick JRD, Hirsch U, Jensen E, Sjolander NO (1959 b) 6-Demethyltetracyclines and methods of preparing the same. US Patent 2,878,289

McCormick JRD, Hirsch U, Sjolander NO, Doerschuk AP (1960) Cosynthesis of tetracyclines by pairs of *Streptomyces aureofaciens* mutants. J Am Chem Soc 82:5006

McCormick JRD, Arnold N, Hirsch U, Miller PA, Sjolander NO (1961 a) Process of producing an antibiotic of the tetracycline series. US Patent 2,970,947

McCormick JRD, Arnold N, Hirsch U, Miller PA, Sjolander NO (1961 b) Cosynthetic factor I and its production. US Patent 2,996,499

McCormick JRD, Sjolander NO, Hirsch U (1961 c) Production of tetracycline. US Patent 2,998,352

McGhee WJ, Megna JC (1957) Process for the production of tetracycline. US Patent 2,776,243

Meshkov AN, Slugina MD, Makarevich VG (1973) Effect of iron and other inorganic elements on the biosynthesis of tetracycline. Antibiotiki 18:493–496

Mikulik K, Blumauerova M, Vanek Z, Ludvik J (1971 a) Characterization of ribosomes of a strain of *Streptomyces aureofaciens* producing chlortetracycline. Folia Microbiol (Praha) 16:24–30

Mikulik K, Karnetova J, Quyen N, Blumauerova M, Komersova I, Vanek Z (1971 b) Interaction of tetracycline with the protein synthesizing system of *Streptomyces aureofaciens*. J Antibiotics 24:801–809

Mikulik K, Karnetova J, Kremen A, Tax J, Vanek Z (1971 c) Protein synthesis and production of tetracycline in *Streptomyces aureofaciens*. Radiat radioisotop ind microorganism, Proc Symp 1971. IAEA, Vienna, Austria, pp 201–222

Miller PA (1961) Production of tetracycline. US Patent 3,005,023

Miller PA, McCormick JRD (1960) Biological transformation of anhydrotetracyclines to 5a(11a)-dehydrotetracyclines. US Patent 2,952,587

Miller PA, McCormick JRD, Doerschuk AP (1956) Studies of chlortetracycline and the preparation of chlortetracycline-C^{14}. Science 123:1030–1031

Miller PA, Sjolander NO, Nalesnyk N, Arnold N, Johnson S, Doerschuk AP, McCormick JRD (1960) Cosynthetic factor I. A factor involved in hydrogen-transfer in *Streptomyces aureofaciens*. J Am Chem Soc 82:5002–5003

Miller PA, Goodman JJ, Sjolander NO, McCormick JRD (1961) Enhancement of 7-chlortetracycline production. US Patent 2,987,449

Miller PA, Saturneli A, Martin JH, Mitscher LA, Bohonos N (1964) A new family of tetracycline precursors: *N*-demethylanhydrocyclines. Biochem Biophys Res Comm 16:285–291

Mindlin SZ, Kubyshkina TA, Alikhanian SI (1961 a) The use of mutants of *Streptomyces rimosus* for studying the biosynthesis of oxytetracycline. Antibiotiki 6:623–629

Mindlin SZ, Alikhanian SI, Vladimirov AV, Mikhailova GR (1961 b) A new hybrid strain of an oxytetracycline-producing organism, *Streptomyces rimosus*. Appl Microbiol 9:349–353

Minieri PP, Sokol H, Firman H (1956) Process for the preparation of tetracycline and chlortetracycline. US Patent 2,734,018

Minieri PP, Firman H, Sokol H (1958) Deionized corn steep liquor in production of tetracycline. US Patent 2,866,738

Minieri PP, Firman MC, Mistretta AG, Abbey A, Bricker CE, Rigler NE, Sokol H (1953–1954) A new broad spectrum antibiotic of the tetracycline group. Antibiotics Annual, pp 81–87

Molinari R (1964) Tetracycline biosynthesis in chemically defined media. Chem Abstr 64:11586

Mostafa MA, Osman HG, Abou-Zeid AA (1972) Production of tetracyclines by *Streptomyces aureofaciens*. Chem Abstr 76:43746

Mracek M, Blumauerova M, Paleckova F, Hostalek Z (1969) Regulation of biosynthesis of secondary metabolites. XI. Induction of variants in *Streptomyces aureofaciens* and the specificity of mutagens. Mutat Res 7:19–24

Neidleman SL (1962) Process for the production of demethyltetracyclines. US Patent 3,061,522

Neidleman SL, Bientstock E, Bennett RE (1963 a) Biosynthesis of 7-chloro-6-demethyltetracycline in the presence of aminopterin and ethionine. Biochim Biophys Acta 71:199–201

Neidleman SL, Albu E, Bienstock E (1963 b) Biosynthesis of 7-chloro-6-demethyltetracycline in the presence of certain homocysteine derivatives and methoxinine. Biotechnol Bioeng 5:87–89

Neshataeva EV, Yakimov PA, Baldina AV (1963) Formation of chlortetracycline and vitamin B_{12} by *Streptomyces aureofaciens* in the presence of different carbohydrates. Chem Abstr 58:6155

Niedercorn JG (1952) Process for producing aureomycin. US Patent 2,609,329

Niedzwiecka-Trzaskowska I, Sztencel M (1958) Recherches concernant *Streptomyces aureofaciens*. Ann Inst Past 91:72–78

Nikitina TS, Tarasova SS, Nikolushkina VM, Bylinkina ES (1974) Effect of dissolved carbon dioxide concentration on the respiration rate of microorganisms-producers of tetracycline and oleandomycin. Chem Abstr 81:36398

Nitelea I, Ardeleanu V, Onu M, Alupei G, Magazin M (1968) Culture media for *Streptomyces* strains producing tetracycline. Chem Abstr 69:42791

Nitescu S, Gheorghiu T, Krupenschi A, Dogaru M (1962) Benzyl thiocyanate, stimulating agent in tetracyclines synthesis. Chem Abstr 57:1379

Novotny K, Herold M (1960) The production of chlortetracycline containing feed supplement by direct enrichment of wheat bran. Antibiotiki 5:42–46

Nyiri L (1961) Variability in *Streptomyces rimosus*. Acta Microbiol Acad Sci Hung 7:257–273

Nyiri L (1962) Comparative studies on the specific characteristics of oxytetracycline producing and non-producing *Streptomyces rimosus* strains. Antibiotiki 7:11–18

Nyiri L, Lengyel ZL, Erdely A (1963) The effect of oxytetracycline on the carbohydrate metabolism of *Streptomyces rimosus* variants. J Antibiotics A 16:80–85

Oblozhko LS, Orlova NV (1975) Effect of aeration conditions on biosynthesis of oxytetracycline and production of organic acids by *Streptomyces rimosus*. Antibiotiki 20:209–212

Oblozhko LS, Borisova TG, Orlova NV (1974) Effect of aeration conditions on the quality of inoculum of an oxytetracycline-producing organism. Antibiotiki 19:873–877

Oblozhko LS, Orlova NV, Borisova TG (1977) Oxygen requirement of an *Actinomyces rimosus* culture in relation to the composition of the medium. Antibiotiki 22:17–21

Orlova NV (1959) The importance of certain organic acids in the biosynthesis of oxytetracycline. Antibiotiki 4:34–39

Orlova NV (1961) The effect of oils upon tetracycline biosynthesis by *Actinomyces rimosus*. Mikrobiologiia 30:710–716

Orlova NV (1968) Biosynthesis of 2-acetyl-2-decarbamoyloxytetracycline by *Actinomyces rimosus*. Antibiotiki 13:291–297

Orlova NV (1971) Media for inoculum cultivation of oxytetracycline-producing organisms. Antibiotiki 16:258–262

Orlova NV, Prokofieva-Belgovskaya AA (1961) The effect of amount and age of culture material on the development of *Actinomyces rimosus* and on the production of oxytetracycline. Antibiotiki 6:15–20

Orlova NV, Pushkina ZT (1972) Oxytetracycline production by *Actinomyces rimosus* under conditions of addition of nutrients during biosynthesis. Antibiotiki 17:108–114

Orlova NV, Verkhovtseva TP (1957) Comparative investigation of the physiological properties of terramycin and biomycin producers. Mikrobiologiia 26:565–572

Orlova NV, Verkhotseva TP (1959) The significance of the phosphorus, nitrogen and lactic acid of corn extract for the biosynthesis of oxytetracycline. Mikrobiologiia 28:514–521

Orlova NV, Zaitseva ZM (1960) Studies on production conditions of oxytetracycline by *Actinomyces rimosus*, LS-T-118. Chemotherapia 1:353–363

Orlova NV, Zaitseva ZM, Khokhlov AS, Cherchess BZ (1961) Some physiological properties of nonactive mutants of *Actinomyces rimosus* the producer of oxytetracycline. Antibiotiki 6:629–635

Orlova NV, Smolenskaya NM, Zaitseva ZM (1964) Distribution among actinomycetes, fungi and bacteria of substances stimulating the formation of oxytetracycline by the *Actinomyces rimosus* T-572 mutant. Mikrobiologiia 33:1032–1041

Orlova NV, Surikova EI, Gracheva IV, Gorskaya SV, Makarevich VG, Laznikova TN, Listvinova SN, Pushkina ZT, Upiter GD (1978) Biosynthesis of antibiotics during culturing with the addition of supplementary nutrients. Chem Abstr 89:178003

Paleckova F, Hostalek Z, Rehacek Z (1969) Method of producing tetracycline. US Patent 3,434,930

Parada JL (1981) Growth inhibition of *Streptomyces* species by L-serine and its effect on tetracycline biosynthesis. Appl Environ Microbiol 41:366–370

Paskova J, Smolek K (1967) Modification of concentrated corn steep liquor. Chem Abstr 66:114490

Pecak V, Cizek S, Musil J, Cerkes L, Herold M, Belik E, Hoffman J (1958) Stimulation of chlortetracycline production by benzyl thiocyanate. J Hyg Epidemiol Microbiol Immunol 2:111–115

Perlman D (1962) Process for preparing 6-demethyltetracyclines. US Patent 3,028,311

Perlman D, Heuser LJ, Dutcher JD, Barrett JM, Boska JA (1960) Biosynthesis of tetracycline by 5-hydroxytetracycline-producing cultures of *Streptomyces rimosus*. J Bacteriol 80:419–420

Perlman D, Heuser LJ, Semar JB, Frazier WR, Boska JA (1961) Process for biosynthesis of 7-chloro-6-demethyltetracycline. J Am Chem Soc 83:4481

Pestereva GD, Baturina RM (1973) Effect of fermentation conditions on cytological features of the development of antibiotic-producing actinomycetes. Antibiotiki 18:432–437

Pettko EF, Kiss P, Kramli A (1956) Effect of metals on respiration and oxidation-reduction potential of *Streptomyces aureofaciens*. Chem Abstr 50:7226

Petty MA (1955) Production of chlortetracycline. US Patent 2,709,672

Petty MA (1961) An introduction to the origin and biochemistry of microbial halometabolites. Bacteriol Rev 25:111–130

Petty MA (1968) Effect of temperature on the coproduction of chlortetracycline and tetracycline by *Streptomyces aureofaciens*. Appl Microbiol 16:1285–1287

Petty MA, Matrishin M (1950) The utilization of chlorine in the fermentation medium by *Streptomyces aureofaciens* in the production of aureomycin. 118th Meeting Am Chem Soc 18A (abstract)

Petty MA, Goodman JJ, Matrishin M (1953) Studies on the nutrition of *Streptomyces aureofaciens* with respect to growth and the biosynthesis of aureomycin and vitamin B_{12}. Proc VI Int Congr Microbiology, Rome 1:248–249

Phillips DH (1964) Process for reducing foam in submerged aerobic fermentations. US Patent 3,142,628

Pierrel SpA (1964) Oxytetracycline. Netherlands Patent 6,400,925

Pivnyak IG (1962) Biosynthesis of oxytetracycline at increased temperatures. Antibiotiki 7:23–27

Pivnyak IG (1963) Temperature conditions for biosynthesis of oxytetracycline. Antibiotiki 8:27–29

Plakunova VG (1961) Possibility of regulation of pH of the medium during the development of microorganisms by ion-exchange resins. Dokl Akad Nauk SSSR 137:189–191

Plakunova VG (1967) Effect of excess aeration on biomycin synthesis by *Actinomyces aureofaciens* cultures. Chem Abstr 67:20570

Plakunova VG (1969) Heterotrophic fixation of carbonic-^{14}C acid by submerged cultures of antibiotic-producing actinomycetes. Antibiotiki 14:14–17

Plakunova VG, Kiseleva SA (1965) Effect of excessive aeration on the biosynthesis of biomycin. Chem Abstr 63:14003

Plichon B, Decq A, Guillaume JB (1976) Oxygen injection during protease and oxytetracycline productions by *Streptomyces*. J Ferm Technol (Jpn) 54:393–395

Polsinelli M, Beretta A (1966) Genetic recombination in crosses between *Streptomyces aureofaciens* and *Streptomyces rimosus*. J Bacteriol 91:63–68

Popova LA, Levitov MM, Belozerova OP (1962) The effect of fats on the biosynthesis of chlortetracycline. Antibiotiki 6:989–994

Prave P, Huber G (1967) Production of metabolic products of gram-positive bacteria and *Streptomyces* by the addition of kinetin to the fermentation broth. US Patent 3,317,404

Preobrazhenskaya TP, Bobkova TS, Gavrilina GV, Lavarova MF, Konstantinova NV (1961) A new producer of oxytetracycline – *Actinomyces aureofaciens* var *oxytetracyclini* var nov. Antibiotiki 6:675–680

Prokofieva-Belgovskaya AA, Kats LN (1960) Volutin in actinomycetes and its chemical character. Microbiologiia 29:826–833

Prokofieva-Belgovskaya A, Popova L (1959) The influence of phosphorus on the development of *Streptomyces aureofaciens* and on its ability to produce chlortetracycline. J Gen Microbiol 20:462–472

Qadeer MA, Ghafoor A, Chughtai MI (1970) Use of penicillin waste mycelium in fermentation media. I. Production of chlortetracycline by *Streptomyces aureofaciens*. Pak J Biochem 3:41–44

Queener SW (1976) Use of mutants in the study of secondary metabolite biosynthesis. Microbiology (ASM) 1976 pp 512–516

Queener SW, Sebek OK, Vezina C (1978) Mutants blocked in antibiotic synthesis. Ann Rev Microbiol 32:593–636

Rakyta J, Frimm R, Welward L, Lacko L, Lukasikova E (1980) Antioxidant stabilization of antifoaming agents used in fermentation. Antibiotiki 25:12–16

Rokos J, Prochazka P (1962) The relation of the metabolism of various carbohydrates to the production of chlortetracycline by *Streptomyces aureofaciens*. Chem Abstr 56:1839

Rolland G, Sensi P (1955) Direct production of tetracycline by fermentation. Farmaco Sci Tech (Pavia) 10:37–46

Rosova N, Zelinka J (1968) Localization of chlortetracycline and vitamin B_{12} in subcellular fractions of *Streptomyces aureofaciens*. J Antibiot 21:363–364

Rudaya SM, Soloveva NK (1960) Comparative study of *Actinomyces rimosus* (oxytetracycline producer) and experimentally induced variants. Mikrobiologiia 29:433–440

Ryabushko TA (1972) Comparative characteristics of pigmented and non-pigmented variants of *Actinomyces aureofaciens* LSB-2201. Antibiotiki 17:981–986

Ryabushko TA (1976) Physiological characteristics of pigmented and pigmentless variants of tetracycline antibiotic producers. Chem Abstr 85:157887

Scotti T, Zocchi P (1955) Studio della struttura del micelio di *Streptomyces aureofaciens* in coltura sommersa. G Microbiol 1:35–43

Sekizawa Y (1955) A biochemical chlorination in *Streptomyces*. J Biochem (Tokyo) 42:217–219

Sekizawa Y (1956a) Studies on a biochemical chlorination in *Streptomyces*. I. J Jpn Biochem Soc 27:698–706

Sekizawa Y (1956b) Studies on a biochemical chlorination in *Streptomyces*. II. J Jpn Biochem Soc 27:706–712

Sekizawa Y (1959) Biogenesis of tetracycline antibiotics I. Sci Rep Meiji Seiki Kaisha 65–75

Sekizawa Y (1960) On the biogenesis of tetracycline antibiotics. Sci Rep Meiji Seiki Kaisha 1960:12–22

Selenkow HA, Collaco FM (1961) Clinical pharmacology of antithyroid compounds. Clin Pharmacol Ther 2:191–219

Sensi P, DeFerrari GA, Gallo GG, Rolland G (1955) Brometetracycline – a new antibiotic. Farmaco Sci Ed 10:337–345
Shaposhnikov VN, Plakunova VG (1964a) Stimulation of the biosynthesis of chlortetracycline by antagonists of aromatic amino acids. Izvest Akad Nauk SSSR Ser biol 1:132–136
Shaposhnikov VN, Plakunova VG (1964b) Stimulation of chlortetracycline biosynthesis by *N*-methylanthranilic acid. Microbiologiia 33:753–757
Shaposhnikov VN, Zaitseva ZM, Orlova NV (1958) A synthetic medium for the biosynthesis of oxytetracycline (Terramycin) in the culture of *Actinomyces rimosus*. Dokl Akad Nauk SSSR 121:366–369
Shen SC (1962) Inhibition of chlortetracycline production by ionic iron during fermentation and control by chelation. Chem Abstr 56:14738
Shen SC, Shan WT (1957) A preliminary study of the effect of conjoint cultivation of *Streptomyces aureofaciens* strains upon the growth of mycelium and aureomycin production. Mikrobiologiia 26:458–463
Shen SC, Chen C (1959) Influence of orthophosphate on the pathways of carbohydrate metabolism in *Streptomyces aureofaciens* in connection with the synthesis of chlortetracycline. Antibiotiki 4:3–6
Shen SC, Chang YP (1960) Pentose metabolism and the effect of orthophosphate on the path of degradation of sugars in *Streptomyces aureofaciens*.Biochimiia 25:523–531
Shen SC, Shan WT, Hung MM, Zia JP, Chen JP, Soong Hy, Yin HC (1955) Physiology of *Streptomyces aureofaciens* and the production of aureomycin. 1. Influence of the inoculation medium on the metabolism of the fungus and the production of antibiotic. Sci Sin 4:313–326
Sherstobitova TS, Bylinkina ES, Makarevitch VG, Upiter GD (1976) Effect of dissolved carbon dioxide on the biosynthesis of tetracycline. Antibiotiki 21:291–295
Shtoffer LD, Biryukov VV, Nikolushkina VM (1973) Control of aeration and agitation in antibiotic fermentations. Pure Appl Chem 36:357–363
Shu P (1966) Development of a cross-flow fermentation process with special reference to chlortetracycline production. Biotechnol Bioeng 8:353–369
Shulo S, Zelinka J (1970) Role of biotin in the metabolism of *Streptomyces aureofaciens*. Mikrobiologiia 39:5–10
Skerman UBD, McGowan V, Sneath PHA (eds) (1980) Approved lists of bacterial names. Int J Syst Bacteriol 30:225–420
Slezak J, Sikyta B (1964) Chlortetracycline and pigment formation by *Streptomyces aureofaciens* in continuous culture. In: Malek I (ed) Proc 2nd Symp Continuous cultivation of microorganisms, Prague 1962. Czech Acad Sci Pub House, Prague, pp 185–192
Smekal F, Zajicek J (1976) Fermentation production of tetracycline antibiotics. Chem Abstr 85:121811
Smolek K, Hodinar F, Kubec K, Ulrych F, Krizek P (1961) Streptomycin or oxytetracycline. Chem Abstr 55:18010
Stoudt TH, Tausig F (1963) Fermentative production of oxytetracycline by a new species of *Streptomyces*. US Patent 3,113,077
Szczesniak T, Karabin L, Kotiuszko D, Ostrowska B, Tyc M, Wituch K, Wolf J (1975) Antibiotics of the tetracycline group. Chem Abstr 83:41523
Szumski S (1957) Employment of peroxide formation inhibitor in nutrient media containing triglyceride oil. US Patent 2,793,165
Szumski SA (1959a) Chlortetracycline fermentation. US Patent 2,871,167
Szumski SA (1959b) Selection of corn steep liquor by measurement of oxidation-reduction potential. US Patent 2,904,473
Szumski SA (1960) Composition of matter for the control of foam. US Patent 2,923,688
Szumski SA (1961) Production of 7-chloro-6-demethyltetracycline. US Patent 3,012,946
Szumski SA (1964) Fermentation preparation of tetracycline and 7-chlortetracycline. US Patent 3,121,670
Szumski SA (1967) *Streptomyces aureofaciens* fermentation process using glyceride oil and casein. US Patent 3,317,403
Tanner FW (1960) Tetracycline process. US Patent 2,940,905

Tarasova SS, Biryukov VV, Makarevich VG, Gerasimova TM (1976) Mathematical model of the effect of inorganic phosphorus on tetracycline biosynthesis. Antibiotiki 21:211–214

Ter-Karapetyan MA, Avakyan SA (1963) Amino acids in the culture medium for *Streptomyces aureofaciens* in chlortetracycline synthesis. Chem Abstr 58:13087

Tokodi I (1962) Flavone utilization by *Streptomyces rimosus*. Chem Abstr 56:5213

Tresner HD, Hayes JA, Backus EJ (1967) Morphology of submerged growth of streptomycetes as a taxonomic aid. 1. Morphological development in *Streptomyces aureofaciens* in agitated liquid media. Appl Microbiol 15:1185–1194

Uzkurenas A (1969) Influence of cobalt, manganese, copper and zinc on synthesis of chlortetracycline and vitamin B_{12} by *Actinomyces aureofaciens (Streptomyces aureofaciens)*. Chem Abstr 71:20890

Van Dyck P, DeSomer P (1952) Production and extraction methods of aureomycin. Antibiot Chemother 2:184–198

Vanek Z (1958) Compounds stimulating the biosynthesis of chlortetracycline in a low-producing strain of *Streptomyces aureofaciens*. Chem Abstr 50:4099

Vanek Z, Hostalek Z (1972) Some aspects of the genetic control of the biosynthesis of chlortetracycline. Postepy Hig Med Dosw 26:445–467

Vanek Z, Cudlin M, Blumauerova M, Hostalek Z (1971) How many genes are required for the synthesis of chlortetracycline? Folia Microbiol (Praha) 16:225–240

Vanek Z, Hostalek Z, Blumauerova M, Mikulik K, Podojil M, Behal V, Jechova V (1973) The biosynthesis of tetracycline. Pure Appl Chem 34:463–486

Vanek Z, Behal V, Jechova V, Curdova E, Blumauerova M, Hostalek K (1978) Formation of tetracycline antibiotics. In: Hutter R, Leisinger T, Nuesch J, Wehrli W (eds) Antibiotics and other secondary metabolites. Fems Symp No 5. Academic Press, London

Vecher AS, Babitskaya VG, Ryabushko TA (1969) Effect of the composition of the culture media on the hydrolytic activity of *Actinomyces (Streptomyces) aureofaciens* LSB-2201. Mikrobiologiia 38:825–827

Vecher AS, Paromchik II, Skachkov EN, Reshetnikov VN, Zaboronok VU, Akimova LN, Tsarenkova IS (1978) Use of proteinless potato juice concentrate in tetracycline production. Antibiotiki 23:963–965

Verkhovtseva TP, Orlova NV (1960) Amino acid metabolism in oxytetracycline production. Antibiotiki 5:37–42

Veselova SI (1969) Combined effect of nitrous acid, ultraviolet light, streptomycin, and chlortetracycline on *Actinomyces aureofaciens*. Antibiotiki 14:698–702

Veselova SI (1978) Mutation of tetracycline producers under the combined effect of mutagens and antibiotics. Chem Abstr 89:174358

Veselova SI, Komarova LV (1968) Use of oxytetracycline as the selective agent in the course of selection of highly productive variants of *Actinomyces (Streptomyces) rimosus*. Genetika 4:100–104

Vining LC (1979) Antibiotic tolerance in producer organisms. Adv Appl Microbiol 25:147–168

Wang EL (1957) Cultural and cytological studies on *Streptomyces aureofaciens*. J Antibiot (Tokyo) A 10:254–259

Welward L, Halama D (1974) Effect of *p*-(dimethylamino)benzaldehyde on chlortetracycline production. Antibiotiki 19:126–128

Welward L, Halama D (1978) Influence of antimicrobial agents on contamination and chlortetracycline production. Folia Microbiol (Praha) 23:12–17

Welward L, Frimm R, Kosalko R (1975) Use of wastes from L-lysine fermentation production for other fermentation products. Chem Abstr 83:76930

Welward L, Frane J, Hudec M, Kvetkova M (1976a) Criteria for estimation of calcium carbonate from the viewpoint of chlortetracycline biosynthesis. Antibiotiki 21:23–26

Welward L, Kosalko R, Frimm R (1976b) Medium for submersed fermentation of tetracycline antibiotics. Chem Abstr 85:121813

Whittenburg JV (1970) Microbiological patents in international litigation. Adv Appl Microbiol 13:383–398

Williams ST, Entwhistle S, Kurylowicz W (1977) The morphology of streptomycetes growing in media used for commercial production of antibiotic. Microbios 11A:47–60

Yakimov PA, Neshateva EV (1961) The use of potatoes in nutrient media for tetracycline production. Antibiotiki 6:891–899

Zaitseva ZM, Mindlin SS (1964) The methods of isolation and properties of 6-demethylchlortetracycline synthesizing mutants of *Actinomyces aureofaciens*. In: Herold M, Gabriel Z (eds) Antibiotics. Advances in research, production and clinical use. Proc Congr antibiotics, Prague. Butterworths, London, pp 710–712

Zaitseva ZM, Mindlin SZ (1965) Production and properties of *Actinomyces aureofaciens* mutants synthesizing 6-demethylchlortetracycline. Mikrobiologiia 34:91–100

Zaitseva ZM, Orlova NV (1962) A study of the physiological properties of *Actinomyces rimosus* mutant LS-T-572 with regard to the biosynthesis of oxytetracycline. Microbiologiia 31:449–453

Zannini E, Piacenza E, Fabbri G (1968a) Process for producing tetracycline. US Patent 3,398,057

Zannini E, Piacenza E, Fabbri G (1968b) Oxytetracycline. South African Patent 68,00,292

Zaslavskaya PL, Makarevich VG, Slugina MD (1977) Morphological study of the development of *Actinomyces aureofaciens* under conditions of controlled and uncontrolled fermentation. Mikrobiologiia 46:283–287

Zelinka J (1968) Regulatory aspects of chlortetracycline fermentation. Biologia (Bratislava) 23:169–174

Zelinka J, Biely P (1967) Stimulating effect of cadaverine on the production of chlortetracycline. Chem Abstr 67:18724

Zelinka J, Hudec M (1962) Amino acids in fermentation media. VI. The metabolism of amino acids during the fermentation under manufacture-scale conditions by the strain of *Streptomyces aureofaciens*. Chem Abstr 57:2677

Zelinka J, Kovachichova L, Hudec M (1962) The effect of amino acids upon biosynthesis of chlortetracycline. Mikrobiologiia 31:816–818

Zelinkova E, Cajkovska C, Zelinka J (1976a) Effect of acridine orange on chlortetracycline production and the growth of the mycelium of *Streptomyces aureofaciens*. Chem Abstr 85:137944

Zelinkova E, Timko J, Cajkovska C, Zelinka J (1976b) Chlortetracycline and streptomycin distribution between producer mycelium and cultivation medium. Chem Abstr 85:175494

Zilberman L, Nistor I, Crupenski A, Burga V (1978) Biosynthesis of tetracycline. Chem Abstr 89:22295

Zygmunt WA (1961) Oxytetracycline formation by *Streptomyces rimosus* in chemically defined media. Appl Microbiol 9:502–507

Zygmunt WA (1962) Selective inhibition in *Streptomyces rimosus*. J Bacteriol 84:1126–1127

Zygmunt WA (1963) Stimulation of oxytetracycline formation by *N*-acetyl derivatives of certain amino acids. Nature 198:289–290

Zygmunt WA (1964) Nutritional factors relating to growth and oxytetracycline formation by *Streptomyces rimosus*. Can J Microbiol 10:389–395

Zygmunt WA (1967) Inhibition of antibiotic formation by bromthymol blue and other indicators in *Streptomyces rimosus*. Nature 195:1102

CHAPTER 3

Structure Determination and Total Synthesis of the Tetracyclines *

R. K. BLACKWOOD

A. Introduction

It is fitting that the two aspects of structure determination and total synthesis of tetracyclines be placed in a single chapter. The structural elucidation of the original fermentation tetracyclines (chlortetracycline and oxytetracycline) was by essentially classical means involving a multitude of degradation reactions. Thus the contrasting destruction and construction of the tetracyclines have been placed in appropriate juxtaposition. Furthermore, the identity of degradation products was in certain cases proven by synthesis – and in certain cases it has been possible to reconstruct tetracyclines from degradation products, simplifying the problem of total synthesis.

It should be noted in reviewing the literature cited at the end of this chapter that, particularly in the early literature, the registered trademarks for the two earliest fermentation tetracyclines were generally employed in designating these compounds. At the time that both their structures were announced, the name tetracycline was coined for the common nucleus (1) (STEPHENS et al. 1952) and the generic name "oxytetracycline" assigned to the compound trademarked Terramycin. Analogously, "chlortetracycline" was assigned as the generic name for trademarked Aureomycin; see BOOTHE et al. (1953 d).

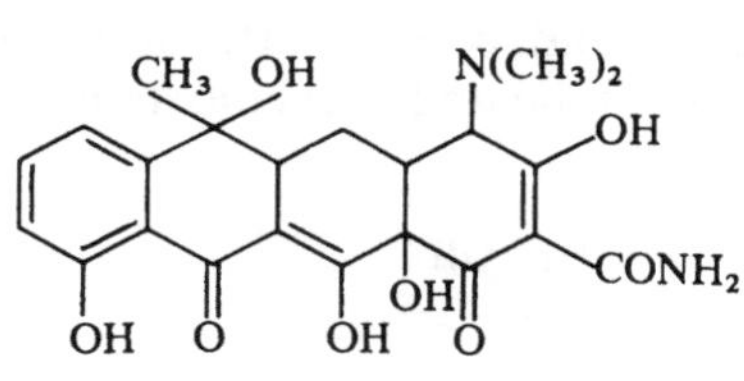

(1)

Certain aspects of the present chapter have been the subject of previous reviews; for example, see BARRETT (1963), BOOTHE (1963), MUXFELDT and BANGERT (1963), CLIVE (1968), MONEY and SCOTT (1968), BLACKWOOD (1969), HLAVKA and BOOTHE (1973), DÜRCKHEIMER (1975), and MITSCHER (1978).

---

* Dedicated to the memory of Robert Burns Woodward (1917–1979) and Hans Muxfeldt (1930–1974) who, each in his own way, contributed so much to the chemistry of the tetracycline antibiotics.

B. Structure Determination

The structure determination of chlortetracycline and oxytetracycline in the early 1950s represented a landmark in the art of structure determination in organic chemistry. Predating the age of high-speed computers and the resultant nearly routine use of X-ray crystallographic methods for the determination of structure of complex molecules, these structural elucidations were essentially based on the classical methods of analysis, degradation, and synthesis of degradation products. Although also predating routine use of mass spectral and nuclear resonance spectral methods, nevertheless a salient feature of this early work is its highly effective use of the infrared, visible, and, most particularly, ultraviolet spectral methods then available. The interest of the scientific community in these structural elucidations was heightened by the fact that two avidly competitive groups, one at Lederle Laboratories and the other at Pfizer working in collaboration with the late Prof. Robert Burns Woodward of Harvard University, vied with each other to be the first to elucidate completely and announce the structure of either chlortetracycline and/or oxytetracycline.

The structure of oxytetracycline was announced by the Pfizer-Woodward group in July of 1952 as (2) (HOCHSTEIN et al. 1952c).

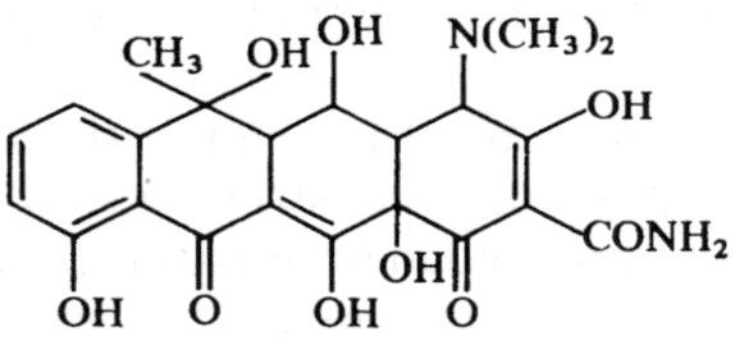

(2)

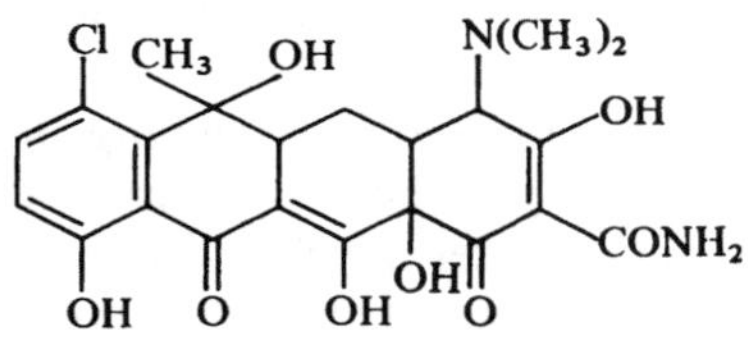

(3)

Three months later the same group announced the structure of chlortetracycline as (3) (STEPHENS et al. 1952), based in part on the published Lederle data. In the same issue of the *Journal of the American Chemical Society*, the Lederle group, but a hair's breadth behind, concurrently announced the further results of their structural studies, which indicated that chlortetracycline was either (3) or (4) (WALLER et al. 1952c, d).

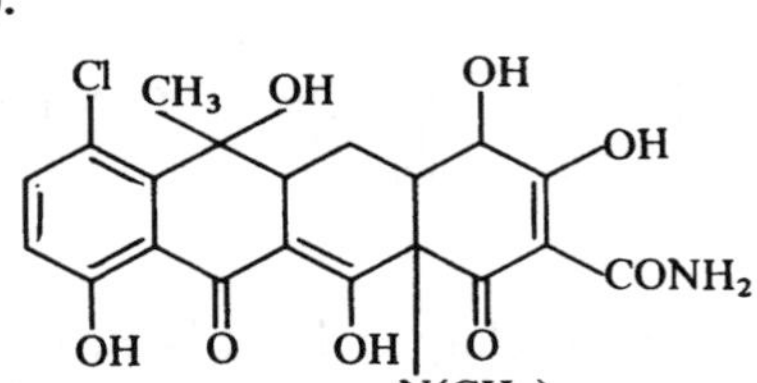

(4)

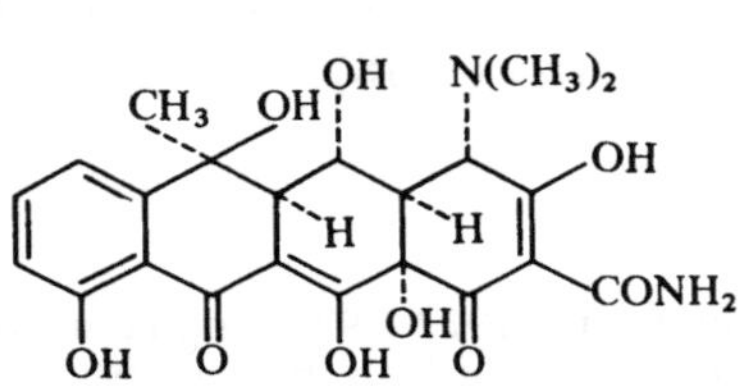

(5)

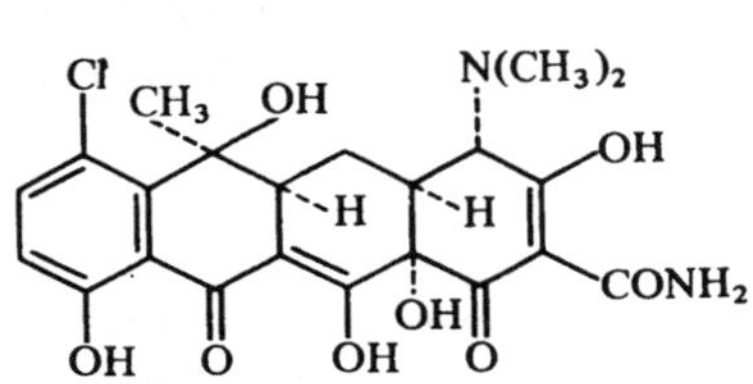

(6)

Ultimately, through a combination of chemical and X-ray crystallographic methods, which are further detailed below, the relative and absolute stereochemistry of oxytetracycline and chlortetracycline were shown to be as depicted by formulae (5) and (6).

There follows a detailed discussion concerning structural determination of the various fermentation tetracyclines, as well as the structural elucidation of certain of their derivatives which are considered to be of particular interest. From the discussion, it will be evident that as the use of modern physical methods such as mass spectroscopy and proton magnetic resonance spectroscopy have become routine, these methods have also been applied to the solution of further structural problems in tetracycline chemistry.

I. Oxytetracycline

1. Gross Structure

The Pfizer-Woodward investigations which led to the assignment of structure to oxytetracycline were first outlined in a series of preliminary communications (Hochstein et al. 1952a–c) and later described in full detail (Hochstein et al. 1953). These publications built upon earlier reports of physical properties by Finlay et al. (1950), Regna and Solomons (1950), and Regna et al. (1951), as well as earlier degradation studies now detailed.

Thus extensive degradation studies reported by Pasternack et al. (1951) included the degradations shown in Fig. 1. Kuhn and Dury (1951a) independently reported alkaline degradation of oxytetracycline to yield ammonia, dimethylamine, and salicylic acid. The molecular weight of oxytetracycline was confirmed by Robertson et al. (1952) using X-ray crystallographic methods.

In a preliminary communication and later full paper, Hochstein and Pasternack (1951, 1952) identified the structure of the "phenolic lactone" derived by

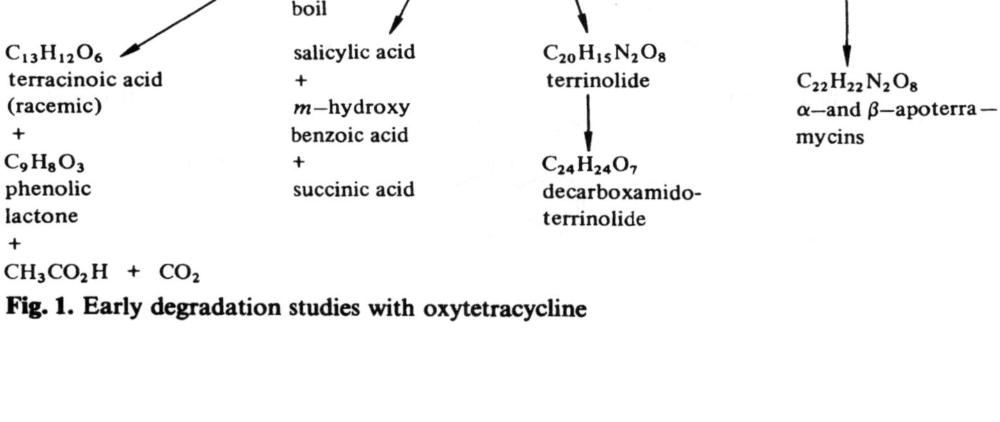

Fig. 1. Early degradation studies with oxytetracycline

basic zinc degradation as 7-hydroxy-3-methylphthalide (7). This assignment was based on the color of the ferric chloride test, alkali fusion to yield salicylic and acetic acids, and methylation of (7) to an ether (8), which in turn was oxidized with permanganate to produce known 3-methoxyphthalic acid (9). The structure of (8) was confirmed by synthesis: viz., pyridine-piperidine condensation of 3-methyoxyphthalic anhydride (10) with malonic acid, hydrolysis/decarboxylation

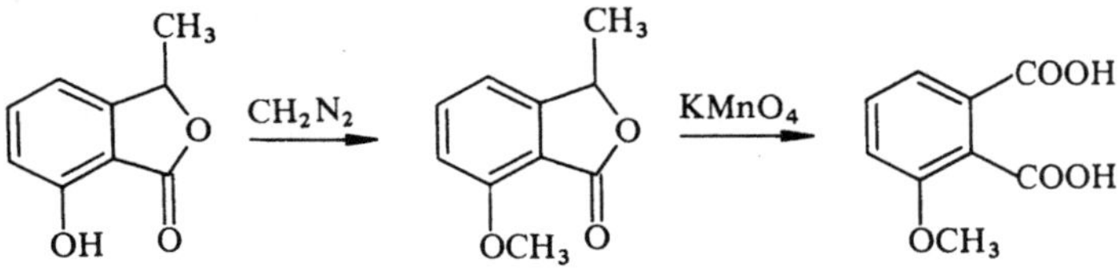

(7) (8) (9)

of the intermediate product, and finally sodium amalgam reduction of the resulting 2-acetyl-6-methoxybenzoic acid (11). Contemporaneously KUHN and DURY (1951 b) independently proved the structure of (7), as well as the further presence of 2-acetyl-6-hydroxybenzoic acid, i.e., the free phenolic form of (11), as an alkaline degradation product of oxytetracycline.

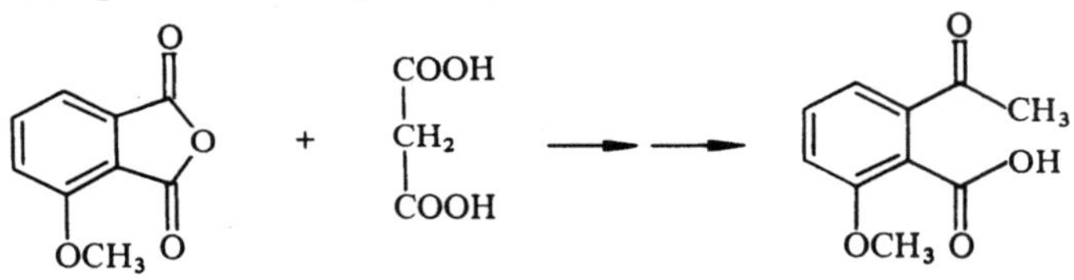

(10) (11)

Two additional publications (PASTERNACK et al. 1952 a, b) further detailed the alkaline degradation of oxytetracycline and the determination of the structure of terracinoic acid as (12). This assignment was on the basis of extensive chemical

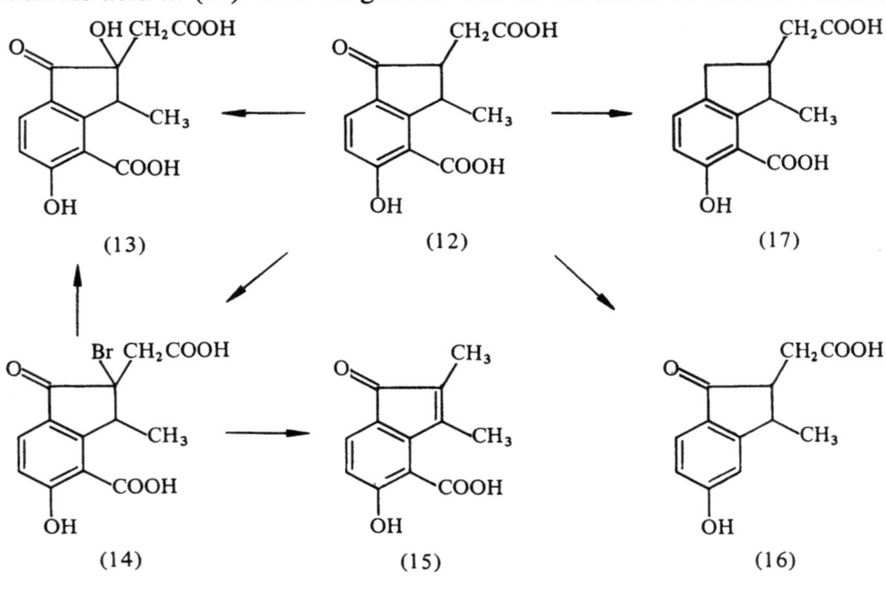

studies including (a) its hydroxylation by alkaline permanganate to yield 2-hydroxyterracinoic acid (13); (b) its bromination to yield 2-bromoterracinoic acid (14), a compound converted to the alcohol (13) by the action of aqueous sodium acetate and readily dehydrobrominated/decarboxylated to (15) in aqueous alkali; (c) its decarboxylation by heating in strong mineral acid to 4-decarboxyterracinoic acid (16); (d) its hydrogenolysis to the methylene derivative (17); and (e) its further degradation to a variety of fragmentary compounds including m-ethylphenol and 6-ethylsalicylic acid; together with pK_a and metal-complexing studies which demonstrated the *ortho* relationship of the aromatic hydroxy and carboxy groups.

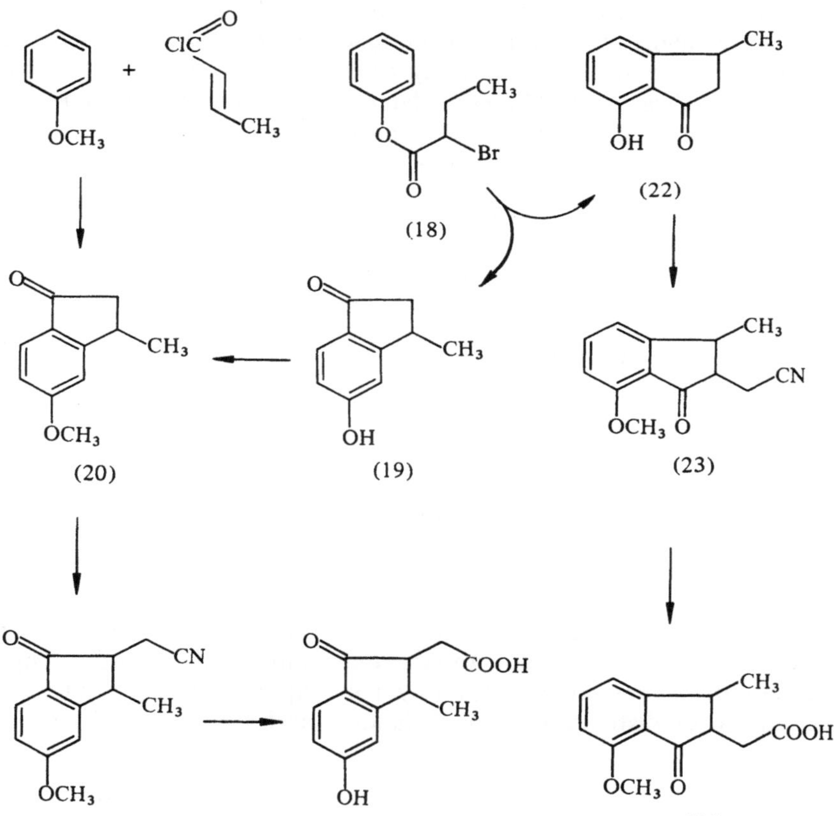

(18) (22) (20) (19) (23) (21) (16) (24)

Subsequent synthetic studies (Conover 1953) confirmed the structure of terracinoic acid (12) and of isodecarboxy terracinoic acid (24), the "bicarbonate soluble fraction" of Pasternack et al. (1952a). Reaction of phenyl α-bromobutyrate with aluminum chloride gave a separable mixture of the phenolic indanones (19) and (22). Methylation of (19) gave the methoxyindanone (20), alternatively prepared by the condensation of anisole with crotonyl chloride. The acetic acid side chain was introduced by formation of a Mannich base with formaldehyde and dimethylamine and conversion of the Mannich base to the nitrile (21). Hydrolysis of (21) gave decarboxyterracinoic acid (16). Analogously, the isomeric phenolic indanone was converted to isodecarboxyterracinoic acid (24) via the nitrile (23).

The coup de grace arrived with three simultaneous preliminary communications (HOCHSTEIN et al. 1962a–c), which assigned structures to the earlier acid degradation products, terrinolide, decarboxamidoterrinolide, α- and β-apoterramycins, and Terramycin (oxytetracycline) itself. These communications were later combined and detailed in a paper, "The Structure of Terramycin" (HOCHSTEIN et al. 1953), which represents a paragon in the determination of organic structure by classical methods.

On the basis of general considerations of microanalysis, pK_a values, infrared analysis (no bands below 6 µm), dimethylation with diazomethane, positive ferric reaction, active hydrogen determination, diacetylation, dimethylamine and ammonia formation on strong alkaline degradation, conversion to nitrile with loss of the elements of water, and C-methyl determination, the structural position, before consideration of degradation reactions, was summarized by the expression (25).

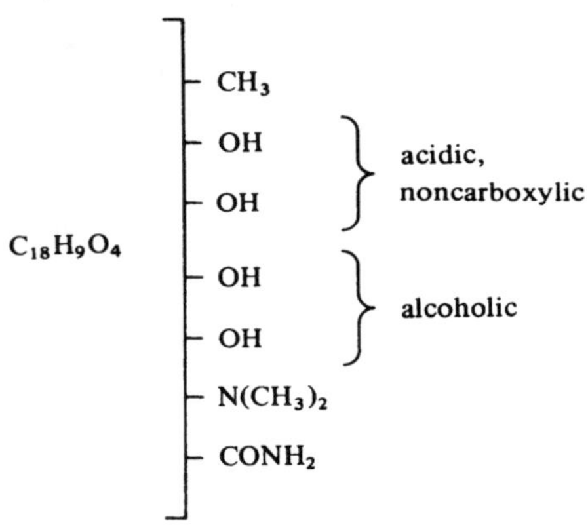

(25)

The structure of further alkaline degradation products, isodecarboxyterracinoic acid (24), terranaphthol (26), and terranaphthoic acid (27), were assigned on the basis of their characteristic 1,8-dihydroxynaphthalene ultraviolet chromophores, zinc dust distillation to naphthalene, and mechanistic considerations

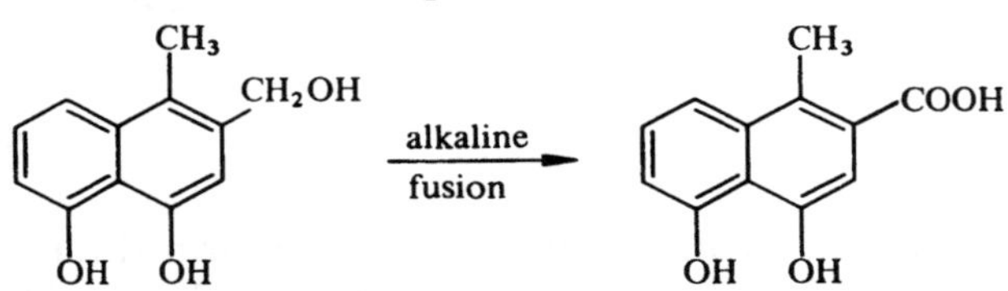

(26) (27)

which permitted the formation of these and the other alkaline degradation products of established structure. The same style mechanistic considerations, in the further light of the structures of terracinoic acid (12) and 7-hydroxy-3-methylphthalide (7) assigned earlier, then permitted formulation of the partial structure (28) for oxytetracycline.

Consideration was then given to the acid degradation of oxytetracycline, whereby partial structure (28) was verified and the partial structures (29)–(32), respectively, were assigned for anhydroterramycin, α- and β-apoterramycins, terrinolide, and decarboxamidoterrinolide. These assignments were based in part on comparison of the ultraviolet chromophores with those of model compounds.

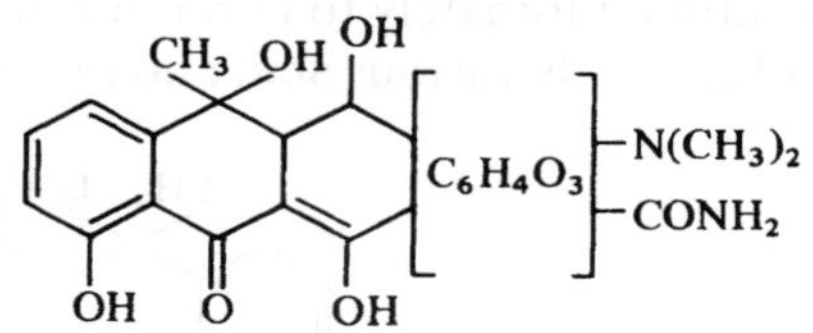

(28)

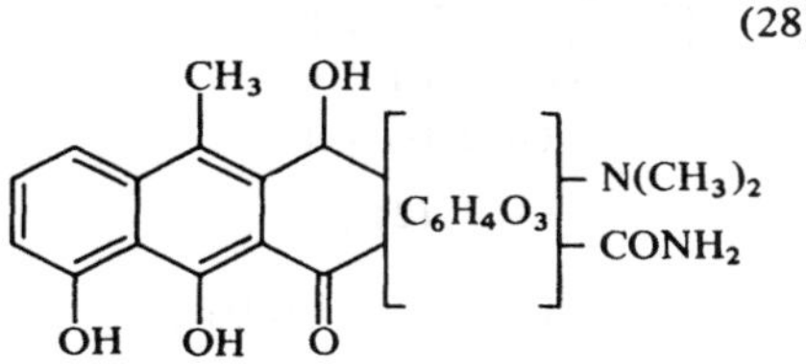

(29)

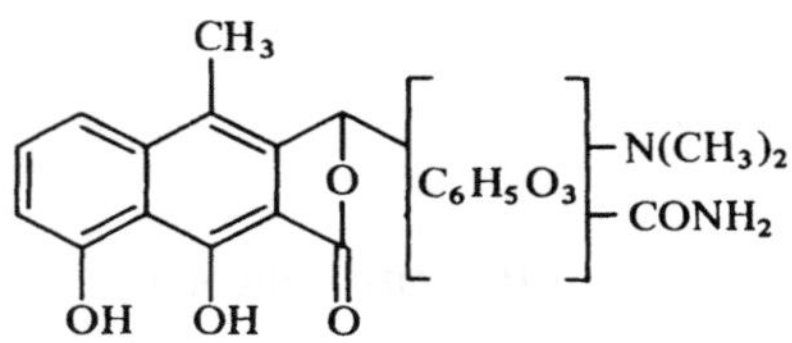

(30)

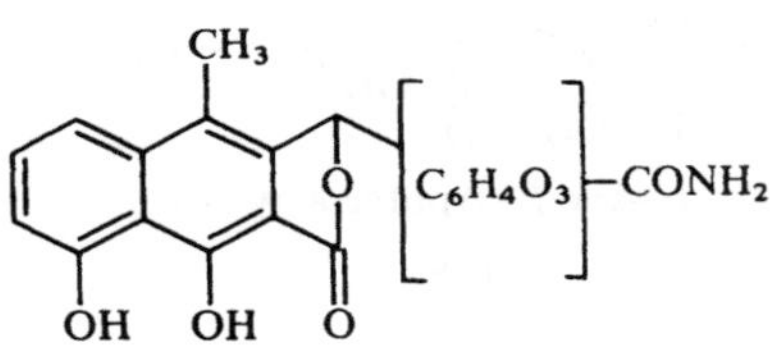

(31)

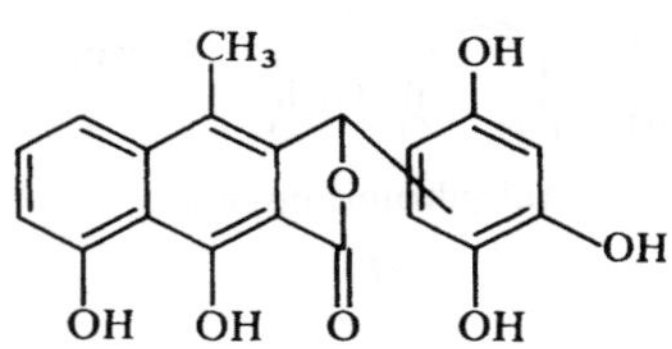

(32)

The marked acidity of terrinolide, again in comparison with the appropriate model compounds, permitted its further formulation as (32a). Additional pK_a and mechanistic considerations permitted the further formulation of α- and β-apoterramycins, anhydroterramycin, and oxytetracycline as (33)–(35) respectively, where X or Y represent OH or $N(CH_3)_2$.

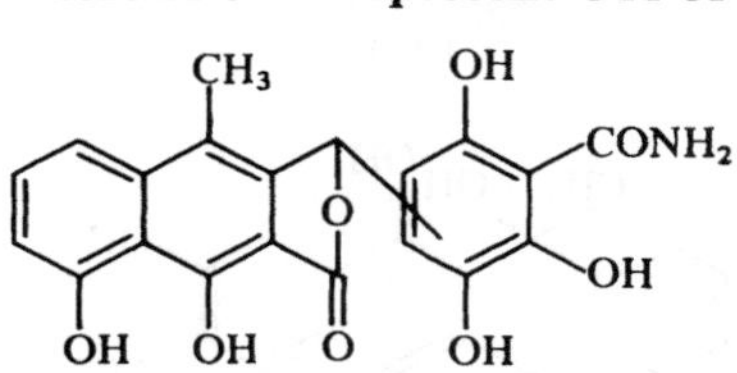

(32a)

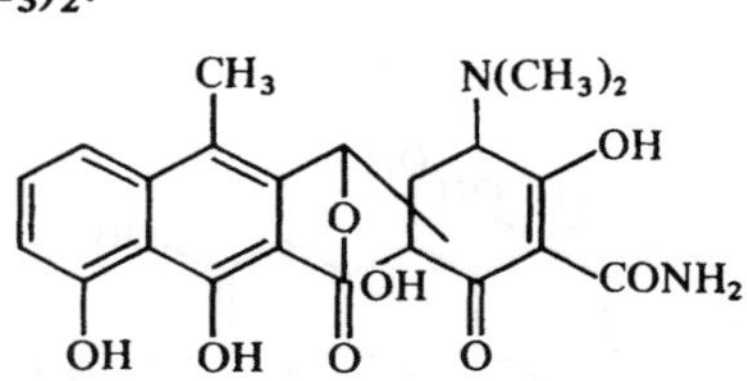

(33)

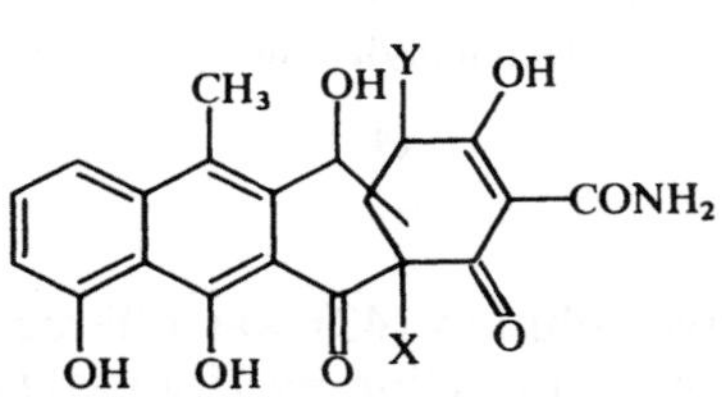

(34)

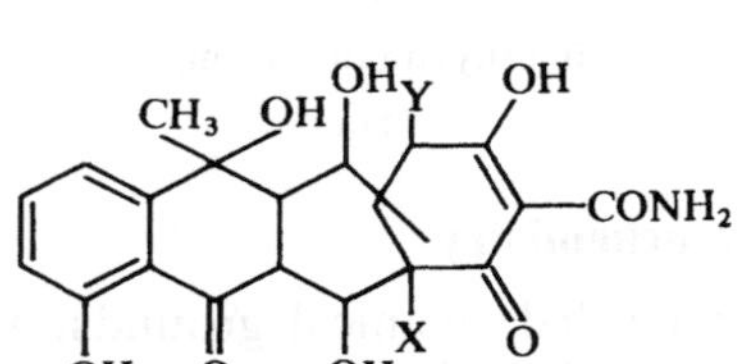

(35)

Finally, reductive degradation studies permitted the unambiguous assignment of structures. Zinc reduction in acetic acid initially gave a dedimethylaminoterramycin, retaining the ultraviolet chromophores of oxytetracycline. Further reduction gave a deoxydedimethylaminoterramycin, having an extended chromophore, leading to the conclusions that in structures (34) and (35) X is OH and Y is $N(CH_3)_2$. Further degradation, ultimately to naphthacene (36), proved the structure of oxytetracycline as (2) and its various acid and reductive degradation products as (37)–(42).

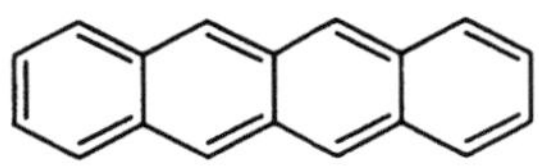

(36)

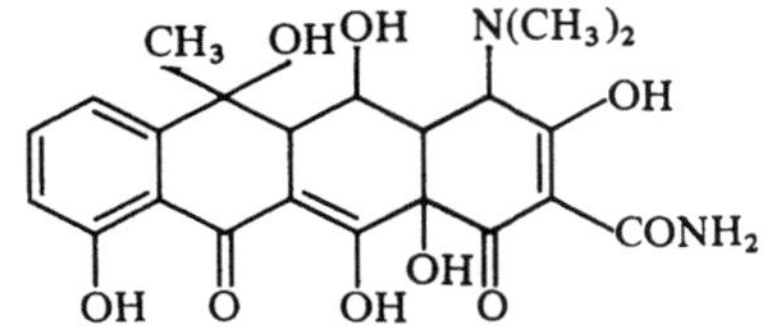

Oxytetracycline

(2)

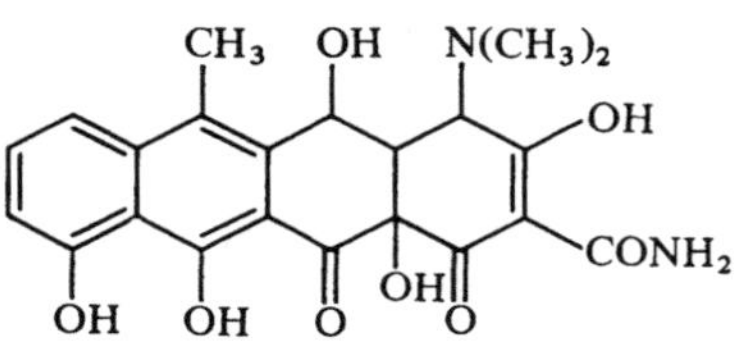

Anhydroterramycin

(37)

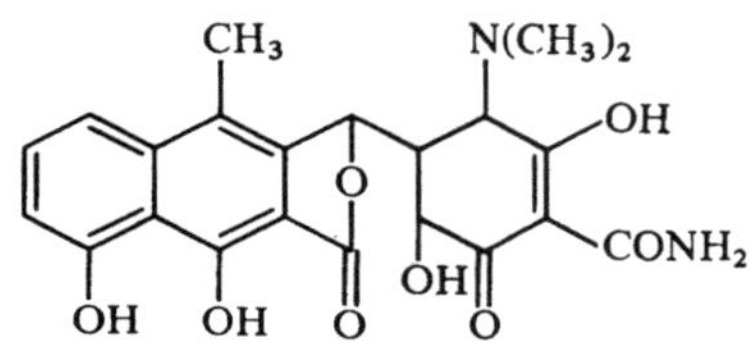

α–and β–Apoterramycins

(38)

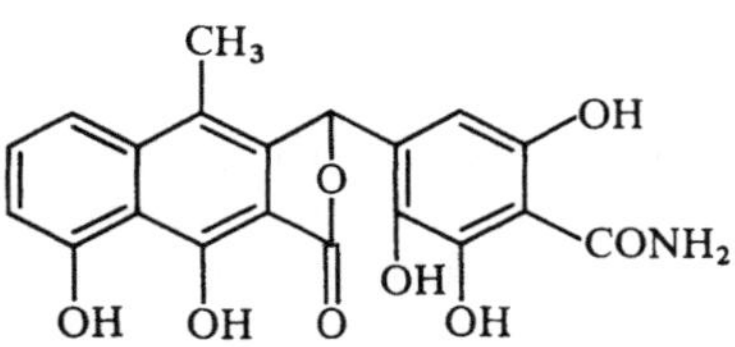

Terrinolide

(39)

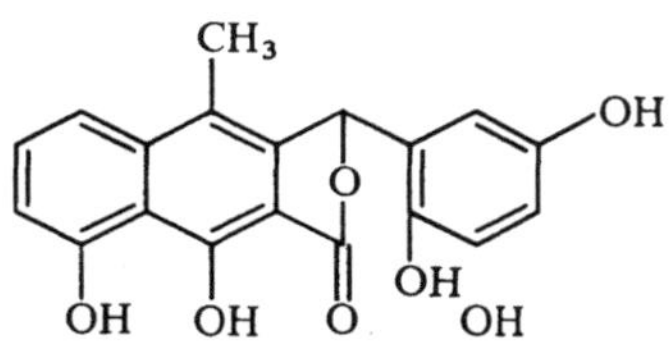

Decarboxamidoterrinolide

(40)

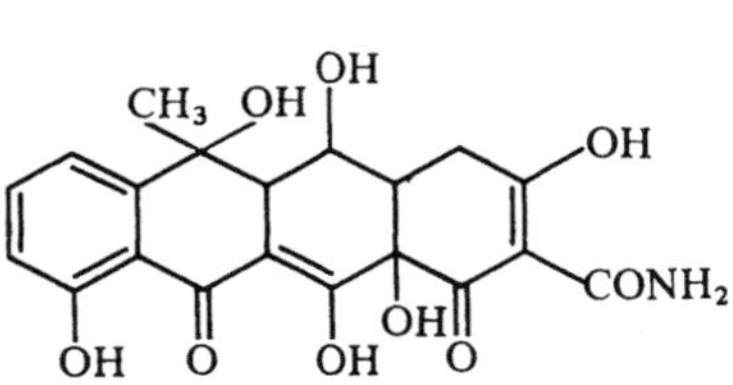

Dedimethylaminoterramycin

(41)

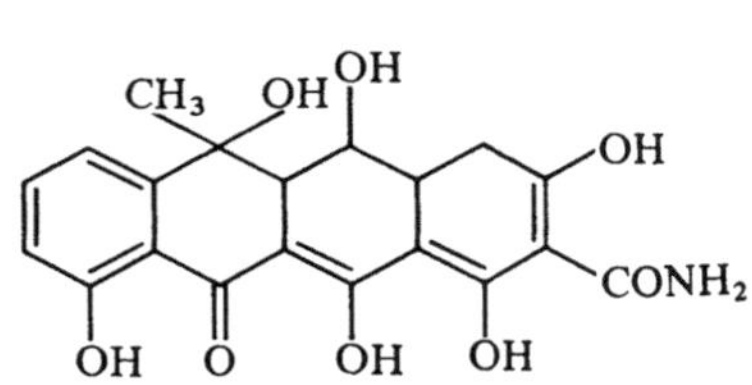

Deoxydedimethylaminoterramycin

(42)

2. Stereochemistry

On unrecorded chemical grounds, a tentative solution (43) was offered to the problem of the relative stereochemistry of oxytetracycline by HOCHSTEIN et al. (1953). Later the facile degradation of oxytetracycline with methyl iodide provided a chemical basis for arguing a *trans* relationship between the 4-dimethylamino group and the 4a-hydrogen (CONOVER 1956). An X-ray crystallographic structural analysis (TAKEUCHI and BUERGER 1960) confirmed the structure of oxytetracycline as (2). Further analysis of their three-dimensional coordinate data indicated that the relative stereochemistry of oxytetracycline was represented by structural formula (5). However, later considerations of crystal geometry by DONOHUE et al. (1963) indicated doubt about the C5 assignment as based on TAKEUCHI and BUERGER, and further suggested, although not unequivocally, that a case could be made for the assignment at C5 as in (43). Doubts were resolved to (5) by a proton nuclear magnetic resonance study by SCHACH VON WITTENAU et al. (1965) and a more detailed X-ray study by CID-DRESDNER (1965).

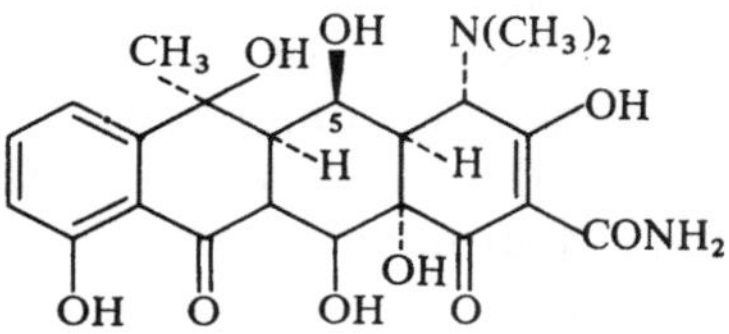

(43)

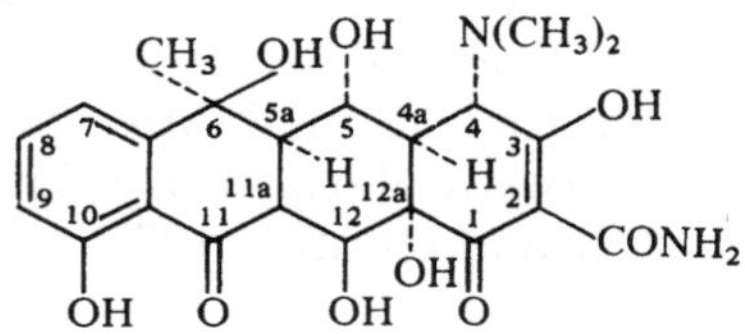

(5)

The absolute stereochemistry of oxytetracycline also corresponds to the structure depicted by formula (5). This assignment was initially made by DOBRYNIN et al. (1962a) as the same as that for chlortetracycline (assigned on the basis of degradation discussed below). These workers noted the common biogenesis and similar activity of these antibiotics and in particular noted the common shift in optical rotation (ca. 100°) on isomerization to the corresponding 4-epimers. A contemporaneous report by MCCORMICK et al. (1962) that 5a,6-anhydrotetracycline (44) was converted biosynthetically to both tetracycline (45) and oxytetracycline effectively confirmed the conclusions of DOBRYNIN et al. Later circular

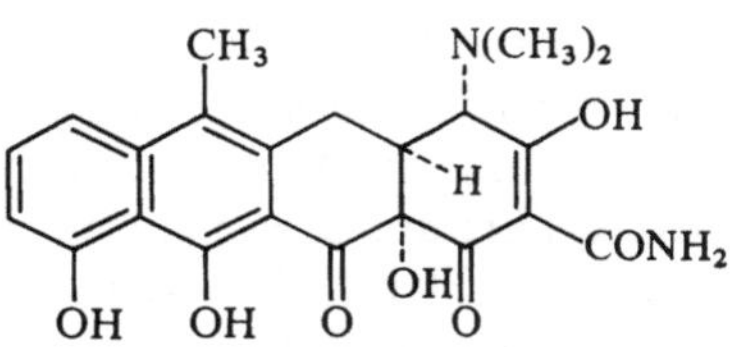

(44)

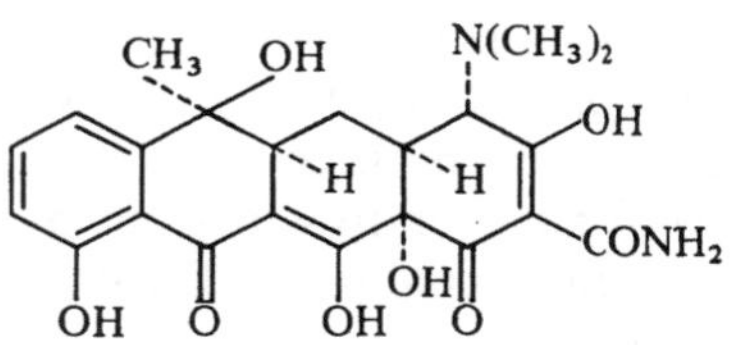

(45)

dichroism studies by MITSCHER et al. (1968) were consistent with these conclusions. The ultimate confirmation of the absolute stereochemistry of oxytetracycline was by X-ray crystallographic studies by STEZOWSKI (1977) on a derivative, α-6-deoxyoxytetracycline (see later in text).

3. Conformation

Proton nuclear magnetic resonance studies on a variety of tetracycline derivatives in such diverse solvents as trifluoroacetic acid, dimethylsulfoxide, chloroform, and pyridine were summarized by SCHACH VON WITTENAU and BLACKWOOD (1966); the assignment of additional protons were made later by ASLESON et al. (1974). Once the full relative stereochemistry of oxytetracycline was established, it was possible to determine the solution conformation of oxytetracycline and several of its derivatives on the basis of proton nuclear magnetic resonance spectral properties (SCHACH VON WITTENAU and BLACKWOOD 1966). For oxytetracycline (5) and a series of derivatives, the apparent coupling constant between the C4 and C4a protons is 9–13 cps. This indicates a *trans* diaxial relationship between these protons. On the other hand, the splitting pattern between the C5 proton in oxytetracyclines and the adjacent 4a and 5a protons indicates no such *trans* diaxial relationship – indicating a pseudoequatorial conformation for the 5a hydrogen. Consideration of Drieding models indicates essentially two possible all-chair conformations for oxytetracycline – one in which the 12a- and 5-hydroxyls occupy closely spaced pseudoaxial positions and the other in which the 4-dimethylamino and the 12a-hydroxy occupy closely spaced pseudoaxial positions. Only in the former conformation do the 4, 4a, and 5 protons possess the steric relationship to account for the ^{1}H-NMR spectra. The solid-state conformation of the O^5,O^{12a}-diacetate of oxytetracycline has been shown by HUGHES et al. (1971) and VON DREELE and HUGHES (1971) to be the same as that noted by ^{1}H-NMR studies.

Subsequent circular dichroism studies by MITSCHER et al. (1968, 1969) suggest that in more dilute concentration, in strong aqueous acid, the conformation of oxytetracycline (as well as other tetracyclines) is neither one of the all-chair conformations discussed above, but rather an intermediate one in which both the 5-hydroxyl and the 4-dimethylamino group occupy pseudoequatorial positions (at the expense of forcing rings A and B into higher-energy boat forms). Such a conformation is consistent with the solid-state conformation earlier evident by X-ray crystallographic methods for chlortetracycline (DONOHUE et al. 1963) and oxytetracycline (CID-DRESDNER 1965).

Later, MITSCHER et al. (1972), based on further circular dichroism studies, concluded that above pH 7.1 there was a divergence of conformation of 5-hydroxytetracyclines and of those not hydroxylated at the 5-position; and furthermore that oxytetracycline, at pH values of 9 and 11 in the presence of magnesium chloride (which both complexes with and stabilizes the antibiotic), has the all-chair conformation in which the 5- and 12-hydroxyl groups are in close proximity, i.e., pseudoaxial to the B-ring, noted in the earlier ^{1}H-NMR studies.

As interpreted by PREWO and STEZOWSKI (1977), later ^{1}H-NMR data on tetracycline-free bases (GULBIS and EVERETT 1975, 1976; WILLIAMSON and EVERETT 1975) are also consistent with other tetracyclines, at least in the free base form in dimethylsulfoxide, having the same conformation as oxytetracyclines, i.e., all-chair with 4-dimethylamino pseudoequatorial. According to X-ray crystallographic analysis, tetracycline and oxytetracycline free-base forms (STEZOWSKI 1976; PREWO and STEZOWSKI 1977), as well as synthetic *N-tert*-butyl-6-deoxy-6-demethyl-8-methoxy tetracycline (GLATZ et al. 1979), also have the same all-chair conformation, while doxycycline hydrochloride exists in the other all-chair conformation (STEZOWSKI 1977).

The overall conclusion to be drawn from all of these studies must surely be that the various possible conformational forms of the tetracyclines must not differ greatly in energy state, and that under appropriate conditions (including those at the ultimate site of action) any one of the indicated conformations can be assumed. Consistent with this view are the many facile transannular chemical interactions seen in the tetracyclines, which variously require the molecule to assume one or another of these conformations. Additional considerations of tetracycline conformation are to be found below in the section on tetracycline metal chelates.

II. Chlortetracycline

1. Gross Structure

The investigations which led to the assignment of structure to chlortetracycline were detailed in a series of communications which culminated in two independent, but concurrent, preliminary reports concerning the structure of chlortetracycline: one by the Pfizer-Woodward group (Stephens et al. 1952) and the other by the Lederle group (Waller et al. 1952c, d). These reports built upon earlier reports of physical properties by Broschard et al. (1949), Dunitz and Leonard (1950), and Pepinsky and Watanabe (1952); an incorrect hypothesis by Dunitz and Robertson (1952), based on X-ray crystallographic studies, that chlortetracycline and oxytetracycline differed only by replacement of chloro with hydroxy at a common position; and degradation studies as detailed below.

Kuhn and Dury (1951a) reported that dimethylamine and 5-chlorosalicylic acid (46) resulted from the alkaline fusion of chlortetracycline, suggesting a relationship between the structure of chlortetracycline and oxytetracycline. Hutchings et al. (1952a) confirmed the formation of these products and reported that, as in the case of oxytetracycline, ammonia was also formed on the alkaline fusion of chlortetracycline. Furthermore, the latter workers reported that methylation and subsequent permanganate oxidation resulted in the formation of a number

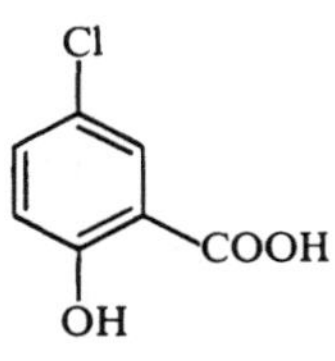

(46)

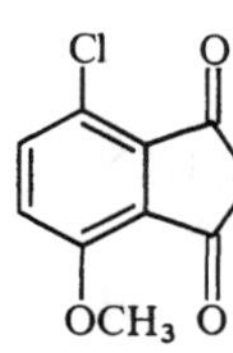

(47)

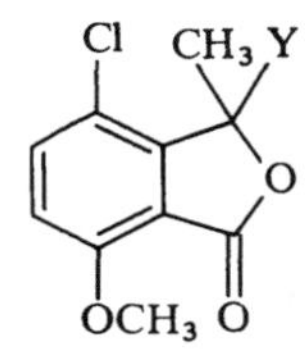

(48) Y = H
(49) Y = OH
(50) Y = COOH
(51) Y = $-\underset{|}{C}HCOOH$ (CH_2COOH)

of p-chloromethoxybenzene derivatives (47)–(51). The structures of these compounds were deduced on the basis of physical and chemical properties and confirmed by synthesis by Kushner et al. (1952). 6-Chloro-3-methoxyphthalic anhydride (47) was synthesized from 3-methoxy-6-chloroanthanilic acid by Sandmeyer replacement of amine with cyano and hydrolysis. The deschloro variants of compounds (48)–(51) were synthesized from 2-amino-3-methoxyacetophenone (52). 7-Methoxy-3-methylphalide (55) was prepared by reduction of the ketone group of (52) to yield the alcohol (53), Sandmeyer replacement of amino with cyano to produce (54), and finally hydrolysis. 3-Hydroxy-7-methoxy-3-methylphthalide (56) was similarly prepared via (57), omitting the reduction step. Addition of hydrogen cyanide to the intermediate 2-cyano-3-methoxyacetophenone (57) gave the *bis*-cyanide (58), which on hydrolysis produced 7-methoxy-3-methyl-3-phthalidecarboxylic acid (59). Reaction of the hydroxyphthalide (56) with phosphorus pentachloride gave the 3-chloro derivative (60), which, when sequentially reacted with sodio diethyl carbethoxysuccinate (to 61), hydrolyzed and decarboxylated, gave 2-(4-chloro-7-methoxy-3-methyl-3-phthalidyl)succinic acid (62).

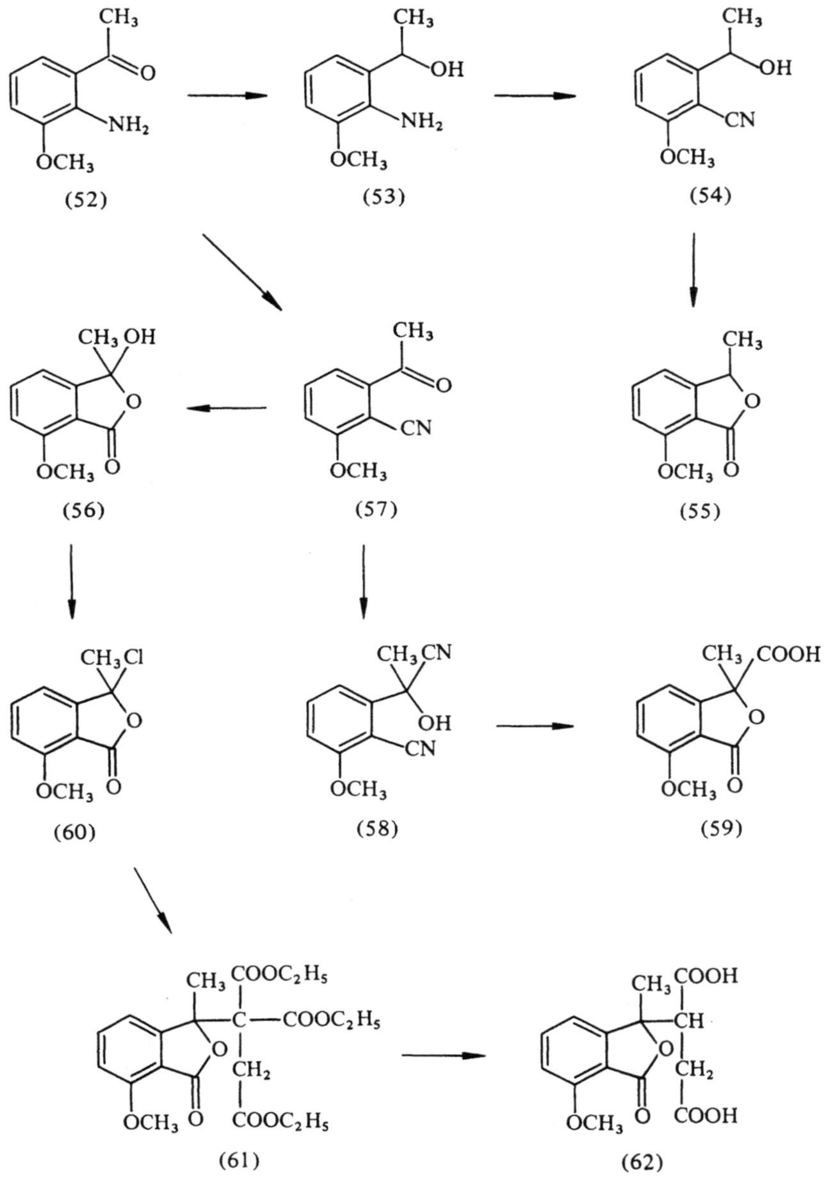

Chlorination of (55), (56), (59), and (62) gave, respectively, chlortetracycline degradation products (48)–(50), and (51), the position of the entering chlorine having already been established by degradation of these compounds to known 5-chloro-2-methoxybenzoic acid. These synthetic studies were described in detail in later reports by BOOTHE et al. (1953 a, b) and KUSHNER et al. (1953). In addition to the compounds whose identity was proved by synthesis, HUTCHINGS et al. (1952 a) also identified 3-(4-chloro-7-methoxy-3-methyl-3-phthalidyl)glutaric acid (63) among the methylation-oxidation degradation products.

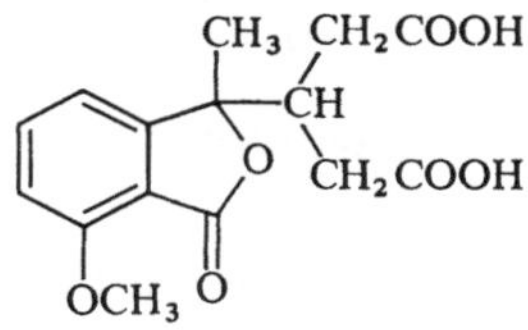

(63)

Given the structure of oxytetracycline reported earlier by HOCHSTEIN et al. (1952 c), the structural relationship between oxytetracycline and chlortetracycline evident from crystallographic studies (DUNITZ and ROBERTSON 1952; PEPINSKY and WATANABE 1952), the degradation studies of the preceding paragraph, and the similarity in pK_as and ultraviolet adsorption, it became a compelling hypothesis that chlortetracycline was a 7-chloro-*x*-deoxy variant of oxytetracycline. STEPHENS et al. (1952) confirmed this hypothesis, assigning the structure (6) to chlortetracycline following reductive degradation studies which paralleled those of

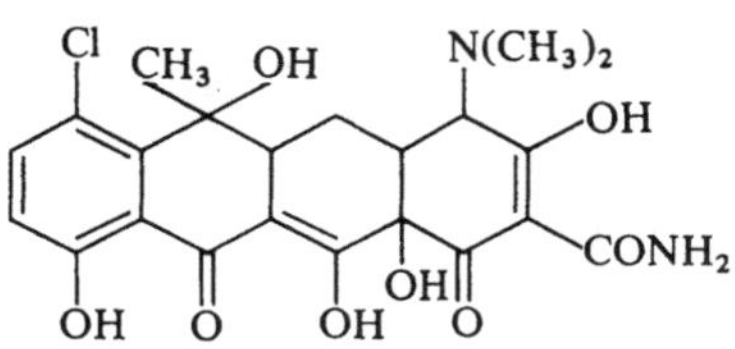

(6)

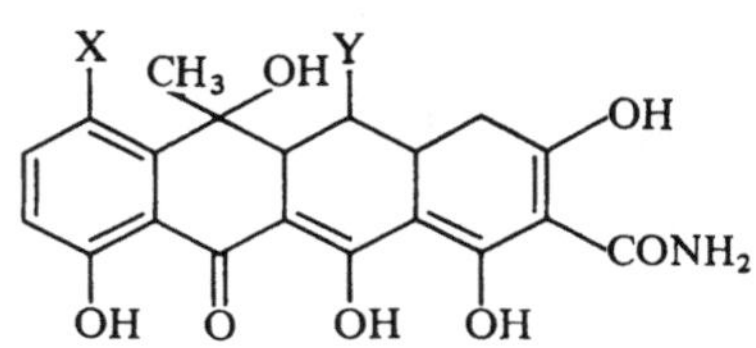

(64) X = Cl, Y = H
(42) X = H, Y = OH

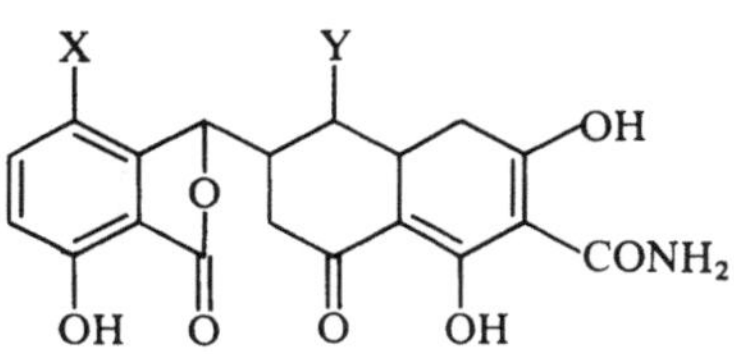

(65) X = Cl, Y = H
(66) X = H, Y = OH

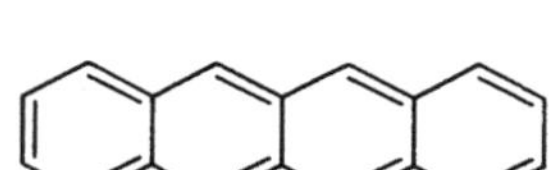

(36)

oxytetracycline, viz., zinc in acetic acid reduction to the dedimethylamino-deoxy derivative (64) and acid degradation of (64) to a "red" compound which gave naphthacene (36) on zinc dust distillation. Furthermore, alkali-induced rearrangement of (64) and (42) gave the substituted phthalides (65) and (66), which on pyrolysis gave, respectively, 4-chloro-7-hydroxy-3-methylphthalide (67) and 7-hydroxy-3-methylphthalide (7).

Concurrent with the report of STEPHENS et al. was a series of reports concerning further degradation studies on chlortetracycline by WALLER et al. (1952 a–d) and HUTCHINGS et al. (1952 b). Degradation of chlortetracycline with 5*N* sodium hydroxide gave dimethylamine and dedimethylaminoaureomycinic acid (68). The

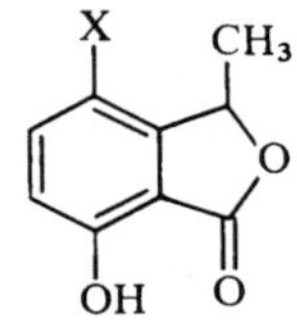

(67) X=Cl
(7) X=H

former was assigned structure on the basis of spectroscopic properties, pK_a considerations, and its further degradation (WALLER et al. 1952 a, b). Oxidative cleavage of (68) gave 3-(4-chloro-7-hydroxy-3-methyl-3-phthalidyl)glutaric acid (69) and 3,4-dihydroxy-2,5-cyclopentanedione-1-carboxamide (70), an alkali-stable compound identified by the further transformations: (a) to 1,3-cyclopentanedione (71), ammonia, and carbon dioxide by the action of hydriodic acid and red phosphorus and (b) to 1,2,4-cyclopentanetrione (72), ammonia, and carbon dioxide by the action of 48% hydrobromic acid. Dehydration of (68) with heat

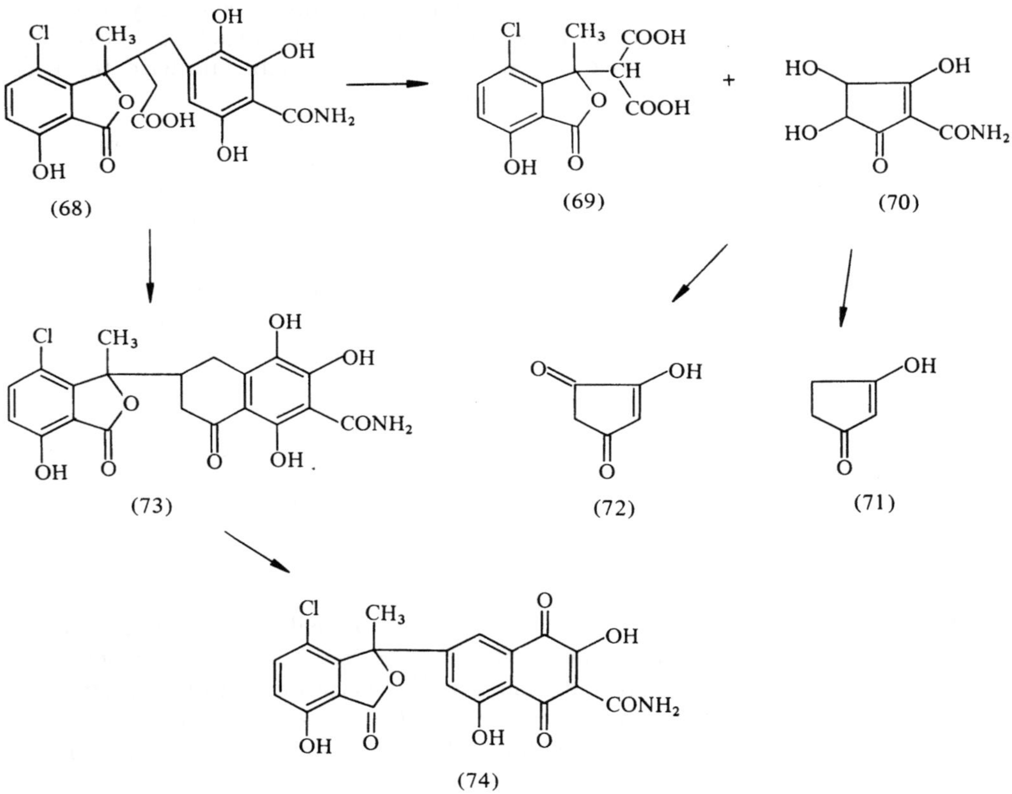

or sulfuric acid gave aureone amide (73), which in turn was air oxidized in alkali to aureoquinone amide (74).

Degradation of chlortetracycline with 5*N* sodium hydroxide containing a reducing agent gave isomeric α- and β-aureomycinic acids (75) (HUTCHINGS et al. 1952b). These compounds were assigned structure on the basis of spectroscopic properties, pK_a considerations, and their further degradation with 5*N* sodium hydroxide, without a reducing agent, to dedimethylaminoaureomycinic acid (68). Reducing agents are understood to prevent the conversion of (75) to (68) by inhibiting initial oxidation of the A-ring by even traces of oxygen, thus preventing an ensuing chain reaction.

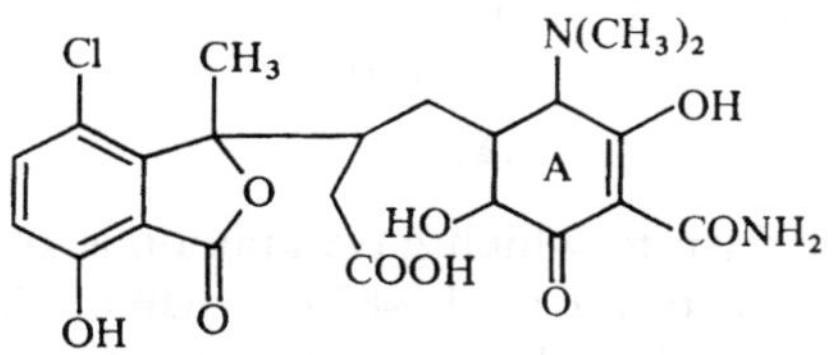

(75)

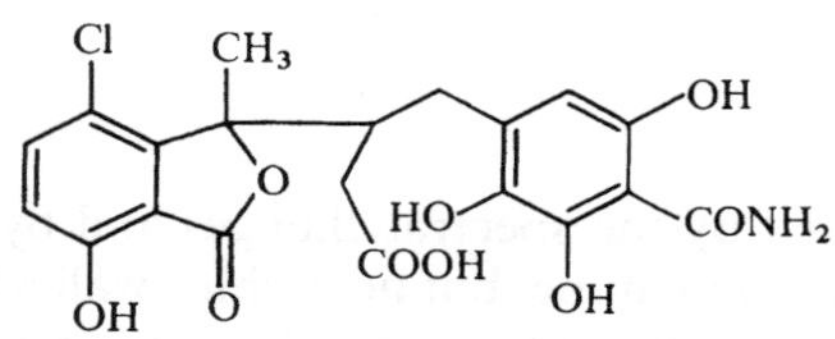

(68)

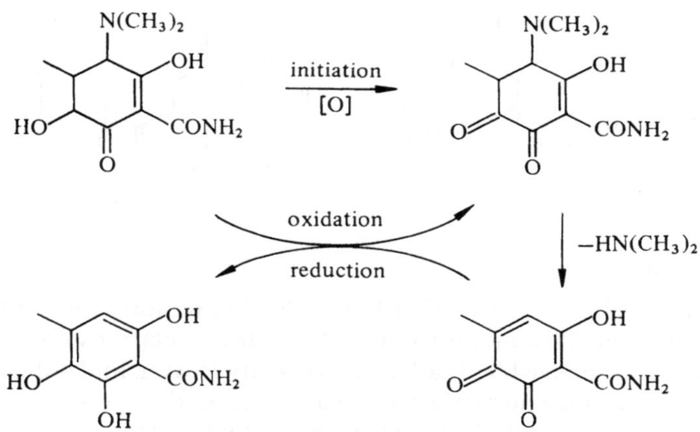

On the other hand, degradation of chlortetracycline in dilute alkali gave an isomeric product, isoaureomycin (76). The infrared and ultraviolet absorption spectra established the presence of the phthalide nucleus as well as the unconjugated ketone and the presence of the same A-ring chromophore as that present in α- and β-aureomycinic acid. Further degradation of isoaureomycin in 5*N* sodium hydroxide in the presence of reducing agents led to α- and β-aureomycinic

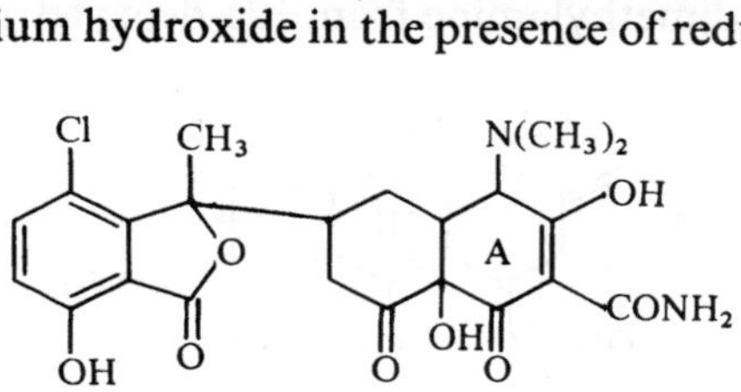

(76)

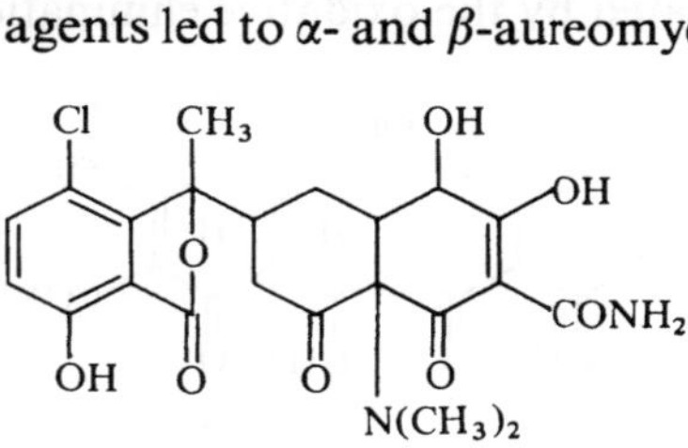

(77)

acids; it was then concluded that isoaureomycin was (76) or (77) and that chlortetracycline was (3) or (4). The structure of the CD-rings was further confirmed by acid dehydration of chlortetracycline to anhydroaureomycin (77a) (WALLER et al. 1952d), also with equivocal assignment of the positions of the dimethylamino and hydroxy groups. The aromatization of the C-ring in (77a) was indi-

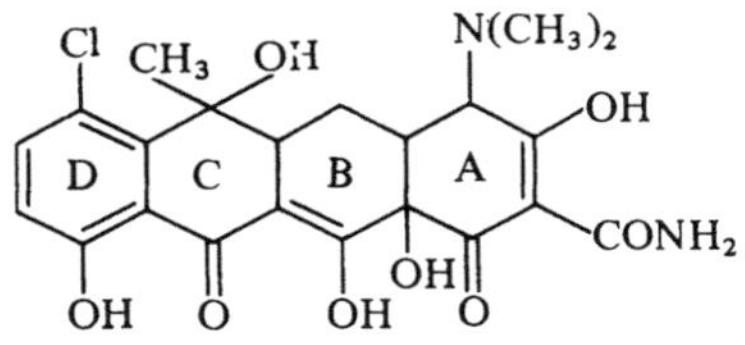

(3)

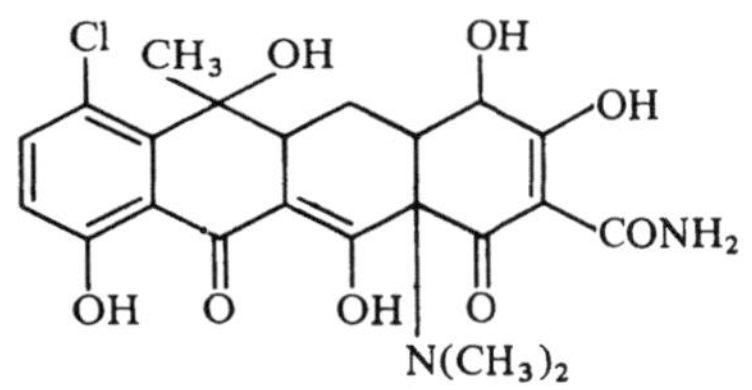

(4)

cated by the spectral changes and by alkaline fusion, which gave ammonia and dimethylamine, but no 5-chlorosalicylic acid. Hydriodic acid (48%) in lieu of hydrochloric acid for the elimination of water gave deschloroanhydroaureomycin [anhydrotetracycline (78)].

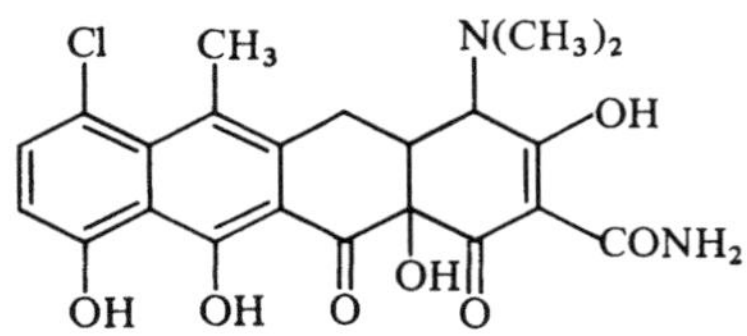

(77a)

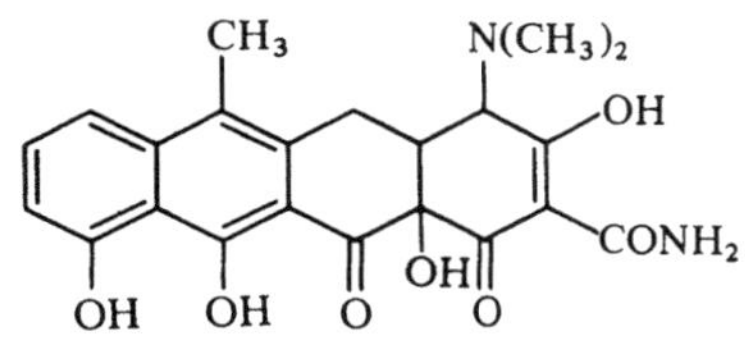

(78)

2. Stereochemistry

WALLER et al. (1952d) suggested that the facile elimination of water from chlortetracycline under acidic conditions indicated a *trans* relationship of 6-hydroxyl and 5a hydrogen groups, while 12a-hydroxyl, 4a hydrogen, and 4-dimethylamino groups were *cis-cis*, since no elimination was noted under the same acidic conditions. The *cis* relationship of 12a-hydroxy and 4a hydrogen was confirmed chemically by the thermal elimination of formic acid from tetracycline 12a-formate (79), producing 4a,12a-anhydrotetracycline (80) (BLACKWOOD et al. 1960a, b); the *trans* relationship of 6-hydroxyl and 5a hydrogen was confirmed by formation of 11a-halotetracycline 6,12-hemiketals (81) (RENNHARD et al. 1961; BLACKWOOD et al. 1963); and the *cis* relationship of 4a hydrogen and 4-dimethylamino further indicated by the oxidative elimination of dimethylamine from 12a-deoxytetracy-

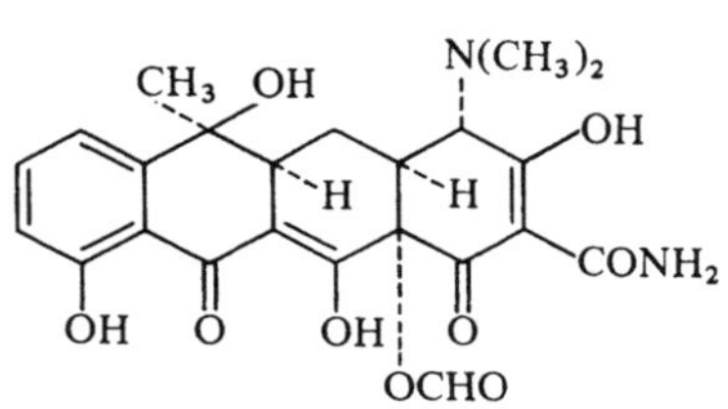

(79)

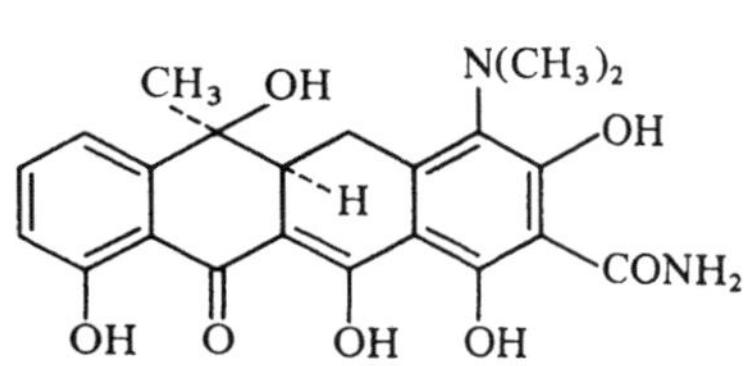

(80)

cline, yielding 4a,12a-anhydro-4-dedimethylaminotetracycline (82) (GREEN and BOOTHE 1960). The complete relative stereochemistry of chlortetracycline was first signaled by the X-ray crystallography studies of HIROKAWA et al. (1959a, b), who confirmed the structure of chlortetracycline as (6), showing relative stereochemistry as indicated. These conclusions were confirmed by the more detailed

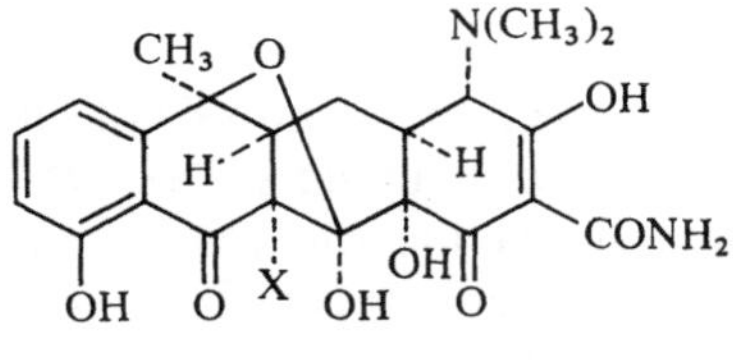

(81)

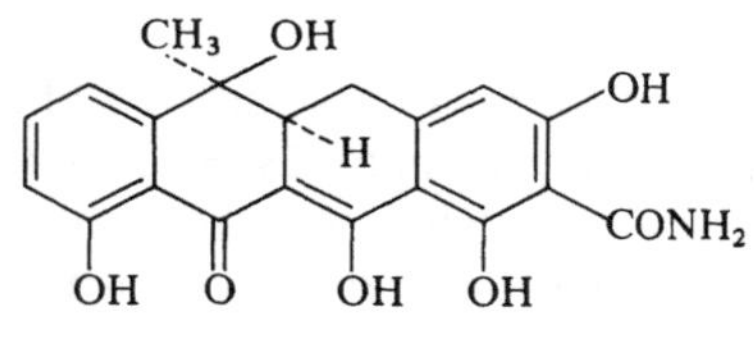

(82)

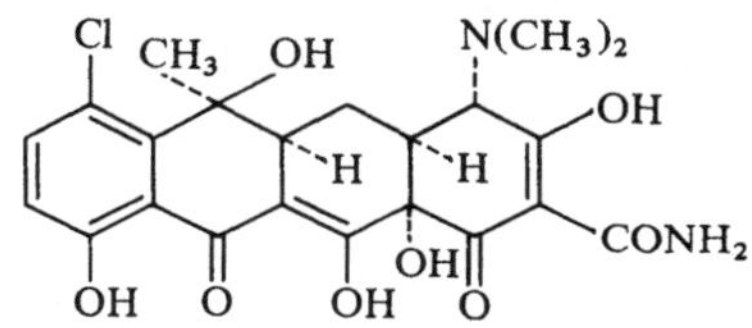

(6)

X-ray crystallography studies of DONOHUE et al. (1963). By chemical methods, DOBRYNIN et al. (1962a, b) and KOLOSOV et al. (1963a, b), demonstrated that the depiction (6) also represented the absolute stereochemistry of chlortetracycline. Thus methylation/permanganate oxidation of chlorotetracycline gave (+)-4-chloro-7-methoxy-3-methyl-phthalide-3-carboxylic acid (50) as described earlier, which was hydrogenolyzed to the corresponding (+) deschloro compound (83). *dl-o*-Acetylaminoatrolactinic acid (84) was resolved. The resulting pure enantiomer was converted to (85) by saponification, diazotization, and replacement of N_2^+ with CN; and then to the (−)enantiomorph of the desmethoxyphthalide (85a) by hydrolysis. The enantiomer (84) was also converted by saponification, diazotization, and H_3PO_2 reduction to (+)-atrolactinic acid (86) of known absolute configuration, thereby determining the absolute stereochemistry of chlorotetracycline. Ultimately, the absolute stereochemistry of chlortetracycline was confirmed by X-ray crystallographic studies on two of its derivatives: 5a,6-anhydrotetracycline (RESTIVO and PALENIK 1969) and tetracycline (KAMIYA et al. 1971).

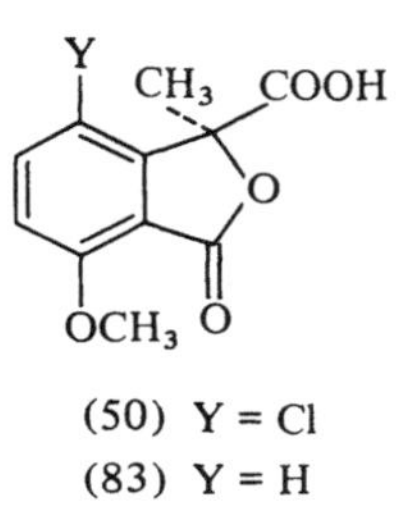

(50) Y = Cl
(83) Y = H

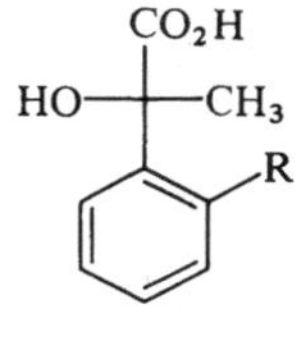

(84) R = NHAc
(85) R = CN
(86) R = H

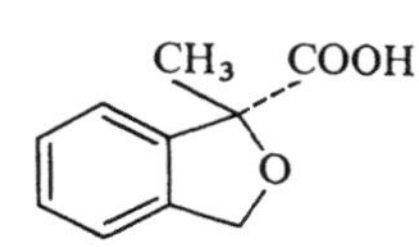

(85a)

3. Conformation

Considerations concerning the conformation of chlortetracycline are essentially as already discussed above in connection with oxytetracycline. See also Sect. IX below concerning tetracycline metal chelates.

III. Tetracycline

Tetracycline (87) was first derived chemically by the hydrogenolysis of chlortetracycline (CONOVER et al. 1953; BOOTHE et al. 1953c, d; STEPHENS et al. 1954). The structural relationship of tetracycline to chlortetracycline was readily apparent from its derivation, molecular formula, pK_a values, and spectral properties. In acid, it degraded to the earlier reported deschloroanhydroaureomycin [5a,6-anhydrotetracycline (78)]. Relative and absolute stereochemistry were established as described in the preceding section. Tetracycline is also derived by fermentation (MINIERI et al. 1953).

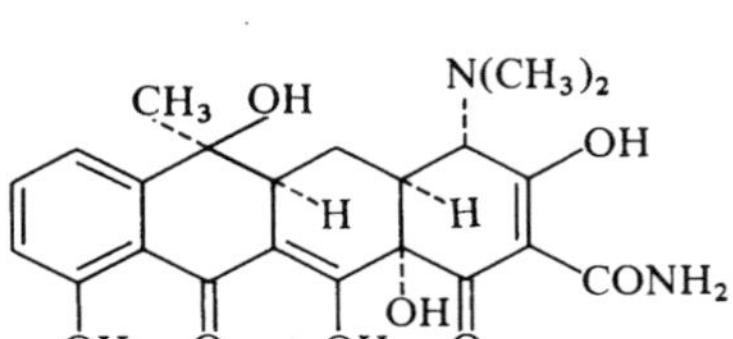

(87)

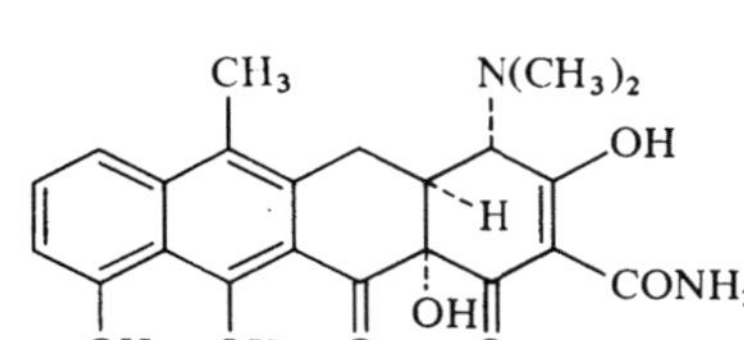

(78)

IV. 6-Demethyltetracyclines

7-Chloro-6-demethyltetracycline [demethylchlortetracycline or demeclocycline (88)] and 6-demethyltetracycline (89) are fermentation-derived tetracyclines first reported by MCCORMICK et al. (1957b). The deschloro compound was also derived at that time by hydrogenolysis of the chloro compound. The enhanced acid

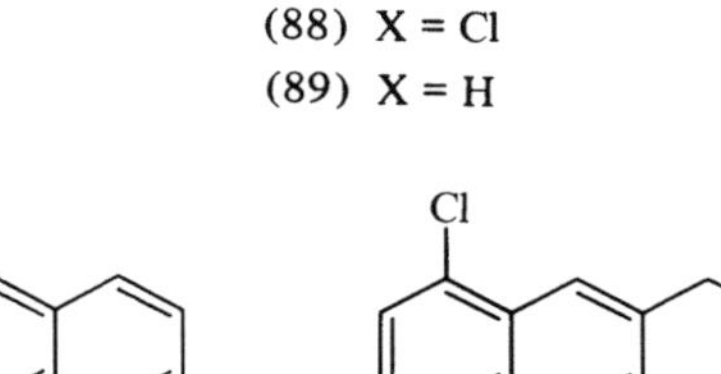

(88) X = Cl
(89) X = H

(90)

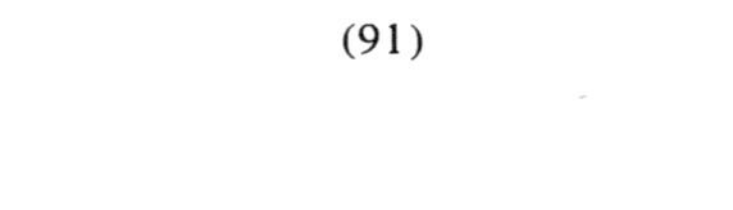

(91)

and base stability of these compounds, together with comparison of their ultraviolet absorption with that of tetracycline, indicated that these compounds differed in the C-ring, possibly at either C5a or C6. Contemporaneous degradation studies (WEBB et al. 1957) led to the indicated structural assignment. Thus zinc dust distillation of the 7-chloro-6-demethyl compound gave only naphthacene, while 7-chlortetracycline under the same conditions gave naphthacene and 5-methylnaphthacene (90). These results, together with the analytical data and zero-value Kuhn-Roth determinations, proved that the 6-methyl group was missing in the new series. That the structure of (88) was the same in all other respects was indicated by further degradation studies. Heating in concentrated hydrochloric acid gave the 5a,6-anhydro compound (91) having the expected spectral

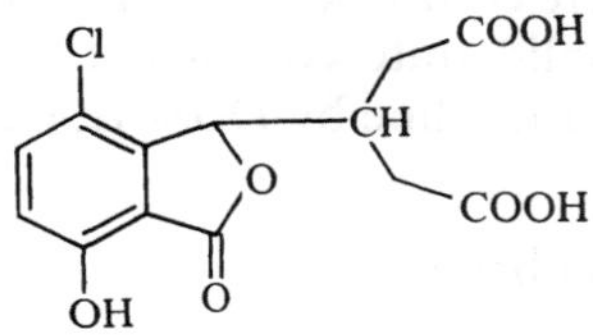

(92)

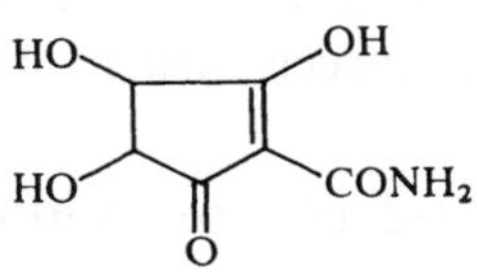

(70)

properties. Basic oxidation, in analogy to chlortetracycline, gave dimethylamine, 3,4-dihydroxy-2,5-dioxocyclopentane-1-carboxamide (70), and β-(4-chloro-7-hydroxyphthalid-3-yl)glutaric acid (92). Zinc in acetic acid gave the 12a-deoxy-4-dedimethylamino compound (93), converted to the corresponding isotetracycline

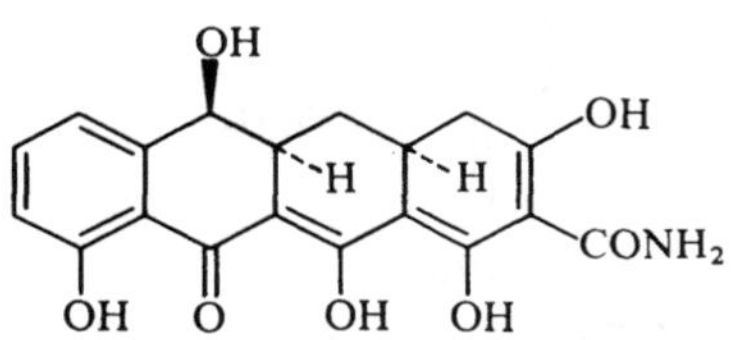

(93)

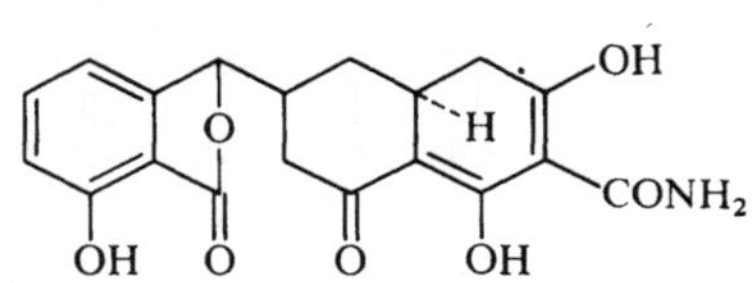

(94)

derivative (94) in alkali. Pyrolysis of the latter gave, in low yield, 4-chloro-7-hydroxyphthalide (95), identified by comparison with a known sample prepared by unambiguous synthesis (BOOTHE et al. 1957). Starting point for the latter synthesis was the previously synthesized chlortetracycline degradation product (49). Oxidation with basic permanganate gave the 3-hydroxyphthalide [also previously derived from chlortetracycline (HUTCHINGS et al. 1952a), but named as its open ketonic tautomer]. Sodium borohydride reduction (3-OH→3-H), pyrolytic decarboxylation, and demethylation in 48% hydrobromic acid gave the desired phthalide (95).

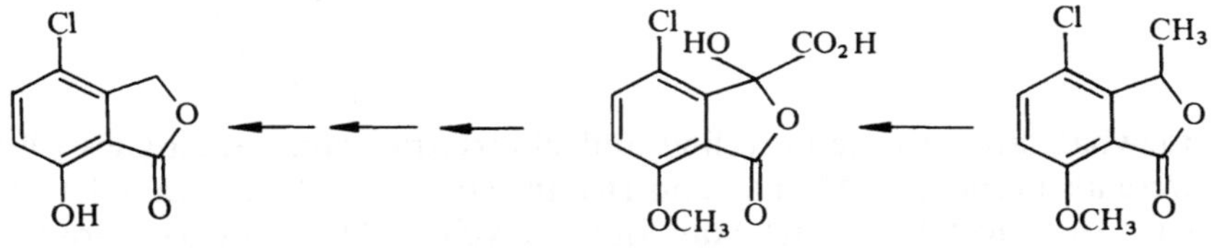

(95) (96) (49)

The relative and absolute stereochemistry of demethylchlortetracycline is as shown in (88). C4 epimerization studies and spectral/optical comparisons with the corresponding 6-methyl-containing tetracyclines indicated that the relative stereochemistry of dimethylamine function is the same in both series (MCCORMICK et al. 1957). Formation of an 11a-fluoro-6,12-hemiketal (RENNHARD et al. 1961) proved the *trans* relationship of 6-hydroxyl and 5a hydrogen. An X-ray structural determination on a derivative of demethylchlortetracycline, viz., 7-chloro-4-hydroxytetracycloxide, proved the relative strereochemistry at C4a, C5a, C6, and C12a (VAN DEN HENDE 1965). Circular dichroism studies (MITSCHER et al. (1969) proved that the demethyltetracyclines are in the same absolute stereochemical family as tetracycline and oxytetracycline. The structure and relative stereochemistra of demethylchlortetracycline were confirmed by X-ray crystallographic studies (PALENIK and MATHEW 1972). Solid-state conformation was noted as identical with that seen earlier for chlortetracycline by DONOHUE et al. (1963).

V. 2-Acetyl-2-decarboxamidotetracyclines

The first of a series of 2-acetyl-2-decarboxamido tetracyclines was reported by HOCHSTEIN et al. (1960). This was the oxytetracycline analogue (97). Structure was assigned on the basis of microanalysis, pK_a values, spectral properties, and degradation studies. The ultraviolet spectral properties pointed to the A-ring

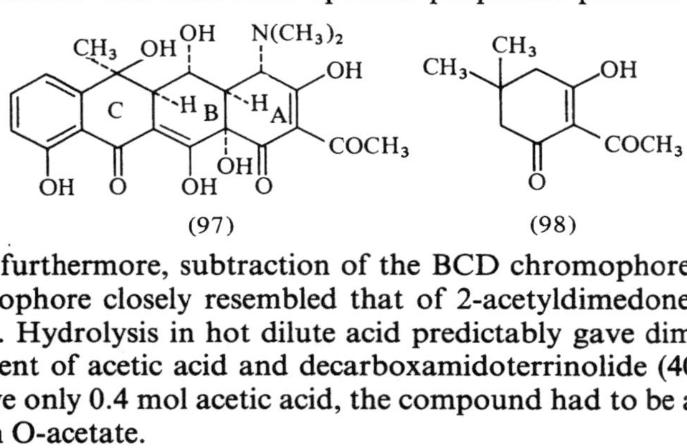

(97) (98)

modification; furthermore, subtraction of the BCD chromophore indicated the A-ring chromophore closely resembled that of 2-acetyldimedone (98), both in acid and base. Hydrolysis in hot dilute acid predictably gave dimethylamine, a molar equivalent of acetic acid and decarboxamidoterrinolide (40). Since basic hydrolysis gave only 0.4 mol acetic acid, the compound had to be a labile methyl ketone, not an O-acetate.

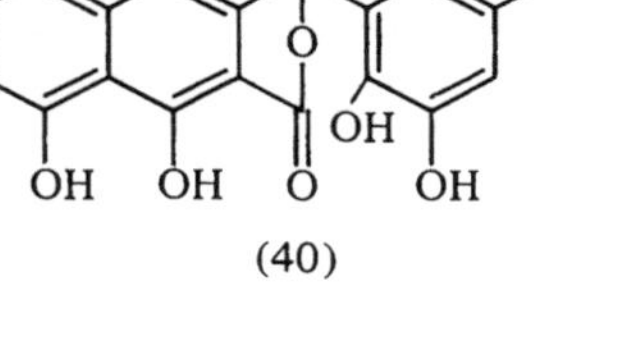

(40)

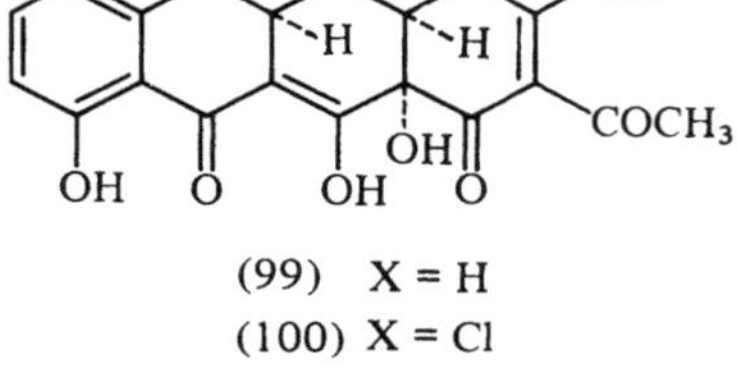

(99) X = H
(100) X = Cl

Somewhat later, the tetracycline and chlortetracycline analogues (99) and (100) were also reported (MILLER and HOCHSTEIN 1962). The ultraviolet spectral properties of 2-acetyl-2-decarboxamidotetracycline (99) matched those of the oxytetracycline analogue (97); the compound likewise gave a full equivalent of acetic acid only on acid hydrolysis. Mild acid degradation gave the 5a,6-anhydro analogue. The 7-chloro analogue (100) differed predictably in ultraviolet absorption from (99); it underwent analogous acid and base degradation; and on hydrogenolysis was dechlorinated to the tetracycline analogue (99).

The relative and absolute stereochemistry of 2-acetyl-2-decarboxamidotetracyclines has not been independently determined. The stereochemistry depicted here is presumed on the basis of analogy to oxytetracycline and tetracycline.

VI. 6-Methylenetetracyclines

The 6-methylenetetracyclines (BLACKWOOD et al. 1961, 1963) are derived chemically from fermentation tetracyclines via 11a-halogenation, exocyclic dehydration, and 11a-dehalogenation. The 11a-halo intermediates demonstrated no ketonic absorption below 6 µm and were thus assigned the hemiketal structure [e.g. (101)]. Dehydration of these hemiketals gave the 11a-halo compounds [e.g. (102)]. This intermediate product now demonstrated the 5.7-µm infrared absorption typical of isolated 12-ketone, and had an extended CD-ring ultraviolet chromophore, suggesting that dehydration had occurred, thus placing a double-bond in conjugation with the D-ring. That exocyclic dehydration, rather than the usual endocyclic dehydration, had occurred was, however, not immediately evident. On chemical reduction or catalytic hydrogenation, the 6-methylene compound (103) was formed, a surprisingly stable compound which rearranges to 5a,6-anhydrotetracycline (78) only under strongly acid conditions, much more vigorous than those required to dehydrate the parent tetracycline. The presence of the 6-methylene group was confirmed by ozonolysis and proton magnetic resonance spectral studies. On hydrogenation, 6-methylenetetracyclines yield epimeric α- and β-6-deoxytetracyclines (SCHACH VON WITTENAU et al. 1962; STEPHENS et al. 1963), as discussed in the next section.

The structure of 7-chloro-6-methylene oxytetracycline (105) (BLACKWOOD et al. 1961, 1963), derived by chlorination of 11a-chloro-6-methylene oxytetracy-

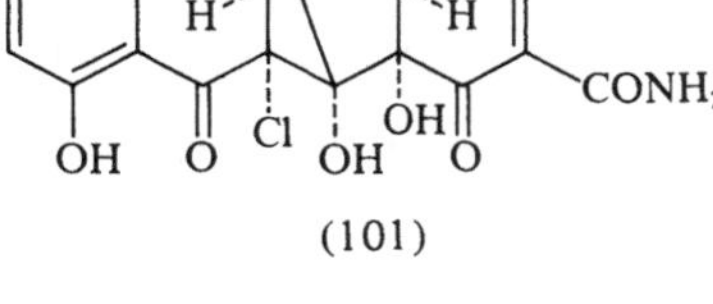

(101)

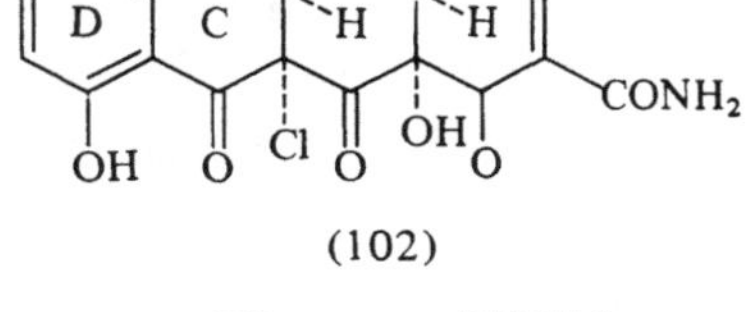

(102)

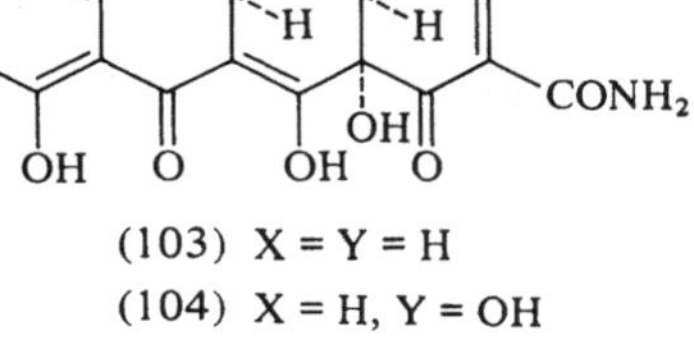

(103) X = Y = H

(104) X = H, Y = OH

(105) X = Cl, Y = OH

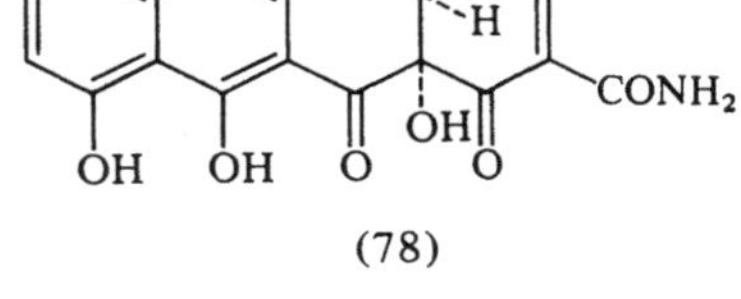

(78)

cline followed by reduction, was assigned on the basis of its exhaustive methylation-oxidation to 6-chloro-3-methoxyphthalic anhydride (47), a compound previously isolated and identified in connection with chlortetracycline structure studies (HUTCHINGS et al. 1952a; KUSHNER et al. 1952).

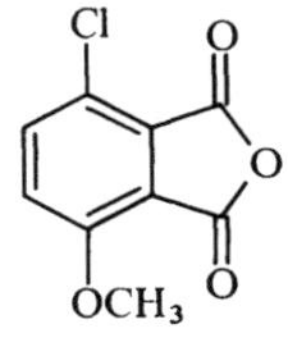

(47)

VII. 6-Deoxytetracyclines and 7- and 9-Substituted 6-Deoxytetracyclines

6-Deoxy-6-demethyltetracycline (106), β-6-deoxytetracycline (107), and β-6-deoxyoxytetracycline (108) were first reported as hydrogenolysis products of the corresponding 6-hydroxylated fermentation tetracyclines (STEPHENS et al. 1958, 1963; MCCORMICK et al. 1960) and later as products of the hydrogenation of the 6-methylenetetracyclines (103) and (104), together with the corresponding epimeric α-6-deoxytetracycline (109) and α-6-deoxyoxytetracycline [doxycycline (110)]. In all cases the gross structure was readily assigned on the basis of their analyses, spectral properties, and stability under even extreme acid conditions. The α- and β-compounds were obviously 6-epimers and the outstanding question related to stereochemistry at C6 relative to the remainder of the molecule, or stated otherwise, the stereochemistry at C6 relative to the parent tetracycline.

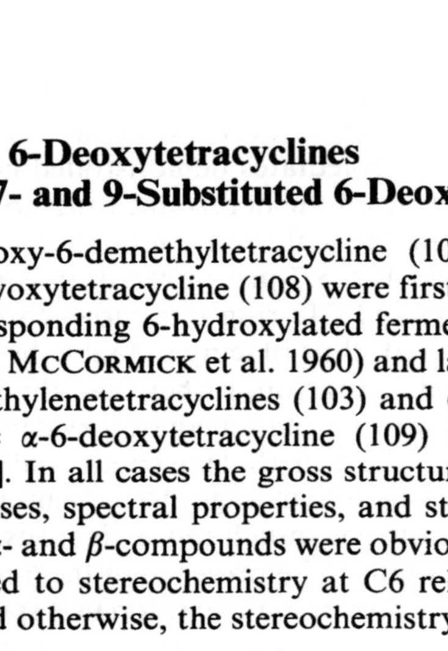

(106) $R = Y = H$
(107) $R = CH_3$, $Y = H$
(108) $R = CH_3$, $Y = OH$

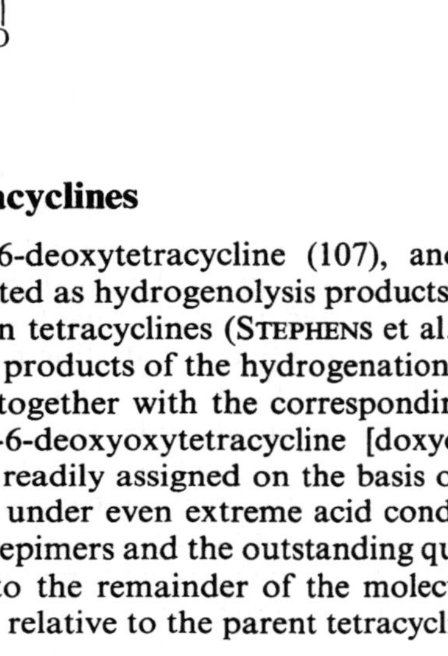

(109) $R = CH_3$, $Y = H$
(110) $R = CH_3$, $Y = OH$
(111) $R = C_6H_5CH_2SCH_2$, $Y = OH$

That inversion had occurred in the hydrogenolysis of fermentation tetracyclines to the β-epimers was first suggested (SCHACH VON WITTENAU et al. 1962) by the facts that:

1. While the hydrogenation of 6-methyleneoxytetracycline (104) gave a more nearly 1:1 mixture of the 6-epimers, hydrogenation of the corresponding 11a-

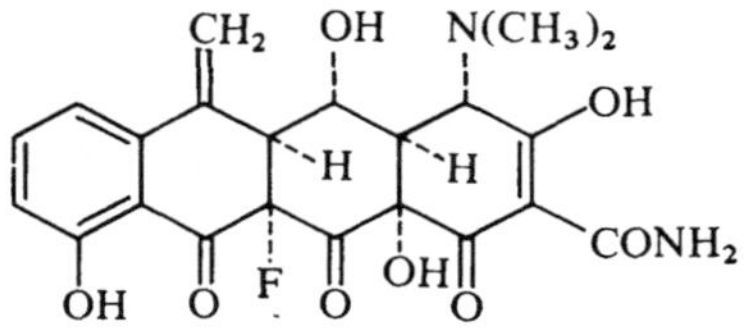

(112)

fluoro intermediate (112) gave the β-epimer in major proportion. Understanding that initial hydrogenation of the double bond was favored in the latter conversion, studies with molecular models indicated the 11a-fluoro side of the molecule to be much less hindered; addition from this side leads to 6-methyl and 5a-hydrogen *trans*, i.e., the stereochemistry indicated for the β-epimer (108).

2. The addition of mercaptans to the 6-methylene compounds (BLACKWOOD and STEPHENS 1962a; BLACKWOOD et al. 1963), followed by Raney nickel desulfurization of the resulting mercaptan adducts [e.g. (111)] provided a stereospecific route to the α-6-deoxytetracyclines. The mercaptan adducts are formed under free radical conditions, generally expected to yield the thermodynamically more stable product. Conformational analysis indicated the more stable form to have the large 6-mercaptomethyl group pseudoequatorial and thus *cis* to the 5a hydrogen, i.e., the stereochemistry indicated for the α-epimer.

At about the same time MUXFELDT (1962a, b) reported his independent conclusion that inversion had occurred in the hydrogenolysis of tetracycline to β-6-deoxytetracycline, based on synthetic studies as detailed in a later section of this chapter. Thus it was indicated by ultraviolet spectral studies that synthetic compounds (113)–(116), as well as the 12a-deoxy-4-dedimethylamino compound

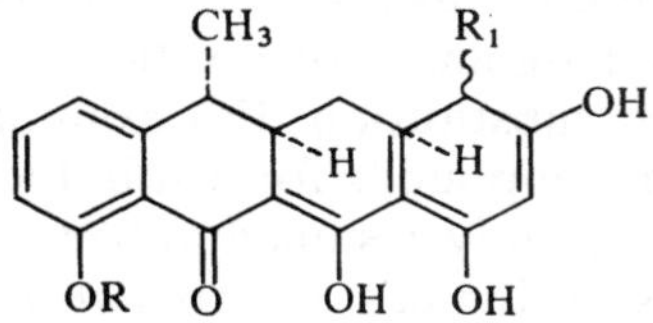

(113) $R = CH_3, R^1 = CO_2CH_3$
(114) $R = CH_3, R^1 = H$
(115) $R = R^1 = H$

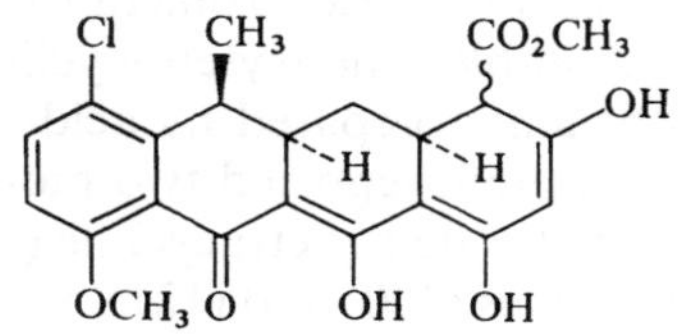

(116)

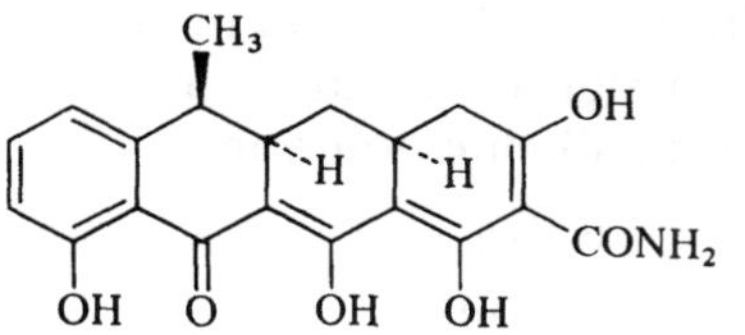

(117)

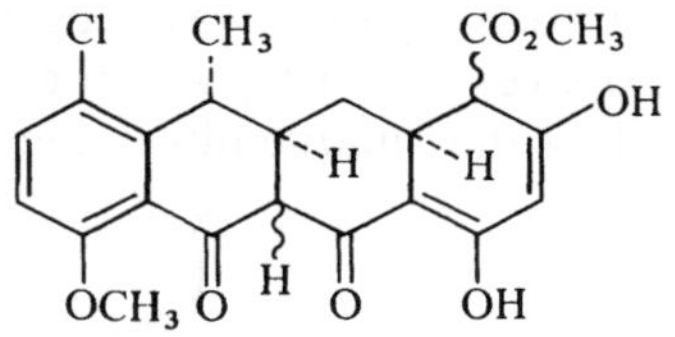

(118)

(117) derived from β-6-deoxytetracycline, are capable of existing in the fully enolized form shown. However, the synthetic compound (118) exists only in the 11a-protonated form indicated. This is attributed to steric interaction between the 6-methyl group and the 7-chlorine atom, an interaction noted to occur only when

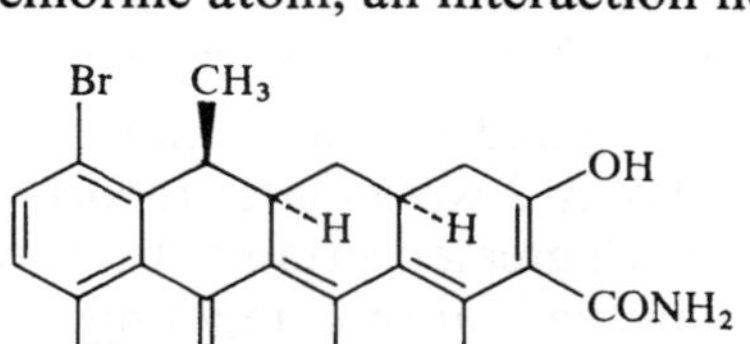

(119)

the 6-methyl group is *cis* to the 5a hydrogen and the 11a-position is enolized. Since the 7-bromo-6-deoxy compound (119) derived from β-6-deoxytetracycline by bromination and zinc reduction is capable of full enolization (Kende 1962, unpublished), it was concluded that it must have 6-methyl and 5a-hydrogen *trans* and that inversion had occurred in the hydrogenolysis of the 6-hydroxy group.

The C6 configuration of α- and β-6-deoxytetracyclines was confirmed by later proton nuclear magnetic resonance studies (SCHACH VON WITTENAU and BLACKWOOD 1966). Thus the β-6-deoxy derivatives show the signal for the C6-methyl group further upfield than the α-analogues. This implies a pseudoaxial position for the C-methyl group in the β-isomer and a pseudoequatorial position in the α-epimer. In corroboration, the C-methyl signal in the β-epimers appears as a doublet (J = 6–8 cps) whereas this peak in the α-isomer is a broadened singlet.

The complete structure, as well as relative and absolute stereochemistry, of α-6-deoxytetracycline [doxycycline (109)], was recently confirmed by X-ray crystallographic analysis (STEZOWSKI 1977). The solid-state conformation of the hydrohalide salts studied appears to be that in which the 12a-hydroxyl and 4-dimethylamino group occupy closely proximate pseudoaxial positions relative to the A-ring.

A further structural problem to arise primarily as a result of the availability of the acid-stable 6-deoxytetracyclines was assignment of position to aromatic ring substituents prepared by acid-catalyzed substitution. For example, BEEREBOOM et al. (1960) reported two mono nitro compounds formed in the nitration of 6-demethyl-6-deoxytetracycline (106), reasonably assumed to be the 7- and 9-nitro derivatives (120) and (121), where substitution has occurred *ortho* and *para* to the phenolic group. Bromination gave the 7-bromo compound (122), assigned structure on the basis of preliminary oxidative degradation studies, which in turn was nitrated to the bromo-nitro compound (123). The nitro group in (123), which was assumed to have entered the open position *ortho* to the phenolic hydroxyl, possesses unusually long wavelength ultraviolet absorption in alkaline solution; the 9-nitro structure (121) was therefore assigned to that mononitro compound showing the same unique ultraviolet shift in alkaline solution.

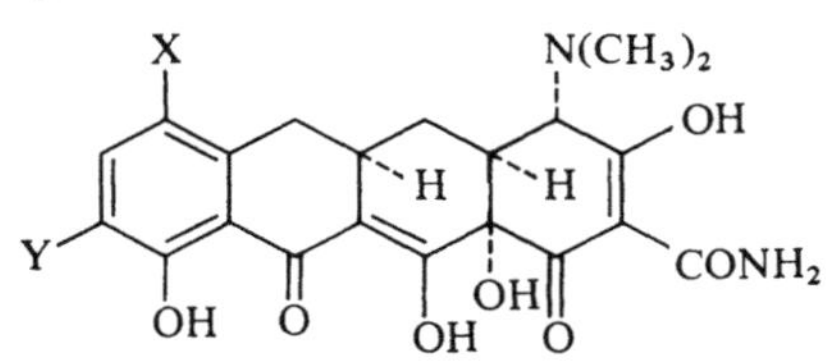

(106) X = Y = H
(120) $X = NO_2$, Y = H
(121) X = H, $Y = NO_2$
(122) X = Br, Y = H
(123) X = Br, $Y = NO_2$
(124) $X = N(CH_3)_2$, Y = H

Having independently prepared the same mononitro compounds (120) and (121), BOOTHE et al. (1960) only 2 weeks later reported assignment of structure to these compounds with much greater certainty by nitrating 7-tritio-6-demethyl-6-deoxytetracycline. Only in the 7-nitro compound had tritium been displaced. These studies were later described in greater detail by PETISI et al. (1962). Ultimately, the structure of the 7-nitro compound was confirmed by an X-ray crystallographic structure analysis of 7-dimethylamino-6-demethyl-6-deoxytetracycline [minocycline (124)], a compound derived from the 7-nitro compound (120) (MARTELL and BOOTHE 1967). These workers report that the X-ray analysis was carried out by VAN DEN HENDE (1965). It is of incidental interest that minocycline (124), produced by reductive methylation, presented a special problem: whether it was a monomethyl or dimethyl derivative. Microanalysis and, for reasons not fully apparent, ^{1}H-NMR studies were not diagnostic. However, mass spectrometry, and ultimately the X-ray studies described above, were definitive in this regard. The mass spectra of other tetracyclines were earlier detailed by HOFFMAN (1966).

The assignment of aromatic substituents to the 7- and/or 9-positions is generally confirmed by ^{1}H-NMR studies, the expected AB-splitting pattern for the *ortho*-proton pair being observed in either case. When 7-deutero precursors are available, in analogy to the 7-tritio studies described above, ^{1}H-NMR studies can be used to determine specifically whether substitution has occurred at the 7-position or the 9-position (Blackwood 1965, unpublished).

VIII. Oxytetracycline Esters

In connection with oxytetracycline structure elucidation (HOCHSTEIN et al. 1953), anhydrous amphoteric oxytetracycline was acetylated with excess acetic anhydride in dioxane to yield the O^{5},O^{12a}-diacetyl derivative (125). Structural assignment was not detailed at that time although we note that its microanalysis (including an acetyl determination), infrared and ultraviolet spectral properties (CONOVER 1956), and pK_a values are consistent with the structure then assigned. Subsequent proton nuclear magnetic resonance studies proved the presence of the O^{5}-acetate (SCHACH VON WITTENAU and BLACKWOOD 1966). Thus in O^{5}-acetates the

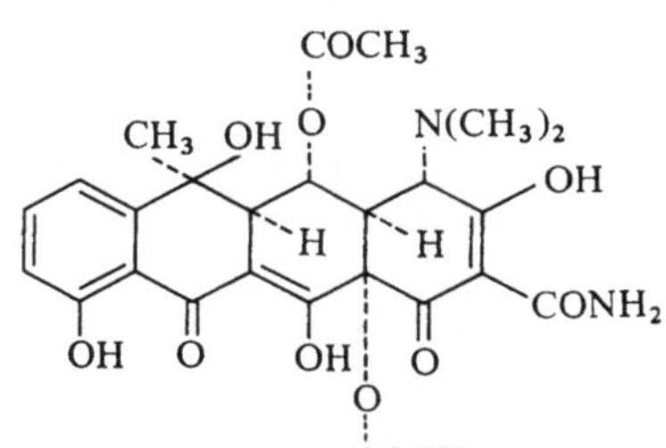

(125)

C5 hydrogen is shifted downfield to about 6.7 ppm from the 5.3- to 5.5-ppm value found in compounds such as oxytetracycline or its O^{12a}-monoacetate. Ultimately the structural assignment of the O^{5},O^{12a}-diacetate was confirmed by X-ray crystallographic analysis (HUGHES et al. 1971; VON DREELE and HUGHES 1971). It is noteworthy that the solid-state conformation is all-chair with the two acetate groups in close proximity and occupying positions pseudoaxial to the B-ring, while the dimethylamine function is pseudoequatorial to the A-ring, i.e., the same conformation which had been noted earlier for this compound by ^{1}H-NMR studies (SCHACH VON WITTENAU and BLACKWOOD 1966). Oxytetracycline has also been acetylated with acetic anhydride in dimethylformamide in the presence of pyridine (BLACKWOOD and STEPHENS 1962b), yielding the O^{10},O^{12a}-diacetate (126). Structure assignment is based on microanalysis (including acetyl determination), infrared and ultraviolet spectral properties (including a somewhat modified ultraviolet BCD-chromophore, but normal shift in the chromophore in the presence of chelating metals, resulting from chelation at O^{11},O^{12}), and the fact that mild hydrolysis with ammonium hydroxide gave the O^{12a}-monoacetate (127). The same monoacetate was reported earlier as an intermediate in the preparation of O^{5},O^{12a}-diacetate (GORDON 1957); it is also formed, to the extent of

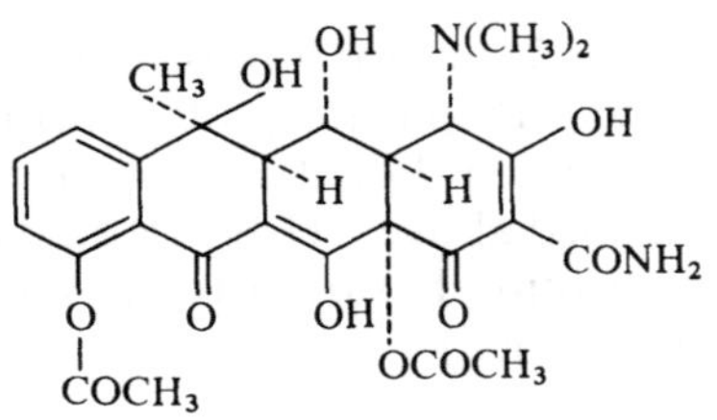

(126)

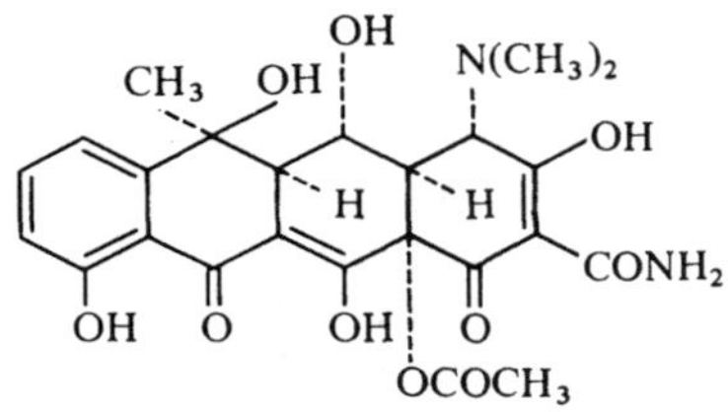

(127)

no more than 50% conversion, by the action of acetyl chloride on anhydrous amphoteric oxytetracycline in dioxane (BLACKWOOD and SCHACH VON WITTENAU 1971). This acetylation probably occurs by intramolecular catalysis, i.e., the dimethylamino group is acetylated and the acetyl group then delivered axially across ring A:

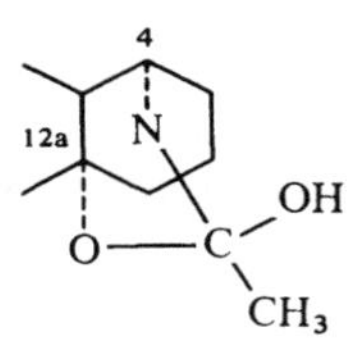

A variety of O^{12a}-esters were reported prepared by this method, not only from oxytetracycline, but also from 6-methyleneoxytetracycline (methacycline) and α-6-deoxytetracycline (doxycycline).

Interestingly, although the O^{10},O^{12a}-diacetate could be partially hydrolyzed by ammonium hydroxide to the O^{12a}-monoacetate, attempted hydrolysis in aqueous sodium hydroxide led to its rearrangement to the O^{5},O^{12a}-diacetate (BLACKWOOD and STEPHENS 1962b). Later rearrangement studies with mixed O^{10},O^{12a}-diesters (cf. BLACKWOOD and SCHACH VON WITTENAU 1971), coupled with ^{1}H-NMR studies, proved unambiguously that this rearrangement was intramolecular, the O^{12a}-acyl group moving axially across the B-ring presumably via the intermediate:

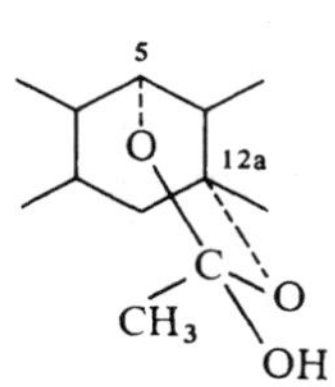

while the O^{10}-acyl group moves to O^{12a}, presumably via the intermediates:

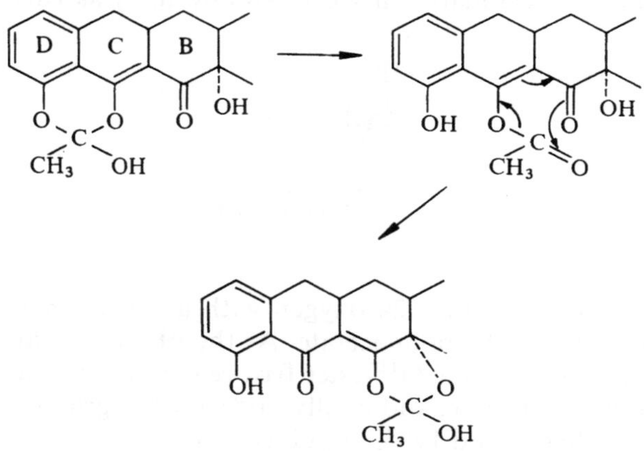

Thus in pyridine the following ^1H-NMR peaks have been noted for various *bis*-esters of oxytetracycline (SCHACH VON WITTENAU and BLACKWOOD 1966, unpublished):

	C5-H	CH_3CO
O^{10},O^{12a}-Diacetate	5.5	2.3, 2.3
O^{10},O^{12a}-Dipropionate	5.5	–, –
O^5,O^{12a}-Diacetate	6.7	2.1, 2.3
O^5-Acetate-O^{12a}-propionate	6.7	2.1, –
O^5,O^{12a}-Dipropionate	6.8	–, –
O^5-Propionate-O^{12a}-acetate	6.8	2.4

Under the same basic conditions employed to rearrange $O^{10},10^{12a}$-diesters, O^{12a}-monoesters are rearranged to O^5-esters (BLACKWOOD and SCHACH VON WITTENAU 1971), such as the O^5-acetate (128). Structure is assigned on the basis of analysis and spectral properties, particularly the ^1H-NMR shift of the C5 hydrogen, diagnostic of the O^5-ester (SCHACH VON WITTENAU and BLACKWOOD 1966).

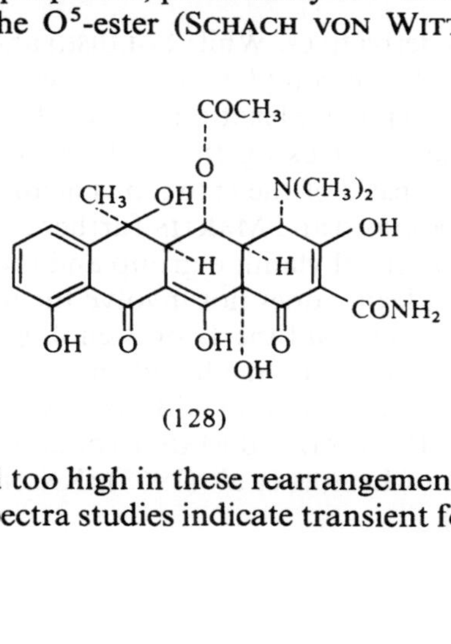

(128)

If the pH is rendered too high in these rearrangement reactions, the esters are degraded. Ultraviolet spectra studies indicate transient formation of a 5a,6-anhydro derivative, a degradation pathway normally seen only in acid. It would appear that this unusual degradation involves an internally assisted dehydration as follows:

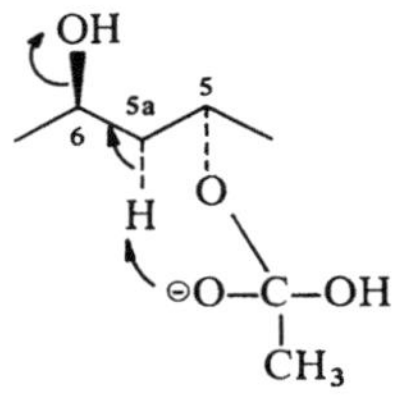

By blocking/deblocking the 12a oxygen with a carbobenzoxy group, it has been possible to make a O^{10}-monoacetate. As the pH of an aqueous solution of this compound is increased, the O^{10}-ester frist rearranges to the isolatable O^{12a}-acetate, then to the O^5-acetate, and finally undergoes degradation via a 5a,6-anhydro compound (Blackwood 1965, unpublished).

IX. Tetracycline Metal Chelates

The tetracyclines are strong chelating agents. The primary site of chelation was first assigned as the 11,12-β-diketone system [e.g. (129)] by CONOVER (1956), based on ultraviolet spectral studies in which modification of chromophore in the presence of nickel chloride in oxytetracycline was compared with that in model

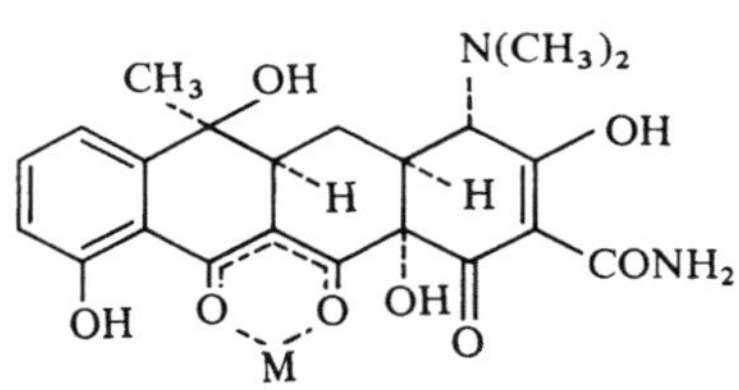

(129)

compounds and various derivatives. While SOLUISIO and MARTIN (1963) concurred with respect to the calcium complex, in the cases of cupric, nickel, and zinc these workers concluded that complexation of the tetracycline A-ring is involved since isochlortetracycline (76) lacking the 11,12-β-diketone system complexed with these metals. On the basis of the erroneous acidity constant assignment of STEPHENS et al. (1956), DOLUISIO and MARTIN further concluded that these A-ring complexes involved the 4-dimethylamino group and the C3-enol or the C12a-hydroxyl. That A-ring complexing does not involve the dimethylamino group, but rather the carboxamido group and the 1- or 3-enol, was suggested by COLAIZZI et al. (1965), based on metal-chelate-mediated enzyme inhibition studies, and by BAKER and BROWN (1966) on the basis of additional spectral evidence and a modified interpretation of the DOLUISIO and MARTIN data using the later, correctly assigned acidity constants of LEESON et al. (1963), KALNINS and BELEN'KII (1964), and RIGLER et al. (1965).

Circular dichroism studies by MITSCHER et al. (1968, 1969) assessed a duality of sites (11,12-β-diketone and A-ring) for metal complexation in the tetracycline series, suggesting that, at low pH, chelation occurs on the BCD-chromophore and that, as pH is increased, the A-ring chromophore becomes involved. Conformation of these complexes at pH values above 7.1 was judged to diverge between 5-hydroxytetracyclines and those tetracyclines lacking a 5-hydroxy group (see Sect. I.3 above); more detailed circular dichroism studies by CASWELL and HUTCHINSON (1971) appear to differentiate further the conformation of the calcium chelate from the magnesium chelate; furthermore, a structure for the calcium chelate is suggested in which the metal ion is simultaneously coordinated with O-11, O-12, and O-3 (or the carboxamide function) within one molecule (see later).

Additional insight into metal-binding sites in the tetracyclines is provided by the proton nuclear magnetic resonance studies on tetracycline and various derivatives in dimethylsulfoxide solution reported by WILLIAMSON and EVERETT (1975) and GULBIS and EVERETT (1976). These workers used a paramagnetic ion probe method and assignment of the exchangeable protons essentially consistent with near-contemporaneous assignment of these protons by ASLESON et al. (1974). Isotopic shifts and broadening of certain tetracycline ^{1}H-NMR signals were observed with several paramagnetic ions, e.g., Cu(II) and Mn(II). Diamagnetic ions, e.g., Ca(II) and Mg(II), also affect some of these signals. It was concluded that A-ring complexing occurred with these various metals, presumably involving the 1- or 3-enol and the carboxamido group, but certainly not the dimethylamino group, since these signal modifications were observed even in the absence of the latter group. Following the complete assignment of the carbon-13 NMR spectra for tetracycline and several of its derivatives by ASLESON and FRANK (1975) a ^{13}C-NMR study of tetracycline in dimethylsulfoxide was carried out employing Nd(III) and La(III) as ion probes (GULBIS and EVERETT 1975). These studies are interpreted as confirming the ^{1}H-NMR conclusions, as are additional ^{1}H- and ^{13}C-NMR studies on the effect of added electrolyte on the binding of tetracycline to paramagnetic ion probes (GULBIS et al. 1976).

Detailed studies by JOGUN and STEZOWSKI (1976a) which concern the shift of the long-wavelength absorption maxima for oxytetracycline as a function of pH in the presence and absence of a variety of metal-chelating agents confirm the general involvement of the BCD-ring chromophore in chelation. These authors further present the X-ray crystallographic strutural analysis for the dipotassium salt of oxytetracycline. In the crystal, four potassium ions are sandwiched between two oxytetracycline *bis*-anions. These anions occupy the all-chair conformation with 12a- and 5-hydroxyl groups oriented in close proximity and pseudoaxial to the B-ring. Potassium ion K_1 (and K_3) is coordinated to O-1, O-12, and O-12a from both of these *bis*-anions while potassium ion K_2 (and K_4) is coordinated to O-1, O-12, and O-11 from the same pair of *bis*-anions. That either of these present suitable model sites for complexing metals is cogently argued by JOGUN and STEZOWSKI (1976a, b). Either type of complexing would account for the variously observed effects of metal ions on both the BCD- and A-ring chromophores. Such structures are similar to that suggested earlier for the calcium chelate by CASWELL and HUTCHINSON (1971) (see above).

C. Partial Synthesis from Derivatives

To a degree, the total synthesis of tetracyclines has been potentially or actually simplified by the availability of methods for the conversion of tetracycline degradation products or biosynthetic precursors to fully active tetracyclines. This section, which describes these conversions, as well as generally describing structural assignment for these various compounds, represents a bridge between the two broad aspects, structure, and synthesis, encompassed by the present chapter.

I. 4-Epitetracyclines

The first 4-epitetracycline disclosed in the literature was 4-epitetracycline itself (130), initially recognized as a reversibly formed isomer of tetracycline and called

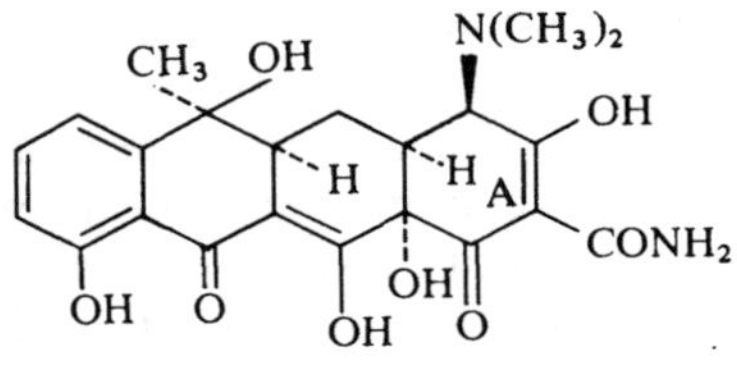

(130)

quatrimycin (DOERSCHUK et al. 1955). Structure was first assigned by STEPHENS et al. (1956a), based on ultraviolet absorption (differs from tetracycline only in the A-ring chromophore), degradation studies comparable to tetracycline, and the fact that the only other viable alternative structure for this isomer, viz., enol tautomers of the type:

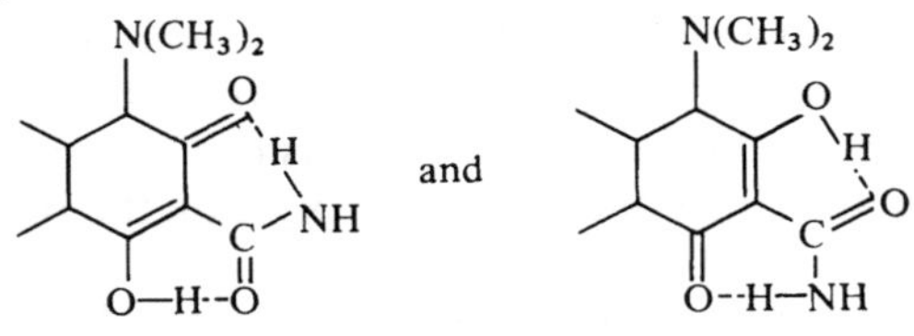

was eliminated, since (a) the epimers yield isomeric nitrile derivatives (131) and (132) when reacted with benzenesulfonyl chloride and (b) 4-dedimethylaminotetracycline undergoes no such isomerization. Structural assignment was confirmed by studies on the methiodide derivatives (MCCORMICK et al. 1956, 1957a). The properties of 4-epitetracycline were also detailed by KAPLAN et al. (1957). The 4-

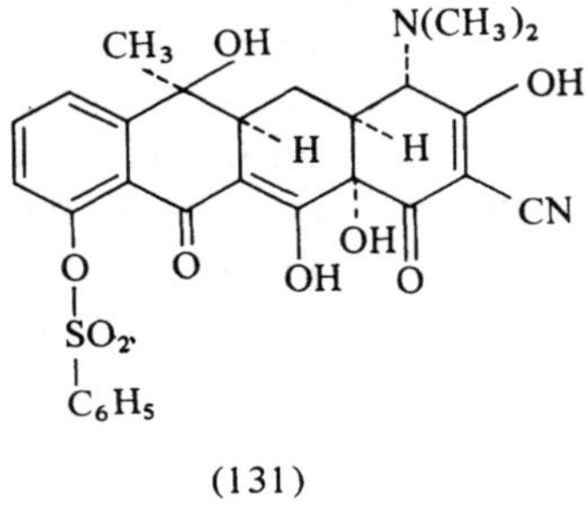

(131)

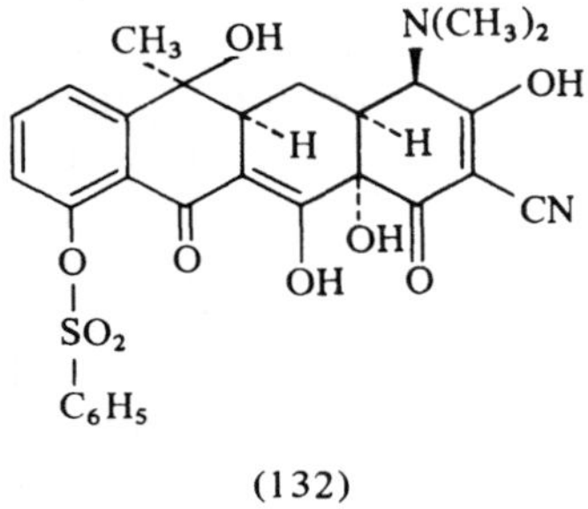

(132)

epimerization has been extensively studied, being extended to other tetracyclines; see for example McCormick et al. (1957a, b, 1960). In the case of 4-epioxytetracycline, structure has been confirmed by X-ray crystallographic analysis (Prewo and Stezowski 1979).

4-Epitetracycline (or mixture of the normal compounds with their 4-epimers) are quantitatively converted to the normal tetracycline by warming in strongly basic solution in the presence of a chelating metal (Noseworthy 1961), a method which has found routine application in the synthesis of tetracyclines; see, for example, Korst et al. (1968).

II. 12a-Deoxytetracyclines

The first 12a-deoxytetracycline to be prepared was 12a-deoxy-4-dedimethylaminotetracycline (42) (Hochstein et al. 1952c, 1953). Structural assignment has already been considered in connection with oxytetracycline structural assignment. Later, two groups independently synthesized 12a-deoxytetracycline (133): Green and Boothe (1960) by zinc/ammonium hydroxide reduction of tetracycline and Blackwood et al. (1960a, b) by the hydrogenolysis of the O^{12a}-formate ester of tetracycline (79). The corresponding 12a-deoxy-6-demethyl-6-deoxytetracycline was also prepared by the latter route.

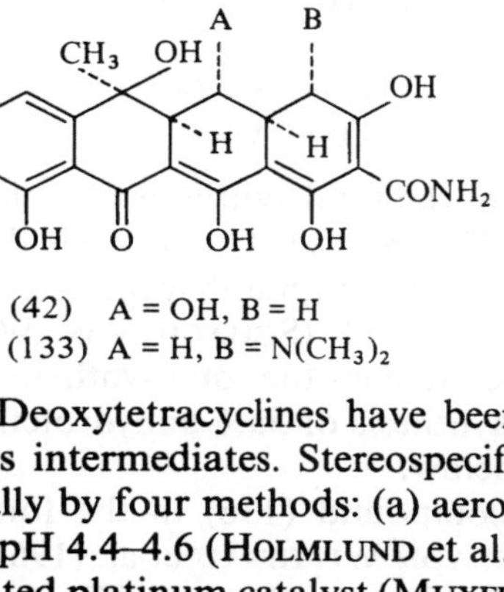

(42) A = OH, B = H
(133) A = H, B = $N(CH_3)_2$

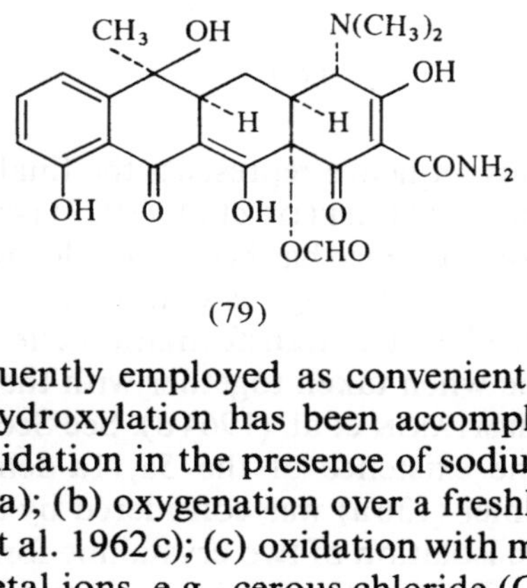

(79)

12a-Deoxytetracyclines have been frequently employed as convenient total synthesis intermediates. Stereospecific rehydroxylation has been accomplished chemically by four methods: (a) aerobic oxidation in the presence of sodium nitrate at pH 4.4–4.6 (Holmlund et al. 1959a); (b) oxygenation over a freshly hydrogenated platinum catalyst (Muxfeldt et al. 1962c); (c) oxidation with molecular oxygen in the presence of chelating metal ions, e.g., cerous chloride (Conover et al. 1962); and (d) base-catalyzed oxygenation (cf. Muxfeldt et al. 1979). 12a-Hydroxylation has also been accomplished microbiologically (Holmlund et al. 1959b).

6-Methylpretramid (134) is readily available by further degradation of 12a-deoxytetracycline (Green and Boothe 1960). This compound, which is a biosyn-

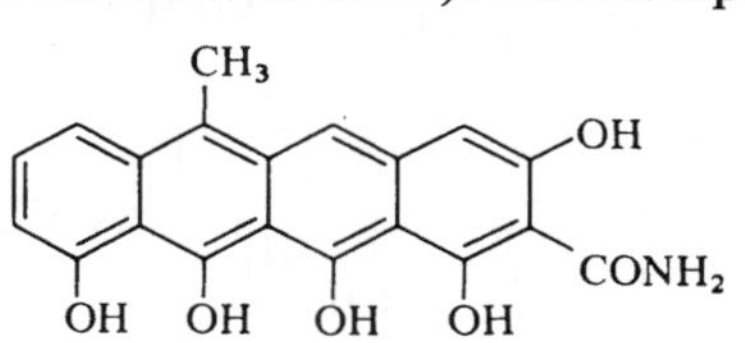

(134)

thetic precursor of tetracycline (McCORMICK et al. 1963 a), has been the subject of total synthesis by BARTON et al. (1971 d). Although (134) has not been converted by other than microbiological methods to tetracycline, steps in this direction have been taken by HASSALL et al. (cf. Sect. D.I.2 below).

III. 5a,6-Anhydrotetracyclines and 5a(11a)-Dehydrotetracyclines

The total synthesis of chlortetracycline and tetracycline was greatly simplified by the chemical reconversion of 5a,6-anhydrochlortetracycline (77) to chlortetracycline by SCOTT and BEDFORD (1962). Photooxygenation gave the 6-hydroperoxy derivative (135) which, on mild catalytic hydrogenation over 5% Pd/C, gave a quantitative yield of 5a(11a)-dehydrochlortetracycline (136), previously isolated as a fermentation product (McCORMICK et al. 1958 a) and converted microbiologically to chlortetracycline (McCORMICK et al. 1958 b, 1962) and by hydrogenation to tetracycline and its 5a-epimer (McCORMICK et al. 1958 a).

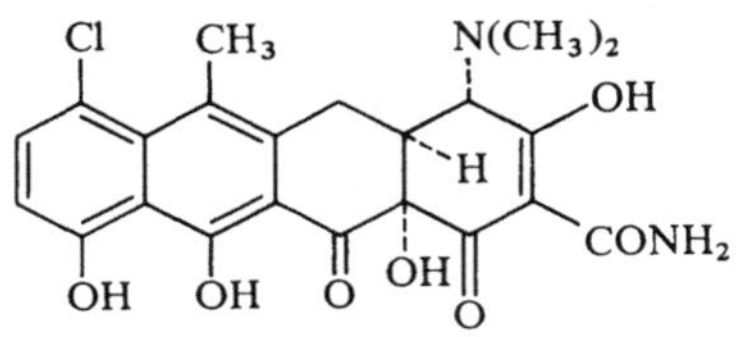

(77)

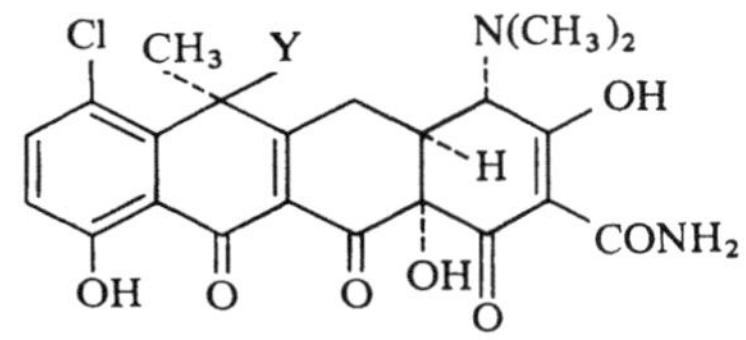

(135) Y = OOH
(136) Y = OH

This sequence represents the final stage of the total synthesis of 7-chlortetracycline by MUXFELDT et al. (1973) (see Sect. F.II below). The photooxidation/reduction sequence has been extended to several other 5a,6-anhydrotetracycline derivatives, including 5a,6-anhydrotetracycline itself (SCHACH VON WITTENAU 1964). The latter transformation effectively completes the total synthesis of tetracycline when taken together with the total synthesis of 5a,6-anhydrotetracycline by SHEMYAKIN et al. (1964 d). See Sect. F.I below.

The existence of the 5a,11a-dehydro compound (136) in the form of its tautomer (136 a) was considered by SCHACH VON WITTENAU et al. (1963), based on the isolation of two crystalline forms of the free base having differing infrared spectral properties, and reactivity which suggested the form (136 a) to exist, at least in solution. Recently, PREWO and STEZOWSKI (1980 a) determined that the structure in fact is (136) even for the crystalline form suggested by infrared to be (136 a). However, on the basis of circular dichroism studies, they suggest that other species [such as (136 a)] exist in solution.

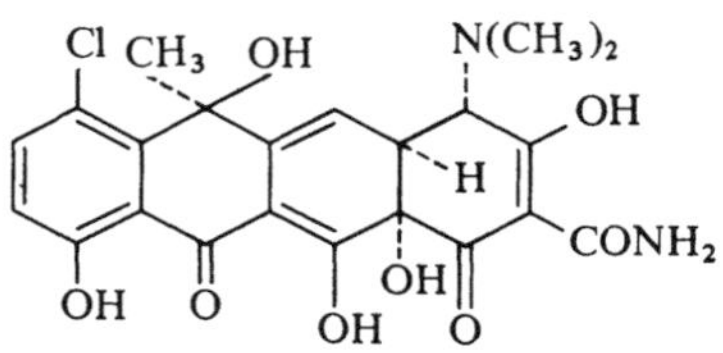

(136a)

IV. 4-Oxotetracycline-4,6-hemiketals and Tetracycloxides

6-Demethyl-4-oxotetracycline-4,6-hemiketal [(137) "4-hydroxytetracycloxide"] was prepared by ESSE et al. (1964a). Structural assignment was based on infrared and ultraviolet spectral properties, as well as the typical ketone reactions of the 4-ketone group. The structure of 7-chloro- and 7-bromo-4-hydroxytetracycloxides (138) and (139) have been confirmed by X-ray crystallographic methods (VAN DEN HENDE 1965).

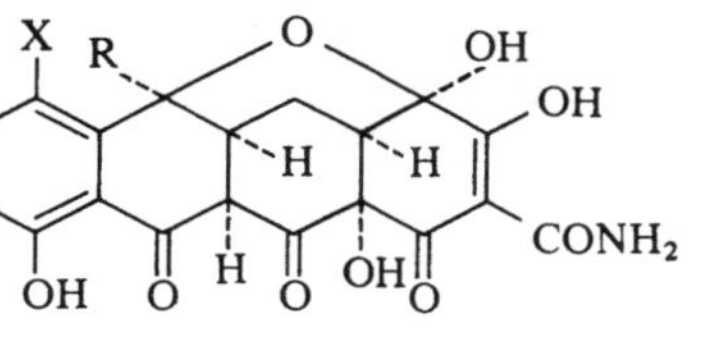

(137) R = X = H
(138) R = H, X = Cl
(139) R = H, X = Br
(140) R = CH_3, X = H

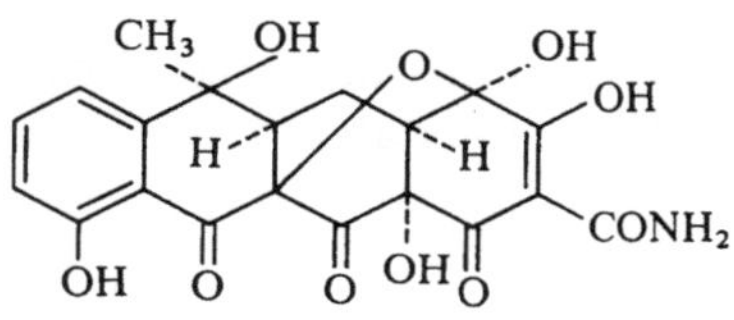

(141)

Independently, BLACKWOOD and STEPHENS (1964, 1965) prepared the corresponding tetracycline analogue by the reaction of tetracycline hydrochloride with *N*-chlorosuccinimide. The product, in the form of its crystalline potassium salt, was also assigned the 4,6-hemiketal structure on the basis of its reactivity and infrared and ultraviolet spectral properties but without the benefit of X-ray crystallographic analyses. Subsequently, GUREVICH et al. (1970) indicated that this reaction in fact gave two products, the major suggested to be the 6,12-hemiketal. More recently, BARTON et al. (1977b) confirmed the formation of two products, the minor one being the 4,6-hemiketal (140), and the major one, as crystallized from methanol, having the unusual bridged structure (141); like the 4,6-hemiketal, this compound has typical ketone reactivity at C4. Although there is no direct evidence bearing on the question, it appears that (140) and (141) represent interconvertible "forms" of 4-oxotetracycline, as is the case with 11a-bromo-4-dedimethylaminotetracycline and its 6,12-hemiketal (BLACKWOOD et al. 1963).

A variety of C4-modified tetracyclines have been synthesized from 4-oxotetracyclines, e.g., 4-amino-4-dedimethylaminotetracycline (142) (BLACKWOOD and STEPHENS 1965) and N^4,6-didemethyltetracycline (143) (ESSE et al. 1964b). 6-Demethyltetracycline (89) has also been resynthesized from the 4-oxo derivative by ESSE et al. (1964b); however, unlike the case of 4-epitetetracyclines, 12a-deoxytetracyclines, and 5a,6-anhydrotetracyclines, there has been no successful total synthesis of a 4-oxotetracycline, although the Barton group has made an effort in this direction (see later).

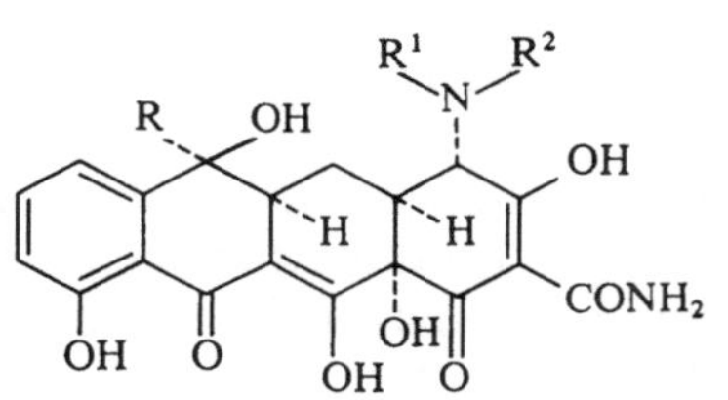

(142) R = CH_3, $R^1 = R^2$ = H
(143) R = R^1 = H, R^2 = CH_3
(89) R = H, $R^1 = R^2$ = CH_3

D. Total Synthesis of Tetracycline Derivatives and Incomplete Syntheses

I. Aromatic A-Ring Compounds

The biosynthetic intermediates, 6-methylpretetramid (134) (McCORMICK et al. 1963a) and 4-hydroxy-6-methylpretetramid (144) (McCORMICK et al. 1965a; McCORMICK and JENSEN 1965) are also available by degradation of tetracyclines (134) from 12a-deoxytetracycline (GREENE and BOOTHE 1960) (see above) and the other (144) by refluxing tetracycline methyl betaine in acetonitrile [to yield (145)], followed by acid-catalyzed dehydration (HLAVKA et al. 1965; McCORMICK et al.

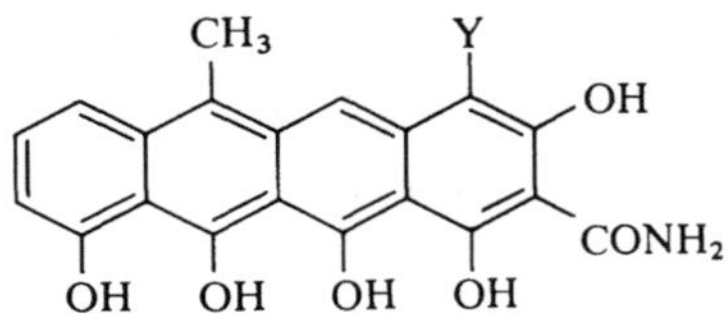

(134) Y = H
(144) Y = OH

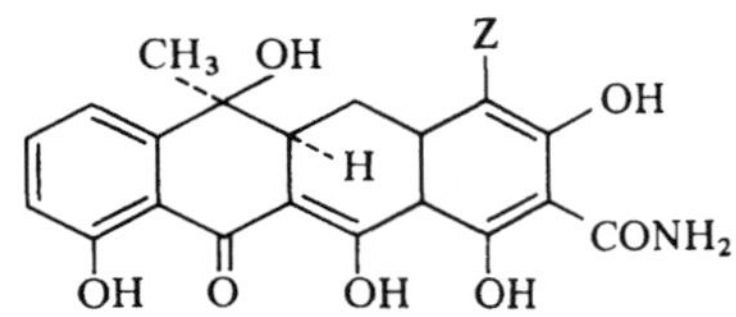

(145) Z = OH
(146) Z = $N(CH_3)_2$
(147) Z = H

1965b; see also HASSALL and WINTERS 1968). In addition the 4a,12a-anhydrotetracyclines (146) and (147) are available through degradation of 12a-deoxytetracyclines (GREEN and BOOTHE 1960; BLACKWOOD et al. 1960a, b). The ready availability of compounds (134) and (144)–(147) has prompted efforts directed to their total synthesis, together with concurrent efforts to convert these compounds back to fully active tetracyclines. To date, although there has been much in the way of model studies, none of these compounds have been reconverted to fully active tetracyclines. However, BARTON et al. (1971d) has prepared 6-methylpretetramid by total synthesis; the earlier chemical conversion of the latter to 5-hydroxy-6-methylpretetramid (HASSALL and WINTERS 1967) effectively extended this synthesis an additional step in the direction of tetracycline. The Barton group has also closely approached the total synthesis of certain 4a,12a-anhydrotetracyclines. There follows below a summary of the work in various laboratories employing this basic approach to the total synthesis of tetracyclines.

1. Barton et al.

As reported in a series of papers, introduced by BARTON and MAGNUS (1971), the Barton group at Imperial College has set as a synthetic objective the 4a,12-anhydrotetracyclines (145) and (146). The approach has been to couple a suitable substituted A-ring moiety, bearing two one-carbon units representing ultimate C5 and C12 carbons, with an appropriately blocked CD moiety, best understood by review of the specific examples given below.

A serendipitious discovery was the formation of the naphthofuran (148), formed when an effort was made to benzoylate 1,5-dihydroxynaphthalene under Friedel-Crafts conditions. Hydrogenation over Raney nickel led to the extremely versatile compound (149), a potential CD-unit which has been uniformly employed by the Barton group in their synthetic studies. After quaternization of the ultimate C6 position, the C10 hydroxy and C11 ketone are to be unmasked by ozonolysis/hydrolysis to yield the phenolic ketone of the type (150) (BARTON et al. 1971 a).

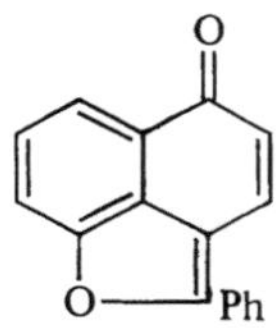

(148)

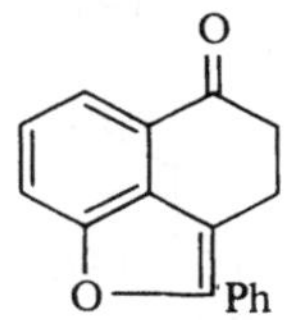

(149)

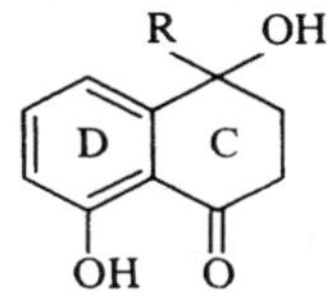

(150)

The promise of the naphthofuran (149) was apparent from the earliest model studies. For example, condensation of (149) with benzaldehyde gave the benzylidene derivative (150 a) converted by hydrogenation over Raney nickel to the benzyl derivative (151). Reaction of (151) with methyl magnesium iodide gave the carbinol (152), which on ozonolysis gave the ketobenzoate (153) (BARTON et al. 1971 a).

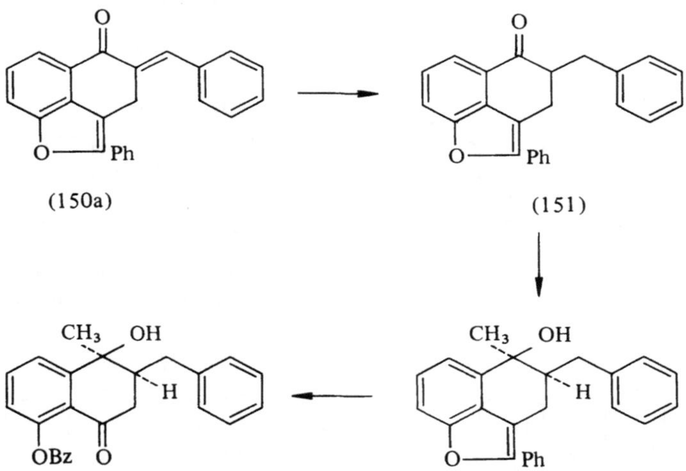

(150a) (151) (153) (152)

Attention was then turned to the synthesis of suitable A-ring precursors. A useful candidate was found in the isoxazole (158), synthesized from methyl p-orsellinate (154) by the classical Gatterman reaction to aldehyde (155), pyrolysis of the oxime (156) to the isoxazole (157), and finally acetylation and Thiele oxidation. The protected aldehyde (158) was condensed with the naphthofuran (149). Failing hydrogenation over Raney nickel, the resulting enone was reduced with hydrogen iodide in acetic acid, producing the benzyl derivative (159). Conversion of the isoxazole to nitrile by treatment with pyridine/acetic anhydride, reaction with methyl Grignard, acetylation, and ozonolysis gave the desired tricyclic nitrile (160). However, cyclization to the desired tetracycline derivative was not achieved. The analogous ester (161) was derived via hydrogenation of the isoxazole to aldehyde, chromic acid oxidation of the aldehyde to acid, esterification of the acid with diazomethane, reduction of the ketone with potassium borohydride, and acetylation. The ester, too, could not be cyclized to the desired tetracyclic compound, and this approach was abandoned in favor of additional approaches discussed below (BARTON et al. 1971 a).

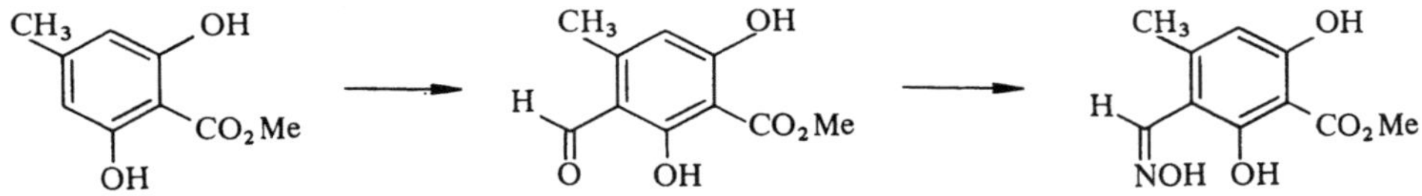

(154) (155) (156)

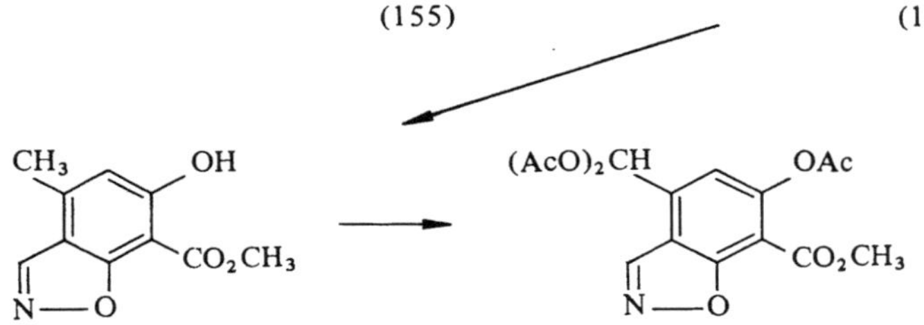

(157) (158)

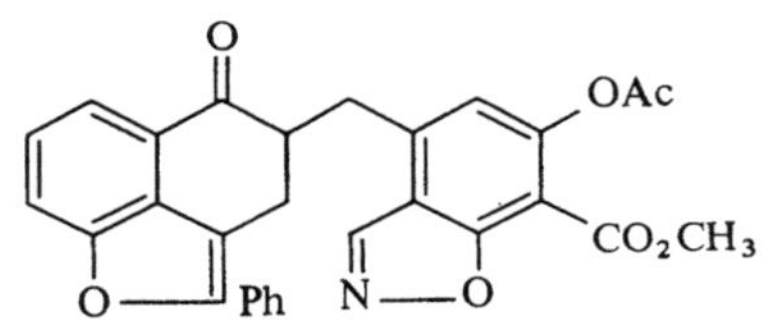

(159)

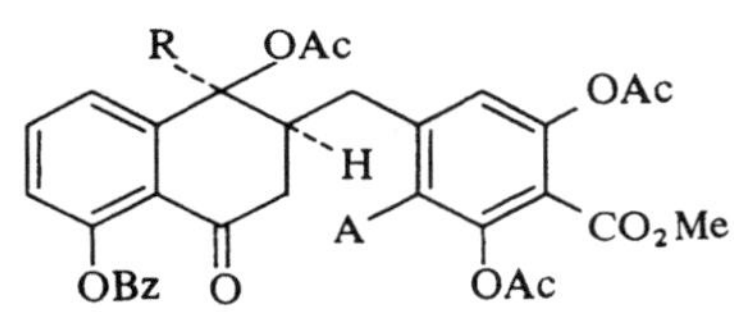

(160) $A = CN$, $R = CH_3$
(161) $A = CO_2Me$, $R = H$

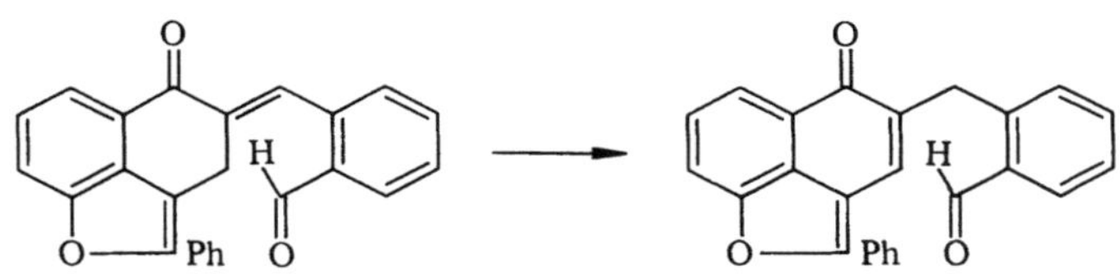

(162) (163)

Michael-type cyclization was then investigated as a means of forming Ring B. The naphthacenofuran (149) was condensed with phthalaldehyd to form the benzylidine aldehyde (162). With triethylamine as catalyst, the enone double bond was rearranged into the fully conjugated endocyclic position (163). After considerable study, it was determined that the tetrahydropyranyl ether of the cyanohydrin (164) was well suited for cyclization in ether, using sodium *t*-butoxide as catalyst. The cyclized product (165) was reduced and acetylated to the carbinol (166), using tri-*t*-butoxyaluminum hydride under controlled conditions as the reducing agent. Finally, ozonolysis, hydrolysis, and chromatography on alumina gave the desired diketone (167). With some effort the corresponding A-ring-substituted cyanohydrin tetrahydropyranyl ether (169) was prepared via the aldehyde (168). Disappointingly, all efforts to cyclize the compound (169) failed (AUFDERHAAR et al. 1971).

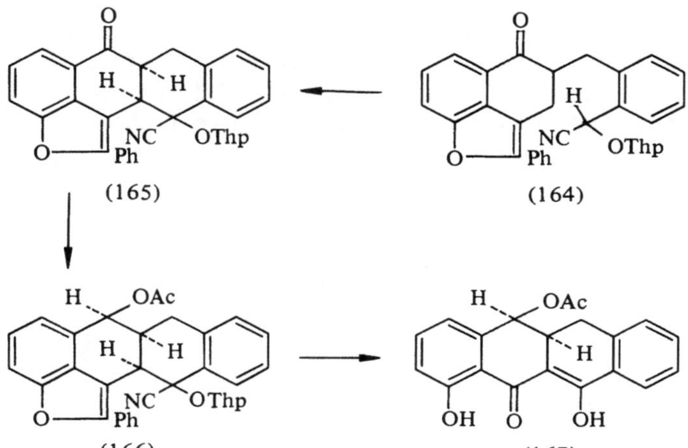

(165) (164) (166) (167)

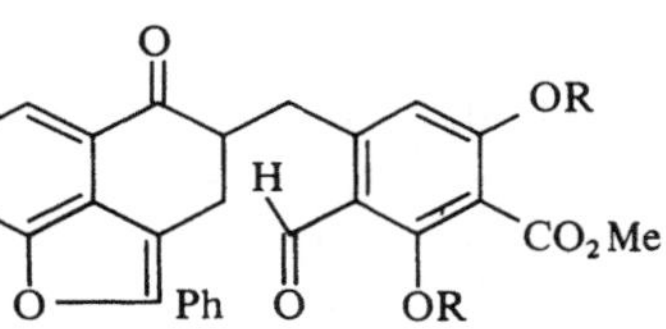

(168) R = Me
(170) R = Ac

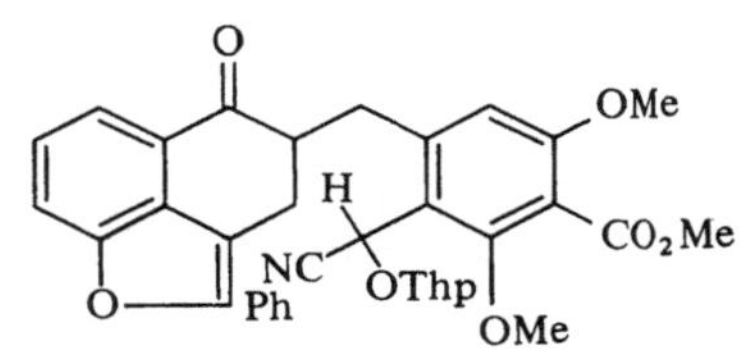

(169)

A third approach to B-ring formation, 1,3-dipolar addition, was then developed. The aldehyde (168) was treated with phenylhydroxyl amine to yield the bridged adduct (171). Zinc/acetic acid couple gave (172) and the 5a-deoxy compound (173), which was rearranged to the *cis* compound (174). Unfortunately, attempts to utilize these intermediates for further elaboration of 4a,12a-anhydrotetracyclines were abortive (BALDWIN et al. 1971).

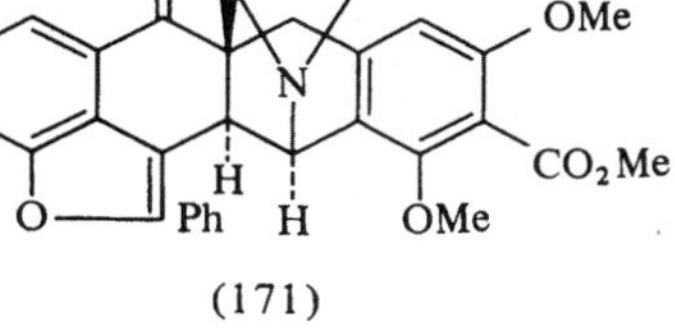

(171)

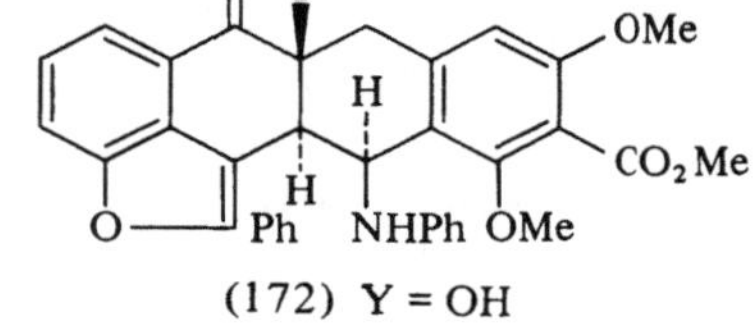

(172) Y = OH
(173) Y = H

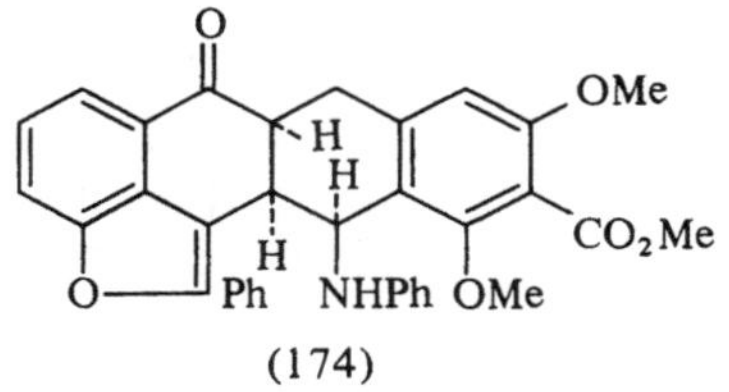

(174)

The Barton group then turned to photocyclization methods to form Ring-B. The model aldehyde (163) was converted to the acetal (175), which on photolysis gave the cyclized acetal (176) in good yield when a tungsten lamp was employed as the source of radiation. Although it was possible to synthesize the 6-demethyl analogue (177) from (176), the closest approaches to the corresponding 6-methyl analogue were the ketone (178) and the acetal (179) (BARTON et al. 1971 b). Subsequently, model studies have provided an oxidative method for deblocking ketone acetals, of possible utility in the present instance, reported by BARTON et al. (1972 a).

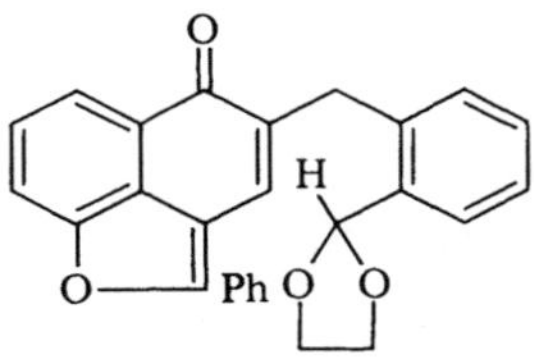

(175)

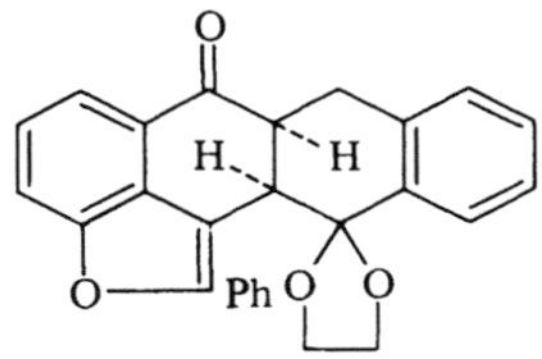

(176)

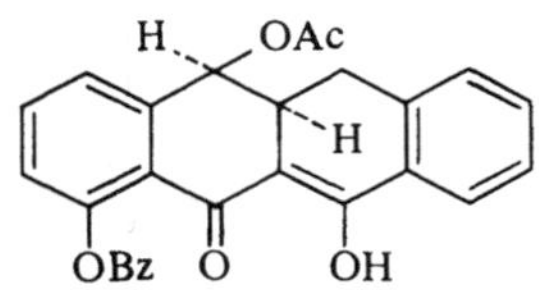

(177)

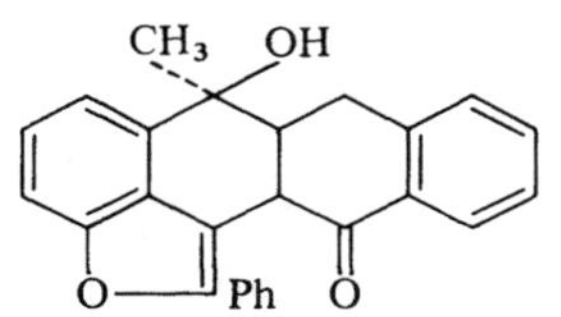

(178)

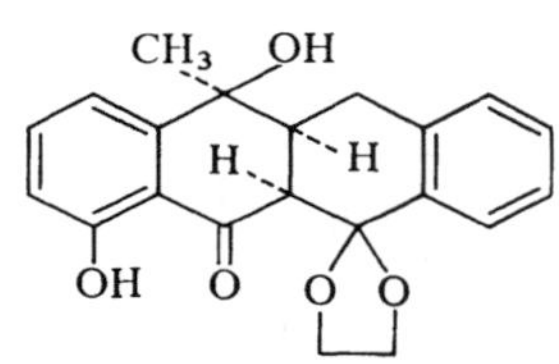

(179)

The photocyclization route was then applied to compounds having suitable A-ring substituents, affording a facile synthesis of 6-methylpretetramide (134). The aldehyde (168) was converted to the acetal and photocyclized to yield (180) which, after conversion to the amide (181), was treated with ethereal methyllithium to yield the carbinol (182). Boiling with hydrogen iodide in phenol led to si-

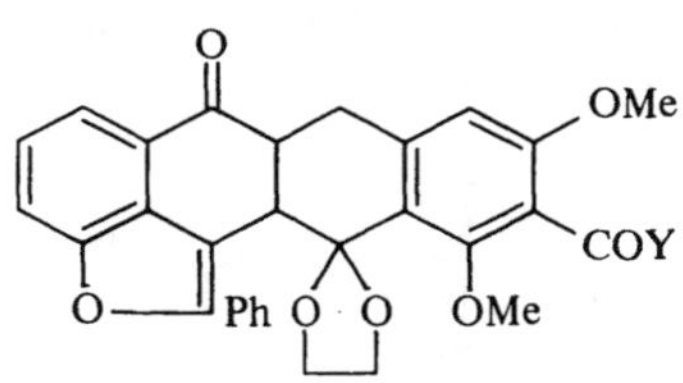

(180) Y = OMe
(181) Y = NH_2

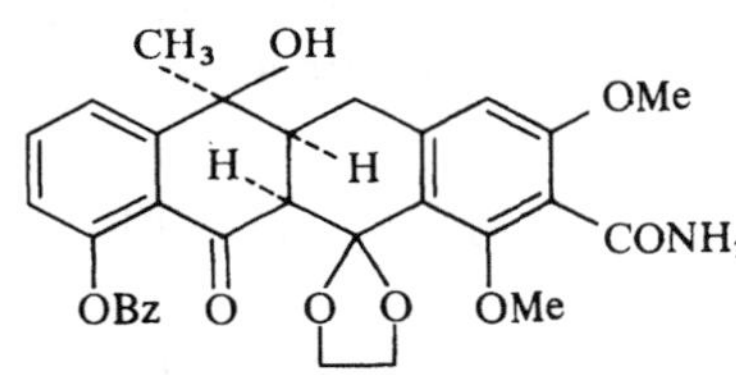

(182)

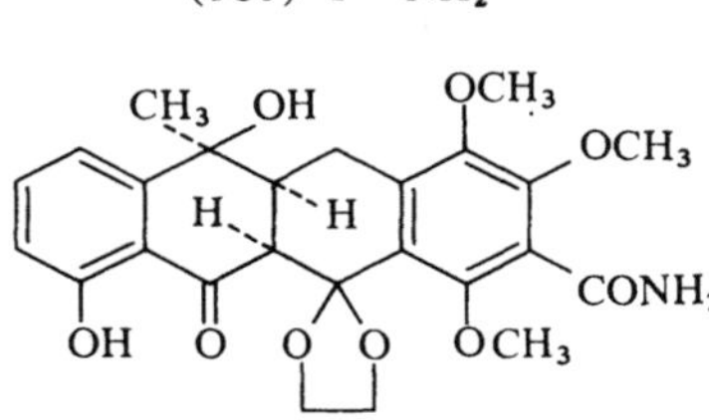

(183)

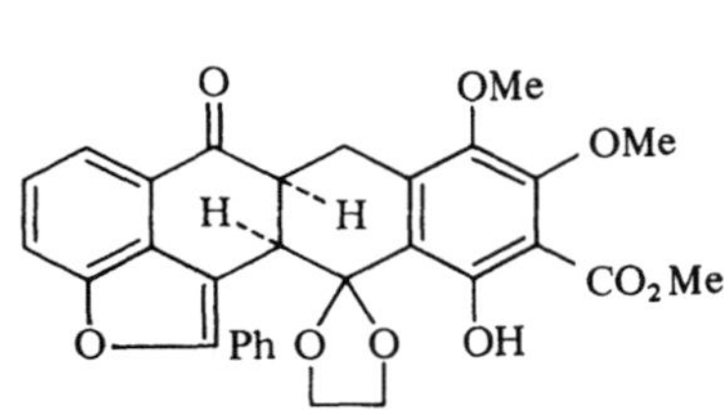

(184)

multaneous demethylation, dehydration, and deacetalization, yielding 6-methylpretetramide (134) directly (BARTON et al. 1971 d). There has been further elaboration of potential tetracycline precursors, e.g., (183) and (184) (BARTON et al. 1971 e, g) by the photocyclization process, as well as further elaboration and improvement of the reaction per se (BARTON et al. 1972 b, 1976).

Concurrent with the studies described above, extensive A-ring model studies have been carried out which have as their ultimate objective the conversion of one or another of the 4a,12a-anhydrotetracyclines to tetracycline (BARTON et al. 1971 c, 1975, 1977 a).

2. Hassall et al.

Synthetic work by the Hassall group carried out primarily at the University College of Swansea, but later at Roche Products Limited, has emphasized the resynthesis of tetracycline from 6-methylpretetramid (134), which, if successful and taken together with BARTON's work, would represent a total synthesis.

As a step in this direction HASSALL and WINTERS (1967, 1968) simulated a step in tetracycline biosynthesis. Thus the quinone (185) was formed by the action of Fremy's salt (potassium nitrosodisulfonate) at pH 10 on 6-methylpretetramide (134). The quinone (185) was converted to 4-hydroxy-6-methylpretetramide (144) by brief contact with phenolic hydrogen iodide, as described earlier by McCORMICK and JENSEN (1965).

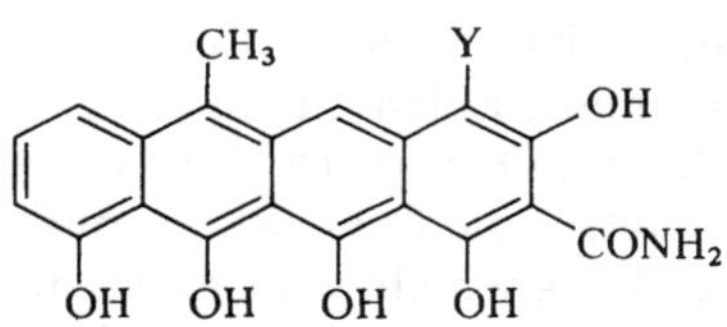

(134) Y = H
(144) Y = OH

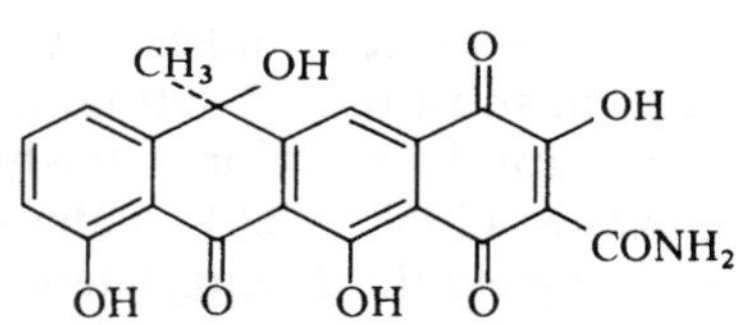

(185)

Oxygenation of 6-methylpretetramide (134) in 0.1 *M* potassium hydroxide-dimethylformamide took a different course. Hydroxylation occurred at 6- and 12a- to yield (186), shown in one of its several tautomeric forms (HASSALL and THOMAS 1970 b, 1978). In alkali, in the presence of air (186) was further oxidized to (185), believed to involve attack of hydroxyl at C4, with elimination of hydroxyl at C12a, with air oxidation of the resulting hydroquinone to quinone. Trimethylsilyl derivatives of the various tautomers of (186) were also prepared (cf. HASSALL and THOMAS 1970 a).

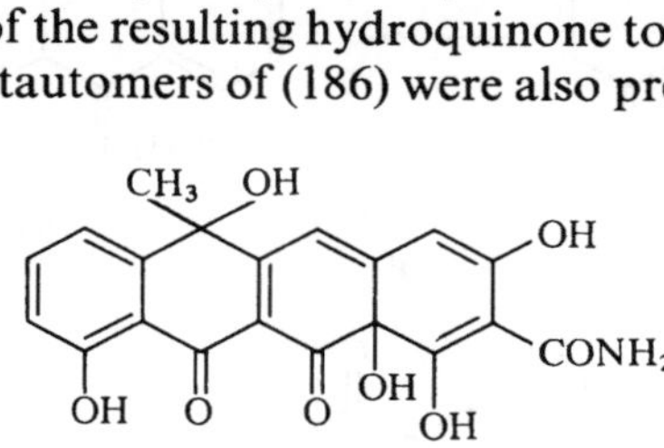

(186)

HASSALL and WOOTTON (1969), HASSALL and MORGAN (1973), and BROADHURST et al. (1977) have also synthesized anthracene-anthraquinone models of the tetracycline antibiotics.

3. McCormick et al.

Pretetramid (189) has also been prepared by total synthesis (MCCORMICK et al. 1963 b). 3-Hydroxyphthalic anhydride was condensed with the naphthalene amide (187) to yield the quinone (188). The latter was converted to (189) by the action of aqueous phenolic hydroiodic acid and potassium hypophosphite.

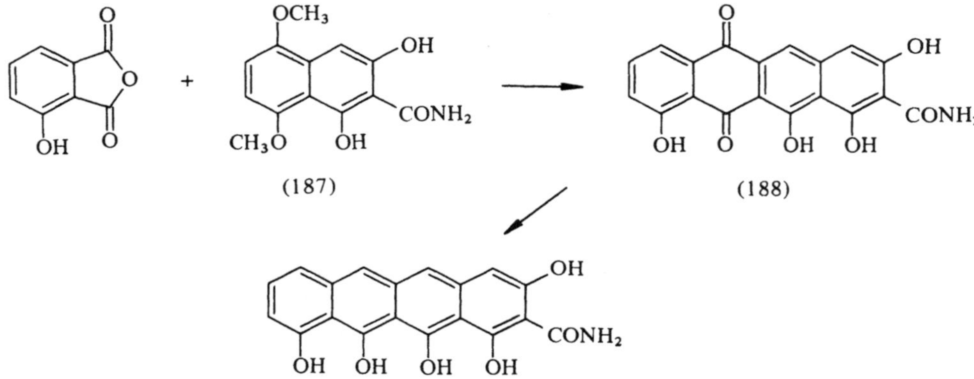

(187) (188) (189)

4. Kulkarni et al.

In extensively reported studies, KULKARNI et al. have studied the condensation of a variety of substituted 1-tetralones with aromatic aldehydes to yield variously substituted naphthacenediones in which the A- and D-rings are aromatic. PANDIT and KULKARNI (1958, 1960) condensed the 1-tetralone (190) with o-phthalaldehydic acid to yield the 2-benzylidenetetralone (191), which was cyclized to the tetrahydronaphthacenedione (192) in poor yield. Alternatively, 1-tetralone-3-carboxylic acids were condensed with aldehydes. In this manner, SESHADRI and KULKARNI (1959) and PANDIT et al. (1960) prepared the 2-benzylidene derivative (193), which was hydrogenated to (194) over Raney nickel, and then cyclized to the hexahydronaphthacene (195) with phosphorus pentoxide.

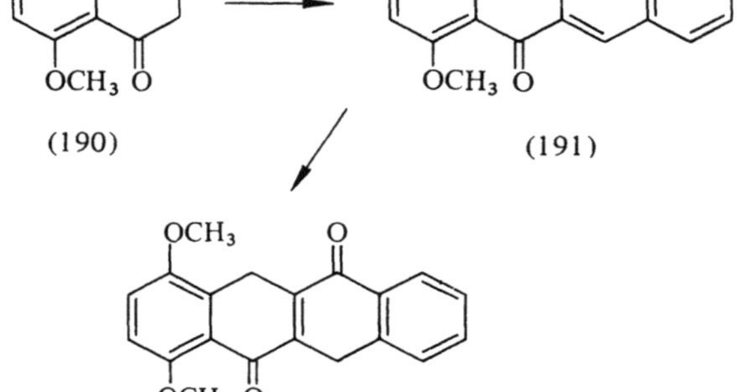

(190) (191) (192)

The same reaction sequence has been applied to the preparation of a variety of related naphthacenes (SESHADRI and KULKARNI 1960; BAKSHI and KULKARNI 1962, 1963), including the 7-chloro-1,3,10-trimethoxy analogue (196) (HOSANGADI et al. 1964), the 6-methyl-2-carboxylic analogue (197) (PANDIT and KULKARNI 1964), and compounds having free hydroxyl groups in rings A and D (HOSANGADI et al. 1969). However, introduction of A-ring amine functionality by this route has failed (SAMANT et al. 1974).

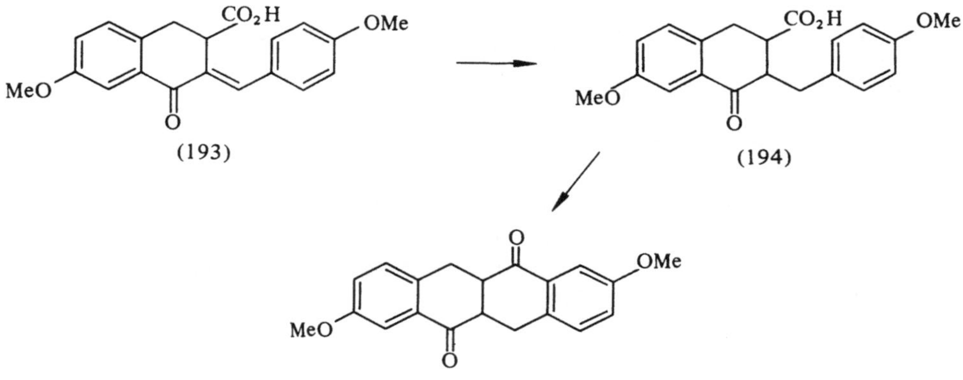

(193) (194) (195)

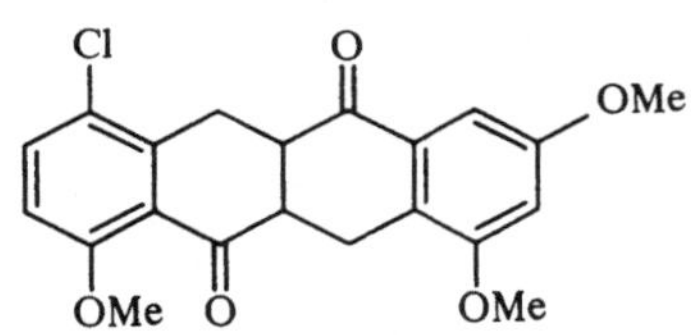

(196)

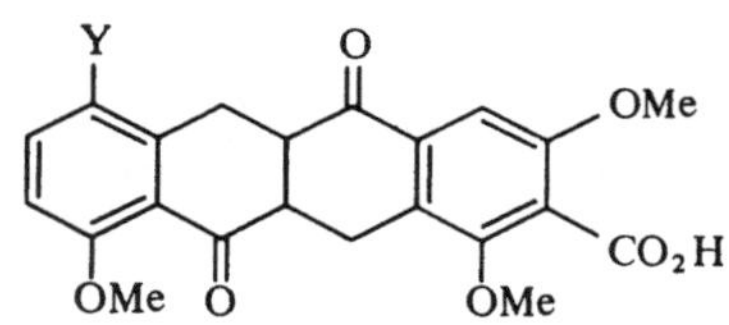

(197) Y = OMe
(198) Y = Cl

By sodium borohydride reduction and then acetylation the dimethoxy compound (196) was converted to the diol diacetate (199). Further oxygen functionality was then introduced into rings B and C by chromic acid oxidation (200) (HOSANGADI et al. 1974). This sequence failed, however, on the two carboxylic acid analogues (197) and (198).

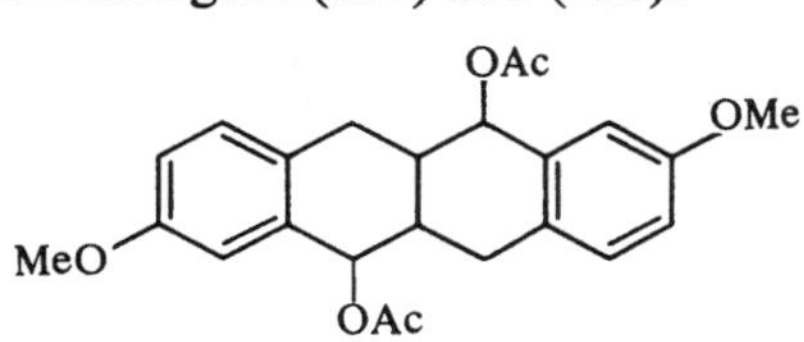

(199)

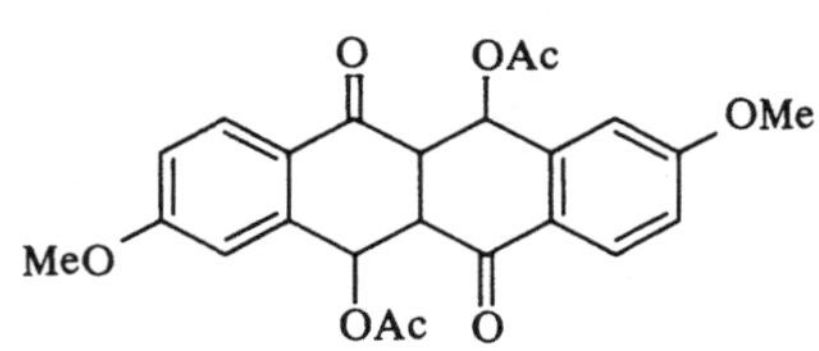

(200)

More recent publications in this series (HOSANGADI and KULKARNI 1975; MAHAJAN and KULKARNI 1975; BARDE and KULKARNI 1978) have dealt with stereochemical questions concerning the various products of these reaction sequences. Much elaboration will be required if the synthesis of a 4,12-anhydrotetracycline is to be achieved using this approach.

5. Kametani et al. and Amaro et al.

As yet another route to ring systems related to those of tetracyclines, KAMETANI et al. (1974) proposed benzocyclobutenes as intermediates for the synthesis of tetracyclines. On heating, the benzocyclobutenes yield reactive dienophilies, viz., o-quinodimethanes. To this end model studies were reported wherein a benzocyclobutene such as (201) was reacted with naphthoquinone, via the diene (202), to yield the naphthacenedione (203).

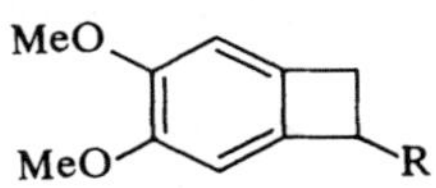

(201) R = CN
(201a) R = OH

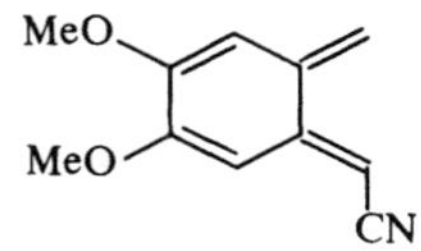

(202)

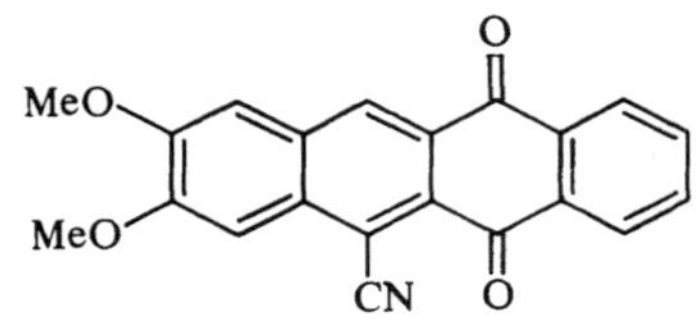

(203)

This work was extended by KAMETANI et al. (1978 a, b) in work directed to the synthesis of Adriamycin, structurally related to tetracycline. Exemplary is the coupling of the alcohol (204), via diene, with the quinoidal compound (205), affording the naphthacanedione (206).

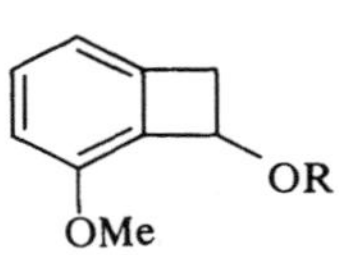

(204) R = H

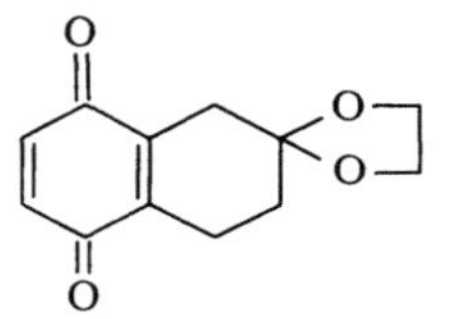

(205)

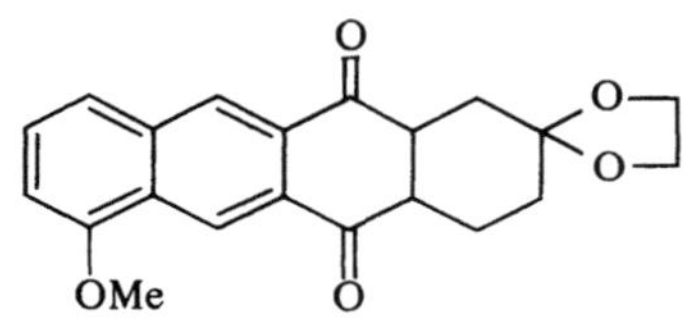

(206)

AMARO et al. (1979) have also reported recent studies along similar lines. Thus refluxing benzocyclobutenol (201a) with naphthazirin (5,8-dihydroxynaphthoquinone) or its diacetate gave the adducts (207) and (208). Yields are relatively low because of facile aromatization of these compounds to (209) and (210). A better yield of adducts is obtained when the alcohol (204) is condensed with the tetrahydronaphthoquinone (211), producing (212).

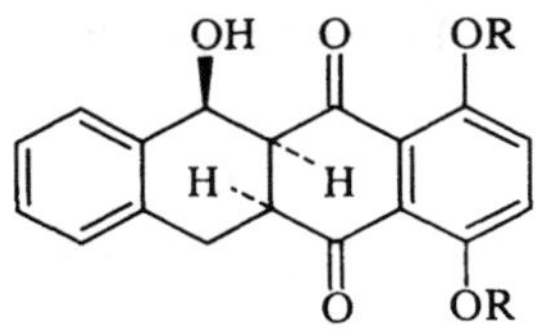

(207) R = H
(208) R = Ac

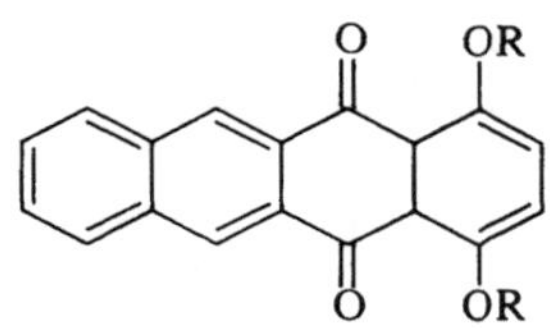

(209) R = H
(210) R = Ac

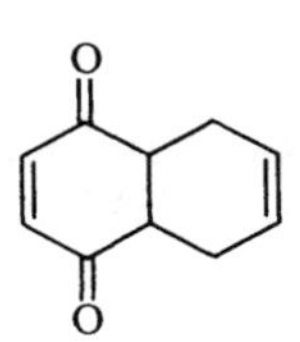

(211)

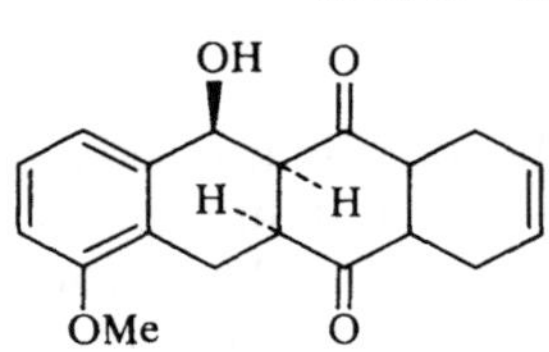

(212)

AMARO et al. (1979) further extended their work to the irradiation of 2-alkyl-substituted aryl carbonyl compounds, e.g., (213) and (214), known to yield the same type of (E)-dienol species, e.g., (215) and (216). Irradiation of 2-methylacetophenone (213) in acetone or benzene in the presence of naphthazarin gave a mixture of (217) and the corresponding aromatized adduct, (218), although the

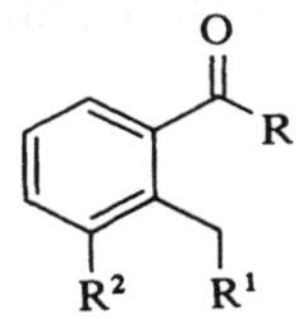

(213) $R = Me, R^1 = R^2 = H$

(214) $R = H, R^1 = OMe, R^2 = OH$

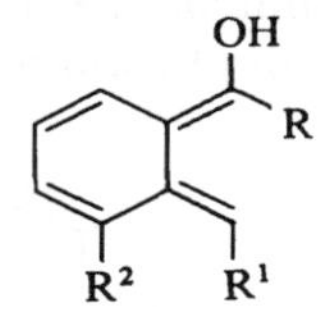

(215) $R = Me, R^1 = R^2 = H$

(216) $R = H, R^1 = OMe, R^2 = OH$

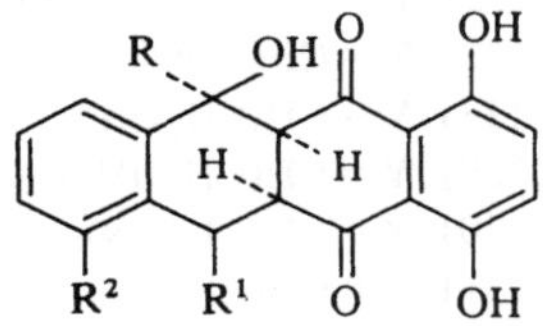

(217) $R = Me, R^1 = R^2 = H$

(220) $R = H, R^1 = OMe, R^2 = OH$

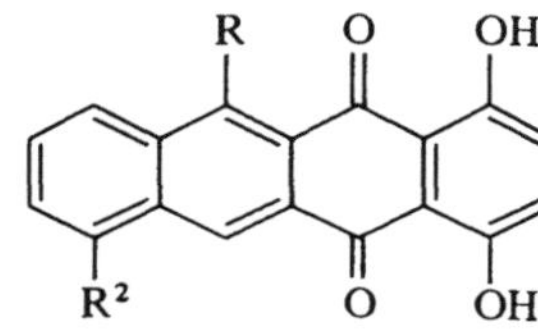

(218) $R = Me, R^2 = H$

(219) $R = H, R^2 = OH$

latter was isolated in pure state only when benzene was employed as solvent. Irradiation of 2-methoxymethyl-3-hydroxybenzaldehyde (214) and trapping the photoenol with naphthazarin gave, after chromatography, the aromatized derivative (219); the intermediate adduct (220) could not be characterized. The structure of (219) was confirmed by independent synthesis. The tribromide (221) was converted with NaI/DMF to the o-quinodimethane (222) and condensed with naphthazarin diacetate to yield the triacetate (223). The same triacetate resulted from acetylation of (219).

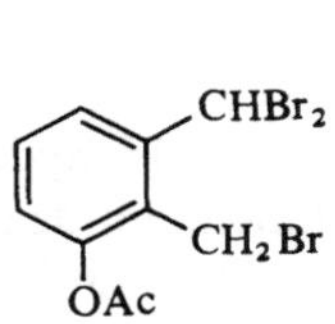

(221)

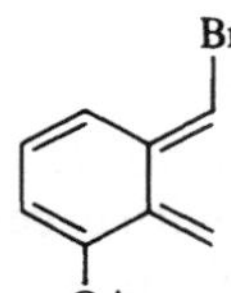

(222)

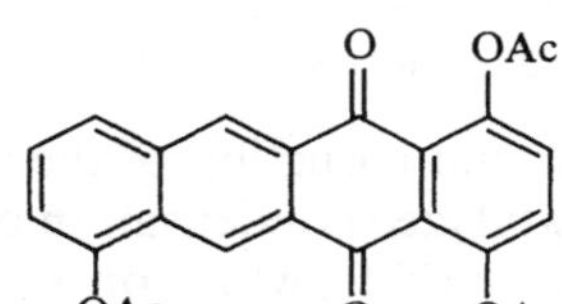

(223)

The use of benzocyclobutenes in the synthesis of linear tricyclic and tetracyclic compounds has been reviewed (KAMETANI and FUKUMOTO 1979, 1980).

II. Analogues Lacking the Dimethylamino Group or Other Key Functionality

1. Boothe et al.

The first total synthesis goal to be met by the BOOTHE et al. group at the Lederle Laboratories Division of the American Cyanamid Company was the synthesis of

(±)-dedimethylamino-12a-deoxy-6-demethylanhydrotetracycline (224) (BOOTHE et al. 1959; KENDE et al. 1961). Starting material was 4-chloro-3-methylanisole (225). Bromination gave the bromide (226), then condensed with diethyl malonate to yield the benzylmalonate (227). Lithium aluminum hydride reduction gave the corresponding 1,3-diol (228), mesylated to the *bis*-sulfonate ester (229), and then converted to the dinitrile (230). Alkaline hydrolysis to the glutaric acid (231) and ring closure with polyphosphoric acid gave the tetralone acetic acid (232).

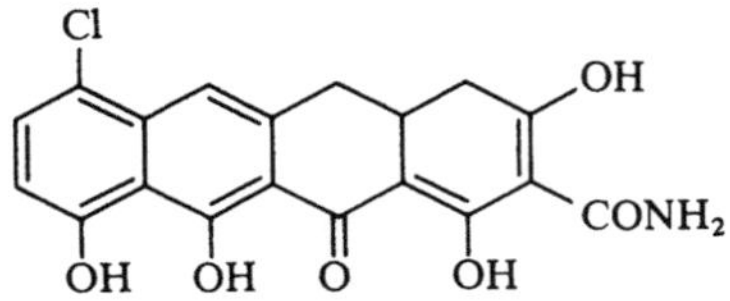

(224)

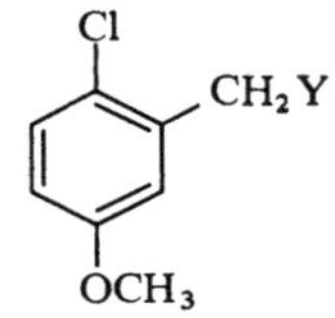

(225) Y = H, (226) Y = Br
(227) Y = CH(COOEt)$_2$
(228) Y = CH(CH$_2$OH)$_2$
(229) Y = CH(CH$_2$OMes)$_2$
(230) Y = CH(CH$_2$CN)$_2$
(231) Y = CH(CH$_2$CO$_2$H)$_2$

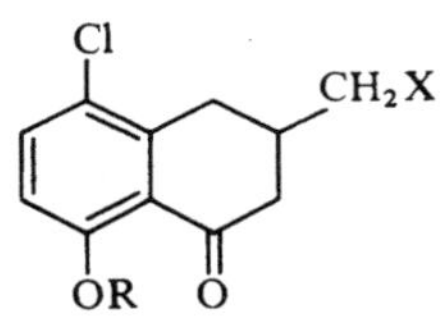

(232) R = Me, X = COOH
(233) R = Me, X = COCl
(234) R = Me, X = CHO
(235) R = Me
X = CH(CHCNCONH$_2$)$_2$
(236) R = H, X = CH(CH$_2$COOH)$_2$
(237) R = Bz, X = CH(CH$_2$COOMe)$_2$

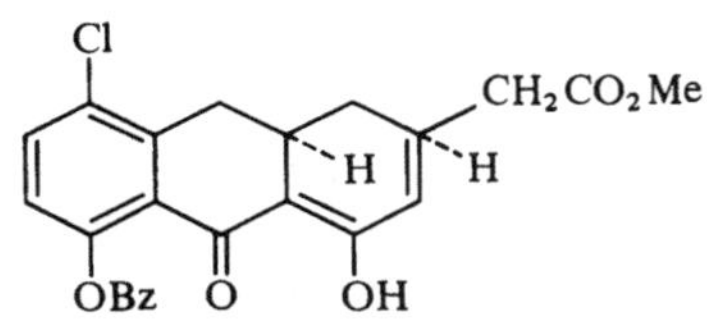

(238)

Rosenmund reduction of the acid chloride (233) gave the aldehyde (234). Piperidine-catalyzed condensation of (234) with excess cyanoacetamide gave the dicyanodiamide (235), which on acid hydrolysis was demethylated and decarboxylated to the phenolic acid (236), then benzylated and esterified to yield (237). Cyclization of the latter by sodium hydride in toluene gave the tricyclic ester (238).

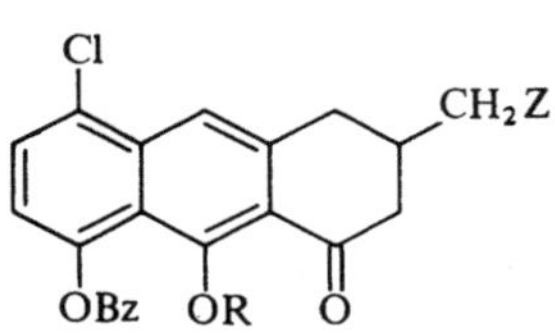

(239) R = H, Z = CO$_2$Me
(240) R = CH$_3$, Z = CO$_2$Me
(241) R = CH$_3$, Z = COOH
(242) R = CH$_3$, Z = CH(CO$_2$Et)$_2$

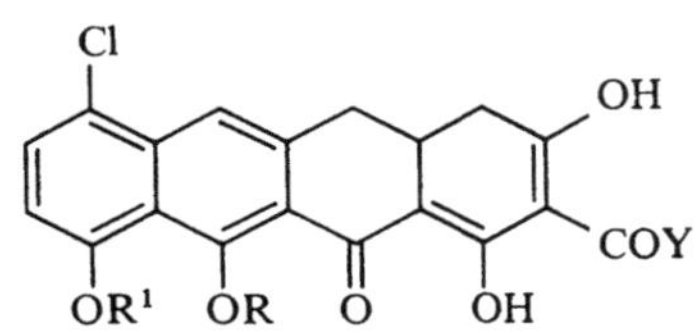

(243) R = Me, R^1 = Bz, Y = OMe
(224) R = R^1 = H, Y = NH$_2$

Angular bromination followed by dehydrobromination in collidine converted (238) into the phenol (239), then methylated to the *bis*-ether (240) and hydrolyzed to the acid (241). Conversion of the acid to the acylmalonate (242) and cyclization, again by sodium hydride in toluene, gave the tetracyclic ester (243). Finally, fusion of the ester with ammonium formate, and dealkylation with hydrogen chloride in acetic acid gave the desired (±)-amide (224).

From the same bicyclic acid chloride (233), WILKINSON et al. (1961) also elaborated the tricyclic model compound (248). The acid chloride was condensed with sodio malonic ester to (244), then cyclized without isolation by additional basic catalyst to the tricyclic ester (245). Methanolic ammonia at 80 °C gave the carboxamide (246), having a C3 vinyl amine group, which was first hydrolyzed in hydrochloric acid to the enolic triketone (247) and finally hydrolyzed in hydrobromic acid-acetic acid to the tricyclic model compound (248).

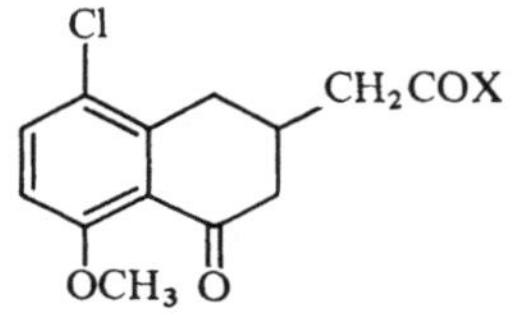

(233) X = Cl
(244) X = $CH(COOEt)_2$

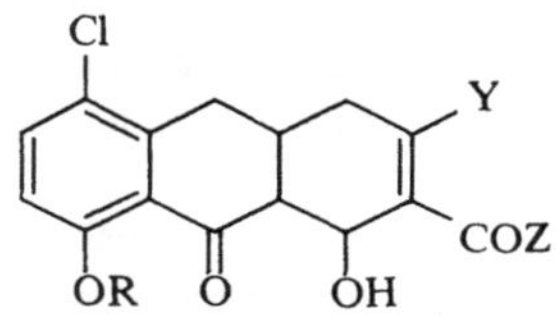

(245) R = Me, Y = OH, Z = OCH_3
(246) R = Me, Y = Z = NH_2
(247) R = Me, Y = OH, Z = NH_2
(248) R = H, Y = OH, Z = NH_2

Finally, the Lederle group employed the acid (236) as a precursor for totally synthetic (±)-dedimethylymino-6-demethyl-6,12a-dideoxy-7-chlorotetracycline (249) (FIELDS et al. 1960, 1961). The derived anhydride (250) was converted to the diastereomeric monoesters (251), which were cyclized using sodium methoxide as base to yield the 3,4-*syn* acid (252), separated by crystallization from its epimeric

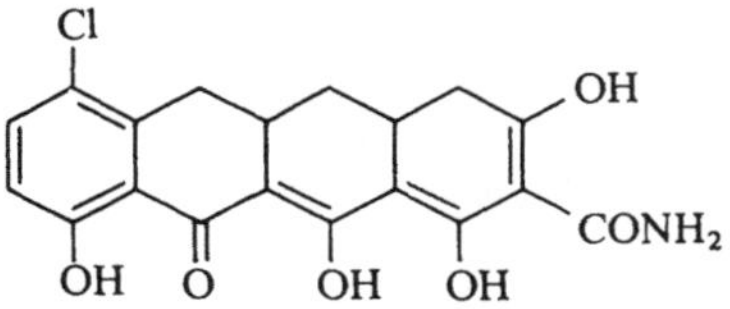

(249)

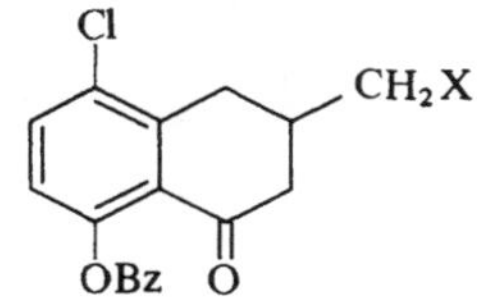

(236) X = $CH(CH_2COOH)$
(250) X = $CH(CH_2CO)_2O$
(251) X = $CH(CH_2CO_2Me)-CH_2CO_2H$

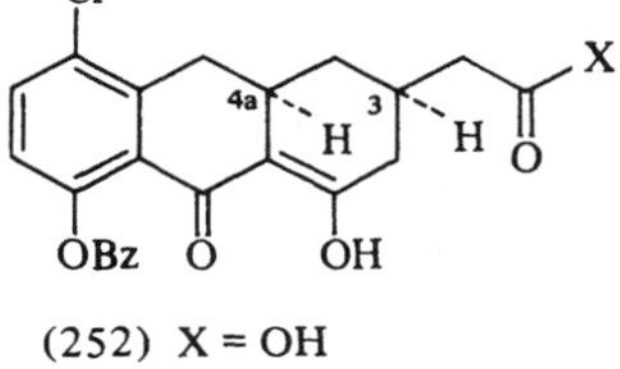

(252) X = OH
(253) X = $CH(CO_2Et)_2$

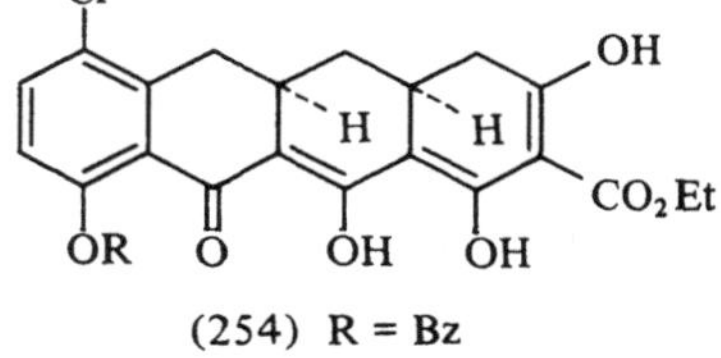

(254) R = Bz
(255) R = H

3,4-*anti* isomer formed in about the same yield. Relative stereochemistry was assigned on the basis of subsequent more rapid cyclization of the *syn* isomer. The acid (252) was converted to the acylmalonate (253) and cyclized to the tetracyclic ester (254) by sodium hydride in toluene. Hydrogenolysis of the benzyl group and fusion of the resulting phenol (255) with ammonium formate gave the desired (±)-amide (249).

2. Muxfeldt et al.

The initial synthetic efforts by MUXFELDT et al. of the Technische Hochschule Braunschweig, the University of Wisconsin, and Cornell University were directed to the synthesis of the epimeric 6-deoxytetracyclines having a methyl group at C6. These early efforts led to the synthesis of a number of 6-deoxytetracycline analogues (MUXFELDT 1962a, b; MUXFELDT et al. 1962a, b, c), as well as the synthesis of dedimethylaminoanhydrochlortetracycline (MUXFELDT 1959, 1962a, b; MUXFELDT and KREUTZER 1959, 1961; MUXFELDT et al. 1960; MUXFELDT and INHOFFEN 1958).

The starting material for these synthetic studies was m-methoxybenzophenone (256), initially condensed with diethyl succinate to yield the *cis-trans* isomers (257) and (258), the first as a crystalline solid, the second as an oil. The

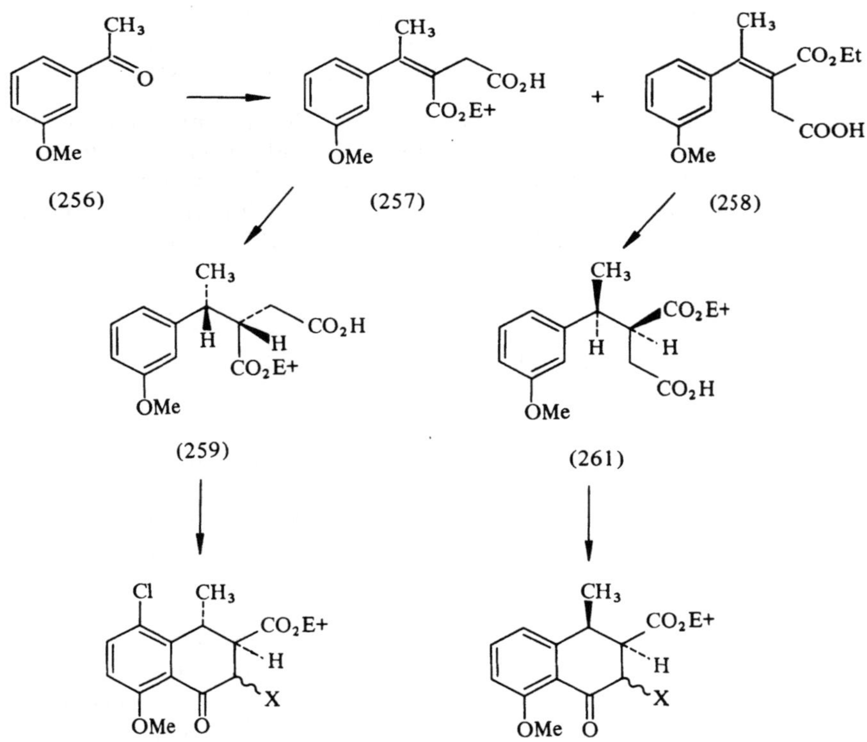

(256) (257) (258)

(259) (261)

(260) X = H
(263) X = Br

(262) X = H
(264) X = Br

isomer (257) was hydrogenated to the saturated acid (259), chlorinated, and cyclized with polyphosphoric acid to the potential α-6-deoxytetracycline precursor (260). In like manner, the isomer (258) was converted via (261) to the potential β-6-deoxytetracycline precursor (262).

Both isomers (260) and (262) represented precursors useful for the synthesis of dedimethylaminoanhydrochlorotetracycline. Thus photocatalyzed bromination of either compound to the corresponding bromo compounds (263) and (264) followed by dehydrobromination with 10% sodium hydroxide gave the same naphtholcarboxylic acid (265). Treatment of the latter with dimethyl sulfate gave the dimethoxy ester (266), then reduced to the alcohol (267) with lithium aluminum hydride, and converted to the bromide (268) with phosphorus tribromide. Treatment with sodio di-*tert*-butyl ethoxycarbonylmethylmalonate gave the *tris*-ester (269), selectively hydrolyzed to the acid (270).

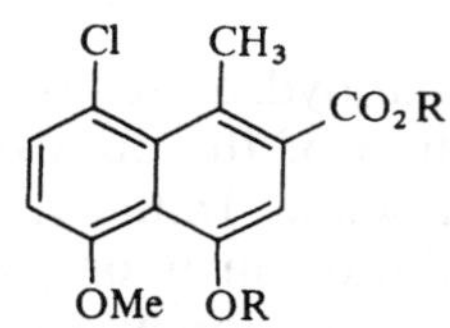

(265) R = H
(266) R = CH_3

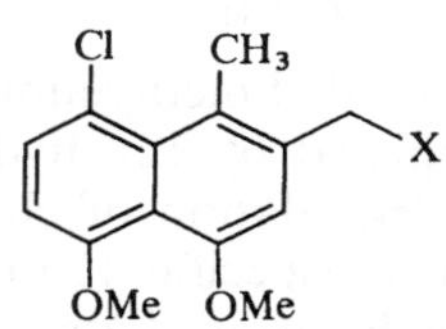

(267) X = OH
(268) X = Br

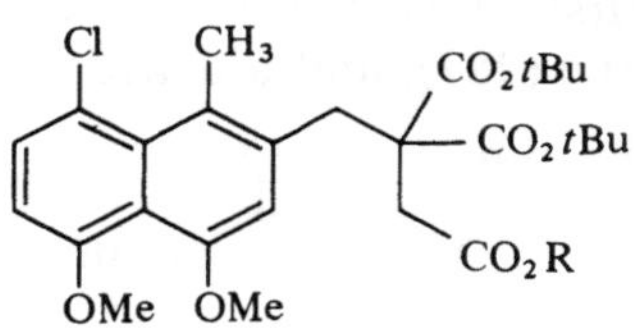

(269) R = Et
(270) R = H

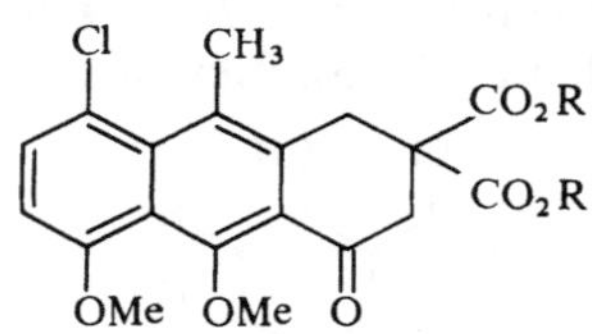

(271) R = *t*Bu
(272) R = H

Cyclization gave the tricyclic diester (271), now readily hydrolyzed to the diacid (272), and subsequently decarboxylated to the monoacid (273) by heating. The latter was easily converted to the diazoketone (274), which under forcing conditions in hot benzyl or preferably cyclohexyl alcohol/dimethylaniline gave the esters (275) or (276), then hydrolyzed to the acid (277). Via acid chloride (278), the acid was coupled with malonic ester to yield to acylmalonate (279). After

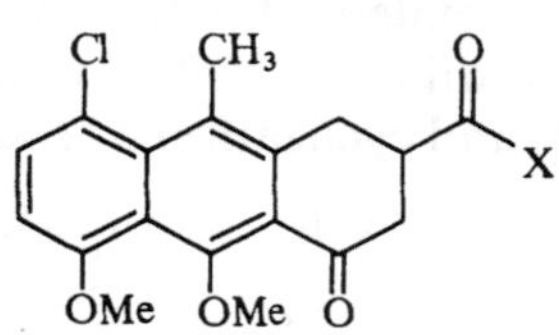

(273) X = OH
(274) X = CH_2N_2

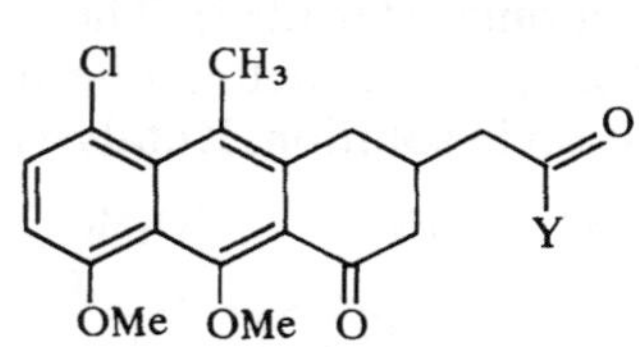

(275) Y = OBz
(276) Y = OC_6H_{11}
(277) Y = OH
(278) Y = Cl
(279) Y = $CH(COOEt)_2$

much experimentation, (279) was successfully cyclized to the naphthacene (280) by sodium hydride in anisole or 1,4-dimethoxybenzene. Methanolic ammonia gave the corresponding amide (281) in low yield. Finally, the amide was smoothly hydrolyzed to the desired crystalline (±)-4-demethylamino-12-deoxy-5a,6-anhydro-7-chlorotetracycline (282).

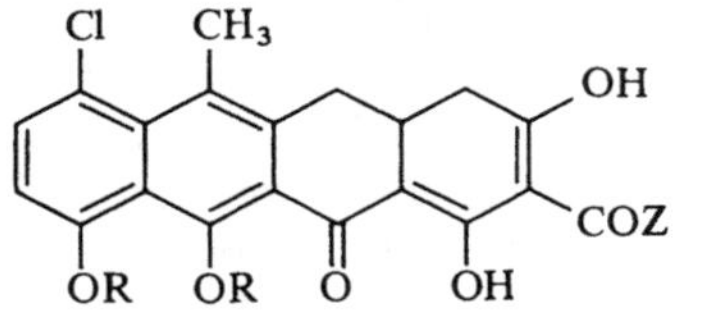

(280) R = Me, Z = Et
(281) R = Me, Z = NH_2
(282) R = H, Z= NH_2

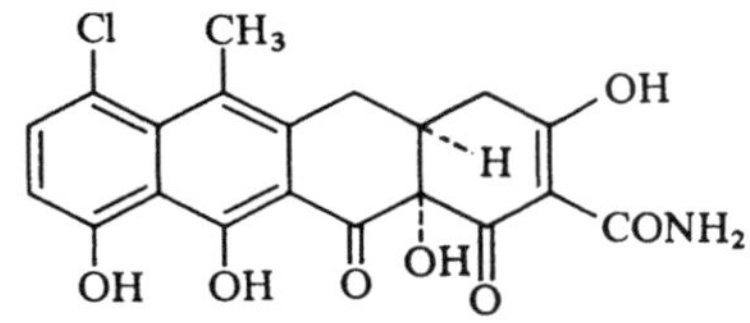

(283)

The synthesis of 4-dedimethylamino-5a,6-anhydro-7-chlorotetracycline (283) was formally completed by 12a hydroxylation of the optically active form of (282), derived by degradation of chlortetracycline. Initially, this was via O^{10}-methylation, nonstereospecific 12a-hydroxylation in poor yield by perbenzoic acid, and O^{10}-demethylation. Later, 12a-hydroxylation was achieved directly, in the desired stereospecific manner, using platinum-catalyzed oxygenation.

Synthetic studies directed to α-6-deoxytetracyclines began with the intermediate bicyclic ketone-ester (260), which was first converted to the ketal (284) and then, via alcohol (285), mesylate (286), nitrile (287), and aldehyde (288), to the

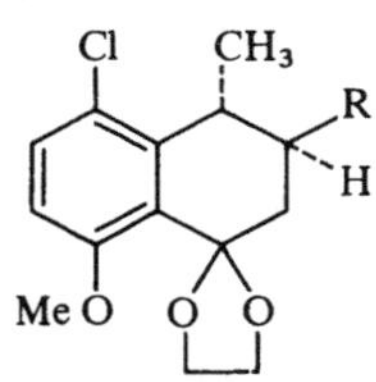

(284) R = CO_2Et
(285) R = CH_2OH
(286) R = CH_2OSO_2Me
(287) R = CH_2CN
(288) R = CH_2CHO

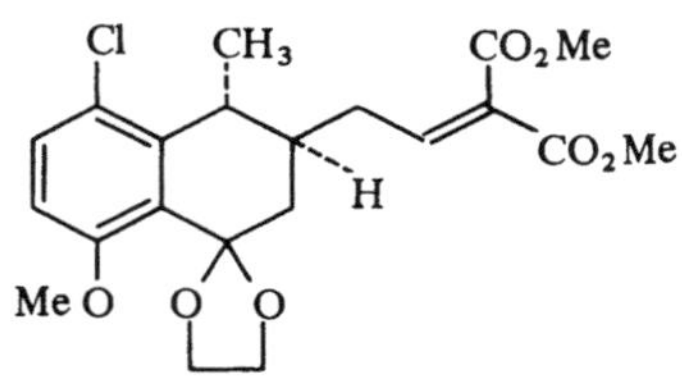

(289)

alkylidene malonic ester (289). The latter was condensed with sodio or potassio methyl acetoacetate in methanol-ether to the diketone (290), subject to rapid tautomerization in solution. Ketalysis to (291) and cyclization by sodium hydride

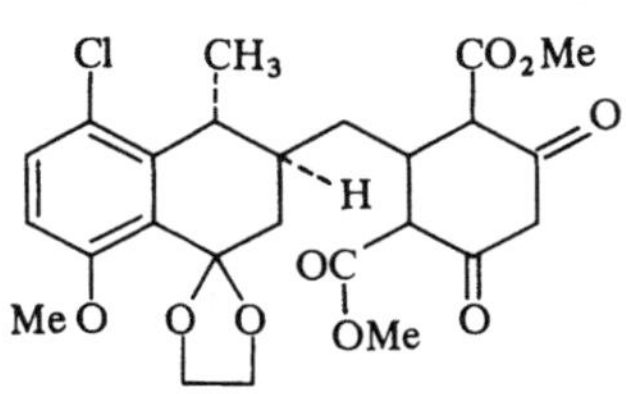

(290)

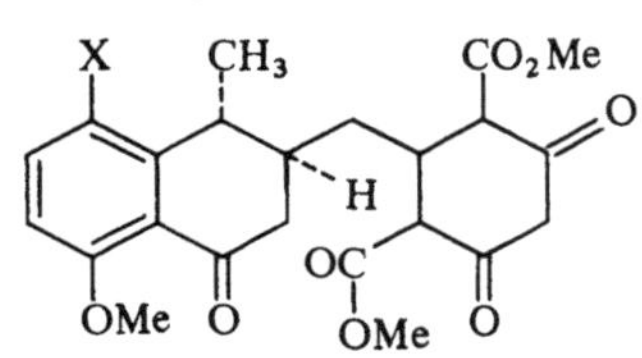

(291) X = Cl
(292) X – H

in anisole gave the tetracyclic compound (118), hydrogenolized to (113); alternatively (291) was dechlorinated to (292) and then cyclized to (113). On mild hydrolysis (113), was converted to the decarboxylated ether (114), while more vigorous hydrolysis gave the decarboxylated phenol (115).

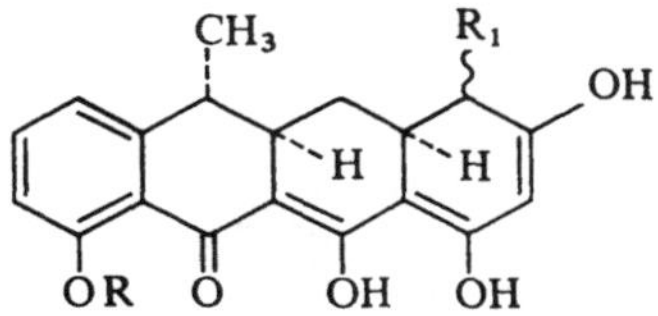

(113) $R = CH_3$, $R^1 = CO_2CH_3$
(114) $R = CH_3$, $R^1 = H$
(115) $R = R^1 = H$

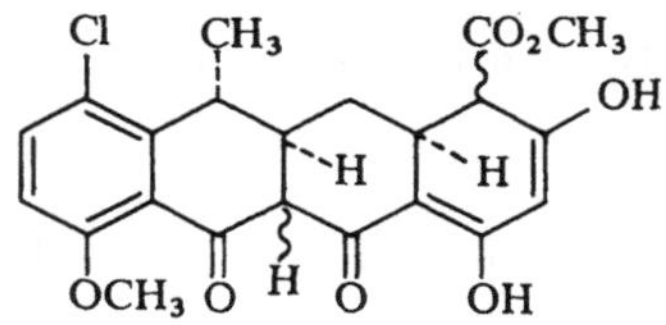

(118)

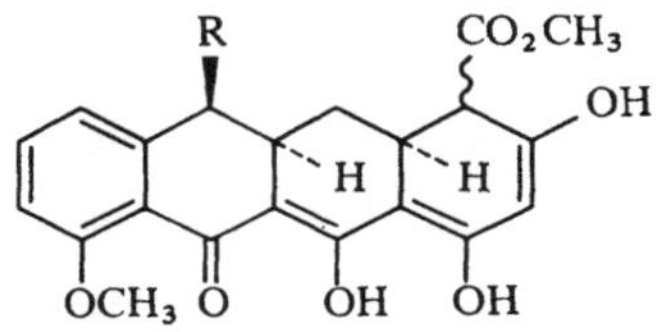

(117) $R = CH_3$
(293) $R = H$

By analogous procedures, the isomeric bicyclic ketone ester (262) was converted to the β-6-deoxytetracycline analogue (117). The 6-demethyl-6-deoxytetracycline analogue (293) was also prepared by similar methods. The use of the ultraviolet spectral properties of the compounds (118) and (117) in the assignment of stereochemistry to α- and β-6-deoxytetracyclines is discussed above.

Muxfeldt et al. (1966), through model studies with dimedone, also provided a method improved over that of Shemyakin et al. (1960 a), which in principle can be used to introduce the 2-carboxamide groups into the compounds such as (113)–(118).

3. Shemyakin et al.

Prior to their successful synthesis of tetracycline, described in detail below, the Shemyakin group carried out extensive studies concerned with potential BCD-ring precursors. For example, generally following condensation, Grignard additions, and hydride reductions also delineated by Inhoffen et al. (1957), juglone ethers were condensed with butadiene or a derivative thereof to yield anthraquinones (294)–(297), reacted with methyl Grignard to yield such compounds as

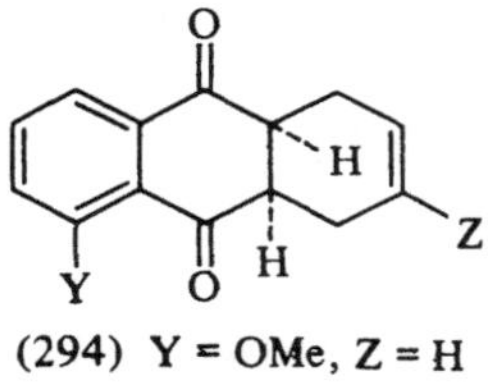

(294) Y = OMe, Z = H
(295) Y = Z = OMe
(296) Y = Z = H

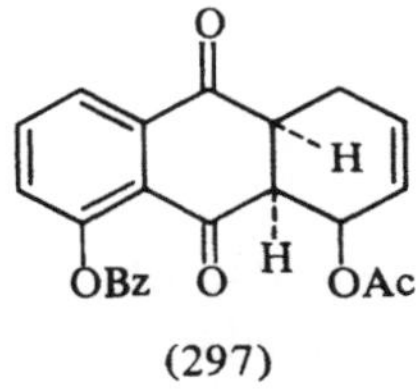

(297)

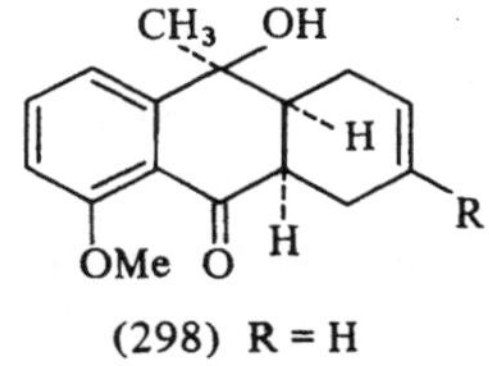

(298) R = H
(299) R = OMe

(298)–(300), and reacted with hydride to yield such compounds as (301) and (302). These compounds were further transformed into numerous other derivatives including (303)–(305) (SHEMYAKIN et al. 1957, 1959 a, c, 1964 a, b; KOLOSOV et al. 1963 a, b, 1964 a, b, c). Analogous *trans* fused compounds such as (306) were prepared by cyclizing *trans*-2-benzyl-5-cyclohexanone-1-carboxylic acid (BOLESOV et al. 1963 a, b; ARBUZOV et al. 1965).

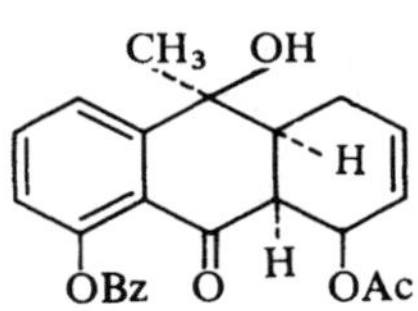

(300)

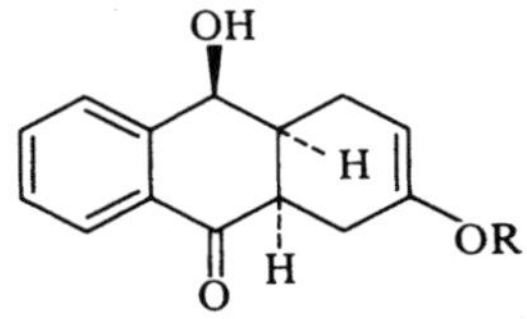

(301)

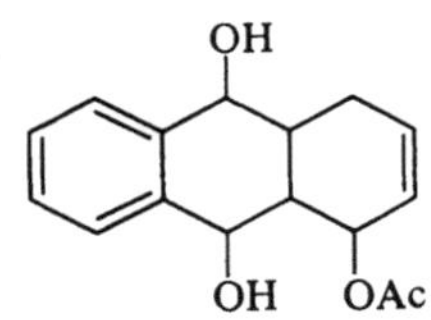

(302)

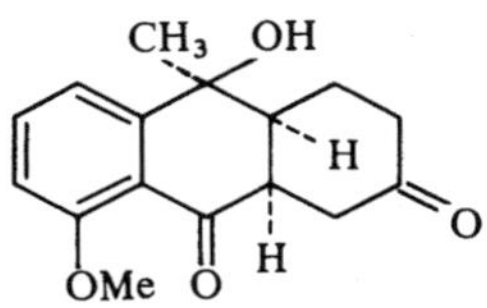

(303)

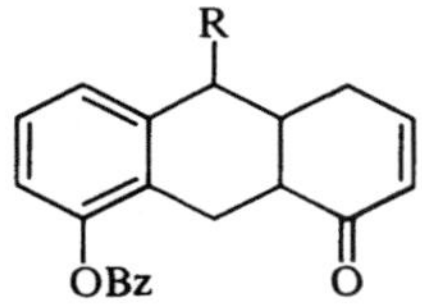

(304) $R = CH_3$
(305) $R = H$

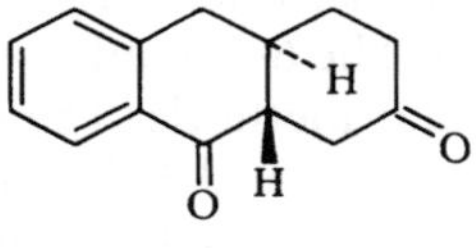

(306)

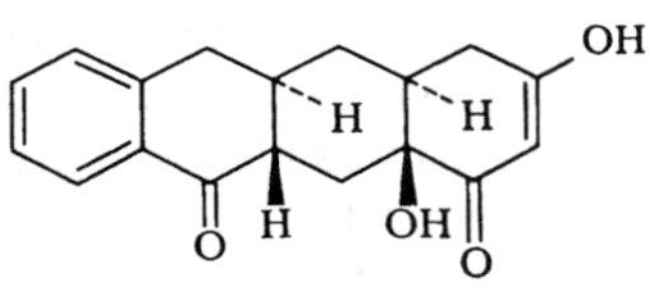

(307)

In addition to the derivation of tetracycline from compound (297), detailed below, a variety of other tetracycline analogues, lacking key groups, were synthesized from these various precursors. Exemplary are (a) preparation of the model compound (307) from (306) by two methods (BOLESOV et al. 1963 a, b, 1965), (b) preparation of (308) from the epoxide of (296) (SHEMYAKIN et al. 1964 c), and (c) preparation of the anhydrotetracycline analogues (309) and (310) from (304) and (305) (GUREVICH et al. 1964 a, b, c, 1965 a, b; KOLOSOV et al. 1965).

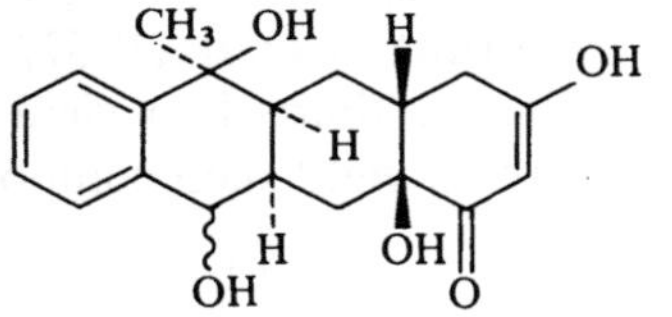

(308)

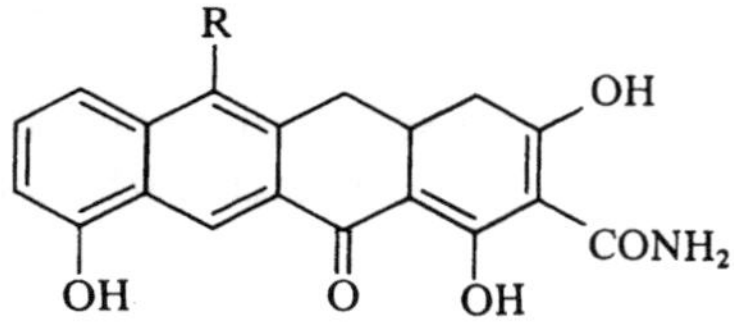

(309) $R = CH_3$
(310) $R = H$

Concurrent with the early studies described above, the SHEMYAKIN group carried out extensive model studies directed to construction of the tetracycline A-ring (SHEMYAKIN et al. 1958, 1959 b, 1960 a, b; KOLOSOV and BERLIN 1962; BERLIN et al. 1964 a, b; GUREVICH et al. 1964 c).

E. Total Synthesis of 6-Demethyl-6-deoxytetracycline

I. Woodward; Conover et al.

The first total synthesis of a fully active tetracycline was that of 6-demethyl-6-deoxytetracycline by WOODWARD of Harvard and a group led by CONOVER at the Medical Research Laboratories of Pfizer Inc. The synthesis was reported preliminarily by CONOVER et al. (1962) and WOODWARD (1963), and in detail by KORST et al. (1968).

Like all successful syntheses, this synthesis began with the aromatic D-ring of tetracycline as a foundation stone on which the more complicated rings were elaborated. Although alternatives were identified, the optimal route for the earliest stages of the synthesis was to condense methyl m-methoxybenzoate (306) with diethylsuccinate to yield the methyl benzoylacetate (307), which without isolation

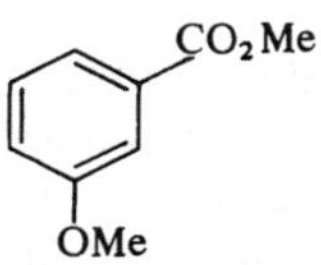
(306)

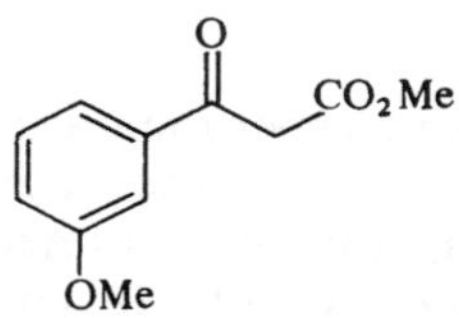
(307)

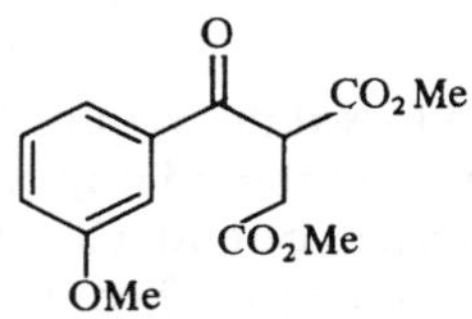
(308)

was alkylated with methyl chloroacetate to the dimethyl benzoyl succinate (308), both reactions carried out by sodium hydride in dimethylformamide. There followed Michael condensation of the keto diester (308) with methyl acrylate, by Triton B in dioxan, affording the keto-triester (309). Hot aqueous acetic/sulfuric acids brought about hydrolysis and decarboxylation to the keto-diacid (310), purified by distillation of the dimethyl ester (311). In principle, a variety of ultimate C6 substituents could be incorporated at this point in the synthesis via reactions of the ketone group; however, moving forward with the simplest possible construction, the ketonic diester (311) was hydrogenolized over Pd/C. The result-

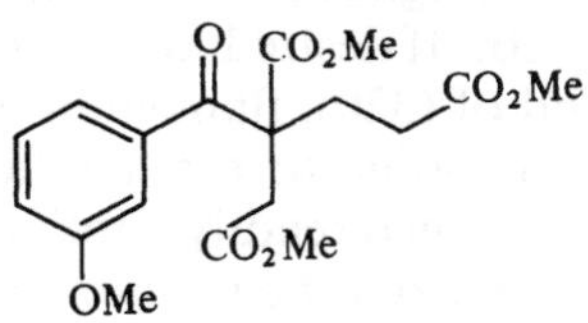
(309)

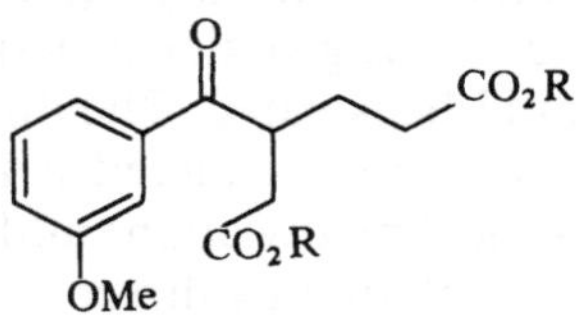
(310) R = H
(311) R = CH_3

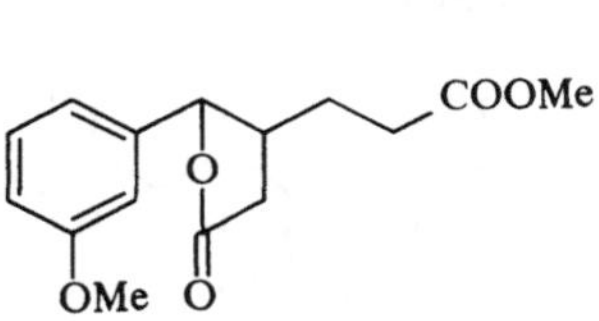
(312)

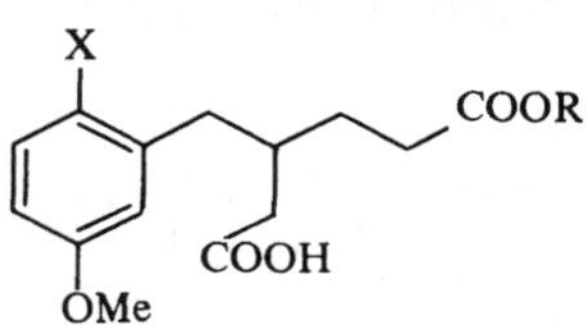
(313) X = H, R = Me
(314) X = R = H
(315) X = Cl, R = H

ing monoester (313), evidently formed via the lactone (312), was hydrolyzed to the diacid (314) and then chlorinated in order to block the position *para* to the methoxy group.

The chloro diacid (315) was cyclized to the tetralone (316) by liquid hydrogen fluoride, then converted to the methyl ester (317). Alternatively, the monoester (313) was chlorinated and cyclized to yield the methyl ester directly. The next phase of the synthesis, construction of the C-ring by condensation of (317) with

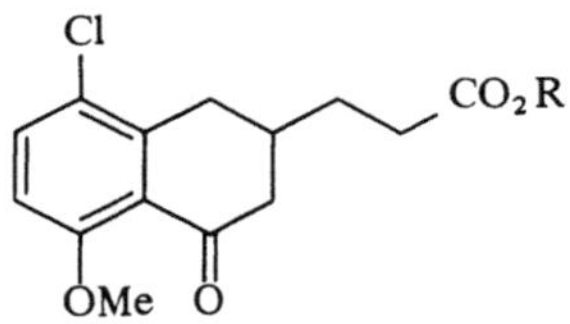

(316) R = H
(317) R = Me

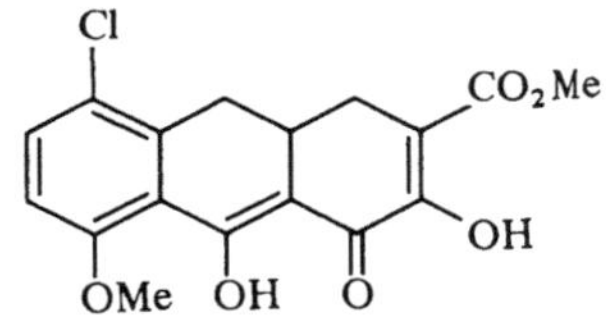

(318)

dimethyl oxalate, required extensive experimentation in order to obtain the desired six-membered ring compound (318) as the major product. The condensation was carried out at elevated temperature in dimethylformamide employing 4 equivalents NaH, 2 equivalents MeO_2CCO_2Me, and 1 equvalent methanol. Hydrolysis/decarboxylation afforded the hydroanthracene ketone (319), a key intermediate in the present synthesis.

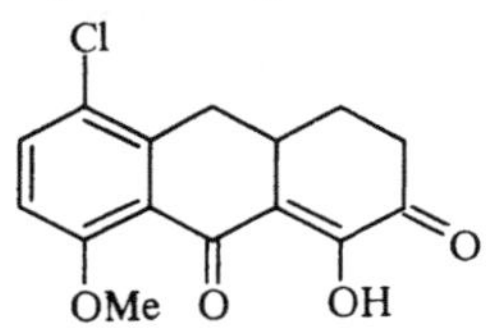

(319)

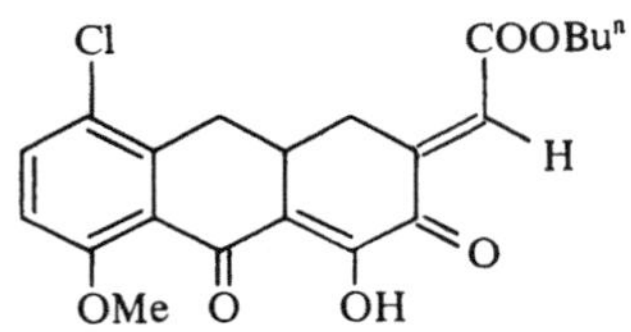

(320)

The highly reactive methylene group in (319) permitted facile condensation of this compound with n-butyl glyoxylate by magnesium methoxide in boiling toluene, yielding the glyoxidene derivative (320). If desired, the intermediate alcohol (321) could be isolated. The double bond of (320), flanked by electron-withdrawing substituents, rendered it highly susceptible to the addition of nucleophiles. Thus the dimethylamine adduct (322) formed readily, albeit reversibly, necessitating its isolation by direct crystallization from the reaction mixture. While this reversibility rendered (322) difficult to handle, it did assure that the indicated, desired stereochemistry was obtained, i.e., the bulky side chain undoubtedly in the stable equatorial disposition. In the next stage of the synthesis, the destabiliz-

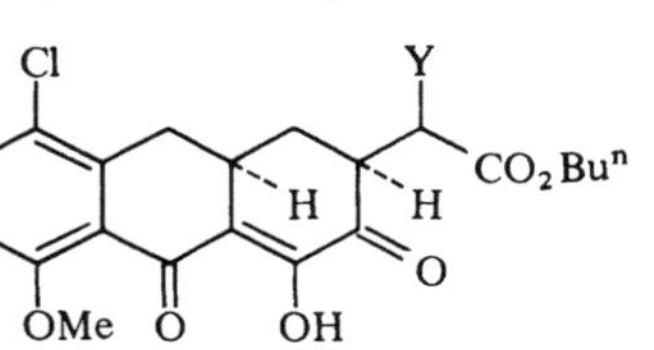

(321) Y = OH
(322) Y = NMe_2

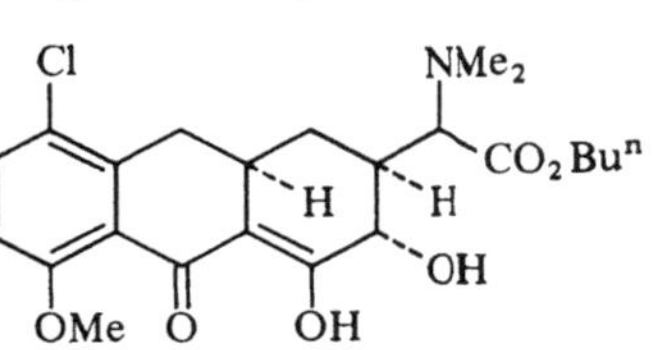

(323)

ing influence of the ketone was removed through its reduction to the alcohol (323), converted to the lactone (324) in boiling toluene in the presence of a generous portion of p-toluenesulfonic acid catalyst. The lactone was readily reduced by zinc/acid couple to (325) and dechlorinated by hydrogenation over Pd/C to (326).

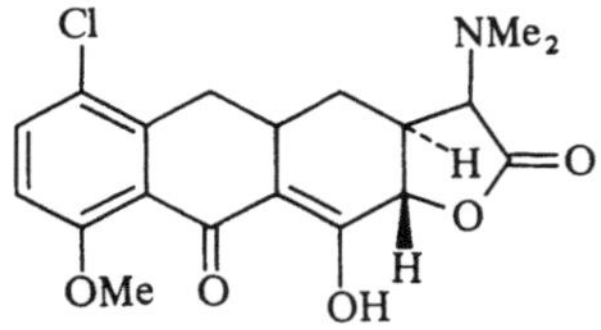

(324)

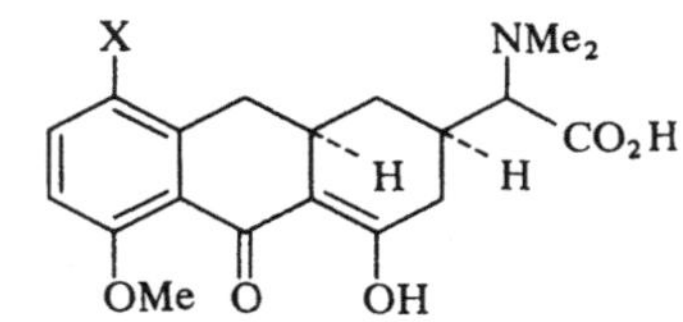

(325) X = Cl
(326) X = H

Via the mixed anhydride (327), which could be optionally isolated, the amino acid (326) was condensed with the ethoxymagnesio derivative of ethyl *N*-*t*-butylmalonamate (derived from ethyl cyanoacetate and isobutylene in the presence of sulfuric acid). The resulting crude product (328) was cyclized to the desired hydronaphthacene (329) by sodium hydride in DMF in the presence of a small amount

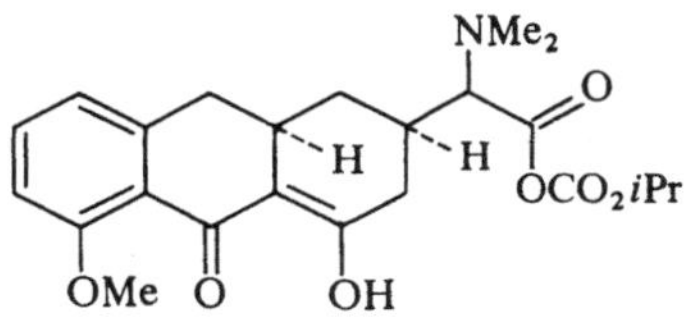

(327)

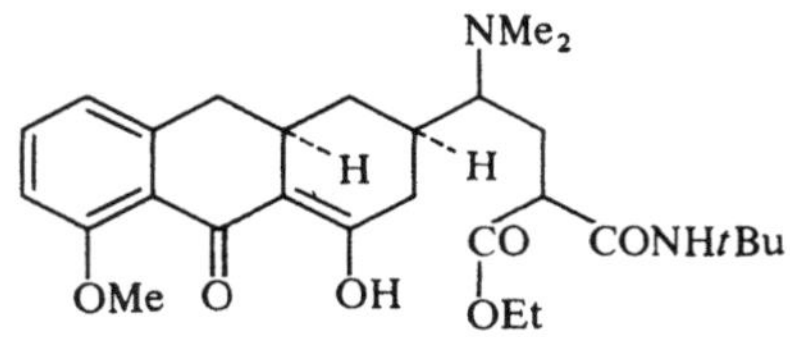

(328)

of methanol, conditions found only after extensive experimentation. This cyclization is considered quite remarkable, in view of the fact that a *tris*-anion is required, and the carbonyl group involved in the cyclization is deactivated in the formation of one of these anions. The methyl and *t*-butyl groups were readily cleaved by short exposure to hot aqueous hydrobromic acid to yield the *dl* form of 6,12a-dideoxy-6-demethyltetracycline (330), identical in all expected respects with the optically active variant derived by 12a-deoxygenation of 6-demethyl-6-deoxytetracycline (cf. BLACKWOOD et al. 1960b).

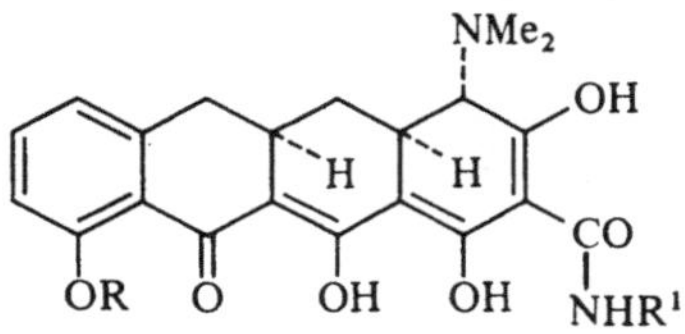

(329) R = Me, R^1 = *t*Bu
(330) R = R^1 = H

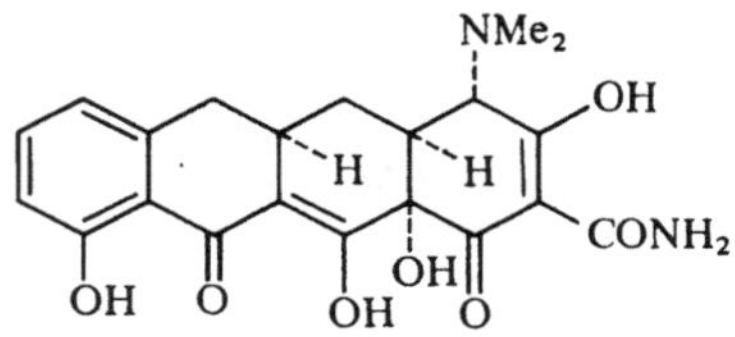

(105)

First identifying more favorable conditions by studies employing the optically active form, the *dl* form of (330) was stereospecifically oxygenated in buffered methanol/DMF, in the presence of cerous ion, to yield *dl*-6-demethyl-6-deoxytetracycline (105). While chromatography indicated that the initially formed product was the C4 *normal* isomer, considerable epimerization occurred in this process and during isolation. This was conveniently equilibrated to the all *normal* isomer by warming in basic, 1-butanolic calcium chloride (cf. NOSEWORTHY 1961).

The resulting *dl*-6-demethyl-6-deoxytetracycline was identical in all expected respects with the optically active variant derived by hydrogenolysis of 6-demethyltetracycline (see above); it possessed exactly half of the bioactivity of the asymmetric compound.

II. Muxfeldt et al.

Subsequent to the synthesis of *dl*-6-demethyl-6-deoxytetracycline described above, an alternative synthesis was reported by MUXFELDT and ROGALSKI (1965), suggested to be more amenable to large-scale operation. The starting point for this synthesis was the bromomethyl compound (226) of BOOTHE et al. (1959) and KENDE et al. (1961). Condensation with dimethyl carbomethoxysuccinate gave the adduct (331), which was hydrolyzed to the triacid (332), decarboxylated to the diacid (333), and cyclized by polyphosphoric acid to the tetralone acid (334).

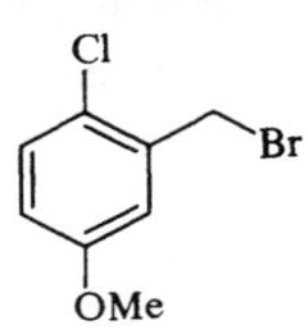

(226) X = Br

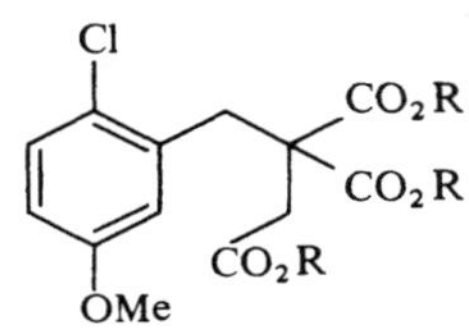

(331) R = Me
(332) R = H

Following procedures reported earlier (MUXFELDT 1962c; MUXFELDT et al. 1962b), the derived ester (335) was converted to the acetal, and then via alcohol (336), mesylate (337), and nitrile (338) transformed into the aldehyde (339) [cf. the BOOTHE et al. (1959) and KENDE et al. (1961) synthesis of the corresponding non-ketalized aldehyde (234)]. Condensation of the aldehyde (339) with hippuric acid in acetic anhydride with lead acetate as catalyst gave the oxazolone derivative (340), which was carefully deketalized to yield ketone.

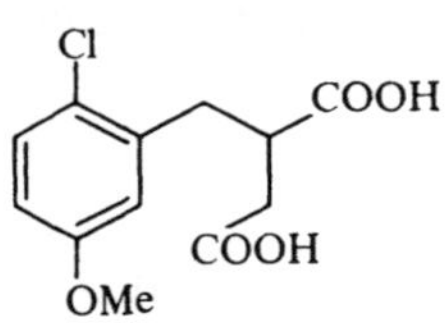

(333)

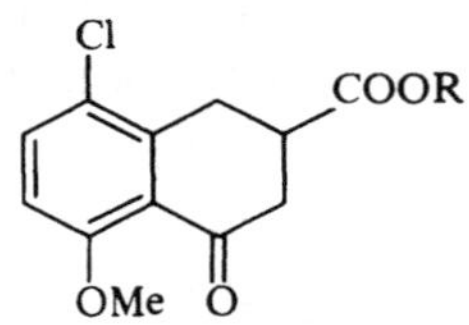

(334) R = H
(335) R = CH_3

In an unusual and rather complex reaction, studied separately in detail (MUXFELDT 1962c; MUXFELDT and HARDTMANN 1963; MUXFELDT et al. 1964, 1967), the ketone-oxazolone (340a) was condensed with methyl *N*-*t*-butyl-3-oxoglutaramate (341) to yield the tetracycline *bis*-amide (342), together with its 4- and 4a-epimers. Equilibration gave only two isomers, from which the single isomer (342) was isolated, treated with Meerwein's reagent and then acetic acid to yield the amine (343), and then treated with HBr in acetic acid to yield the phenolic amide

(344), as a C4 epimeric mixture. Simultaneous hydrogenolytic dechlorination and reductive methylation over Pd/C gave epimeric *dl*-6,12a-dideoxy-6-demethyltetracyclines (330), converted earlier to *dl*-6-demethyl-6-deoxytetracycline (105) as detailed in the preceding section, optionally using the oxygen-platinum method of MUXFELDT et al. (1962c) for the oxygenation step.

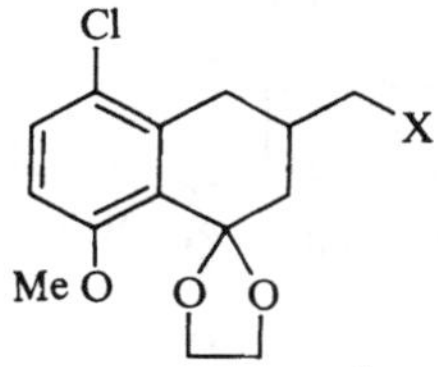

(336) X = OH
(337) X = OSO_2Me
(338) X = CN
(339) X = CHO

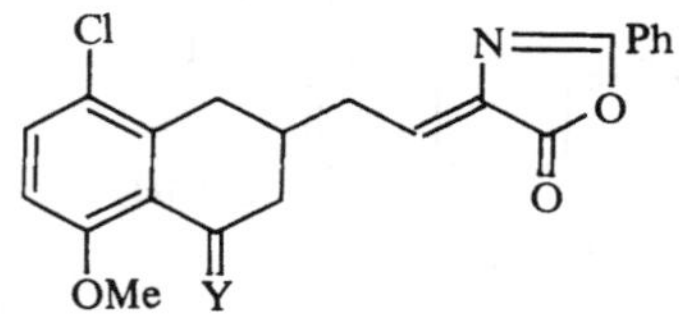

(340) Y = CH_2–O– / CH_2–O– (ethylenedioxy)
(340a) Y = O

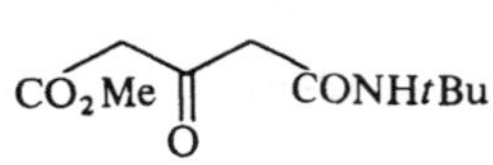

(341)

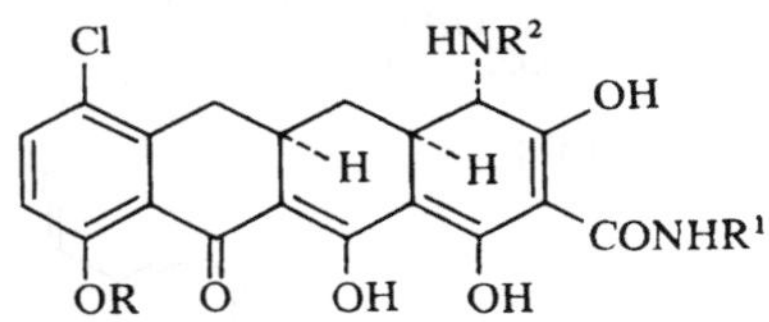

(342) R = Me, R^1 = *t*Bu, R^2 = COPh
(343) R = Me, R^1 = *t*Bu, R^2 = H
(344) R = R^1 = R^2 = H

MUXFELDT and ROGALSKI (1965) also reported that the tetralone (334) had been resolved into its optical isomers and that the synthesis of optically active 6-demethyl-6-deoxytetracycline would be reported at a later date.

MUXFELDT et al. (1973) by related methods also accomplished the total synthesis of a *dl*-7-chloro-β-6-deoxytetracycline precursor, detailed below as part of the total synthesis of chlortetracycline, while MARTIN et al. (1973) have extended this synthetic approach to a number of α- and β-6-deoxytetracycline analogues described in Sect. G.I below.

F. Total Synthesis of Fermentation Tetracyclines

I. Tetracycline: Shemyakin et al.

The first formal total synthesis of a fermentation tetracycline was that by the SHEMYAKIN group, working at the Institute for Chemistry of Natural Products, USSR Academy of Sciences, Moscow. This synthesis took advantage of the resynthesis of tetracycline from 12a-deoxy-5a,6-anhydrotetracycline (345).

The total synthesis of the latter compound was reported preliminarily by SHEMYAKIN et al. (1964d). The conversion of anhydrotetracycline (78) to tetracycline (87) via the hydroperoxide (346) was contemporaneously reported by SCHACH VON WITTENAU (1964) using the method of SCOTT and BEDFORD (1962).

Employing 12a-deoxy-5a,6-anhydrotetracycline (345) derived from tetracycline according to GREEN and BOOTHE (1960), the total synthesis of tetracycline was formally completed by hydroxylation of the latter to 5a,6-anhydrotetracycline (78) (GUREVICH et al. 1966), following essentially the method of MUXFELDT et al. (1962).

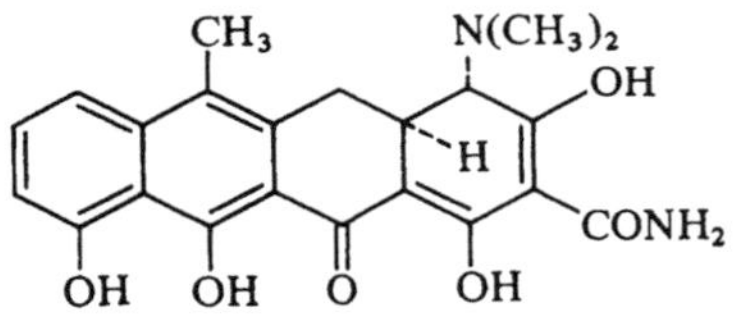

(345)

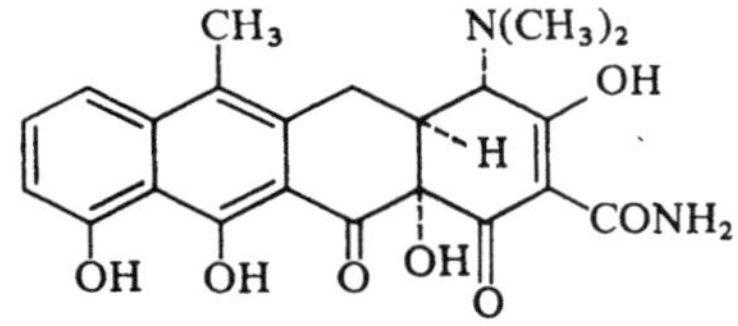

(78)

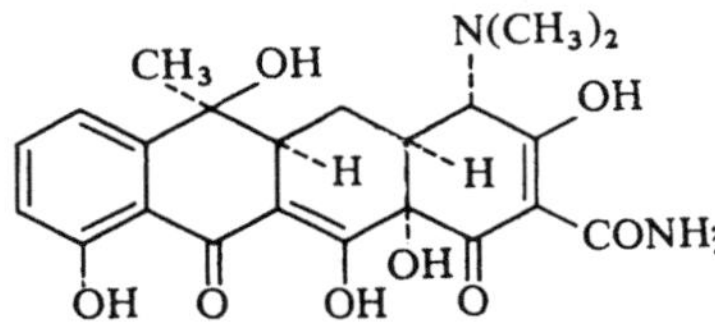

(87)

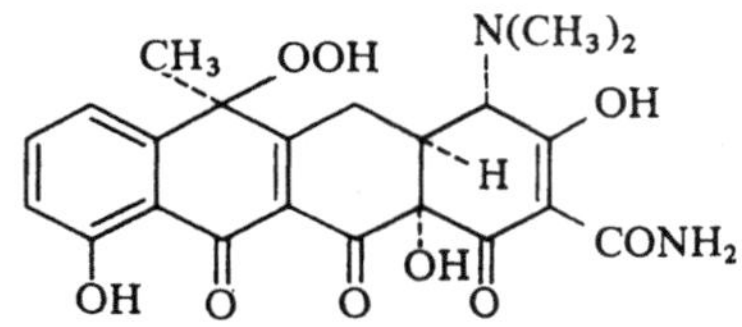

(346)

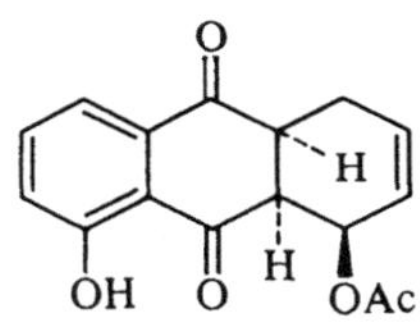

(297)

The early stages of the present synthesis have been detailed by KOLOSOV et al. (1963 b, c, 1964 a, b, c). The starting point was the anthraquinone (297) prepared earlier by INHOFFEN et al. (1957) through condensation of juglone with 1-acetoxybutadiene. Lithium aluminum hydride reduction gave (347) as the preferential ketonic alcohol. The phenolic group of (347) was benzylated to the ether (348), which was then converted to the methyl carbinol (349) with methylmagnesium io-

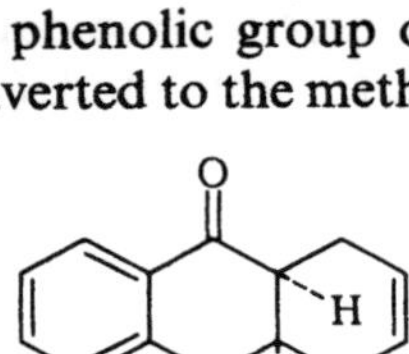

(347) R = H
(348) R = Bz

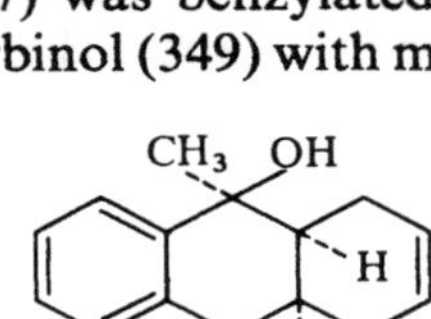

(349) R = Ac
(350) R = H

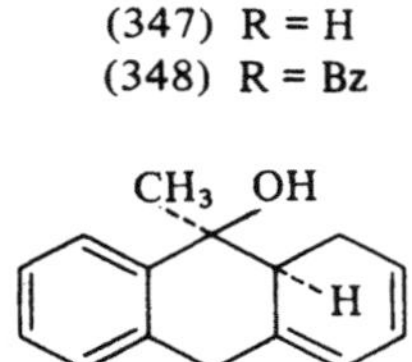

(351)

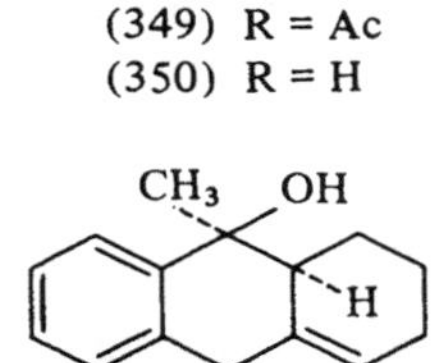

(352)

dide; interestingly, the acetate rearranged during the latter process. Following hydrolysis of the acetate ester, the *tris* alcohol (350) was oxidized with chromic acid in acetone to yield the enolized β-diketone (351). Of incidental interest was the hydrogenation of (351) to the tetracycline BCD-model compound (352).

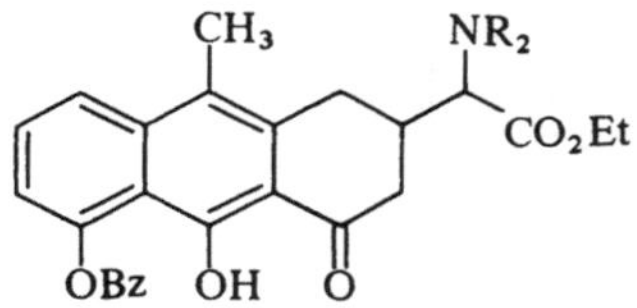

(352a) R = O
(353) R = H
(354) $R_2 = o{-}C_6H_4(CO)_2$

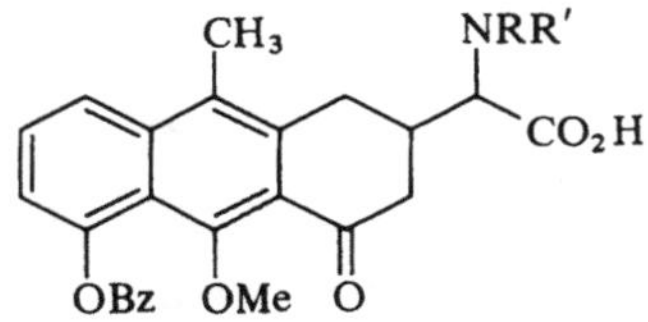

(355) $R = o{-}HOOCC_6H_4CO$
$R' = H$
(356) $RR' = o{-}C_6H_4(CO)_2$

The later stages of the present synthesis have been detailed by GUREVICH et al. (1967a, b, 1968b). The β-diketone (351) was condensed with ethyl nitroacetate, then dehydrated to yield the nitroester (352a), reduced to the aminoester (353) with zinc dust in acetic acid, and converted to the phthalimidoester (354) by reaction with carbethoxyphthalimide. Methylation with methyl iodide/silver oxide, followed by saponification and recrystallization of intermediate phthalamide (355) from hot diglyme, gave the methyl ether-acid (356). Treatment of (356) with phosphorus pentachloride-formamide, followed by $EtOMgCH(CO_2Et)CONH_2$, gave the *N*-phthaloylglycylomalonamate (357), which was cyclized by dimsyl anion in dimethylsulfoxide to the hydronaphthacene (358), in turn hydrolyzed with hydrogen bromide in acetic acid and methylated with methyl iodide in tetrahydrofuran to ($\pm$)-12-deoxy-5a,6-anhydrotetracycline (345).

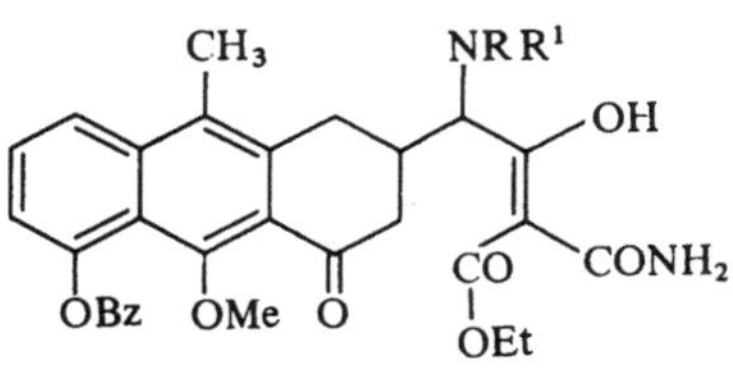

(357) $RR^1 = o{-}C_6H_4(CO)_2$

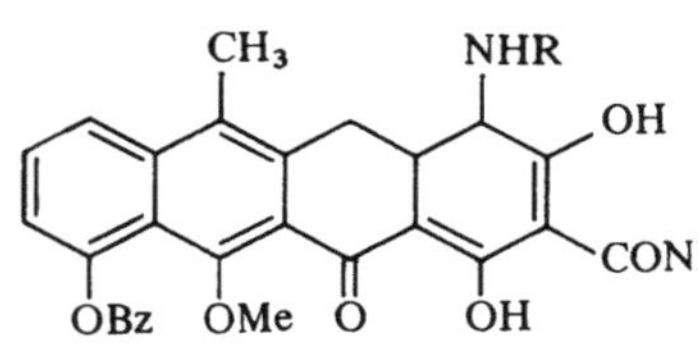

(358) $R = o{-}HOOCC_6H_4CO$

The Shemyakin group has also synthesized 4-dedimethylamino-5a,6-anhydrotetracycline from the juglone derivative (297) (GUREVICH et al. 1968b).

Furthermore, using considerably different synthetic intermediates, this group has made a close approach to the synthesis of 6-demethyltetracycline (GUREVICH et al. 1968c, 1969). Thus the 6-demethyltetracycline analogue (359) was synthe-

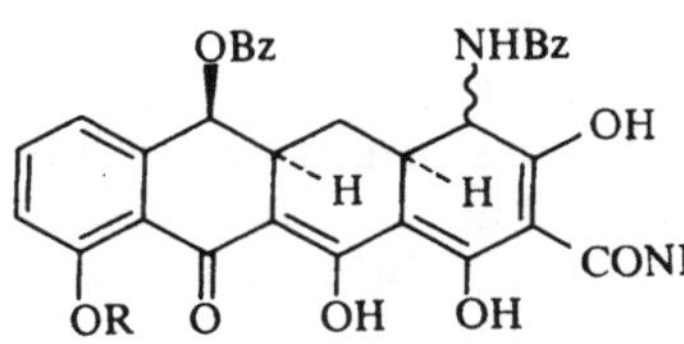

(359) R = H
(360) R = Bz

sized from the naphthalene triol (361), first converted to the allyl ether (362), and then pyrolyzed to the 2-allylquinone (363) and acetylated. Lithium aluminum hydride reduction of the acetate (364) gave the desired *cis* isomer (365) in generous

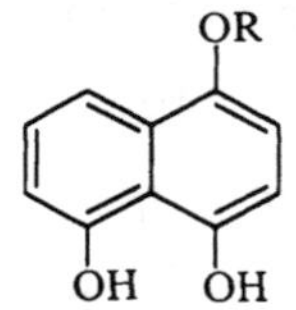

(361) R = H
(362) R = $CH_2CH{=}CH_2$

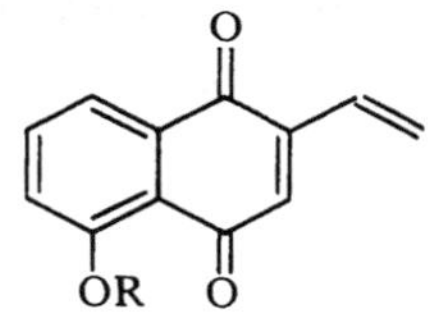

(363) R = H
(364) R = $COCH_3$

portion. Its benzyl derivative (366) was oxidized with osmium tetroxide/meta-periodic acid to the aldehyde (367). Then, following the Muxfeldt approach as detailed below, (367) was condensed with 2-phenyl-5-oxazolone to yield the azlactone (368), then condensed with the sodium salt of ethyl 3-oxoglutaramate to yield (369), cyclized using sodium dimsylate to the tribenzyl compound (360), and O^{10}-debenzylated to (359) in low yield with trifluoroacetic acid.

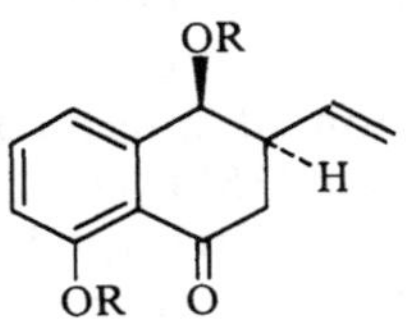

(365) R = H
(366) R = Bz

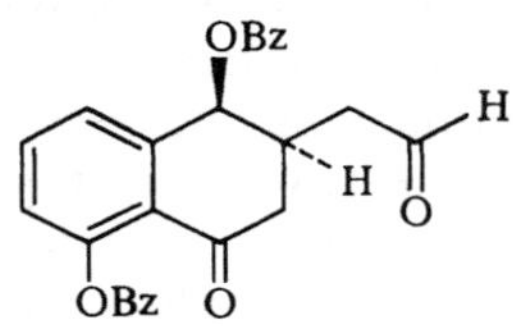

(367)

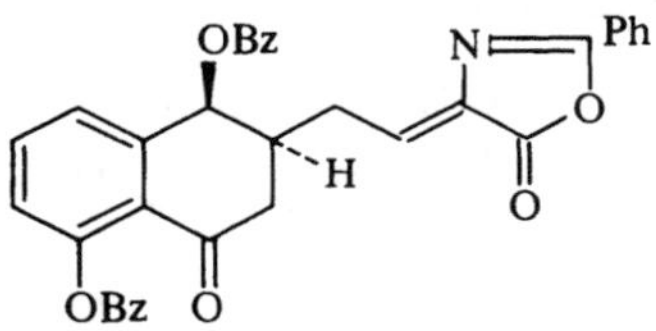

(368)

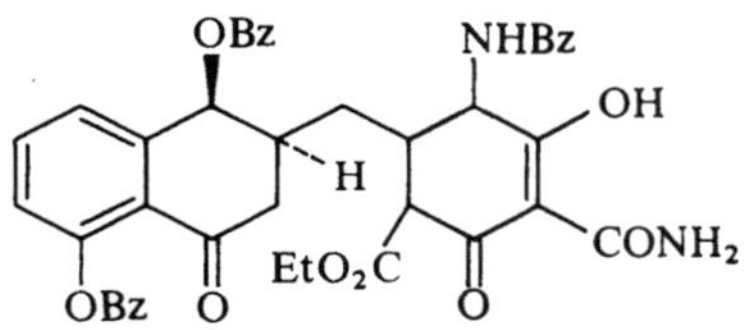

(369)

II. Chlortetracyclines: Muxfeldt et al.

The honor of the first and only formal total synthesis of chlortetracycline belongs to MUXFELDT et al. (1973), through their synthesis of *dl*-anhydrochlortetracycline, a compound earlier converted in its optically active form into chlortetracycline by photooxidation and reduction (SCOTT and BEDFORD 1962).

The earlier described nitrile (369a) (MUXFELDT et al. 1962b) (see above) was reduced with diisopropylaluminum hydride, using acid work-up, to yield the ketone-aldehyde (370). The latter was condensed with hippuric acid with lead acetate in acetic anhydride, affording the oxazolone (371). Condensation with methyl *N*-*t*-butyl-3-oxoglutaramate (342) gave a tautomeric mixture of four 4- and 4a-epimeric compounds, equilibrated to the simpler mixture of 4,4a-*bis*-epimeric compounds (372) and (373) in pyridine, compounds now readily separated by crystallization and chromatography.

While pointing out that either (372) or (373) can be converted to anhydrochlortetracycline, only the conversion of the latter was detailed. *cis*-Hydroxylation of (373) was accomplished by oxygenation at −9 °C in dimethylformamide/triethyl phosphite in the presence of potassium *t*-butoxide, affording the *dl*-12a-hydroxylated compound [(374), equivalent structures shown]. There followed alkylation to (375) with excess Meerwein's reagent in methylene chloride in the

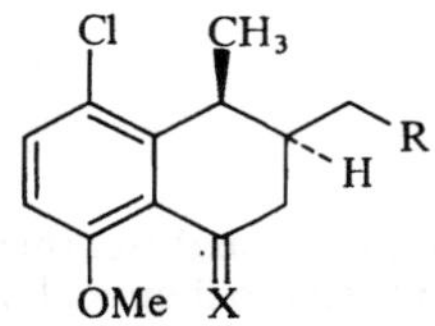

(369a) X = (CH_2–O–/CH_2–O–), R = CN
(370) X = O, R = HCO

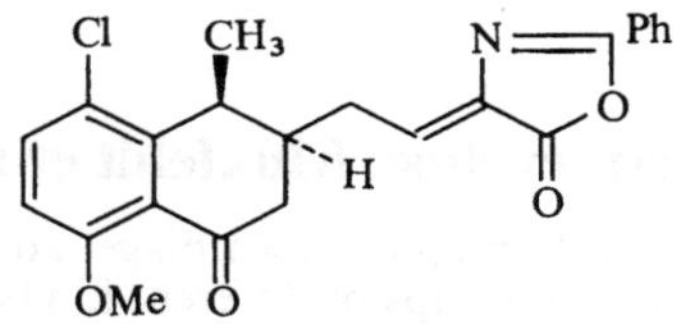

(371)

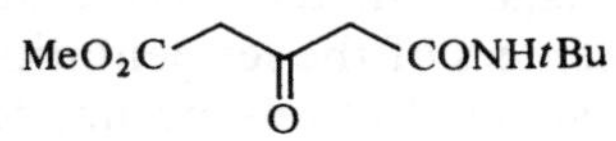

(342)

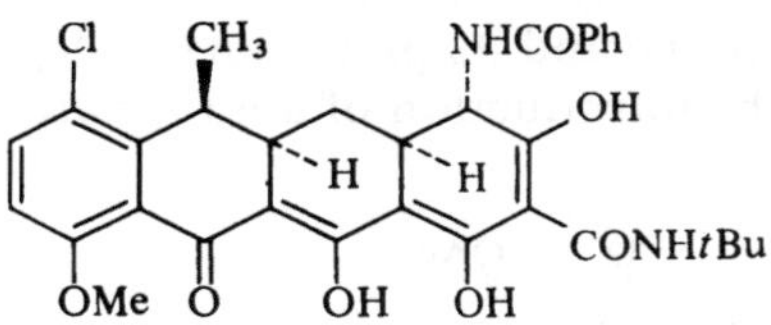

(372)

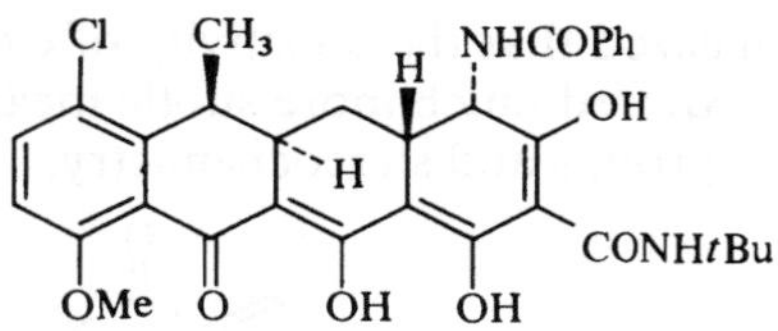

(373)

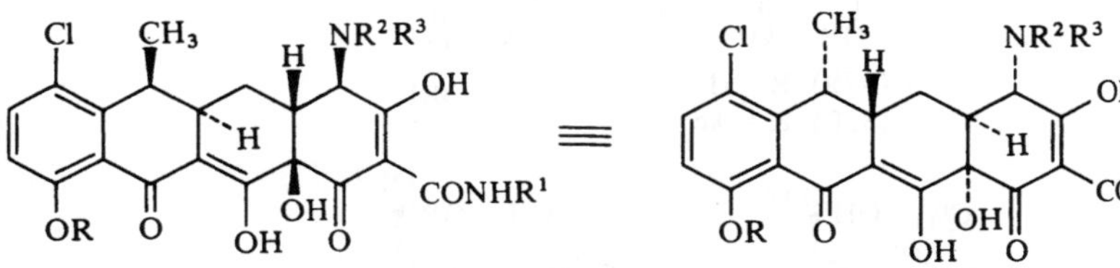

(374) R = Me, R^1 = *t*Bu, R^2 = H, R^3 = COPh
(375) R = Me, R^1 = *t*Bu, R^2R^3 = EtO(Ph)C=
(376) R = Me, R^1 = *t*Bu, R^2 = R^3 = H
(377) R = Me, R^1 = *t*Bu, R^2 = R^3 = Me
(378) R = R^1 = H, R^2 = R^3 = Me

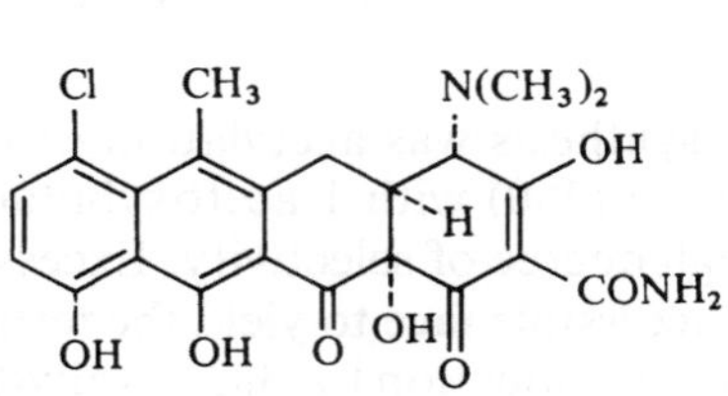

(77a)

presence of tetra-*N*-methyl-1,8-naphthalenediamine and methanolysis to the amine (376). The latter was dimethylated to (377) by treatment with sodium cyanoborohydride and formaldehyde in the presence of excess Hunig's base and the protecting groups R and R^1 removed by the action of 48% hydrobromic acid to produce *dl*-5a-epi-α-6-deoxytetracycline (378). Finally, dehydrogenation by dichlorodicyanobenzoquinone in dioxane gave the desired *dl*-anhydrochlortetracycline (77a).

III. Oxytetracycline: Muxfeldt et al.

The complicated tetracyclic assemblage, adorned with an unusual number of contiguous reactive functional groups of different kinds, replete with stereochemical imperatives, has presented a synthetic challenge to which many have responded (WOODWARD 1963).

The elegant synthesis of oxytetracycline, having the most complicated tetracyclic assemblage with the largest number of reactive functional groups and asymmetric centers of the fermentation tetracyclines, by MUXFELDT et al., represents the crown jewel of tetracycline total syntheses. The synthesis was reported preliminarily by MUXFELDT et al. (1968) and in detail by MUXFELDT et al. (1979). While principles evolved in their earlier prototype syntheses were used, it must be emphasized that the sensitivity of oxytetracycline and its precursors to degradation required much more subtle means for the introduction of appropriate functional groups and stereochemistry.

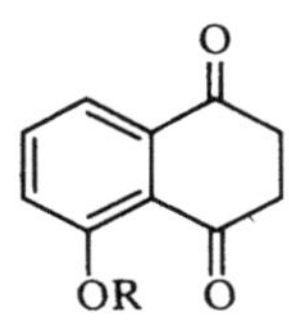

(379) R = H
(380) R = Ac

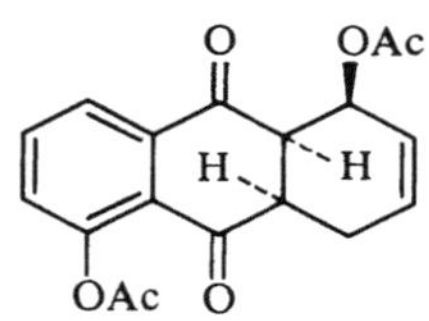

(381)

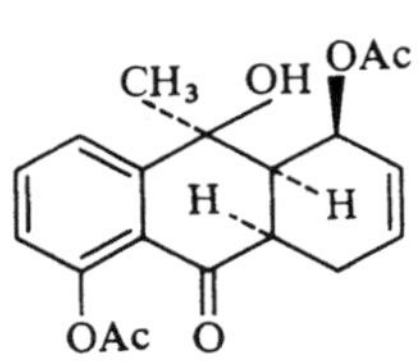

(382)

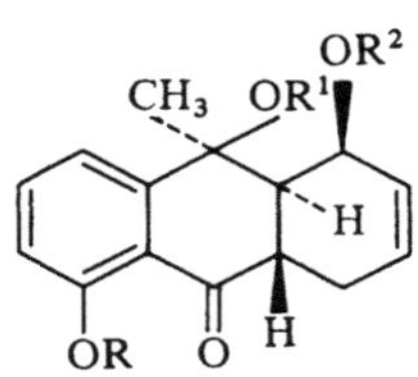

(383) R = R^1 = R^2 = H
(384) R = H, R^1R^2 = CH_3 CH_3
(385) R = Ac, R^1R^2 = CH_3 CH_3

The first step of the synthesis was acetylation of juglone (379), followed by condensation of the acetate (380) with 1-acetoxybutadiene to yield the tricyclic diacetate (381) with a high degree of selectivity. Excess methylmagnesium iodide attacked from the more accessible face to yield the tertiary alcohol (382), epimerized at ultimate C11a on saponification to (383). Anhydrous copper sulfate in acetone gave the acetonide (384), which was acetylated to (385) and the isolated double bond then oxidized to a mixture of *cis*-glycols (386), which were cleaved to the dialdehyde (387) with lead tetraacetate. At the time that this synthetic effort was initiated, MUXFELDT considered it likely that the dialdehyde (387) had appropriate stereochemistry at ultimate C5, cf. DONOHUE et al. (1963). Subsequent resolution of this question (SCHACH VON WITTENAU et al. 1965) necessitated further elaboration of these early intermediates.

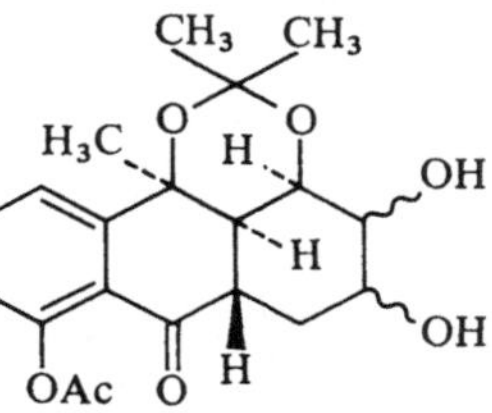

(386)

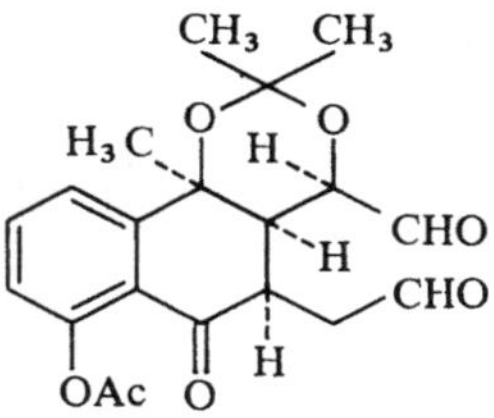

(387)

To obtain the required stereochemistry at C5 the dialdehyde was subjected to intramolecular Mannich reaction and elimination, affording (388). The latter sequence was accomplished by a mixture of diazabicyclooctane, catalytic amounts of piperidine, and acetic acid in refluxing toluene, avoiding isomerization of the double bond into conjugation with the ketone function. Ozonolysis of (388) produced a crystalline ozonide, cleaved with water to the crude diketodialdehyde (389), which was readily cleaved by alkali to the phenolic monoaldehyde (390) and also epimerized to the isomer having the more stable, required C5 stereochemistry when somewhat more vigorous alkaline conditions were employed. Purification was achieved via the base stable enamine (391), then converted to the methoxymethyl ether (392) with chloromethyl methyl ether by sodium hydride, and hydrolyzed back to the desired ether aldehyde (393) on moist silica gel.

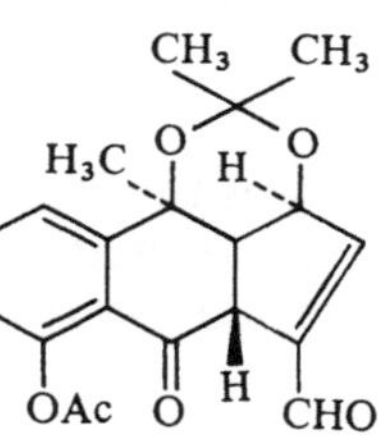

(388)

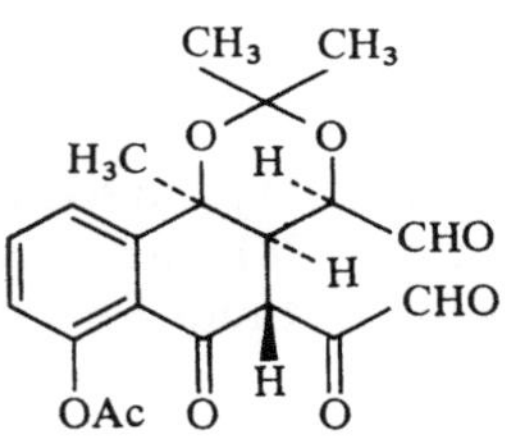

(389)

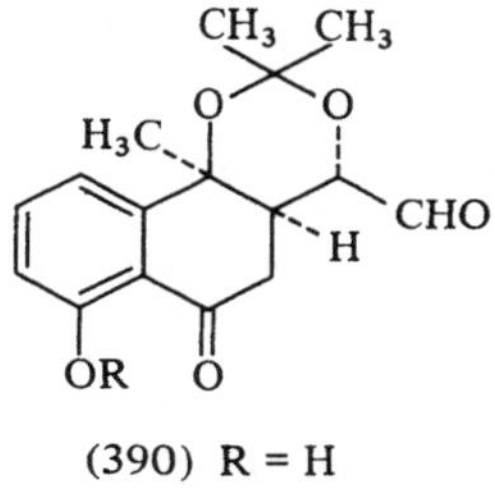

(390) R = H
(393) R = CH_2OMe

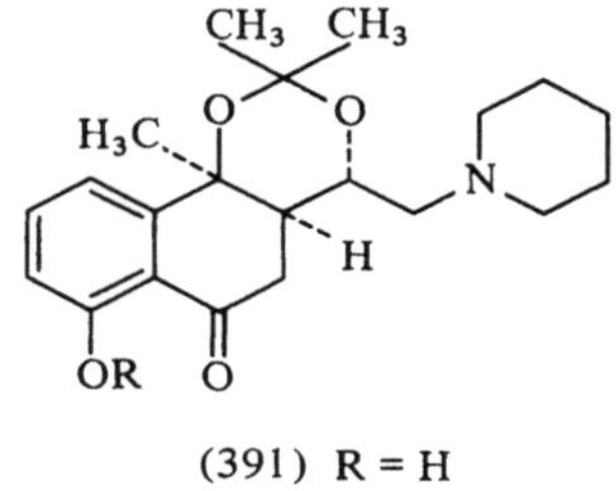

(391) R = H
(392) R = CH_2OMe

In remarkably direct manner, the aldehyde was condensed with 2-phenylthiazole-5-one (394) in the presence of basic lead acetate to yield the thiazolone

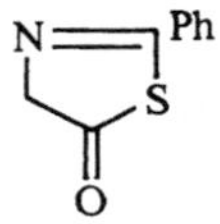

(394)

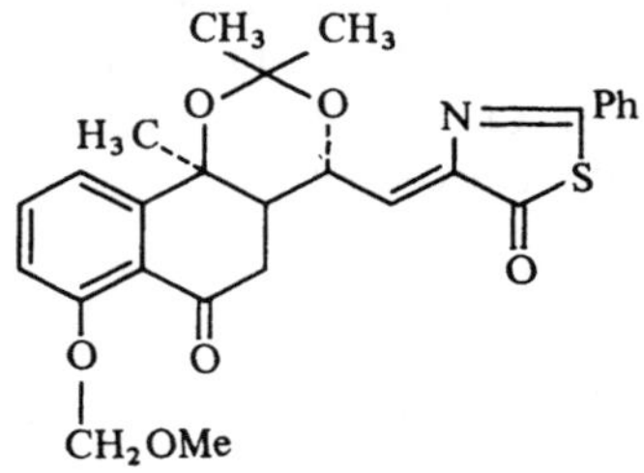

(395)

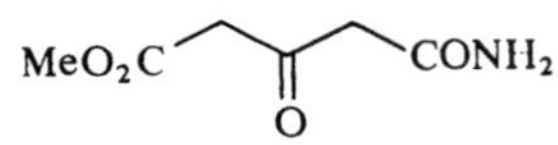

(396)

(395), then condensed with the lithio salt of 3-oxoglutaramate (396) in tetrahydrofuran to yield a mixture including (397); further addition of strong base (lithium or potassium *t*-butoxide) and heating led to B-ring closure and isolation of the crystalline 12a-deoxytetracycline analogue (398) in modest (27%) overal yield.

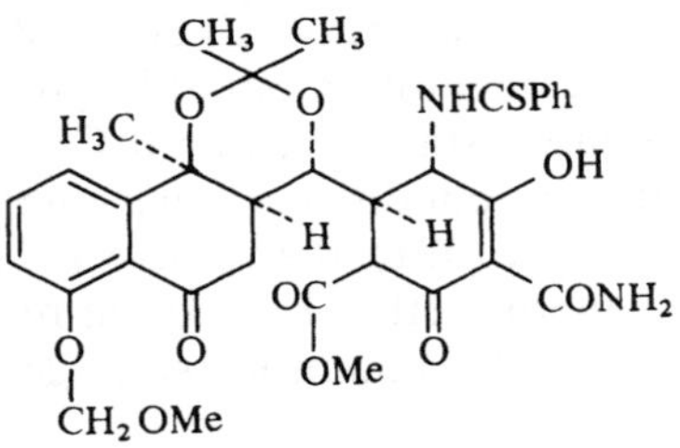

(397)

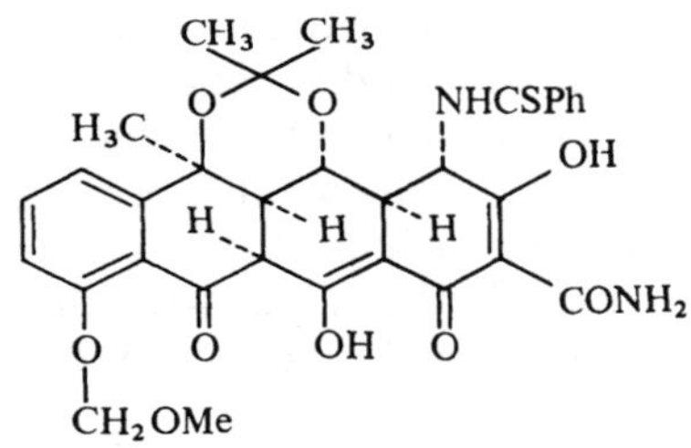

(398)

Of great concern in the synthesis at this point was the fact that acid would not cleave the actonide of (398) without concomitant aromatization of the C-ring. Furthermore, existing methods for stereospecific 12a-hydroxylation proved un-

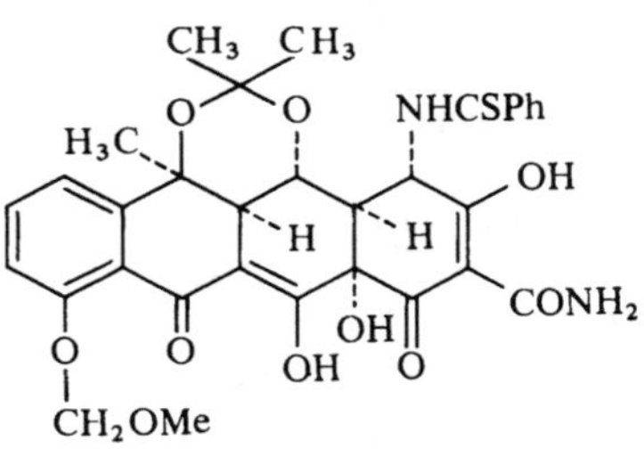

(399)

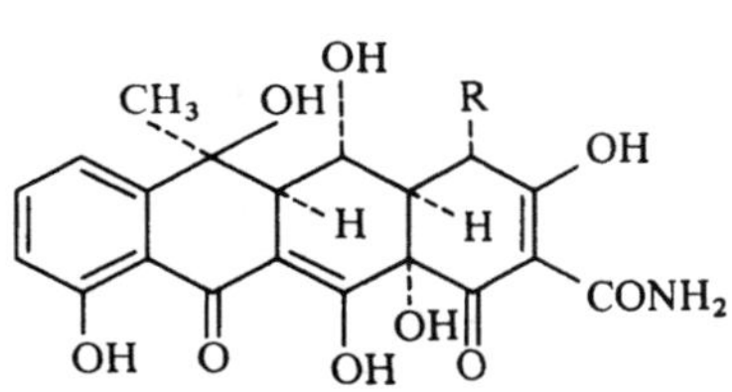

(400) R = NHCSPh

(401) R = $\overset{+}{\underset{H}{N}}$=C(Ph)SMe

(402) R = NH_2

(5) R = NMe_2

satisfactory. Ultimately, 12a-hydroxylation was accomplished by gaseous oxygen in tetrahydrofuran/triethylphosphite in the presence of sodium hydride, a novel and highly reproducible method discovered by necessity (the mother of invention). Providently, the acetonide group of the 12a-hydroxy compound (399) was readily hydrolyzed without significant 5a,6-dehydration, yielding the thioamide (400). The latter was methylated at sulfur by methyl iodide to produce (401), then hydrolyzed to the amine (402) in hydrochloric acid under conditions sufficiently mild to avoid significant 5a,6-dehydration. Finally, alkylation of the amine hydrochloride with dimethylsulfate in the presence of diisopropylethylamine (Hunig's base) gave the long-sought synthetic *dl*-oxytetracycline (5).

G. Total Synthesis of Tetracycline Analogues

The original tetracyclines, oxytetracycline and chlortetracycline, were derived by fermentation. These compounds were followed by a trickle of highly active tetracyclines made either biosynthetically by blocked mutants (notably demethyltetracyclines) or chemically (notably tetracycline itself, also available by fermentation). The discovery of the 6-deoxytetracyclines and 6-methylenetetracyclines were keys to a large number of active tetracyclines and much insight into structure-activity relationships; and furthermore led to the clinical use of superior tetracyclines such as α-6-deoxytetracycline (doxycycline) and 4-dimethylamino-6-demethyl-6-deoxytetracycline (minocycline).

Although it is unlikely that the fermentation tetracyclines, or their derivatives, will ever be prepared commercially by total synthesis, the future nevertheless belongs to tetracycline analogues prepared by total synthesis, permitting the rational design and preparation of clinically advantageous tetracycline antibiotics. While some of the early efforts in this direction appear disappointing, already a viable candidate for clinical use is seen in 6-thiatetracycline, whose synthesis is described in the final section below.

I. *dl*-7-Chloro-6-deoxytetracyclines

Extending work reported earlier by Muxfeldt and Rogalski (1965) and Muxfeldt et al. (1973), Martin et al. (1973) have reported the synthesis of a number of racemic 7-chloro-6-deoxytetracycline analogues prepared from the compounds (342), (372), (373), and (403). In this case 12a-oxygenation was accomplished by base-catalyzed autoxidation, yielding compounds (374) and (404)–(406). Hydrolysis of the latter compounds in hot 48% HBr gave the deprotected 4-amino analogues (407)–410), reported to possess unspecified biological activity.

Removing the benzoyl group selectively by treatment with Meerwein's reagent and hydrolysis of the intermediate iminoether, the benzamides (374) and (404)–(406) were converted to the protected amines (376) and (411)–(413). Compounds (411)–(413) were alkylated with dimethyl or diethylsulfate, as appropriate, to yield the tertiary amines (414)–(416), then deprotected to yield the dialkyl amines (417)–(419), also reported to have unspecified bioactivity.

The intermediate (342) was earlier reported in the total synthesis of *dl*-6-demethyl-6-deoxytetracycline by Muxfeldt and Rogalski (1965); the byproduct (403) was at that time misidentified as the 4-epimer of (342). The intermediates (372)–(376) were previously reported as intermediates in the total synthesis of *dl*-anhydrochlortetracycline by Muxfeldt et al. (1973).

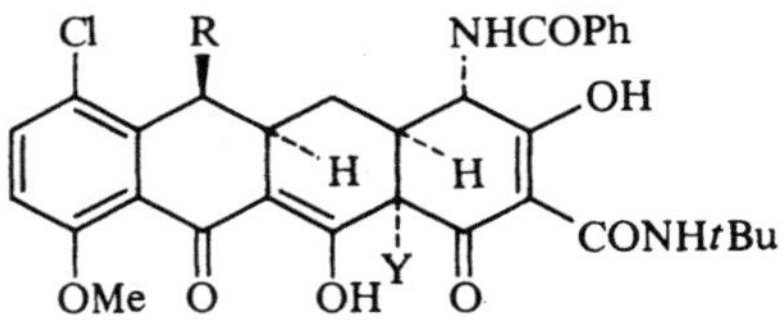

(342) R = Y = H
(372) R = CH_3, Y = H
(404) R = H, Y = OH
(405) R = CH_3, Y = OH

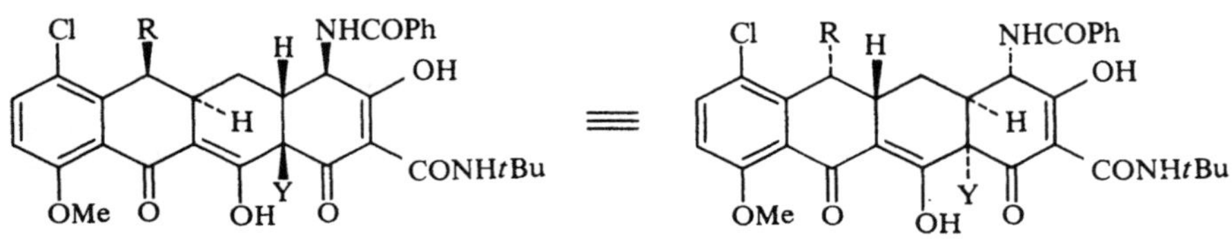

(403) R = Y = H
(373) R = CH_3, Y = H
(406) R = H, Y = OH
(374) R = CH_3, Y = OH

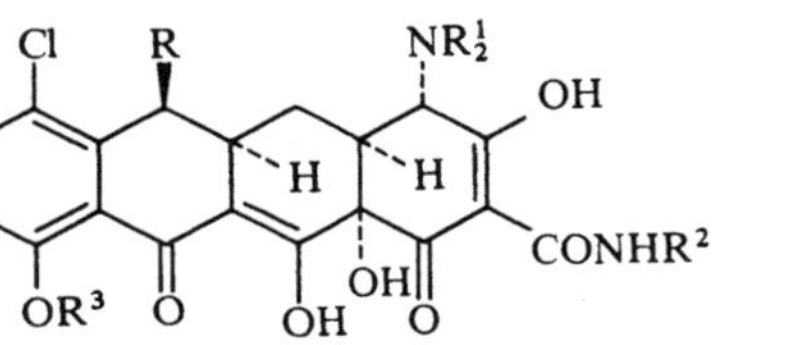

(407) R = R^1 = R^2 = R^3 = H
(408) R = Me, R^1 = R^2 = R^3 = H
(411) R = R^1= H, R^2 = *t*Bu, R^3 = Me
(412) R = R^3 = Me, R^1 = H, R^2 = *t*Bu
(414) R = H, R^1 = R^3 = Me, R^2 = *t*Bu
(415) R = R^1 = R^3 = Me, R^2 = *t*Bu
(417) R = R^2 = R^3 = H, R^1 = Me
(418) R = R^1 = Me, R^2 = R^3 = H

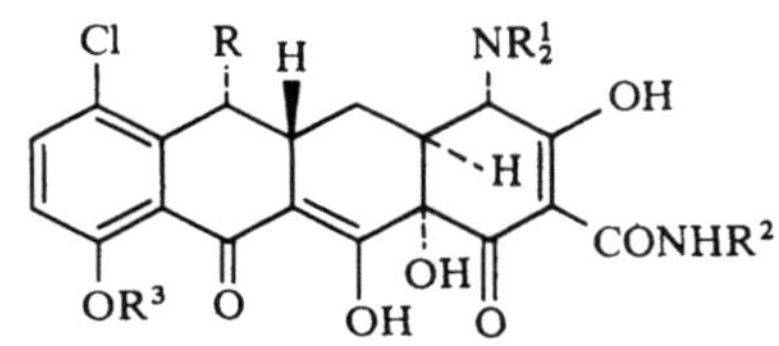

(409) R = R^1 = R^2 = R^3 = H
(410) R = Me, R^1 = R^2 = R^3 = H
(413) R = R^1 = H, R^2 = *t*Bu, R^3 = Me
(376) R = R^3 = Me, R^1 = H, R^2 = *t*Bu
(416) R = H, R^1 = E+, R^2 = *t*Bu, R^4 = Me
(419) R = R^2 = R^3 = H, R^2 = Et

II. *dl*-8-Hydroxy-6-demethyl-6-deoxytetracycline

Essentially substituting 3,5-dimethoxybenzoate for m-methoxybenzoate, the synthetic sequence used by Muxfeldt and Rogalski (1965) to prepare *dl*-6,12a-dideoxy-6-demethyltetracycline (330), Glatz et al. (1979) synthesized *dl*-8-hydroxy-6-demethyl-6-deoxytetracycline (420). The activity of this compound, unavailable from fermentation tetracyclines by any known route, was of considerable theoretical interest, in the light of the biosynthetic origin of the tetracyclines. Disappointingly, however, the compound was reported to have only limited in vitro antibacterial activity and no in vivo activity.

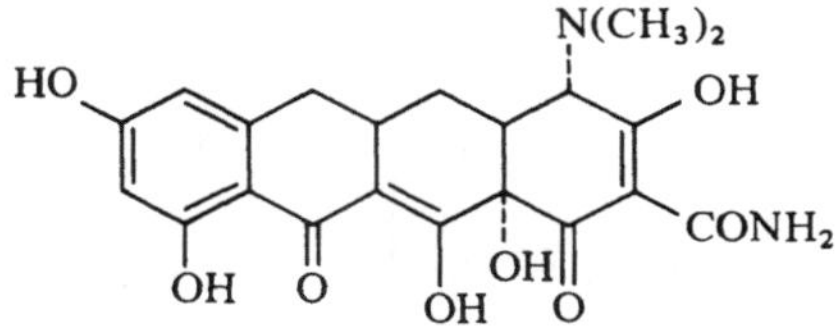

(420)

The condensation of the azlactone (421) with methyl 3-oxoglutaramate, paralleling the earlier synthetic sequence, gave no useful yields of tetracyclic compounds. However, substitution of thioazlactone (422) provided the expected mixture of four 4,4a-epimeric products, from which the 4-epimeric compounds having the required 4a,5a stereochemistry could be isolated by chromatography. One

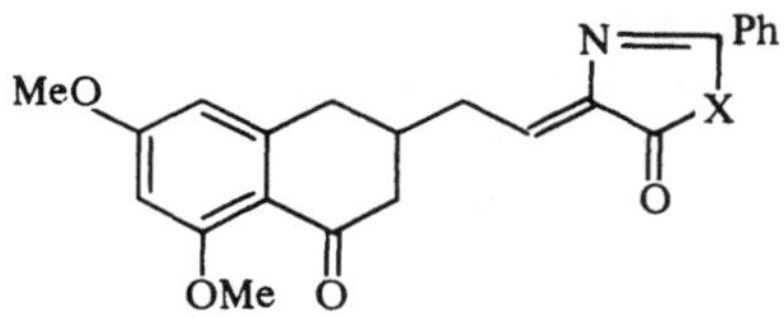

(421) X = O
(422) X = S

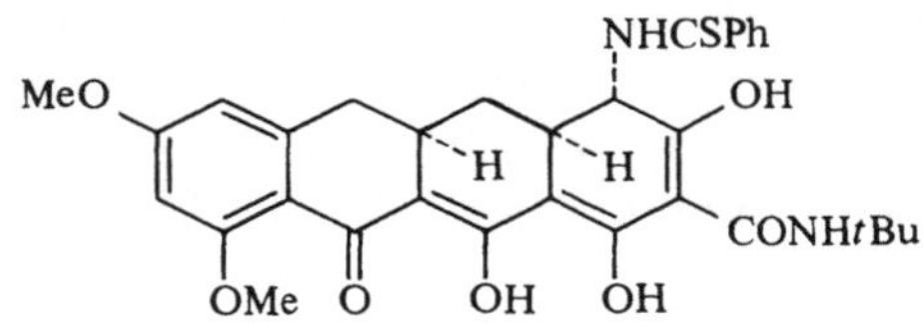

(423)

of these (423) was 12a-hydroxylated (oxygen in basic dimethylformamide/tetrahydrofuran containing sodium hydride and triethylphosphite) to (424); the thioamine alkylated with triethyloxonium fluoroborate (Meerwein's reagent) and hydrolyzed to the amine (425) with aqueous acid, reductively methylated with formaldehyde and sodium cyanoborohydride to yield the dimethylamine (426), and readily epimerized to (427) on silica gel.

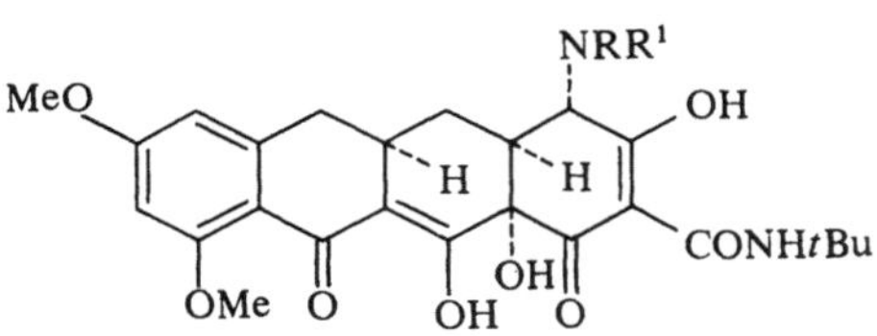

(424) $R = H, R^1 = CSPh$
(425) $R = R^1 = H$
(426) $R = R^1 = Me$

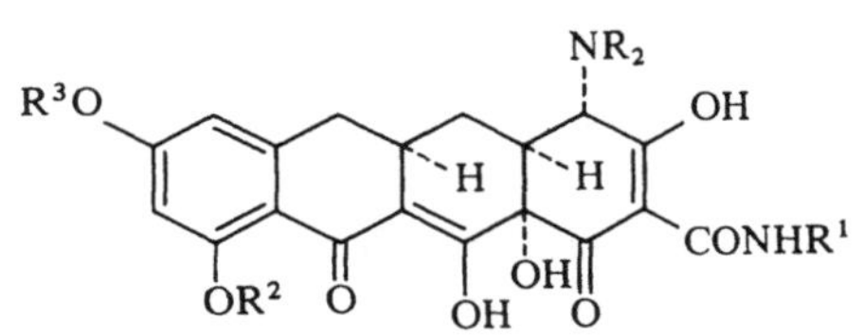

(427) $R = R^2 = R^3 = Me, R^1 = t\mathrm{Bu}$
(428) $R = R^3 = Me, R^2 = H, R^1 = t\mathrm{Bu}$
(420) $R = Me, R^1 = R^2 = R^3 = H$

The *dl*-dimethylamino compound of requisite stereochemistry was selectively hydrolyzed to the monophenol (428) by boron tribromide. Its structure was fully confirmed by X-ray crystallographic analysis. Treatment of (427) with hot conc. hydriodic acid gave the completely deprotected compound (420).

III. *dl*-6-Thiatetracycline

Following the basic strategy of MUXFELDT et al., KIRCHLECHNER and ROGALSKI (1980) have recently reported the preparation of the heterocyclic tetracycline analogue (429), dubbed "6-thiatetracycline." This compound, available only by total synthesis, is reported to be superior in its antibacterial spectrum to all known tetracyclines.

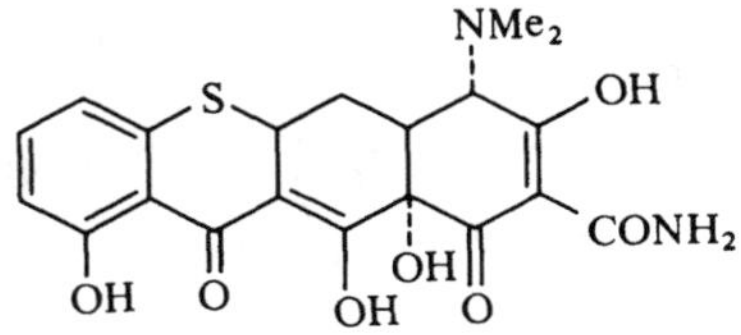

(429)

2-Chloro-5-methoxy-thiophenol (430), derived from the corresponding aniline by standard methods, was condensed with the unsaturated ester (431), hydrolyzed to the diacid (432), and then cyclized in anhydrous hydrogen fluoride to the bicyclic acid (433). In contrast to the MUXFELDT strategy of waiting to the last stages of the synthesis, the ether was cleaved to the phenol (434) in the next step. The chlorine, originally present to direct the cyclization *ortho* to the phenol, was then removed by hydrogenation, affording (434), and the acid converted to the aldehyde (436) via the acid chloride and the Rosenmund reduction.

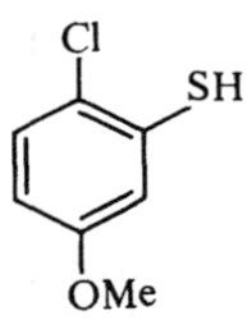

(430)

+

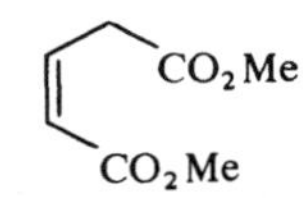

(431)

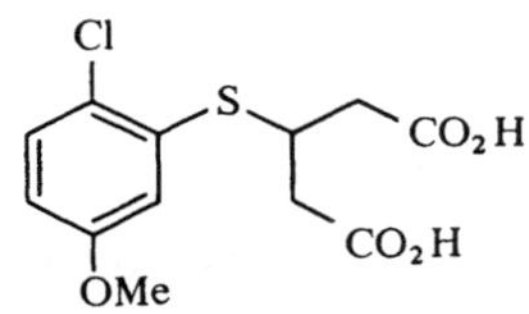

(432)

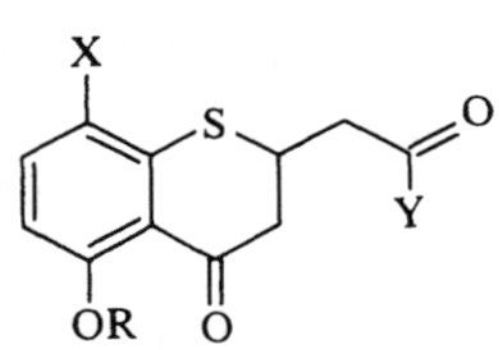

(433) X = Cl, Y = OH, R = Me
(434) X = Cl, Y = OH, R = H
(435) X = R = H, Y = H
(436) X = R = Y = H

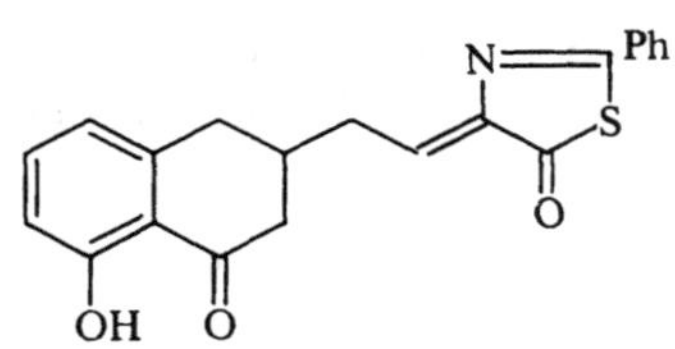

(437)

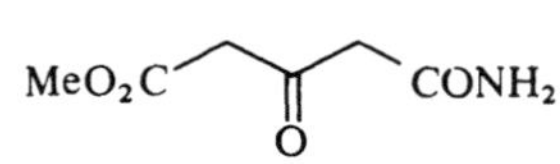

(396)

Following the methods of MUXFELDT et al., the aldehyde (436) was converted to the thioazlactone (437), which was condensed with methyl 3-oxoglutaramate (396) in two steps, without isolation of the intermediate, producing a mixture of three tetracyclic compounds, only one of which (438) had the required C4, C4a, and

C5a stereochemistry. However, when maintained in piperidine at 50 °C for 1 h both of the other isomers epimerized to the desired compound, i.e., not only epimerization at C4, but also the conversion of the 4a,5a-*anti* isomer to its *syn* analogue.

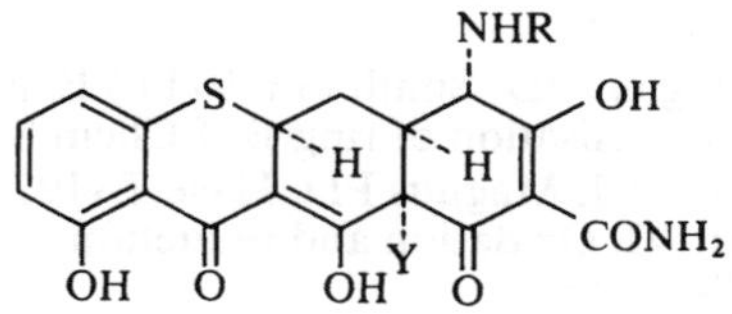

(438) Y = H, R = CSPh
(439) Y = OH, R = CSPh
(440) Y = OH, R = H

The 12a-deoxy analogue (438) was hydroxylated by base-catalyzed oxygenation, affording (439). Treatment with Meerwein's reagent and aqueous acid hydrolysis of the intermediate imino ether gave the amine (440). The latter was reductively methylated with formaldehyde and sodium cyanoborohydride to produce *dl*-6-thiatetracycline (429).

The full structure of 6-thiatetracycline has been confirmed by X-ray crystallography (PREWO and STEZOWSKI 1980b; PREWO et al. 1980).

References

Amaro A, Carreño MC, Fariña F (1979) Synthesis of tetracyclic hydroxyquinones by cycloaddition reactions with dienols. Tetrahedron Lett 1979:3383–3386

Arbuzov YA, Bolesov IG, Ahuze AL, Koslov MN, Osanova LK, Shemyakin MM (1965) Tetracyclines. XXXIII. Synthesis of 8-chloro-5-methoxy-3,10-dioxo-1,2,3,4,4a,9,9a,10-octahydroanthracene (in Russian). Izv Akad SSSR [Khim] 1965:806–810

Asleson GL, Frank CW (1975) Carbon-13 nuclear magnetic resonance spectral analysis of tetracycline hydrochloride and related antibiotics. J Am Chem Soc 97:6246–6248

Asleson GL, Frank CW (1976) pH dependence of carbon-13 nuclear magnetic resonance shifts of tetracycline. Microscopic dissociation constants. J Am Chem Soc 98:4745–4749

Asleson GL, Stoel LJ, Newman EC, Frank CW (1974) NMR spectra of tetracyclines: assignment of additional protons. J Pharm Sci 63:1144–1146

Aufderhaar E, Baldwin JE, Barton DHR, Faulkner DJ, Slayton M (1971) Experiments on the synthesis of tetracycline. Part III. Michael-type cyclisation in the formation of ring B. J Chem Soc [C] 1971:2175–2183

Baker WA Jr, Brown PM (1966) Metal binding in tetracyclines. Cobalt (II) and nickel (II) complexes. J Am Chem Soc 88:1314–1317

Bakshi VM, Kulkarni AB (1962) Tetracyclines. V. Synthesis of hexahydronaphthacenes having different substituents in ring D. J Sci Ind Res (India) 21B:542–546

Bakshi VM, Kulkarni AB (1963) Tetracyclines. VI. Synthesis of naphthacenequinones. Indian J Chem 1:215–217

Baldwin JE, Barton DHR, Gutteridge NJA, Martin RJ (1971) Experiments on the synthesis of tetracycline. Part IV. Ring B formation through 1,3-dipolar additions. J Chem Soc [C] 1971:2184–2192

Barde DP, Kulkarni AB (1978) Tetracyclines. Part XIV. Stereochemistry of isomeric 5,5a,6,11,11a,12-hexahydronaphthacene-6,12-diones and diols. Indian J Chem [Sect B] 16B:959–962

Barrett H (1963) Synthesis of tetracycline analogs. J Pharm Sci 52:309–330
Barton DHR, Magnus PD (1971) Experiments on the synthesis of tetracycline. Part I. Introduction to the series. J Chem Soc [C] 1971:2164–2166
Barton DHR, Halpern B, Porter QN, Collins DJ (1971 a) Experiments on the synthesis of tetracycline. Part II. The synthesis of potential ring A and ring C–ring D components. J Chem Soc [C] 1971:2166–2174
Barton DHR, Clive DLJ, Magnus PD, Smith G (1971 b) Experiments on the synthesis of tetracycline. Part V. Photocyclisation of ring B. J Chem Soc [C] 1971:2193–2203
Barton DHR, Bould L, Clive DLJ, Magnus PD, Hase T (1971 c) Experiments on the synthesis of tetracycline. Part VI. Oxidation and reduction of potential ring A precursors. J Chem Soc [C] 1971:2204–2215
Barton DHR, Magnus PD, Hase T (1971 d) Experiments on the synthesis of tetracycline. Part VII. The total synthesis of 6-methylpretetramid. J Chem Soc [C] 1971:2215–2225
Barton DHR, Magnus PD, Pearson MJ (1971 e) Experiments on the synthesis of tetracycline. Part VIII. An attempted synthesis of 4-hydroxy-6-methylpretetramid. J Chem Soc [C] 1971:2225–2231
Barton DHR, Magnus PD, Pearson MJ (1971 f) Experiments on the synthesis of tetracycline. Part IX. The synthesis and rearrangement of 6-acyloxycyclohexa-2,4-dienones. J Chem Soc [C] 1971:2231–2241
Barton DHR, Challis JA, Magnus PD, Marshall JP (1971 g) Experiments on the synthesis of tetracycline. Part X. Synthesis of a tetracycline compound suitable for 12a α-hydroxylation. J Chem Soc [C] 1971:2241–2243
Barton DHR, Magnus PD, Smith G, Streckert G, Zurr D (1972 a) Experiments on the synthesis of tetracycline. Part XI. Oxidation of ketone acetals and ethers by hydride transfer. J Chem Soc Perkin Trans I 1972:542–552
Barton DHR, Magnus PD, Okogun JI (1972 b) Experiments on the synthesis of tetracycline. Part XII. Extension of the acetal photocyclisation process. J Chem Soc Perkin Trans I 1972:1103–1105
Barton DHR, Magnus PD, Quinney JC (1975) Experiments on the synthesis of tetracycline. Part XIII. Oxidation of ring A model phenols to *p*-hydroxycyclohexadienones. J Chem Soc Perkin Trans I 1975:1610–1614
Barton DHR, Bateson JH, Datta SC, Magnus PD (1976) Experiments on the synthesis of tetracycline. Part 14. Closure of ring B by base-catalysed photocyclisation. J Chem Soc Perkin Trans I 1976:503–507
Barton DHR, Ley SV, Magnus PD, Rosenfeld MN (1977 a) Experiments on the synthesis of tetracycline. Part 15. Oxidation of phenols and ring A model phenols to *o*-hydroxydienones with benzene-selenic anhydride. J Chem Soc Perkin Trans I 1977:567–572
Barton DHR, Ley SV, Meguro K, Williams DJ (1977 b) Reaction of tetracycline hydrochloride with *N*-chlorosuccinimide: X-ray crystal structure of the major product. J Chem Soc Chem Commun 1977:790–791
Beereboom JJ, Ursprung JJ, Rennhard HH, Stephens CR (1960) Further 6-deoxytetracycline studies: effect of aromatic substituents on biological activity. J Am Chem Soc 82:1003–1004
Berlin YA, Volkov YP, Kolosov MN, Ovchinnikov YA, Yeh C-T, Shemyakin MM (1964 a) Tetracyclines. XXIII. New paths for construction of ring A in dedimethylaminotetracyclines (in Russian). Zh Obshch Khim 34:790–798
Berlin YA, Kolosov MN, Shemyakin MM (1964 b) Tetracyclines. XXIV. Construction of ring A of tetracyclines (in Russian). Zh Obshch Khim 34:798–807
Blackwood RK (1969) Tetracyclines. In: Kirk-Othmer Encyclopedia of chemical technology, 2nd edn, vol 20. Wiley, New York, pp 1–33
Blackwood RK, Schach von Wittenau M (1971) Esters of 5-hydroxytetracyclines. US Patent 3,579,564
Blackwood RK, Stephens CR (1962 a) 6-Methylenetetracyclines. II. Mercaptan adducts. J Am Chem Soc 84:4157–4158
Blackwood RK, Stephens CR Jr (1962 b) Alkanoic acid esters of 5-hydroxytetracyclines and process for preparation US Patent 3,047,617

Blackwood RK, Stephens CR (1964) Novel C-4 modified tetracycline derivatives. J Am Chem Soc 86:2736–2737

Blackwood RK, Stephens CR (1965) Some transformation of tetracycline at the 4-position. Can J Chem 43:1382–1388

Blackwood RK, Rennhard HH, Stephens CR (1960a) Some transformations at the 12a-position of the tetracyclines. J Am Chem Soc 82:745

Blackwood RK, Rennhard HH, Stephens CR (1960b) Some transformations at the 12a-position in the tetracycline series. J Am Chem Soc 82:5194–5197

Blackwood RK, Beereboom JJ, Rennhard HH, Schach von Wittenau M, Stephens CR (1961) 6-Methylenetetracyclines. I. A new class of tetracycline antibiotics. J Am Chem Soc 83:2773–2774

Blackwood RK, Beereboom JJ, Rennhard HH, Schach von Wittenau M, Stephens CR (1963) 6-Methylenetetracyclines. III. Preparation and properties. J Am Chem Soc 85:3943–3953

Bolesov IG, Kolosov MN, Shemyakin MM (1963a) Synthesis of a demethyltetracycline analog. Tetrahedron Lett 1963:1631–1636

Bolesov IG, Kolosov MN, Shemyakin MM (1963b) Synthesis of a demethyltetracycline analog (in Russian). Dokl Akad Nauk SSSR 151:1097–1099

Bolesov IG, Kolosov MN, Shemyakin MM (1965) Tetracyclines. XXXIV. Synthesis of an analog of 6-demethyltetracycline, 2-decarboxamido-4-dedimethylamino-6,10,12,trideoxy-6-demethyl-11a,12-dihydrotetracycline (in Russian). Izv Akad Nauk SSSR [Khim] 1965:1039–1094

Boothe JH (1963) Chemistry and biological activities of the tetracyclines. In: Sylvester JC (ed) Antimicrobial agents and chemotherapy – 1962. American Society for Microbiology, Washington, pp 213–225

Boothe JH, Kushner S, Petisi J, Williams JH (1953a) Synthesis of degradation products of Aureomycin. IV. J Am Chem Soc 75:3261–3263

Boothe JH, Kushner S, Williams JH (1953b) Synthesis of degradation products of Aureomycin. V. J Am Chem Soc 82:3262–3264

Boothe JH, Morton J II, Petisi JP, Wilkinson RG, Williams JH (1953c) Tetracycline. J Am Chem Soc 75:4621

Boothe JH, Morton J II, Petisi JP, Wilkinson RG, Williams JH (1953d) Chemistry of tetracycline. In: Welch H (ed) Antibiotics annual 1953–1954. Medical encyclopedia, New York, pp 46–48

Boothe JH, Green A, Petisi JP, Wilkinson RG, Weller CW (1957) Demethyltetracyclines. Synthesis of a degradation product. J Am Chem Soc 79:4564

Boothe JH, Kende AS, Fields TL, Wilkinson RG (1959) Total synthesis of tetracyclines. I. (±)-Dedimethylamino-12a-deoxy-6-demethylanhydrochlortetracycline. J Am Chem Soc 81:1006–1007

Boothe JH, Hlavka JJ, Petisi JP, Spencer JL (1960) 6-Deoxytetracyclines. I. Chemical modification by electrophilic substitution. J Am Chem Soc 82:1253–1254

Broadhurst MJ, Hassall CH, Thomas GJ (1977) Tetracycline studies. Part 5. New syntheses of anthracenes and anthraquinones through benzophenone carbanions. J Chem Soc Perkin Trans I 1977:2502–2512

Broschard RW, Dornbush AC, Gordon S, Hutchings BL, Kohler AR, Krupka G, Kushner S, Lefemine DV, Pidacks C (1949) Aureomycin, a new antibiotic. Science 109:199–200

Caswell AH, Hutchison JD (1971) Selectivity of cation chelation to tetracyclines: evidence for special conformation of calcium chelate. Biochem Biophys Res Commun 43:625–630

Cid-Dresdner H (1965) The crystal structure of Terramycin hydrochloride, $C_{22}H_{24}N_2O_9 \cdot HCl$. Z Krist 121:170–189

Clive DLJ (1968) Chemistry of tetracyclines. Q Rev Chem Soc 22:435–456

Colaizzi JL, Knevel AM, Martin AN (1965) Biophysical study of the mode of action of tetracycline antibiotics. Inhibition of metalloflavoenzyme NADH cytochrome oxidoreductase. J Pharm Sci 54:1425–1435

Conover LH (1953) Terramycin. IX. The synthesis of indanone degradation products of Terramycin. J Am Chem Soc 75:4017–4020
Conover LH (1956) Progress in the chemistry of oxytetracycline and related compounds. In: Symposium on antibiotics and mould metabolites. Special publication no. 5. The Chemical Society, London, pp 48–81
Conover LH, Moreland WT, English AR, Stephens CR, Pilgrim FJ (1953) Terramycin. XI. Tetracycline. J Am Chem Soc 75:4622
Conover LH, Butler K, Johnston JD, Korst JJ, Woodward RB (1962) The total synthesis of 6-demethyl-6-deoxytetracycline. J Am Chem Soc 84:3222–3224
Dobrynin VN, Gurevich AJ, Karapetyan MG, Kolosov MN, Shemyakin MM (1962a) The absolute configuration of the tetracyclines. Tetrahedron Lett 1962:901–904
Dobrynin VN, Gurevich AI, Karapetyan MG, Kolosov MN, Shemyakin MM (1962b) Absolute configuration of tetracycline antibiotics (in Russian). Izv Akad Nauk SSSR, Otd Khim Nauk 1962:1697
Doerschuk AP, Bitler BA, McCormick JRD (1955) Reversible isomerization in the tetracycline family. J Am Chem Soc 77:4687
Doluisio JT, Martin AN (1963) Metal complexation of the tetracycline hydrochlorides. J Med Chem 6:16–20
Donohue J, Dunitz JD, Trueblood KN, Webster MS (1963) The crystal structure of Aureomycin (chlortetracycline) hydrochloride. Configuration, bond distances and conformation. J Am Chem Soc 85:851–856
Duggar BM (1948) Aureomycin: a product of the continuing search for new antibiotics. Ann NY Acad Sci 51:177–181
Dunitz JD, Leonard JE (1950) X-ray analysis of some antibiotic substances. J Am Chem Soc 72:4276–4277
Dunitz JD, Robertson JH (1952) Relationship between Aureomycin and Terramycin. J Am Chem Soc 74:1108
Dürckheimer W (1975) Tetracyclines: chemistry, biochemistry and structure-activity relations. Angew Chem Int Edit 14:721–774
Esse RC, Lowery JA, Tammoria CR, Sieger GM (1964a) Tetracycloxides. I. A new class of tetracycline derivatives. J Am Chem Soc 86:3874–3875
Esse RC, Lowery JA, Tammoria CR, Sieger GM (1964b) Tetracycloxides. II. Transformations at the C-4 position. J Am Chem Soc 86:3875–3877
Fields TL, Kende AS, Boothe JH (1960) Total synthesis of tetracyclines. II. Stereospecific synthesis of (±)-dedimethylamino-6-demethyl-6,12a-dideoxy-7-chlortetracycline. J Am Chem Soc 82:1250–1251
Fields TL, Kende AS, Boothe JH (1961) Total synthesis of tetracyclines. V. The stereospecific elaboration of the tetracycline ring system. J Am Chem Soc 83:4612–4618
Finlay AC, Hobby GL, P'an Sy, Regna PP, Routien JB, Seeley DB, Schull GM, Sobin BA, Solomons IA, Vinson JW, Kane JH (1950) Terramycin, a new antibiotic. Science 111:85
Glatz B, Helmchen G, Muxfeldt H, Porcher H, Prewo R, Senn J, Stezowski JJ, Stojda RJ, White DR (1979) A total synthesis and structural aspects of racemic 8-oxygenated tetracyclines. J Am Chem Soc 101:2171–2181
Gordon PN (1957) Alkanoic acid esters of tetracycline antibiotics. US Patent 2,812,349
Green A, Boothe JH (1960) Chemistry of tetracycline antibiotics. III. 12a-Deoxytetracycline. J Am Chem Soc 82:3950–3953
Gulbis J, Everett GW Jr (1975) A ^{13}C nuclear magnetic resonance analysis of metal binding site in tetracycline. J Am Chem Soc 97:6248–6249
Gulbis J, Everett GW Jr (1976) Metal binding characteristics of tetracycline derivatives in DMSO solution. Tetrahedron 32:913–917
Gulbis J, Everett GW Jr, Frank CW (1976) Effect of added electrolyte on the binding of tetracycline to paramagnetic ion probes. A ^{13}C and ^{1}H nuclear magnetic resonance study. J Am Chem Soc 98:1280–1281
Gurevich AI, Karapetyan MG, Kolosov MN, Korobko VG, Onoprienko VV, Shemyakin MM (1964a) Tetracyclines. XXXIX. The synthesis of 11,12a-dideoxy-4-dedimethylamino-5a,6-anhydrotetracyclines. Tetrahedron Lett 1964:877–881

Gurevich AI, Karapetyan MG, Kolosov MN, Korobko VG, Onoprienko VV, Shemyakin MM (1964b) Synthesis of hydronaphthacenes related to anhydrotetracyclines (in Russian). Dokl Akad Nauk SSSR 155:125–127

Gurevich AI, Karapetyan MG, Kolosov MN, Onoprienko VV, Shemyakin MM (1964c) A new synthesis of ring A of tetracyclines (in Russian). Izv Akad Nauk SSSR [Khim] 1964:945

Gurevich AI, Kolosov MN, Korobko SA, Popravko SA, Shemyakin MM (1965a) Tetracyclines. XL. Michael reaction with Δ^2-tricycline-DCB derivatives (in Russian). Zh Obshch Khim 35:652–659

Gurevich AI, Karapetyan MG, Kolosov MN, Korobko VG, Shemyakin MM (1965b) Tetracyclines. XLII. Synthesis of 11,12a-dideoxy-4-dedimethylamino-5a,6-anhydrotetracycline (in Russian). Zh Obshch Khim 35:668–673

Gurevich AI, Karapetyan MG, Kolosov MN (1966) Tetracyclines. XLIII. Partial synthesis of anhydrotetracycline (in Russian). Khim Prirodn Soedin, Akad Nauk Uz SSSR 2:141–142

Gurevich AI, Karapetyan MG, Kolosov MN, Korobko VG, Onoprienko VV, Popravko SA, Shemyakin MM (1967a) Studies in the tetracycline series. Part XLIV. The first total synthesis of the naturally occurring tetracycline. Tetrahedron Lett 1967:131–134

Gurevich AI, Karapetyan MG, Kolosov MN, Korobko VG, Popravko SA, Shemyakin MM (1967b) Total synthesis of tetracycline (in Russian). Dokl Akad Nauk SSSR 174:358–361

Gurevich AI, Karapetyan MG, Kolosov MN, Korobko VG, Onoprienko VV, Popravko SA (1968a) Tetracyclines. XLVII. Derivatives of (4-oxo-5,10-dihydroxy-9-methyl-1,2,3,4-tetrahydro-2-anthryl)glycine (in Russian). Zh Obshch Khim 38:50–57

Gurevich AI, Kolosov MN, Korobko VG, Popravko SA (1968b) Tetracyclines. XLVIII. Synthesis of 4-dedimethylamino-5a,6-anhydrotetracycline (in Russian). Zh Obshch Khim 38:57–61

Gurevich AI, Kolosov MN, Nametkina LN (1968c) Tetracyclines. XLIX. Synthesis of diastereomeric 1,5-bis(benzyloxy)-4-tetralone-2-acetaldehyde (in Russian). Zh Obshch Khim 38:1240–1246

Gurevich AI, Kolosov MN, Nametkina LN (1969) Synthesis of 6-demethyltetracycline derivatives (in Russian). Izv Akad Nauk SSSR [Khim] 1969:1401

Gurevich AI, Karapetyan MG, Kolosov MN (1970) Tetracyclines. LIII. Reactions of tetracycloxides and *N*-demethyltetracyclines (in Russian). Khim Prir Soedin 6:247–251

Hassall CH, Morgan BA (1973) Tetracycline studies. Part IV. Some novel cyclisations through benzophenone carbanions, including a new synthesis of anthraquinones. J Chem Soc Perkin I 1973:2853–2861

Hassall CH, Thomas GJ (1970a) Tetracycline studies. Part III. Trimethylsilyl derivatives of tetracyclines. J Chem Soc [C] 1970:636–640

Hassall CH, Thomas GJ (1970b) 6- and 12a-Hydroxylation of 6-methylpretetramid. Chem Commun 1970:1053–1054

Hassall CH, Thomas GJ (1978) Tetracycline studies. Part 6. 6- and 12a-Hydroxylation of 6-methylpretetramid. J Chem Soc Perkin Trans I 1978:145–152

Hassall CH, Winters TE (1967) Simulating a step in tetracycline biosynthesis. Chem Commun 1967:77–78

Hassall CH, Winters TE (1968) Tetracycline studies. Part I. The selective oxidation of 6-methylpretetramid. J Chem Soc [C] 1968:1558–1560

Hassall CH, Wooton G (1969) Tetracycline studies. Part II. Synthesis of 2-carboxyl-1,3,8,9-tetrahydroxy-5-methylanthracene and related compounds. J Chem Soc [C] 1969:2805–2808

Hirokawa S, Okaya Y, Lovell FM, Pepinski R (1959a) On the crystal structure of Aureomycin hydrochloride. Acta Cryst 12:811–812

Hirokawa S, Okaya Y, Lovell FM, Pepinski R (1959b) The crystal structure of Aureomycin hydrochloride. Z Krist 112:439–464

Hlavka JJ, Boothe JH (1973) The tetracyclines. In: Jucker E (ed) Progress in drug research, vol 17. Birkhauser, Basel, pp 210–240

Hlavka JJ, Bitha P, Boothe JH (1965) 4-Hydroxy-6-methylpretetramid. Synthesis *via* quaternary tetracyclines. J Am Chem Soc 87:1795–1797
Hochstein FA, Pasternack R (1951) A degradation product of Terramycin. J Am Chem Soc 73:5008–5009
Hochstein FA, Pasternack R (1952) Structure of Terramycin. IV. 7-Hydroxy-3-methylphthalide. J Am Chem Soc 74:3905–3908
Hochstein FA, Regna PP, Brunings KJ, Woodward RB (1952a) Terramycin. V. Structure of terrinolide, an acid degradation product of Terramycin. J Am Chem Soc 74:3706–3707
Hochstein FA, Stephens CR, Gordon PN, Regna PP, Pilgrim FJ, Brunings KJ, Woodward RB (1952b) Terramycin. VI. The structure of α- and β-apoterramycin, acid rearrangement products of Terramycin. J Am Chem Soc 76:3707–3708
Hochstein FA, Stephens CR, Conover LH, Regna PP, Pasternack R, Brunings KJ, Woodward RB (1952c) Terramycin. VIII. The structure of Terramycin. J Am Chem Soc 74:3708–3709
Hochstein FA, Stephens CR, Conover LH, Regna PP, Pasternack R, Gordon PN, Pilgrim FJ, Brunings KJ, Woodward RB (1953) The structure of Terramycin. J Am Chem Soc 75:5455–5475
Hochstein FA, Schach von Wittenau M, Tanner FW Jr, Murai K (1960) 2-Acetyl-2-decarboxamidoöxytetracycline. J Am Chem Soc 82:5934–5937
Hoffman DR (1966) The mass spectra of tetracyclines. J Org Chem 31:792–796
Holmlund CE, Andres WW, Shay AJ (1959a) Chemical hydroxylation of 12a-deoxytetracycline. J Am Chem Soc 81:4748–4749
Holmlund CE, Andres WW, Shay AJ (1959b) Microbiological hydroxylation of 12a-deoxytetracycline. J Am Chem Soc 81:4750–4751
Hosangadi BD, Kulkarni AB (1975) Tetracyclines. XII. Synthesis of 1,3,9-trimethoxy-6-methyl-5,5a,6,11,11a,12-hexahydronaphthacene-5,11-diol. Indian J Chem 13:218–221
Hosangadi BD, Pandit AL, Kulkarni AB (1964) Tetracyclines. VII. Synthesis of hexahydronaphthacenes having different substituents in ring D and a resorcinol nucleus in ring A. Indian J Chem 2:235–237
Hosangadi BD, Amonkar NS, Kulkarni AB (1969) Tetracyclines. IX. Synthesis of model hexahydronaphthacenes with free phenolic hydroxyl groups in rings A and D. Indian J Chem 7:561–565
Hosangadi BD, Pandit AL, Kulkarni AB (1974) Tetracyclines. XI. Introduction of additional oxygen functions in rings B and C of hexahydronaphthacenes. Indian J Chem 12: 920–922
Hughes RE, Muxfeldt H, Dreele RB von (1971) Conformation of tetracycline ring systems. Structure of 5,12a-diacetyloxytetracycline. J Am Chem Soc 93:1037–1038
Hutchings BL, Waller CW, Gordon S, Broschard RW, Wolf CF, Goldman AA, Williams JH (1952a) Degradation of Aureomycin. J Am Chem Soc 74:3710–3711
Hutchings BL, Waller CW, Broschard RW, Wolf CF, Fryth PW, Williams JH (1952b) Degradation of Aureomycin. V. Aureomycinic acid. J Am Chem Soc 74:4980
Inhoffen HH, Muxfeldt H, Schaefer H, Krämer H (1957) Structural and steric course of organometallic reactions on diene adducts of 1,4-naphthoquinones (in German). Croat Chem Aeta 29:329–345
Jogun KH, Stezowski JJ (1976a) Chemical-structural properties of tetracycline derivatives. 2. Coordination and conformational aspects of oxytetracycline metal ion complexation. J Am Chem Soc 98:6018–6026
Jogun KH, Stezowski JJ (1976b) Oxytetracycline hydrobromide dihydrate, $C_{22}H_{24}N_2O_9 \cdot HBr \cdot 2H_2O$. Cryst Struct Comm 5:381–386
Kalnins K, Belen'skii BG (1964) A study of dissociation of tetracyclines by infrared spectroscopy. Dokl Akad Nauk SSSR 157:619–621
Kametani T, Fukumoto K (1979) Synthesis of linear tetracycline antibiotics. Tetracyclines and anthracyclines (in Japanese). Kagaku Koggo 1979:1023–1031
Kametani T, Fukumoto K (1980) Chemistry of natural products. 1980A. Synthesis of natural products starting from benzocyclobutene. Kogaku no Ryoiki, Zokan 1980:81–116

Kametani T, Takahashi T, Kajiwara M, Hirai Y, Ohtsuka C, Satoh F, Fukumoto K (1974) Studies on the synthesis of tetracycline derivatives. I. Thermolytic cycloaddition of *o*-quinodimethanes with naphthoquimone. Chem Pharm Bull (Jpn) 22:2159–2163

Kametani T, Takeshita M, Nemoto H, Fukumoto K (1978a) Studies on the synthesis of tetracycline derivatives. II. Thermolytic cycloaddition of *o*-quinodimethanes with tetrahydronaphthoquinone and naphthoquinone. Chem Pharm Bull (Jpn) 26:556–562

Kametani T, Chihiro M, Takeshita M, Takahashi K, Fukumoto K, Takano S (1978b) Studies in the synthesis of tetracycline derivatives. III. Synthetic approach to adriamycin synthesis of the linear tetracyclic skeleton having the same BC ring system as adriamycin. Chem Pharm Bull (Jpn) 26:3820–3824

Kamiya K, Hsai M, Wada Y, Nishikawa M (1971) Opposite chirality of pillaromycin A to tetracyclines: the X-ray analysis of Achromycin hydrochloride. Experimentia 27:363–364

Kaplan MA, Granatek AP, Buckwalter FH (1957) Quatrimycin: preparation and properties. Antibiot Chemother 7:569–576

Kende AS, Fields TL, Boothe JH, Kushner S (1961) Total synthesis of tetracyclines. IV. Synthesis of an anhydrotetracycline derivative. J Am Chem Soc 83:439–449

Kirchlechner R, Rogalski W (1980) Synthesis of 6-thiatetracycline, a highly active analogue of the antibiotic tetracycline. Tetrahedron Lett 21:247–250

Kolosov MN, Berlin YA (1962) Tetracyclines. XII. A method of introduction of the *N,N*-dimethylglycine residue into the cyclohexane ring (in Russian). Zh Obshch Khim 32:2893–2905

Kolosov MN, Dobrynin VN, Gurevich AI, Karapetyan MG (1963a) Tetracyclines. XVI. Absolute configuration of tetracyclines (in Russian). Izv Akad Nauk SSSR, Otd Khim Nauk 1963:696–701

Kolosov MN, Gurevich AI, Shvetsov YB (1963b) Tetracyclines. XVII. Asymmetric synthesis of (−)-3-methylphthalide-3-carboxylic acid (in Russian). Izv Akad Nauk SSSR, Otd Khim Nauk 1963:701–705

Kolosov MN, Popravko SA, Shemyakin MM (1963c) Untersuchungen in der Tetracyclinreihe, XXXI. Synthese des DCB-Tricyclins. Liebig's Ann Chemie 668:86–91

Kolosov MN, Popravko SA, Shemyakin MM (1963d) The structure of the DCB tetracycline system (in Russian). Dokl Akad Nauk SSSR 150:1285–1288

Kolosov MN, Popravko SA, Gurevich AI, Korobko VG, Vasina IV, Shemyakin MM (1964a) Tetracyclines. XXVIII. Synthesis and reversible isomerization of 9-oxo-4,5,10-trihydroxy-1,4,4a,9a,10-hexahydroanthracene derivatives (in Russian). Zh Obshch Khim 34:2534–2539

Kolosov MN, Popravko SA, Korobko VG, Shemyakin MM (1964b) Tetracyclines. XXIX. Structure of the DCB tricyclic system of tetracycline antibiotic (in Russian). Zh Obshch Khim 34:2540–2547

Kolosov MN, Popravko SA, Korobko VG, Karapetyan MG, Shemyakin MM (1964c) Tetracyclines. XXX. Structure of the DCB tricyclic system of tetracycline antibiotic (in Russian). Zh Obshch Khim 34:2547–2553

Kolosov MN, Onoprienko VV, Shemyakin MM (1965) Tetracyclines. XLI. Synthesis of 11,12a-dideoxy-4-dedimethylamino-6-demethyl-5a,6-anhydrotetracycline (in Russian). Zh Obshch Khim 35:659–667

Korst JJ, Johnston JD, Butler K, Bianco EJ, Conover LH, Woodward RB (1968) The total synthesis of *dl*-6-demethyl-6-deoxytetracycline. J Am Chem Soc 90:439–457

Kuhn R, Dury K (1951a) Alkalischer Abbau von Aureomycin und Terramycin. Chem Ber 84:563–565

Kuhn R, Dury K (1951b) 6-Acetylsalicylsäure. Chem Ber 84:848–850

Kushner S, Boothe JH, Morton J II, Petisi J, Williams JH (1952) Synthesis of degradation products of Aureomycin. J Am Chem Soc 74:3710

Kushner S, Morton J II, Boothe JH, Williams JH (1953) Synthesis of degradation products of Aureomycin. III. J Am Chem Soc 75:1097–1100

Leeson LJ, Kruger JE, Nash RA (1963) Concerning the structural assignment of the second and third acidity constants of the tetracyclines antibiotics. Tetrahedron Lett 1963:1155–1160

Mahajan AP, Kulkarni AB (1975) Stereochemistry of isomeric 6-methyl-1,3,9-trimethoxy-5,5a,6,11,11a,12-hexahydronaphthacene-5,11-diones. Indian J chem 13:1254–1256
Martell JM Jr, Booth JH (1967) The 6-deoxytetracyclines. VII. Alkylated aminotetracyclines possessing unique antibacterial activity. J Med Chem 10:44–46
Martin W, Hartung H, Urbach H, Dürckheimer W (1973) Totalsynthese von *d,l*-7-Chlor-6-desoxytetracyclinen und *d,l*-7-Chlor-6-desmethyl-6-desoxytetracyclinen der natürlichen, der 5a-epi- und der 6-epi-Reihe. Tetrahedron Lett 1973:3513–3516
McCormick JRD, Jensen ER (1965) Biosynthesis of tetracyclines. VIII. Characterization of 4-hydroxy-6-methylpretetramid. J Am Chem Soc 87:1794–1795
McCormick JRD, Fox SM, Smith LL, Bitler BA, Reichenthal J, Origoni VE, Muller WH, Winterbottom R, Doerschuk AP (1956) On the nature of the reversible isomerization in the tetracycline family. J Am Chem Soc 78:3547–3548
McCormick JRD, Fox SM, Smith LL, Bitler BA, Reichenthal J, Origoni VE, Muller WH, Winterbottom R, Doerschuk AP (1957a) Studies of the reversible epimerization occurring in the tetracycline family. The preparation, properties and proof of structure of some 4-epitetracyclines. J Am Chem Soc 79:2849–2858
McCormick JRD, Sjolander NO, Hirsch U, Jensen ER, Doerschuk AP (1957b) A new family of antibiotics: the demethyltetracyclines. J Am Chem Soc 79:4561–4563
McCormick JRD, Miller PA, Growich JA, Sjolander NO, Doerschuk AP (1958a) Two new tetracycline-related compounds: 7-chloro-5a(11a)-dehydrotetracycline and 5a-*epi*-tetracycline. A new route to tetracycline. J Am Chem Soc 80:5572–5573
McCormick JRD, Sjolander NO, Miller PA, Hirsch U, Arnold NH, Doerschuk AP (1958b) The biological reduction of 7-chloro-5a(11a)-dehydrotetracycline to 7-chlorotetracycline by *Streptomyces aureofaciens*. J Am Chem Soc 80:6460
McCormick JRD, Jensen ER, Miller PA, Doerschuk AP (1960) The 6-deoxytetracyclines. Further studies on the relationship between structure and antibacterial activity in the tetracycline series. J Am Chem Soc 82:3381–3386
McCormick JRD, Miller PA, Johnson S, Arnold N, Sjolander NO (1962) Biosynthesis of the tetracyclines. IV. Biological rehydration of 5a,6-anhydrotetracyclines. J Am Chem Soc 84:3023–3025
McCormick JRD, Johnson S, Sjolander NO (1963a) Biosynthesis of the tetracyclines. V. Naphthacenic precursors. J Am Chem Soc 85:1692–1694
McCormick JRD, Reichenthal J, Johnson S, Sjolander NO (1963b) Biosynthesis of tetracyclines. VI. Total synthesis of a naphthacenic precursor: 1,3,10,11,12-pentahydroxynaphthacene-2-carboxamide. J Am Chem Soc 85:1694–1695
McCormick JRD, Joachim UH, Jensen ER, Johnson S, Sjolander NO (1965a) Biosynthesis of the tetracyclines. VII. 4-Hydroxy-6-methylpretetramid, an intermediate accumulated by a blocked mutant. J Am Chem Soc 87:1793–1794
McCormick JRD, Sjolander NO, Johnson SJ (1965b) Biological transformation of 1,3,10,11,12-penta hydroxynaphthacene-2-carboxamides to tetracycline antibiotics. US Patent 3,276,305
Miller MW, Hochstein FA (1962) Isolation and characterization of two new tetracycline antibiotics. J Org Chem 27:2525–2528
Minieri PP, Firman MC, Mistretta AG, Abbey A, Bricker CE, Rigler NE, Sokol H (1953) A new broad spectrum antibiotic product of the tetracycline group. In: Welch H (ed) Antibiotics annual 1953–1954. Medical encyclopedic, New York, pp 81–87
Mitscher LA (1978) The chemistry of the tetracycline antiobiotics. Dekker, New York
Mitscher LA, Bonacci AC, Sokoloski TB (1968) Circular dichroism and solution conformation of the tetracycline antibiotics. Tetrahedron Lett 1968:5361–5364
Mitscher LA, Bonacci AC, Sokoloski TD (1969) Circular dichroism and solution conformation of the tetracycline antiobiotics. In: Hobby GL (ed) Antimicrobial agents and chemotherapy – 1968. American Society for Microbiology, Bethesda, pp 78–86
Mitscher LA, Bonacci AC, Slater-Eng B, Hacker AK, Sokoloski TD (1970) Interaction of various tetracyclines with metallic cations in aqueous solutions as measured by circular dichroism. In: Hobby GL (ed) Antimicrobial agents and chemotherapy – 1969. American Society for Microbiology, Bethesda, pp 111–115

Mitscher LA, Slater-Eng B, Sokoloski TD (1972) Circular dichroism measurements of the tetracyclines. IV. 5-Hydroxylated derivatives. In: Hobby GL (ed) Antimicrobial agents and chemotherapy, August 1972. American Society for Microbiology, Bethesda, pp 66–72

Money T, Scott AI (1968) Recent advances in the chemistry and biochemistry of tetracyclines. In: Cook J, Carruthers W (eds) Progress in organic chemistry, vol 7. Butterworths, London, pp 1–34

Muxfeldt H (1959) Synthese tetracylischer Abbauprodukte von Anhydro-tetracyclinen. Chem Ber 92:3122–3150

Muxfeldt H (1962a) Synthesen in der Tetracyclin-Reihe. Angew Chem 74:443–452

Muxfeldt H (1962b) Syntheses in the tetracycline series. Angew Chem Int Ed 1:372–381

Muxfeldt H (1962c) Synthese eines Terramycin-Bausteins. Angew Chem 74:825–828

Muxfeldt H, Bangert R (1963) Die Chemie der Tetracycline. Fortschr Chem Org Naturst 21:80–120

Muxfeldt H, Hardtmann G (1963) Tetracycline. V. Modellversuche zum Aufbau des Terramycins. Liebig's Ann Chem 669:113–121

Muxfeldt H, Inhoffen HH (1958) Synthese von Anhydro-tetracyclinen. Abhandl Braunschweig Wiss Ges 10:1–8

Muxfeldt H, Kreutzer A (1959) Ab- und Aufbauerreaktionen in der Anhydro-tetracyclin-Reihe. Naturwissenschaft 46:204–205

Muxfeldt H, Kreutzer A (1961) Tetracycline. II. Syntheses des Desdimethylamino-anhydro-aureomycins. Chem Ber 94:881–893

Muxfeldt H, Rogalski W (1965) Tetracyclines. V. A total synthesis of (±)-6-deoxy-6-demethyl-tetracycline. J Am Chem Soc 87:933–934

Muxfeldt H, Rogalski W, Striegler K (1960) Aufbau des *β*-Tetracarbonyl-Systems der Tetracycline. Angew Chem 72:170–171

Muxfeldt H, Rogalski W, Striegler K (1962a) Tetracycline. III. Aufbau des Ringsystems von 6-Desoxy-tetracyclinen. Chem Ber 95:2581–2603

Muxfeldt H, Jacobs E, Uhlig K (1962b) Tetracycline. IV. Aufbau der Ringsysteme von 6-Desoxy-6-epi-tetracycline und 6-Desoxy-6-desmethyl-tetracyclin. Chem Ber 95:2901–2911

Muxfeldt H, Buhr G, Bangert R (1962c) Catalytic hydroxylation of 12a-deoxytetracyclines. Angew Chem Int Ed 1:1571

Muxfeldt H, Rogalski W, Kathawala FG, Grethe G, Behling J (1964) Eine neue Reaktion von Azlactonen und ihre Anwendung auf Tetracyclin- und Alkaloid-Synthesen. Angew Chem 76:791–792

Muxfeldt H, Grethe G, Rogalski W (1966) Carboxamidation of *β*-dicarbonyl compounds. J Org Chem 31:2429–2430

Muxfeldt H, Behling J, Grethe G, Rogalski W (1967) Tetracyclines. VI. Some new aspects in the chemistry of oxazolones and their sulfur analogs. J Am Chem Soc 89:4991–4996

Muxfeldt H, Hardtmann G, Kathawala F, Vedejs E, Moorberry JB (1968) Tetracyclines. VII. Total synthesis of *dl*-Terramycin. J Am Chem Soc 90:6534–6536

Muxfeldt H, Döpp H, Kaufman JE, Schneider J, Hansen PE, Sasaki A, Geiser T (1973) Total synthesis of anhydroaureomycin. Angew Chem Int Ed 12:497–499

Muxfeldt H, Haas G, Hardtmann G, Kathawala F, Moorberry JB, Vedejs E (1979) Tetracyclines. 9. Total synthesis of *dl*-Terramycin. J Am Chem Soc 101:689–701

Noseworthy MM (1961) 4-Epitetracycline antibiotic transformation process. US Patent 3,009,956

Palenik GJ, Mathew M (1972) Structure-activity relationships in tetracyclines. Acta Cryst A 28:S47

Pandit AL, Kulkarni AB (1958) Synthesis of 7,10-dimethoxy-5,6,11,12-tetrahydro-6,12-naphthacenedione. Current Sci (India) 27:254–255

Pandit AL, Kulkarni AB (1960) Tetracyclines. I. Synthesis of 7,10-dimethoxy-5,6,11,12-tetrahydronaphthacene-6,12-dione. J Sci Ind Research (India) 19B:138–142

Pandit AL, Kulkarni AB (1964) Tetracyclines. VIII. Synthesis of hexahydronaphthacenes with methyl group and carboxy group in suitable positions. India J Chem 2:327–329

Pandit AL, Seshadri S, Kulkarni AB (1960) Tetracyclines. II. 3-Carboxy-1-tetralones as intermediates for the synthesis of hydronaphthacenes. J Sci Ind Research (India) 19B:155–158

Pasternack R, Regna PP, Wagner RL, Bavely A, Hochstein FA, Gordon PN, Brunings KJ (1951) Degradation of Terramycin. J Am Chem Soc 73:2400

Pasternack R, Bavely A, Wagner RL, Hochstein FA, Regna PP, Brunings KJ (1952a) Terramycin. II. Alkaline degradation. J Am Chem Soc 74:1926–1928

Pasternack R, Conover LH, Bavely A, Hochstein FA, Hess GB, Brunings KJ (1952b) Terramycin. III. Structure of terracinoic acid, an alkaline degradation product. J Am Chem Soc 74:1928–1934

Pepinski R, Watanabe T (1952) Isomorphism of Terramycin and Aureomycin hydrochlorides. Science 115:541

Petisi J, Spencer JL, Hlauka JJ, Boothe JH (1962) 6-Deoxytetracyclines. II. Nitrations and subsequent reactions. J Med Chem 5:538–546

Prewo R, Stezowski JJ (1977) Chemical-structural properties of tetracycline derivatives. 3. The integrity of the conformation of the nonionized free base. J Am Chem Soc 99:1117–1121

Prewo R, Stezowski JJ (1979) Chemical-structural properties of tetracycline derivatives. 8. The interrelationships between oxytetracycline and 4-epioxytetracycline. J Am Chem Soc 101:7657–7660

Prewo R, Stezowski JJ (1980a) Chemical-structural properties of tetracycline derivatives. 9. 7-Chlorotetracycline derivatives with modified stereochemistry. J Am Chem Soc 102:7015–7020

Prewo R, Stezowski JJ (1980b) The crystal and molecular structure of nonionized 6-thiatetracycline free base. Tetrahedron Lett 21:251–254

Prewo R, Stezowski JJ, Kirchlechner R (1980) Chemical-structural properties of tetracycline derivatives. 10. The 6-thiatetracyclines. J Am Chem Soc 102:7021–7026

Regna PP, Solomons IA (1950) The chemical and physical properties of Terramycin. Ann NY Acad Sci 53:229–237

Regna PP, Solomons IA, Murai K, Timreck AE, Brunings KJ, Lazier WA (1951) The isolation and general properties of Terramycin and Terramycin salts. J Am Chem Soc 73:4211–4215

Rennhard HH, Blackwood RK, Stephens CR (1961) Fluorotetracyclines. I. Perchloryl fluoride studies in the tetracycline series. J Am Chem Soc 83:2774–2776

Restivo R, Palenik GJ (1969) Structural relationships in tetracyclines. The crystal structure of anhydrotetracycline hydrobromide. Biochem Biophys Res Commun 36:621–624

Rigler NE, Bag SP, Leyden DE, Sudmeier JL, Reilly CN (1965) Determination of a protonation scheme of tetracycline using nuclear magnetic resonance. Anal Chem 37:872–875

Robertson J, Robertson I, Eiland PF, Pepinsky R (1952) X-ray measurements of Terramycin salts. J Am Chem Cos 74:841

Samant BR, Hosangadi BD, Kulkarni AB (1974) Tetracycline. X. Synthetic approaches for the introduction of amine functions in ring A of hexahydronaphthacenes. Indian J Chem 12:916–919

Schach von Wittenau M (1964) Preparation of tetracyclines by photooxidation of anhydrotetracyclines. J Org Chem 29:2746–2748

Schach von Wittenau M, Blackwood RK (1966) Proton magnetic reasonance spectra of tetracyclines. J Am Chem Soc 31:613–615

Schach von Wittenau M, Beereboom JJ, Blackwood RK, Stephens CR (1962) 6-Deoxytetracyclines. III. Stereochemistry at C-6. J Am Chem Soc 84:2645–2646

Schach von Wittenau M, Hochstein FA, Stephens CR (1963) Tautomerism of 5a,11a-dehydro-7-chlortetracycline. Preparation of 5-alkoxy-7-chloroanhydrotetracyclines. J Org Chem 28:2454–2456

Schach von Wittenau M, Blackwood RK, Conover LH, Gluart RH, Woodward RB (1965) The stereochemistry at C-5 in oxytetracycline. J Am Chem Soc 87:134

Scott AI, Bedford CT (1962) Simulation of the biosynthesis of tetracyclines. A partial synthesis of tetracycline from anhydroaureomycin. J Am Chem Soc 84:2271–2272

Seshadri S, Kulkarni AB (1959) Tetracyclines. II. Synthesis of 2,8-dimethoxy-5,5a,6,11,11a,12-hexahydro-6,12-naphthacenedione. Current Sci (India) 28:65–67

Seshadri S, Kulkarni AB (1961) Tetracyclines. IV. A novel rearrangement of 2-(2-carboxy-benzylidene)-3-carboxy-1-tetralone derivatives. J Sci Ind Research (India) 20B:30–33

Shemyakin MM, Kolosov MN, Karpetyan MG, Chaman ES (1957) Initial stages of the synthesis of tetracyclines. Proc Acad Sci USSR, Sect Chem 112:111–114 (in Russian). Dokl Akad Nauk SSSR 112:669–672

Shemyakin MM, Kolosov MN, Arbuzov YA, Onoprienko VV, Shatenshtein GA (1958) A new path to synthesis of ring A in tetracyclines (in Russian). Izv Akad Nauk SSSR, Oidel Khim Nauk 1958:794–795

Shemyakin MM, Kolosov MN, Arbuzov YA, Karpetyan MG, Chaman ES, Onishchenko AA (1959a) Tetracyclines. IV. Paths of synthesis of the DCB ring system of tetracyclines (in Russian). Zh Obshch Khim 29:1831–1842

Shemyakin MM, Kolosov MN, Arbuzov YA, Berlin YA (1959b) Ways of synthesis of the A ring in tetracyclines – method of introduction of a *N,N*-dimethylglycine residue into the cyclohexanone ring (in Russian). Dokl Akad Nauk SSSR 128:744–747

Shemyakin MM, Kolosov MN, Arbuzov YA, Se Y-Y, Shen KY, Sklobovskiy KA, Guervich AI (1959c) Intermediate stages of synthesis of tetracyclines (in Russian). Dokl Akad Nauk SSSR 128:113–116

Shemyakin MM, Arbuzov YA, Kolosov MN, Shatenshetein GA, Omoprienko VV, Konnova YV (1960a) Tetracyclines. VI. Carboxamidation of dimedone with isocyanates (in Russian). Zh Obshch Khim 30:542–545

Shemyakin MM, Kolosov MN, Arbuzov YA, Omoprienko VV, Hsieh Y-Y (1960b) Tetracyclines. VII. Paths of synthesis of ring A in tetracyclines (in Russian). Zh Obshch Khim 30:545–546

Shemyakin MM, Kolosov MN, Hseih Y-Y, Karapetyan MG, Shen H-Y, Gurevich AI (1964a) Tetracyclines. XXI. Synthesis of 2- and 3-substituted 10-oxo-9-hydroxy-9-methyl-1,2,3,4,4a,9,9a,10-octahydroanthracenes (in Russian). Izv Akad Nauk SSSR [Khim] 1964:1013–1024

Shemyakin MM, Kolosov MN, Karapetyan MG, Hsieh Y-Y, Omoprienko VV (1964b) Tetracyclines. XXII. Stereochemistry of 2- and 3-substituted-10-oxo-9-hydroxy-9-methyl-1,2,3,4,4a,9,9a,10-octahydroanthacenes (in Russian). Izv Akad Nauk SSSR [Khim] 1964:1024–1035

Shemyakin MM, Kolosov MN, Hsieh Y-Y, Omoprienko VV, Karapetyan MG, Korobko VG, Shen H-Y (1964c) Tetracyclines. XXXV. Synthesis of a hydronaphthacene analog of 12a-deoxytetracycline (in Russian). Zh Obshch Khim 34:2553–2564

Shemyakin MM, Kolosov MN, Gurevich AI (1964d) Synthese von Verbindungen, die in Beziehung zum Anhydrotetracyclin stehen. Angew Chem 76:791

Stephens CR, Conover LH, Hochstein FA, Regna PP, Pilgrim FJ, Brunings KJ, Woodward RB (1952) Terramycin. VIII. Structure of Aureomycin and Terramycin. J Am Chem Soc 74:4976–4977

Stephens CR, Conover LH, Pasternack R, Hochstein FA, Moreland WT, Regna PP, Pilgrim FJ, Brunings KJ, Woodward RB (1954) The structure of Aureomycin. J Am Chem Soc 76:3568–3575

Stephens CR, Conover LH, Gordon PN, Pennington FC, Wagner RL, Brunings KJ, Pilgrim FJ (1956a) Epitetracycline – the chemical relationship between tetracycline and "quatrimycin." J Am Chem Soc 78:1515–1516

Stephens CR, Murai K, Brunings KJ, Woodward RB (1956b) Acidity constants of the tetracycline antibiotics. J Am Chem Soc 78:4155–4158

Stephens CR, Murai K, Rennhard HH, Conover LH, Brunings KJ (1958) Hydrogenolysis studies in the tetracycline series – 6-deoxytetracyclines. J Am Chem Soc 80:5324–5325

Stephens CR, Beereboom JJ, Rennhard HH, Gordon PN, Murai K, Blackwood RK, Schach von Wittenau M (1963) 6-Deoxytetracyclines. IV. Preparation, C-6 stereochemistry, and reactions. J Am Chem Soc 85:2643–2652

Stezowski JJ (1976) Chemical-structural properties of tetracycline derivatives. 1. Molecular structure and conformation of the free base derivatives. J Am Chem Soc 98:6012–6018

Stezowski JJ (1977) Chemical-structural properties of tetracycline antibiotics. 4. Ring A tautomerism involving the protonated amide substituent as observed in the crystal structure of α-6-deoxytetracycline hydrohalides. J Am Chem Soc 99:1122–1129
Takeuchi Y, Buerger MJ (1960) The crystal structure of Terramycin hydrochloride. Proc Nat Acad Sci USA 46:1366–1370
Urbach H, Hartung H, Martin W, Dürckheimer W (1973) Totalsynthese von *d,l* 4-Amino-7-chlor-2-*N*-methylcarbamyl-2-descarbamyl-4-desdimethylamino-6-desmethyl-6-desoxytetracylin. Tetrahedron Lett 1973:4907–4910
Van den Hende JH (1965) The crystal and molecular structures of 7-chloro- and 7-bromo-4-hydroxytetracycloxide. J Am Chem Soc 87:929–931
Von Dreele RB, Hughes RE (1971) Crystal and molecular structure of 5,12a-diacetyloxytetracycline. J Am Chem Soc 93:7290–7296
Waller CW, Hutchings BL, Wolf CF, Broschard RW, Goldman AA, Williams JH (1952a) Degradation of Aureomycin. III. 3,4-Dihydroxy-2,5-dioxocyclopentane-1-carboxamide. J Am Chem Soc 74:4978–4979
Waller CW, Hutchings BL, Goldman AA, Wold CF, Boschard RW, Williams JH (1952b) Degradation of Aureomycin. IV. Desdimethylaminoaureomycinic acid. J Am Chem Soc 74:4979–4980
Waller CW, Hutchings BL, Wolf CF, Goldman AA, Broschard RW, Williams JH (1952c) Degradation of Aureomycin. VI. Isoaureomycin and Aureomycin. J Am Chem Soc 74:4981
Waller CW, Hutchings BL, Broschard RW, Goldman AA, Stein WJ, Wolf CF, Williams JH (1952d) Degradation of Aureomycin. VII. Aureomycin and anhydroaureomycin. J Am Chem Soc 74:4981–4982
Webb JS, Broschard RW, Cosulich DB, Stein WJ, Wolf CF (1957) Demethyltetracyclines. Structure studies. J Am Chem Soc 79:4563–4564
Wilkinson RG, Fields TL, Booth JH (1961) Total synthesis of tetracyclines. III. Synthesis of a tricyclic model system. J Org Chem 26:637–643
Williamson DE, Everett GW Jr (1975) A proton nuclear magnetic resonance study of the site of metal binding in tetracycline. J Am Chem Soc 97:2397–2405
Woodward RB (1963) The total synthesis of a tetracycline. Pure Appl Chem 6:561–573

CHAPTER 4

Biosynthesis of the Tetracyclines

Z. Hošťálek and Z. Vaněk

A. Introduction

Research on the biosynthesis of tetracyclines, which has developed rapidly since the discovery of chlortetracycline (Duggar 1948), oxytetracycline (Finlay et al. 1950), and the biological synthesis of tetracycline (Minieri et al. 1954), can be divided into several historical phases. The first tempestuous phase of the study of the technology of tetracycline fermentation occurred in the fifties; the results of studies from this period are surveyed in an excellent review by Di Marco and Pennella (1959). The sixties were characterized by the study of the building blocks and biosynthetic intermediates of tetracycline antibiotics; significant contribution in this field is due to the research team of the Lederle Laboratories headed by McCormick. Pertinent results from this period were published in several review articles (Hlavka and Boothe 1973; McCormick 1967, 1969: Mitscher 1968). In the following decade, the study of tetracycline biosynthesis was focused on the elucidation of regulatory mechanisms in the biosynthesis and on deciphering the molecular nature of these processes.

Both the development of production technology and the elucidation of the biosynthesis pathway of tetracyclines were greatly aided by genetic manipulation with production strains, in the former case due to the improvement of high-production variants and in the latter due to the isolation and evaluation of mutants blocked in the biosynthetic pathway. The genetic problems of the biosynthesis of tetracyclines are summarized in a review by Hošťálek et al. (1974). An extensive survey of the literature dealing with all aspects of the biosynthesis was published by Turley and Snell (1966) and more recently by Hošťálek et al. (1979), Podojil et al. (1984), and Hutchinson (1981).

B. Production Strains

I. Taxonomy

Apart from the species *Streptomyces aureofaciens* producing chlortetracycline and *S. rimosus* producing oxytetracycline, a number of other *Streptomyces* species have been reported to produce tetracycline antibiotics (for review see Di Marco and Pennella 1959; Hošťálek et al. 1979). The patent literature contains reports on many tetracycline-producing species. After a thorough taxonomic evaluation, some of these species have been stated to be identical with *S. aureofaciens* (Hütter 1967) while others were confirmed as independent species in the International *Streptomyces* Project (SHIRLING and GOTTLIEB 1968, 1969, 1972). However, the classification system of Actinomycetales is still in a disappointing state since the criteria for physiological characteristics are inadequate and obsolete (PRIDHAM 1977). A mutagenic treatment can alter substantially the physiological properties used as taxonomic criteria (VILLAX 1962) and the isolated variants can then be declared as new species different from the parent strain. Modern criteria such as the sensitivity to a specific phage (WEINDLING et al. 1961) or genetic homology determined by the method of DNA association (KOIKE et al. 1977) have shown, however, that producers of tetracycline declared as independent species are identical with *S. aureofaciens*.

II. Growth

Submerged cultivation of *S. rimosus* and *S. aureofaciens* proceeds in several phases (DOSKOČIL et al. 1958, 1959). The first, *preparatory* phase extending up to the 10th h is characterized by intensive RNA synthesis. The protein-synthesizing system of *S. aureofaciens* is at this stage sensitive to exogenous tetracycline (MIKULÍK et al. 1971 a). The subsequent *vegetative* phase, setting in after the 10th h, is characterized by intensive protein synthesis and vegetative growth; first traces of produced antibiotic appear in the culture. Low-production strains terminate the antibiotic production after the termination of culture growth, no synthesis taking place in the *stationary* phase. In high-production variants, on the other hand, the antibiotic biosynthesis is extended into a subsequent, *production* phase after the 48th h of cultivation (MAKAREVICH and LAZNIKOVA 1963). A characteristic feature of the vegetative growth phase is the formation of thick hyphae containing homogeneous basophile cytoplasm with a high RNA content. The mycelium from the production phase grows in thin filaments with differentiated cytoplasm; the basophile character is attenuated. These difference are typical of high-production strains of *S. aureofaciens* (PROKOFIEVA-BELGOVSKAYA and ORLOVA 1956) as well as *S. rimosus* (PROKOFIEVA-BELGOVSKAYA et al. 1956). The transition to production phase is given by the concentration of phosphate ion in the medium. With excess orthophosphate no thin "secondary" mycelium is formed and antibiotic formation ceases (BORETTI et al. 1955). The production phase can be extended by continuous addition of nutrients during the cultivation of both *S. aureofaciens* (MAKAREVICH et al. 1976) and *S. rimosus* (ORLOVA and PUSHKINA 1972).

III. Genetics

A mutagenic treatment of the producers of tetracyclines yields relatively easily blocked strains which produce mostly antibiotically inactive substances – intermediates or shunt metabolites of the biosynthetic pathway (BLUMAUEROVÁ et al. 1969 a, b). The mutations are pleiotropic and alter the morphology, pigmentation, and biochemical activity as well as the spectrum of produced metabolites in the treated strains (HOŠŤÁLEK et al. 1976 a).

The metabolites of mutants blocked in the biosynthetic pathway greatly aided in the elucidation of the biosynthetic sequence of tetracyclines (MCCORMICK

1967, 1969). A useful tool was the method of cosynthesis (McCormick et al. 1960), i.e., a mixed cultivation of pairs of blocked mutants in a submerged culture.

Delič et al. (1969) studied the cosynthetic effect and identified the character of mutants blocked in the biosynthetic pathway using a contact cultivation of two strains on a solid medium with a subsequent biological detection of inhibition zones. This approach made it possible to find out whether the mutant under study is the source of the enzyme system transforming a given substance (a convertor) or whether it produces the transformed substance (a secretor).

Studies concerned with the genome topology (construction of a linkage chromosome map) of the producers of tetracycline antibiotics were concentrated mostly on *S. rimosus*. Attempts at genetical mapping of *S. aureofaciens* were unsuccessful mainly because of low stability and difficulty in obtaining suitable auxotrophic mutants (Blumauerová et al. 1972).

The genetic map of the *S. rimosus* chromosome was constructed by Alačević (1973, 1976) and by Friend and Hopwood (1971). The work was performed independently in two laboratories on different strains, with the mapping of different nutritional markers. Even so the identical position of some markers indicates a similarity between the two maps. The sequence of markers is also similar to that found in the linkage map of *Streptomyces coelicolor* A3 (Hopwood 1967).

C. Building Units of Tetracyclines

The molecule of tetracycline antibiotics has functional groups arranged in a complex pattern located upon the characteristic hydroxynaphthacene ring. The presence of a chain of potential carbonyl groups in mutual β-positions indicates a biogenetic relationship to other ketide metabolites of microbial origin. The structure of the tetracycline molecule, especially of 2-acetyl-2-decarboxyamidotetracyclines (Hochstein et al. 1960), resembles that of molecules of aglycones of anthracyclines such as aklavinone, ε-pyrromycinone, rhodomycinones, or daunomycinones (Vaněk et al. 1977). A structural relationship with tetracyclines is also found in viridicatumtoxin [Table 1 (49)], a toxic substance produced by *Penicillium viridicatum* Westling (Kabuto et al. 1976). The occurrence of this type of substance in eukaryotes is interesting from the viewpoint of chemotaxonomy.

The localization of substituents on the tetracenequinone skeleton of tetracyclines confirms the earlier hypothesis of Birch (1957) on the biosynthesis of natural products by head-to-tail condensation of acetate units with the participation of coenzyme A (CoA), similar to that in derivatives of naphthacenequinone, anthraquinone, or macrolides. The polycarbonyl chain of these substances arises by condensation of malonyl CoA with simultaneous decarboxylation, as proved, e.g., in the biosynthesis of 6-methylsalycylic acid (Lynen and Tada 1961; Dimroth et al. 1970). This mechanism was indeed experimentally confirmed by Gatenbeck (1961), who studied the mechanism of oxytetracycline biosynthesis.

In the first experiments concerning the fate of the building blocks of tetracycline antibiotics, Miller et al. (1956) proved that acetate-1-[^{14}C] and acetate-2-[^{14}C] are precursors of labeled chlortetracycline. Identical incorporation of the two substances suggested that the whole acetate group was incorporated. Snell et al. (1956) also found an incorporation of acetate-2-[^{14}C] into the oxytetracycline molecule. A partial degradation showed that labeled acetate was probably directly incorporated into rings B, C, and D; the activity of ring A was negligible. A detailed degradation study of oxytetracycline synthesized on a medium containing acetate-2-[^{14}C] showed that rings B, C, and D (between C5 and C12, with the exception of the 6-methyl group) arise by condensation of acetate units (Snell et al. 1960; Birch et al. 1962).

Miller et al. (1956) found a high and, probably, direct incorporation of the labeled methyl group of glycine and methionine into the chlortetracycline molecule. Differences between the incorporation of glycine labeled on C1 (low activity) and C2 indicate that glycine serves as a donor of a one-carbon group. As found by degradation, the activity is concentrated mostly in the dimethylamino group in position-4. Similar conclusions were made by Snell et al. (1956), who found incorporation of glycine-2-[^{14}C] into the methyl group in position-6 of the oxytetracycline molecule.

Experiments with specific incorporation of glutamic acid-2-[^{14}C] led Snell et al. (1960) to the conclusion that this compound was probably a direct precursor of carbons 2, 3, 4, and 4a of ring A. Degradation of tetracycline synthesized on a medium containing methionine labeled in the methyl group showed that all activity was concentrated in the *N*-methyl groups in position-4 and in the methyl group in position-6. The activity of all methyl groups was identical (Snell et al. 1960; Birch et al. 1962).

The results of Podojil et al. (1973) show that the terminal carboxamide group of the tetracycline molecule differs biogenetically from the building blocks which make up the basic skeleton. Its precursor, malonamoyl CoA, is probably formed by decarboxylation of a C4 unit. Incorporation of U-[^{14}C]-asparagine was tenfold higher into the terminal group than into other positions on the tetracycline skeleton. These conclusions were also confirmed by Běhal et al. (1974).

D. The Biosynthetic Pathway of Tetracyclines

The elucidation of the biosynthetic sequence of tetracyclines was greatly aided by the immense variability of *S. aureofaciens* (Backus et al. 1954), which made it possible to isolate a set of mutants blocked in almost all the biosynthetic steps (McCormick 1966). This facilitated the isolation and identification of intermediates or shunt products.

A significant contribution was due to the so-called cosynthesis technique (McCormick et al. 1960). Mixed cultivation of a pair of blocked mutants leads to an intercellular transfer of biosynthetic intermediates or essential cofactors, resulting in the production of a final substance which is otherwise produced in neither of the pure cultures of the two partners. It is usually the transfer of biosynthetic intermediates from the mutant blocked in later steps into the mutant with an earlier block. This mutant carries out the complete synthesis thanks to its enzyme equipment.

The biosynthetic sequence was also studied by the technique of conversion of isolated metabolites of blocked mutants, or proposed intermediates prepared by chemical synthesis, in a culture or suspension of mutant cells of different types (McCormick 1965). An important contribution to the deciphering of the biosynthetic pathway of tetracyclines was also made by the study of conversion of natural or synthetic intermediates by cell-free extracts of *S. aureofaciens* and *S. rimosus* (Miller 1967).

I. The Origin of the Tricyclic Nonaketide

McCormick (1965) assumes that the oligoketide chain of tetracyclines arises by primary condensation of malonyl CoA with malonamoyl CoA, after which the chain extends by linear condensation of another 7 malonyl CoA units. In mutants incapable of malonamoyl CoA formation, the synthesis of 2-acetyldecarboxamidotetracyclines (Hochstein et al. 1960; Miller and Hochstein 1962) is initiated by acetoacetyl CoA.

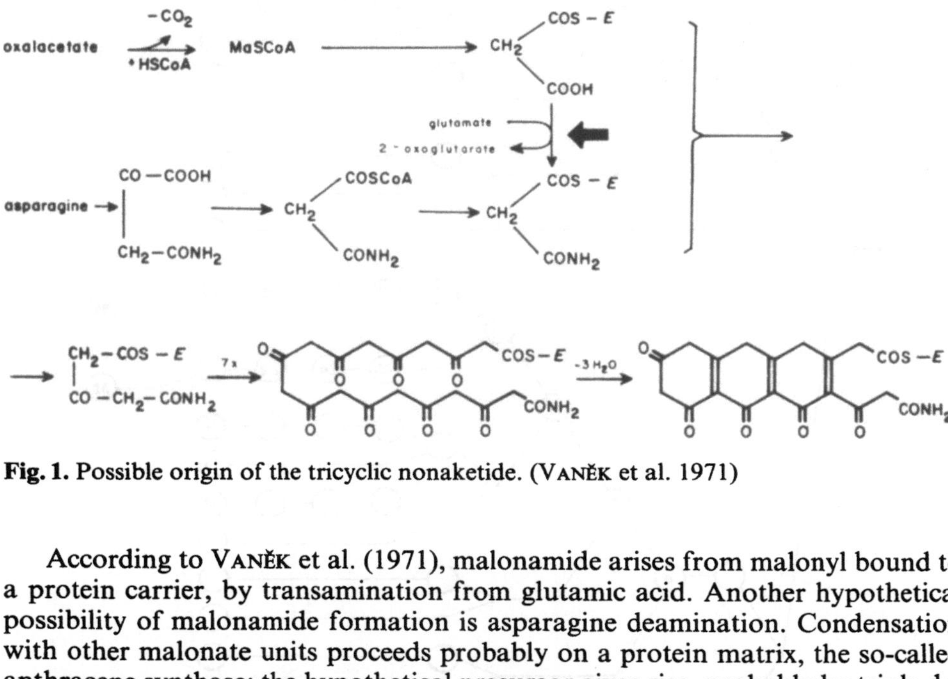

Fig. 1. Possible origin of the tricyclic nonaketide. (Vaněk et al. 1971)

According to Vaněk et al. (1971), malonamide arises from malonyl bound to a protein carrier, by transamination from glutamic acid. Another hypothetical possibility of malonamide formation is asparagine deamination. Condensation with other malonate units proceeds probably on a protein matrix, the so-called anthracene synthase; the hypothetical precursor gives rise, probably by triple dehydration, to a tricyclic nonaketide (Fig. 1). In strains that do not form malonamide the condensation of eight molecules of malonyl CoA with acetoacetyl CoA probably yields a tricyclic decaketide (McCormick 1966).

The summary of biosynthetic steps involved in further transformation of the hypothetical nonaketide and decaketide precursors is given in Fig. 2. Compounds which are presumed to take part in this process are numbered according to the biosynthetic sequence in Table 1.

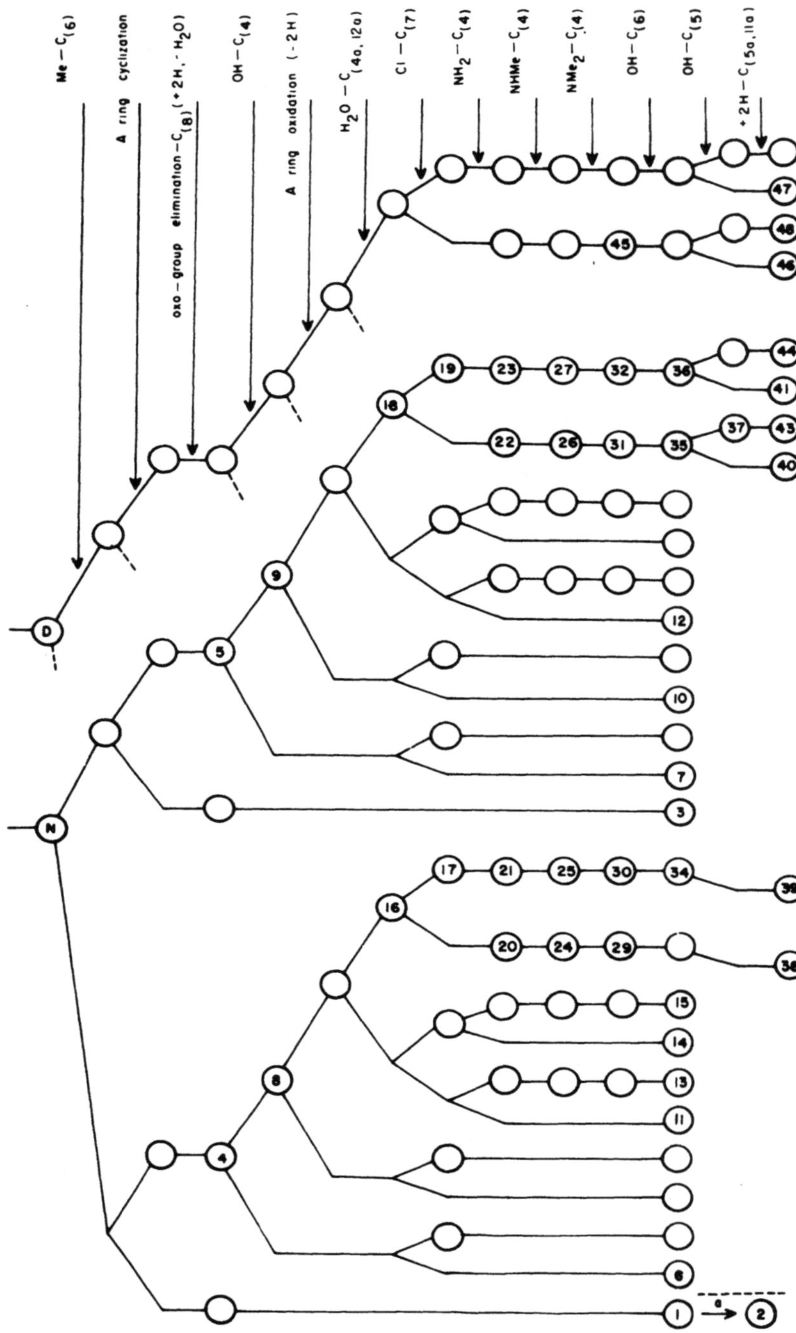

Fig. 2. Summary of the biosynthetic reactions of the tetracyclines. (VANĚK et al. 1971). *D*, the hypothetical decatetide; *N*, the hypothetical nonaketide. *Ascendant lines* indicate that the reaction runs and *descendant lines* that the reaction does not run. *Numbers in circles* represent the numbers of compounds listed in Table 1. *Open circles* indicate hypothetical compounds. Reaction *a* (transformation of compound 1 to compound 2) indicates a reduction and lactonization (PŘIKRYLOVÁ et al. 1978)

Table 1. Tetracycline compounds obtained by biosynthesis including substrates or products of biotransformation[a]

Compound	References
1 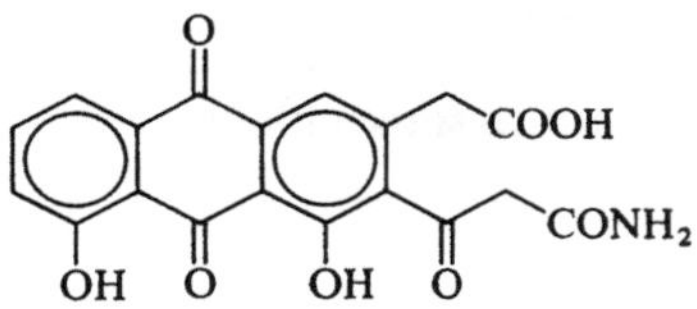 Protetrone	McCormick (1966) McCormick and Jensen (1968)
2 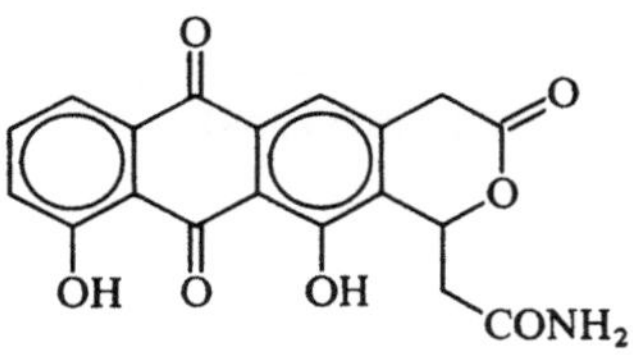 Ekatetrone	Podojil et al. (1978) Přikrylová et al. (1978)
3 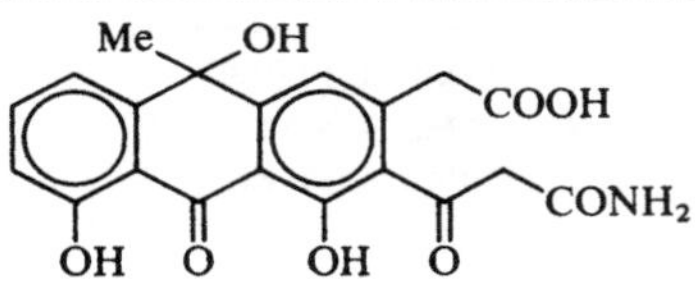 Oxanthranol derivate ("anthrone")	McCormick et al. (1968b)
4 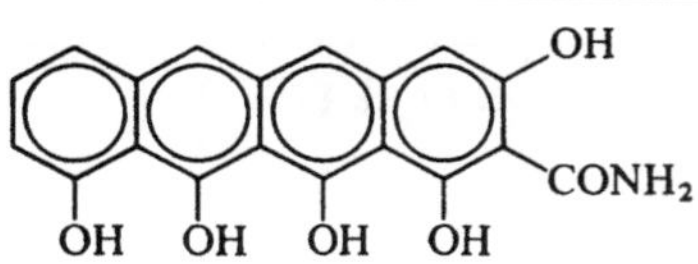 Pretetramid	McCormick (1969) McCormick et al. (1963a)
5 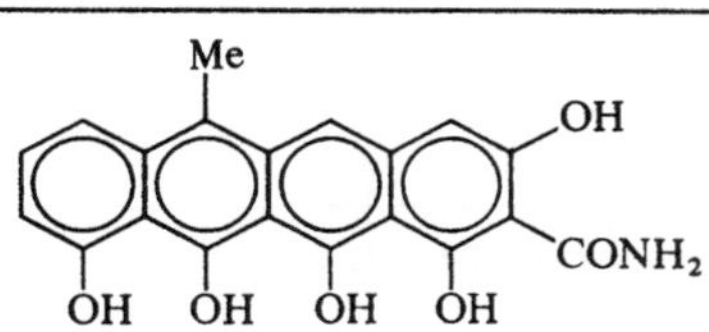 6-Methylpretetramid	McCormick (1969) McCormick et al. (1963a)
6 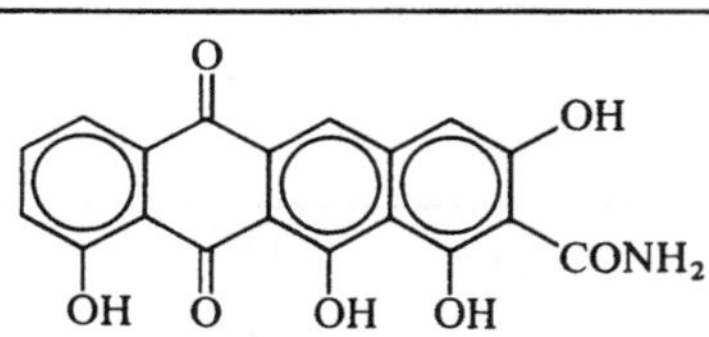 Naphthacenequinone derivative	McCormick (1969)

[a] Compounds are numbered according to the proposed biosynthetic sequence (see Fig. 2), with the exception of 2-acetyl-2-decarboxamidotetracyclines (45, 46, 47, 48) and viridicatumtoxin (49)

Table 1 (continued)

Compound	References
7 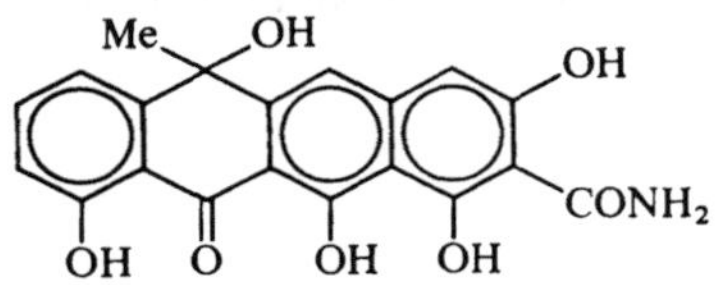 6-Hydroxy-6-methyl-pretetramid	McCormick (1969)
8 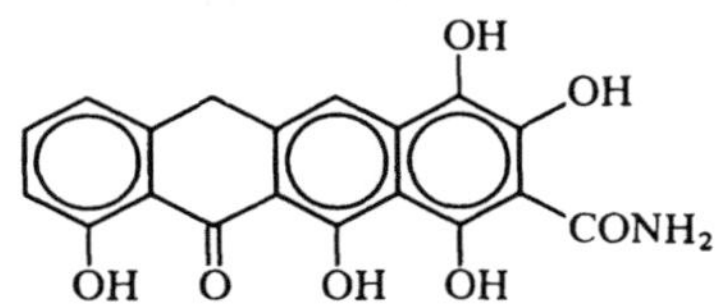 4-Hydroxypretetramid	McCormick (1969)
9 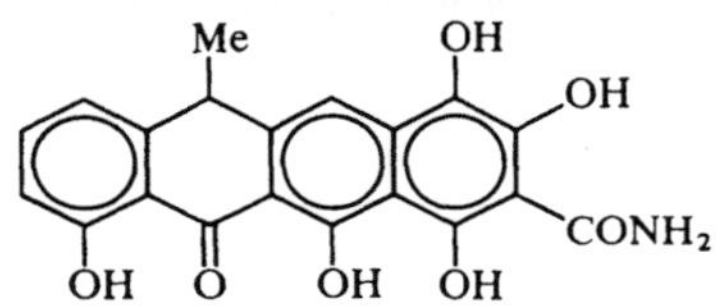 4-Hydroxy-6-methyl-pretetramid	McCormick (1969) McCormick and Jensen (1965) McCormick et al. (1965)
10 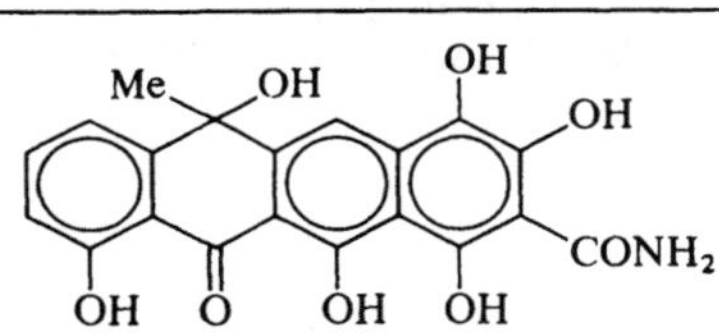 Aureovocidin (4,6-dihydroxy-6-methyl-pretetramid)	Vaněk et al. (1971)
11 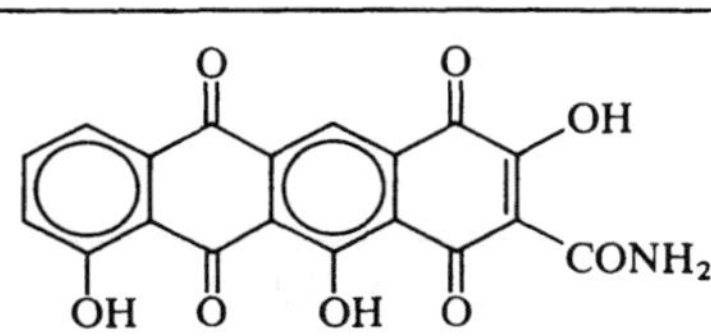 A-C-Diquinone	McCormick (1969)
12 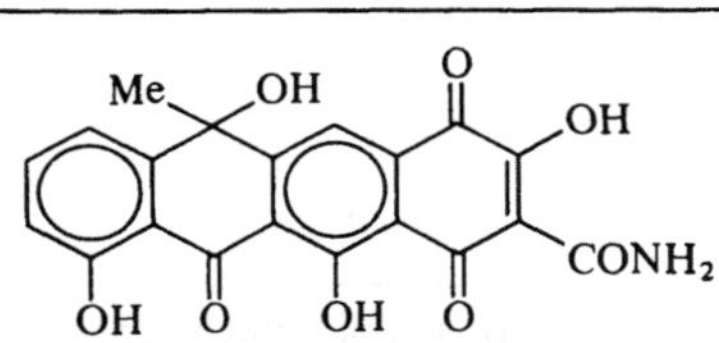 Tetramid-green	McCormick (1969)

Table 1 (continued)

Compound	References
13 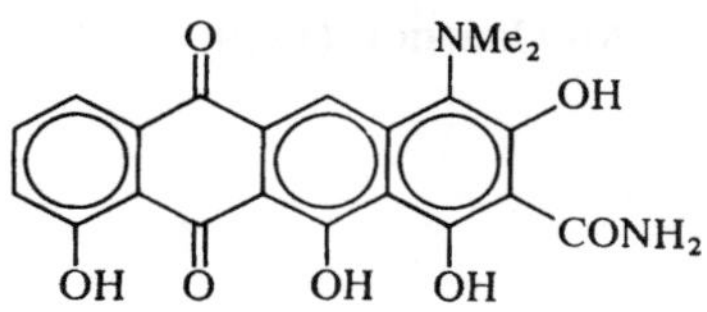 Tetramid-blue	McCormick (1969)
14 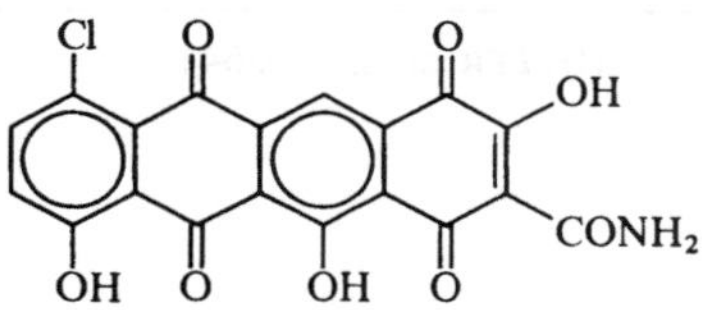 Chloro-A-C-diquinone	McCormick (1969)
15 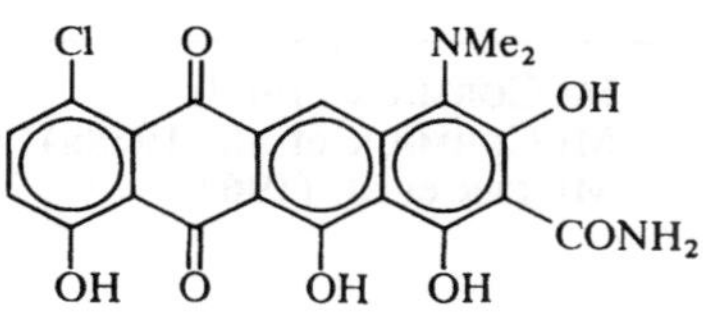 Chlortetramid-blue	McCormick (1969)
16 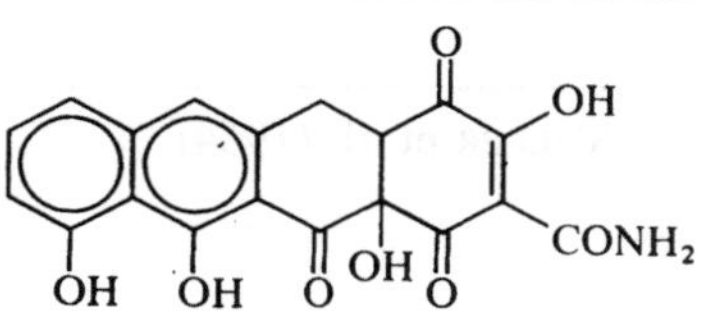 4-Oxo-6-demethyl-anhydrotetracycline	McCormick (1969)
17 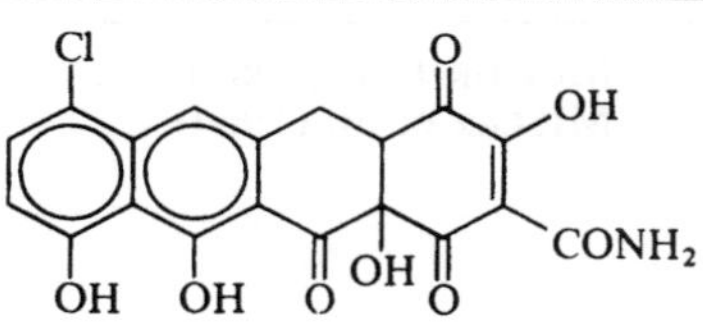 4-Oxo-6-demethylanhydro-chlortetracycline	McCormick (1969)
18 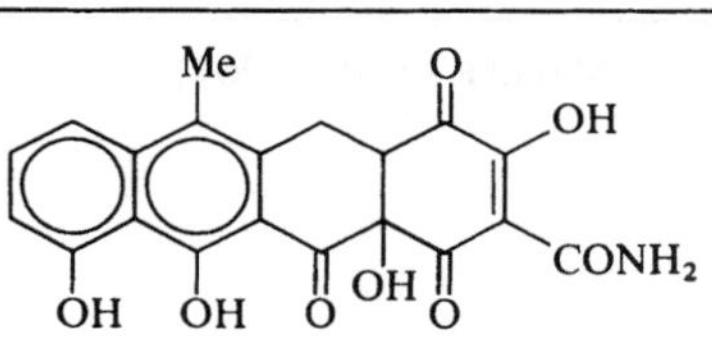 4-Oxoanhydrotetracycline	McCormick (1967, 1969)

Table 1 (continued)

Compound		References
19	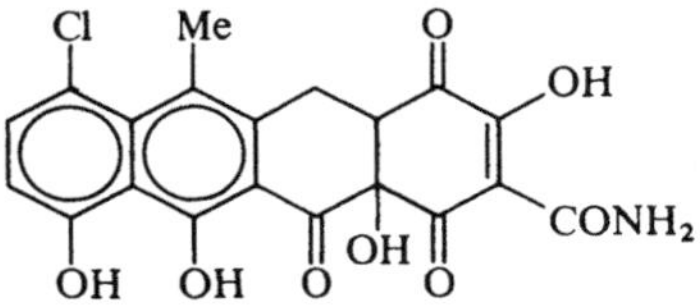 4-Oxoanhydro-chlortetracycline	McCORMICK (1969)
20	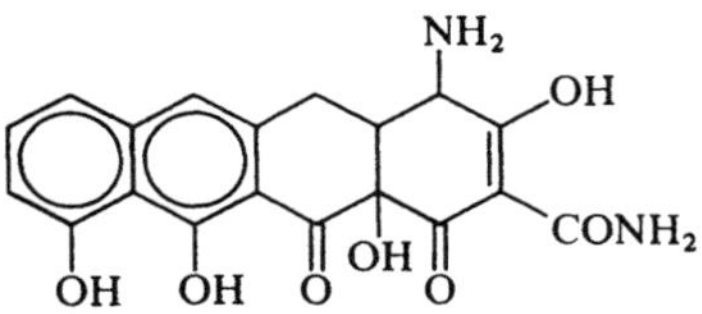 4-Amino-6-demethyl-anhydrotetracycline	MILLER et al. (1964)
21	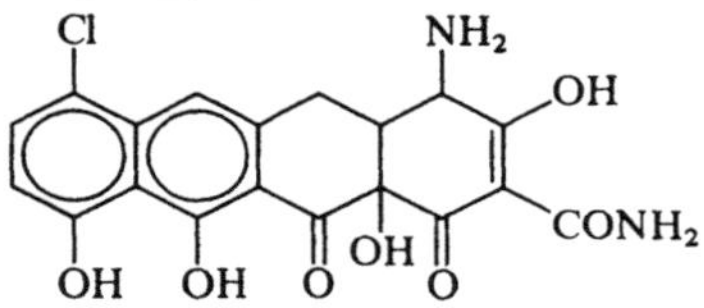 4-Amino-6-demethylanhydro-chlortetracycline	McCORMICK (1969) McCORMICK et al. (1968a) MILLER et al. (1964)
22	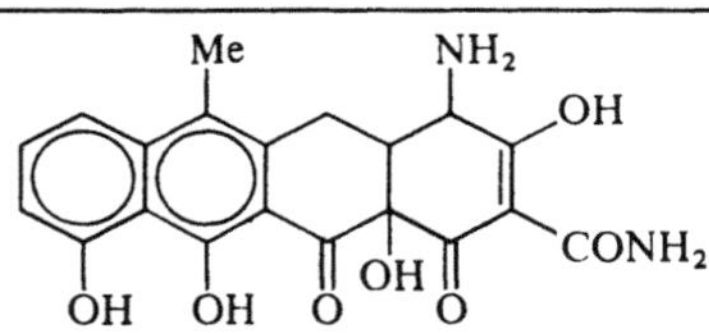 4-Amino-anhydrotetracycline	MILLER et al. (1964)
23	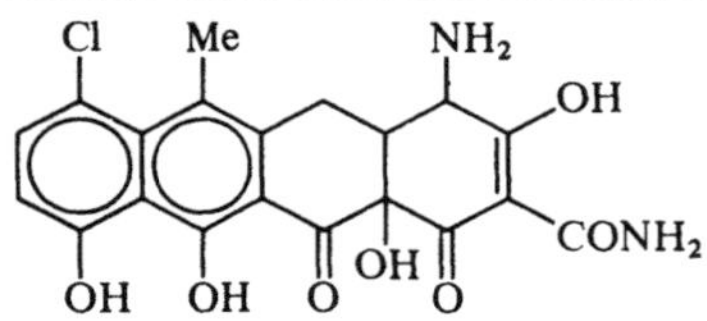 4-Amino-anhydro-chlortetracycline	McCORMICK (1969) MILLER et al. (1964)
24	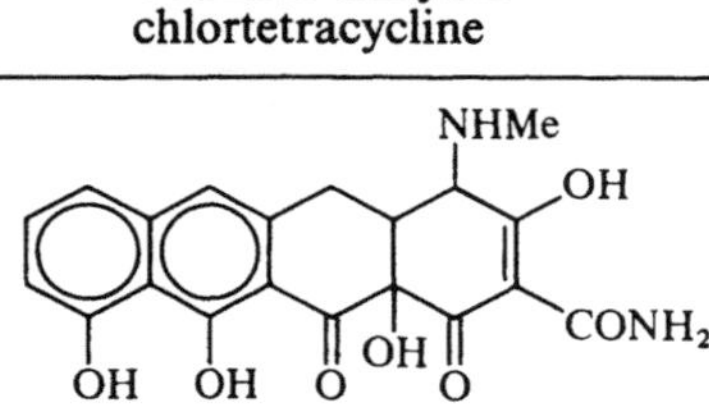 4-Methylamino-6-demethyl-anhydrotetracycline	MILLER et al. (1964)

Table 1 (continued)

	Compound	References
25	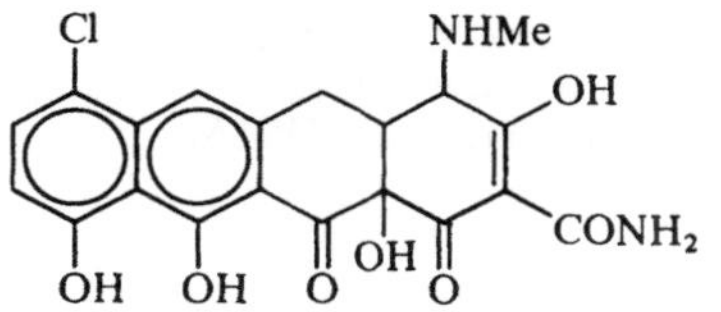 4-Methylamino-6-demethyl-anhydrochlortetracycline	MILLER et al. (1964)
26	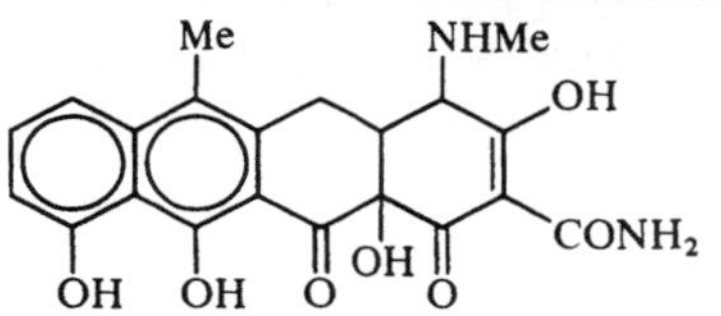 4-Methylamino-anhydrotetracycline	MILLER et al. (1964)
27	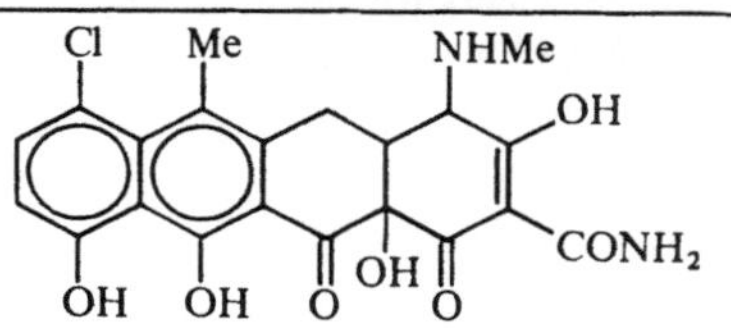 4-Methylamino-anhydrochlortetracycline	MILLER et al. (1964)
28	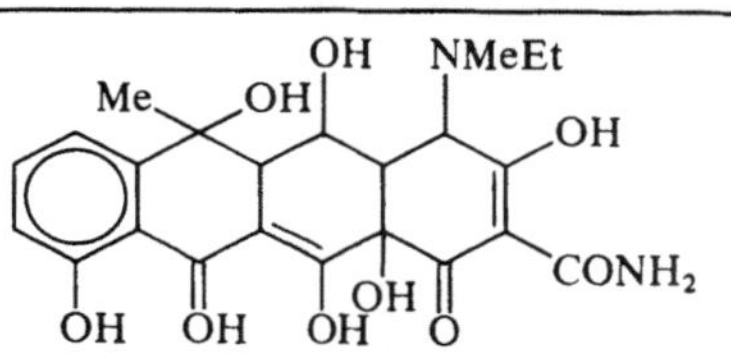 4-Methylethyloxytetracycline	DULANEY et al. (1962)
29	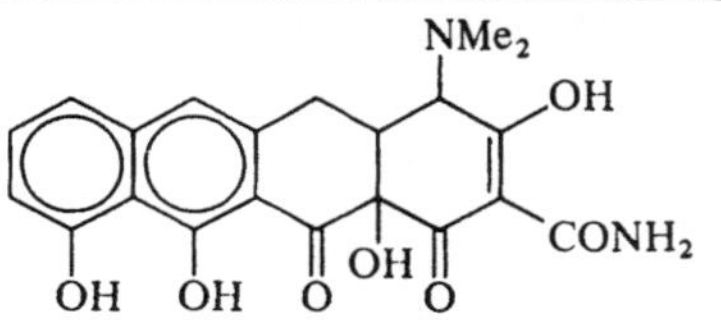 6-Demethylanhydro-tetracycline	MCCORMICK et al. (1962) MILLER et al. (1964)
30	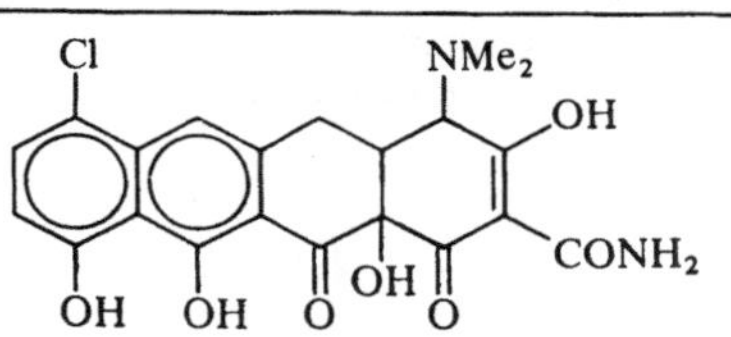 6-Demethylanhydro-chlortetracycline	MCCORMICK et al. (1962) MCCORMICK and JENSEN (1969)

Table 1 (continued)

Compound	References
31 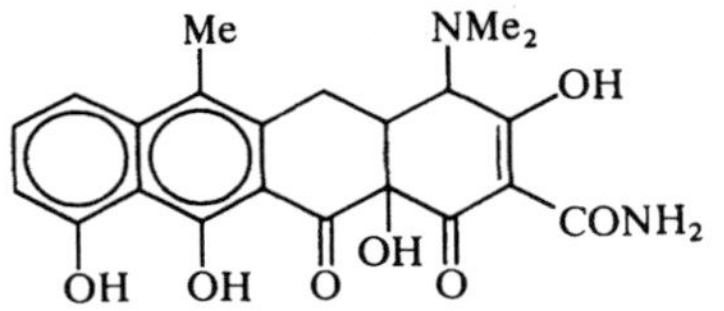 Anhydrotetracycline	McCormick et al. (1962) Miller et al. (1964) Miller et al. (1965)
32 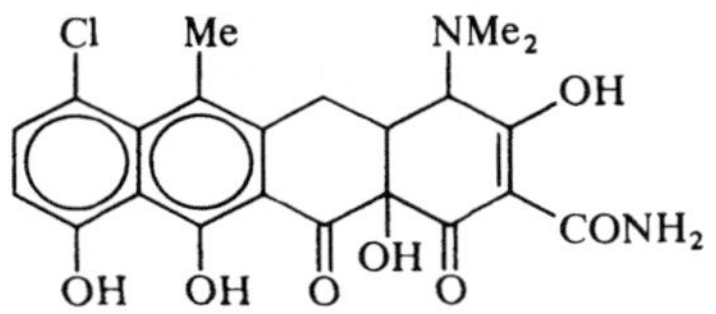 Anhydrochlortetracycline	McCormick (1969) McCormick et al. (1962)
33 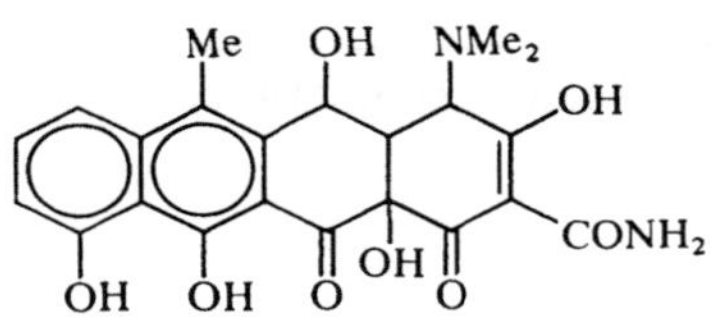 Anhydrooxytetracycline	McCormick et al. (1962) McCormick (1965)
34 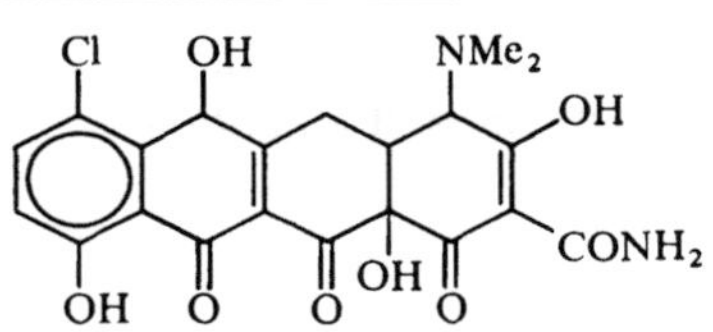 6-Demethyldehydro-chlortetracycline	McCormick (1969)
35 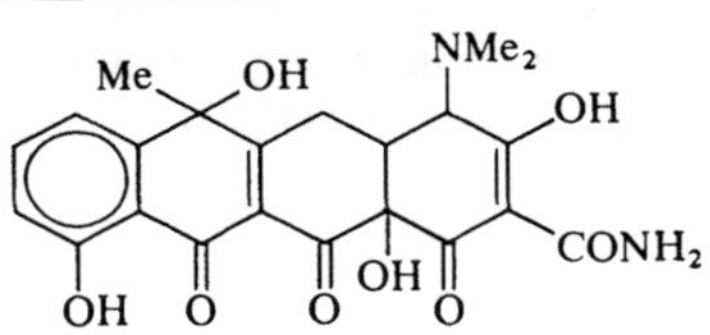 Dehydrotetracycline	Miller et al. (1965)
36 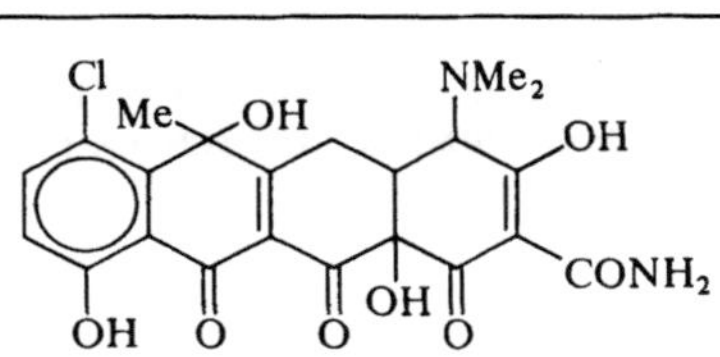 Dehydrochlortetracycline	McCormick (1969) McCormick et al. (1958a, 1958b)

Table 1 (continued)

	Compound	References
37	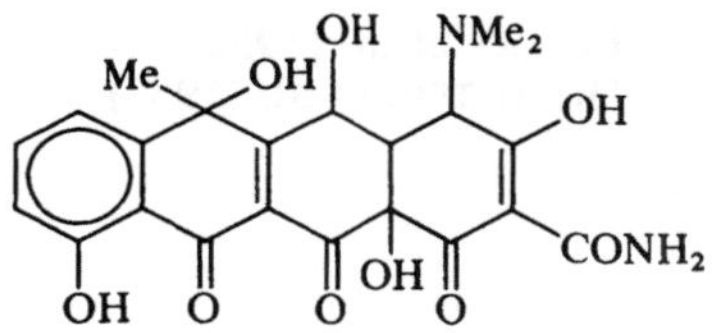 Dehydrooxytetracycline	MILLER (1967)
38	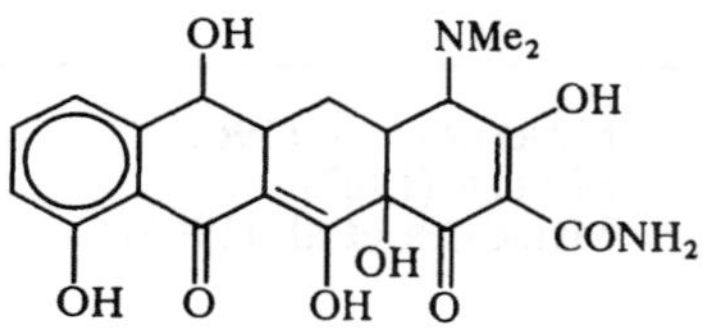 6-Demethyltetracycline	McCORMICK et al. (1957) PERLMAN et al. (1961) McCORMICK et al. (1962)
39	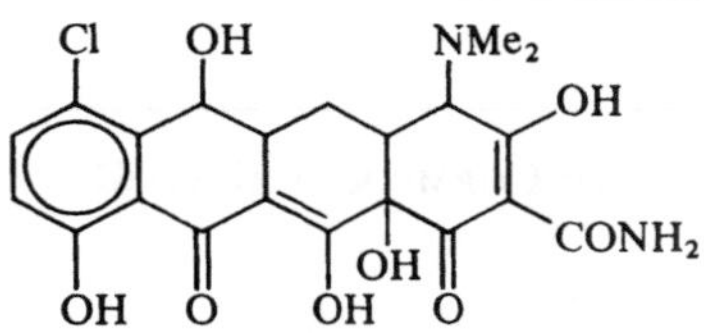 6-Demethylchlortetracycline	McCORMICK et al. (1962) PERLMAN et al. (1961)
40	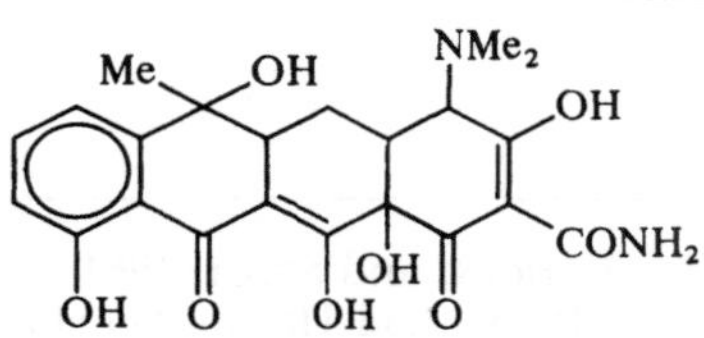 Tetracycline	MINIERI et al. (1954)
41	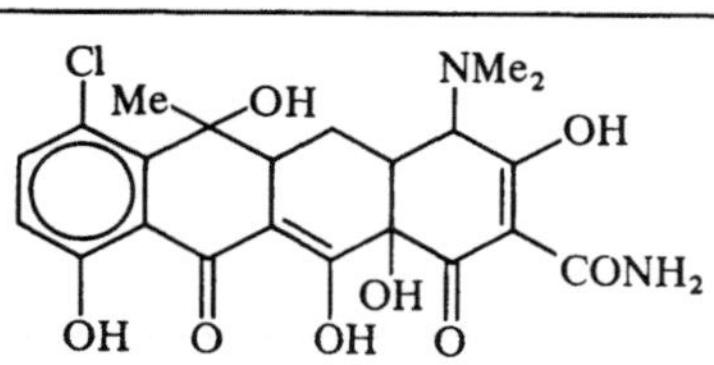 Chlortetracycline	DUGGAR (1948) STEPHENS et al. (1954)
42	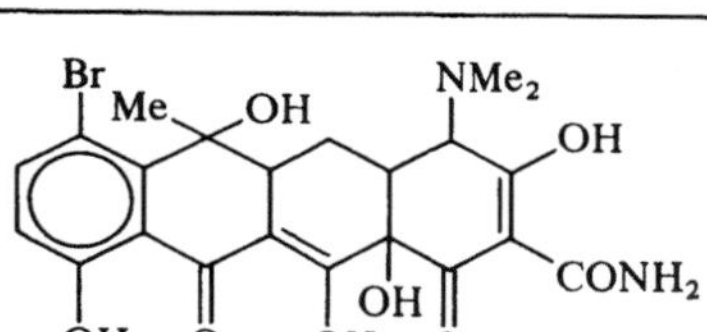 Bromtetracycline	DOERSCHUK et al. (1959)

Table 1 (continued)

Compound	References
43 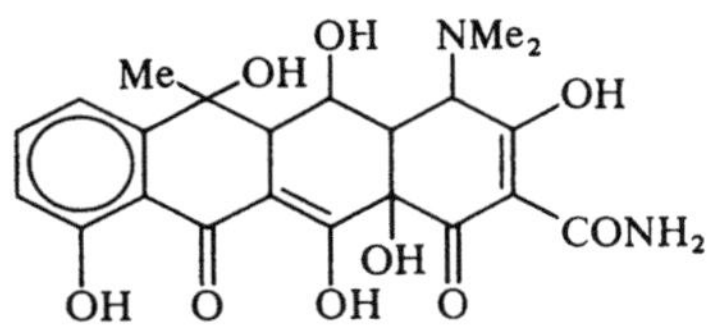 Oxytetracycline (5-hydroxytetracycline)	FINLAY et al. (1950) HOCHSTEIN et al. (1953)
44 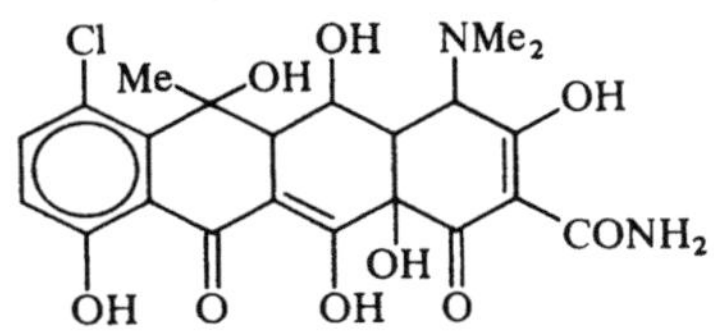 5-Hydroxychlortetracycline	MARTIN et al. (1967) MILLER (1967) MITSCHER et al. (1966)
45 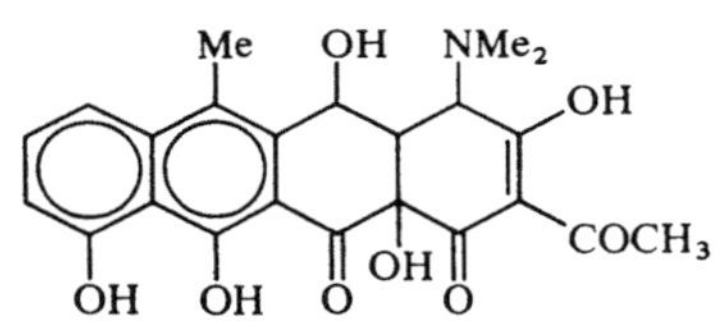 2-Acetyl-2-decarboxamido-anhydrotetracycline	MCCORMICK et al. (1962)
46 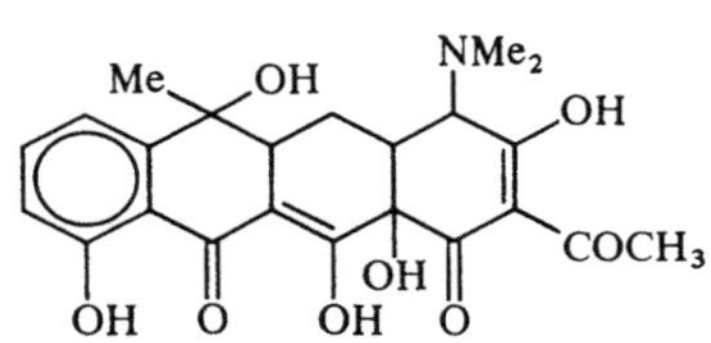 2-Acetyl-2-decarboxamido-tetracycline	LANCINI and SENSI (1964) MILLER and HOCHSTEIN (1962) MCCORMICK (1966)
47 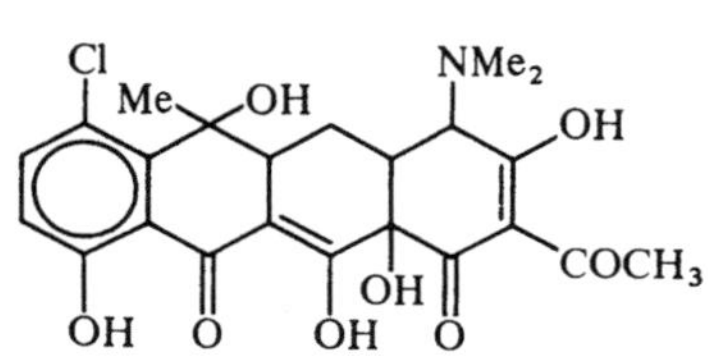 2-Acetyl-2-decarboxamido-chlortetracycline	MILLER and HOCHSTEIN (1962)

Table 1 (continued)

Compound	References
48 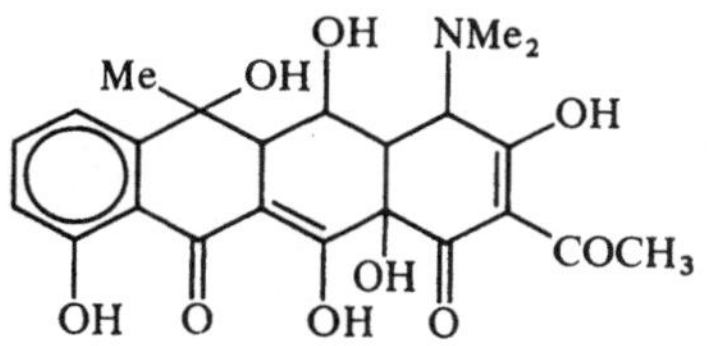 2-Acetyl-2-decarboxamido-oxytetracycline	HOCHSTEIN et al. (1960) McCORMICK (1966)
49 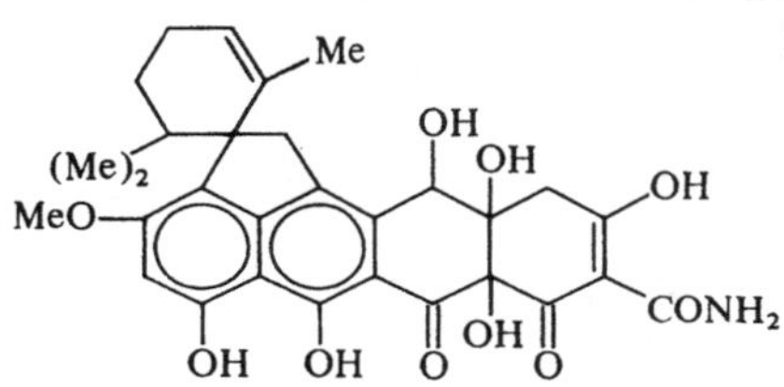 Viridicatumtoxin	KABUTO et al. (1976)

II. Transformations of the Tricyclic Nonaketide

1. *Streptomyces aureofaciens*

The results of McCORMICK (1965, 1969) and MILLER (1967), who, using the technique of conversion of biosynthetic intermediates by different types of blocked mutants, proved the sequence of reactions transforming the tetracycline nucleus, formed a basis for the scheme of the biosynthesis of tetracyclines in *S. aureofaciens* proposed by VANĚK et al. (1971). The scheme includes 72 substances out of which 27 were identified while 45 remain hypothetical. The substances may be formed form a hypothetical tricyclic derivative by a combination of the following 11 reactions: C6 methylation, cyclization of ring A, C4 hydroxylation, oxidation of ring A, removal of the oxo group on C8, C4a,12a hydration, C7 chlorination, C4 transamination, double N-methylation, C6 hydroxylation (and perhaps oxidation to an oxo group), and a final reduction. The proposed biosynthetic scheme for chlortetracycline biosynthesis is given in Fig. 3.

a) C6 Methylation

Identification of shunt metabolites, namely protetrone (1) in *S. aureofaciens* ED 1369 (McCORMICK and JENSEN 1968) and ekatetrone (2) in *S. aureofaciens* 8425 (PODOJIL et al. 1978; PŘIKRYLOVÁ et al. 1978), supports the assumption that the first step in the transformation of the tricyclic nonaketide is C6 methylation.

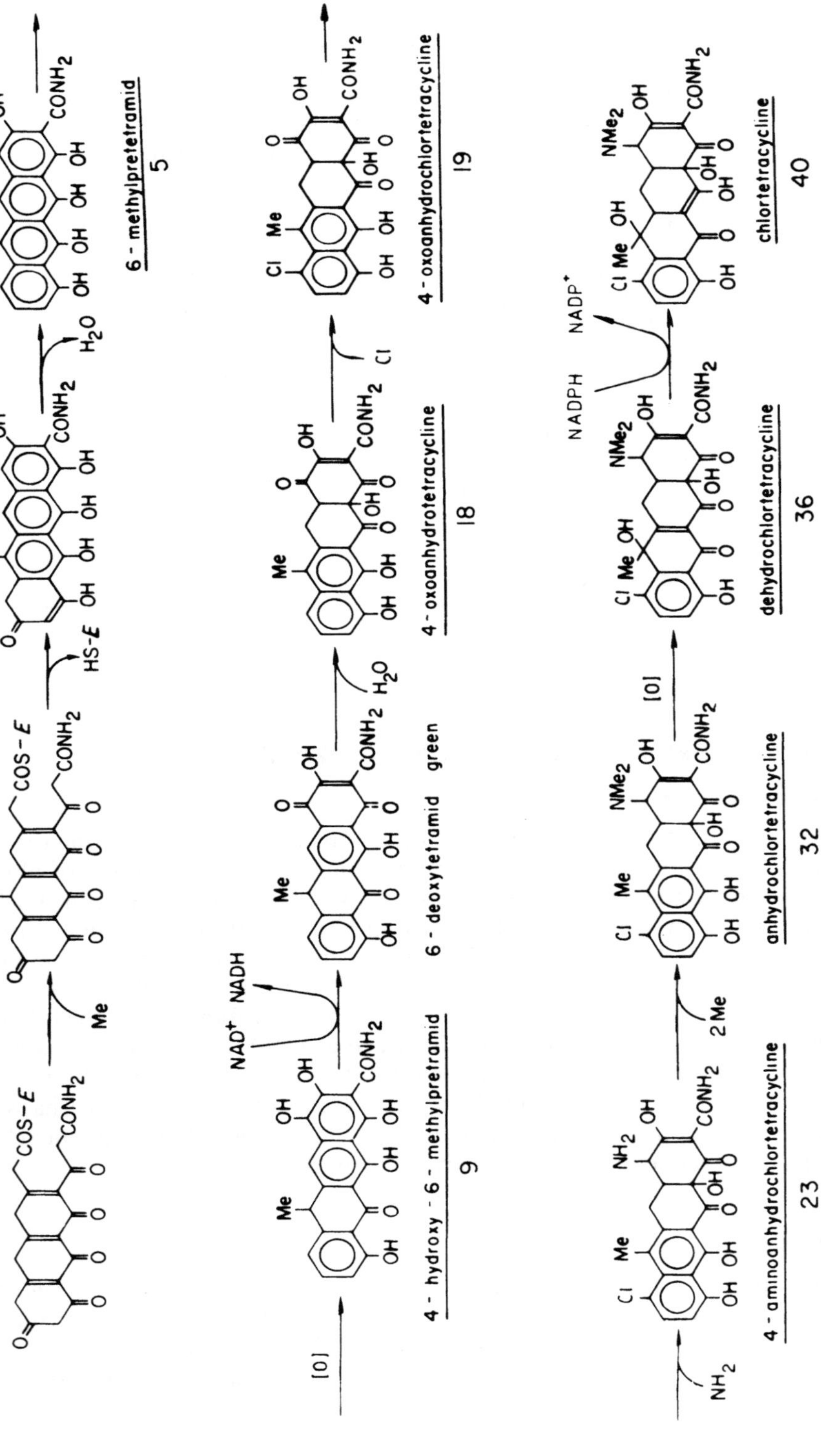

Fig. 3. Biosynthetic scheme of chlortetracycline. (VANĚK et al. 1971)

The hypothetical intermediate has not yet been proved; the methylation thus takes place probably still in the thioester-bound form on the enzyme template.

Demethyltetracyclines were identified by McCormick et al. (1957) as products of biochemical mutant *S. aureofaciens* S 604, which has a block in the C6 methylation. They are also produced in wild strains in which the C6 methylation is inhibited by sulfonamides (Goodman and Matrishin 1961; Perlman et al. 1961) or other analogues of p-aminobenzoic acid (Goodman and Miller 1962) or by ethionine (Hendlin et al. 1962) or norleucine (Goodman and Matrishin 1964). The inhibitory effect of analogues or antimetabolites was usually eliminated by the addition of methionine or p-aminobenzoic acid. Hendlin et al. (1962) assume that the formation of demethyltetracyclines results from insufficient activity of methyltransferase or a suppressed synthesis of methionine. Auxothrophy for p-aminobenzoic acid, however, is not a necessary condition for the biosynthesis of demethyltetracyclines (Zaitseva and Mindlin 1965).

Inhibition of C6 methylation is typical solely for *S. aureofaciens*; in *S. rimosus* an addition of ethionine inhibits oxytetracycline production; however, no 6-demethyloxytetracycline was found in the culture (Zigmunt 1962).

b) Cyclization of Ring A

Vaněk et al. (1971) assume that further reaction after the release from the enzyme template, the cyclization of ring A, provides the possibility of formation of biosynthetic intermediates in both the methylated and in the nonmethylated series. In cases where the cyclization did not take place, the number of resulting metabolites with an open fourth ring is substantially lower.

c) Elimination of the Oxo Group on C8

Metabolites that would be formed from a hypothetical intermediate with a closed ring A by elimination of the oxo group on C8 were also found in none of the cultures of *S. aureofaciens* mutants under study. When these substances, i.e., 6-methylpretetramid (5) in the methylated and pretetramid (4) in the nonmethylated series, prepared by degradation of tetracycline antibiotics as well as by total synthesis (McCormick et al. 1963 b), were added to the culture of blocked mutants of *S. aureofaciens*, they were transformed to corresponding tetracyclines (McCormick et al. 1963 a).

d) C4 Hydroxylation

This biosynthetic step was demonstrated by McCormick et al. (1965) by the identification of 4-hydroxy-6-methylpretetramid (9) in a culture of spontaneous variant *S. aureofaciens* V 655 (McCormick and Jensen 1965). This compound was transformed to chlortetracycline in a culture of a nonmethylating mutant of *S. aureofaciens* ED 1369. In the strain *S. aureofaciens* ED 1424 the authors succeeded in also identifying the nonmethylated analogue 4-hydroxypretetramid (8) (McCormick 1969). Both 4-hydroxypretetramids are accompanied by shunt oxidation products tetramid green (12) and A–C-diquinone (11).

e) Oxidation of Ring A

VANĚK et al. (1971) suggest that this reaction is necessary for further biosynthetic steps of the tetracycline pathway. The corresponding hypothetical intermediate, the so-called "6-deoxytetramid green," however, has not yet been identified in cultures of production strains or their biochemical mutants.

f) C4a,12a Hydration

Further hydration yields 4-oxo-anhydrotetracycline (18), a labile substance which provides another nonstable rearrangement product "metatetrene." 4-Oxo-anhydrotetracycline (18) was found in a culture of *S. aureofaciens* T 219 and S 2308 (MCCORMICK 1967, 1969). The corresponding 6-demethyl derivative 4-oxo-6-demethylanhydrotetracycline (16) was identified in a culture of *S. aureofaciens* T 995 (MCCORMICK 1969).

g) C7 Chlorination

Chlorination of 4-oxo-anhydrotetracycline (18) yields 4-oxo-anhydrochlortetracycline (19), which is also labile and undergoes a rapid contraction of ring B to yield a nontetracycline shunt product (MCCORMICK 1969). In the demethylated series labile 4-oxo-6-demethylanhydrochlortetracycline (17) is formed through chlorination of 4-oxo-6-demethylanhydrotetracycline (16). This metabolite (17) was identified in the mutant *S. aureofaciens* ED 518 (MCCORMICK 1969).

Chlorination of the tetracycline nucleus is competitively inhibited by the presence of bromide ions in the medium (GOUREVITCH et al. 1955); under these conditions some strains produce bromtetracycline (42) (DOERSCHUK et al. 1959; SENSI et al. 1955). Chlorination is inhibited by a number of substances such as 2-thiouracyl or 2-mercaptobenzthiazole; some of them act as chelating agents and inhibit copper-containing oxidases. The effect of these substances may be eliminated by an excess of Cu^{2+} or Ag^{2+} ions (GOODMAN et al. 1959, 1963; JÁRAI and KOLLÁR 1962; LEIN et al. 1959; SEKIZAWA 1955). The chlorination also fails to take place in the absence of chlorides in the fermentation medium (MINIERI et al. 1954).

Tetracycline, which is formed as the final product when the chlorination of the tetracycline nucleus is suppressed, is also produced by *S. aureofaciens* mutants with a reduced chlorination ability (DARKEN et al. 1960; DOERSCHUK et al. 1959; JÁRAI 1965).

h) C4 Transamination

The products of the following biosynthetic step, the C4 transamination, were identified in *S. aureofaciens* cultures supplied with ethionine. MILLER et al. (1964) found 4-amino-anhydrochlortetracycline (23) in a sonic extract from *S. aureofaciens* BC 41 (chlortetracycline producer) on a complex medium with ethionine. The nonmethylating mutant *S. aureofaciens* ED 3636 produced, on a synthetic medium with ethionine, 4-amino-6-demethylanhydrotetracycline (20) and 4-amino-6-demethylanhydrochlortetracycline (21).

The evidence that *N*-demethyl analogues of anhydrotetracyclines are the biosynthetic intermediates of the biosynthetic pathway was also provided by

McCormick et al. (1968a), who isolated 4-amino-6-demethylanhydrochlortetracycline (21) from the blocked mutant *S. aureofaciens* 1E 1407.

i) Double *N*-Methylation

Miller et al. (1964) showed that this process has two steps, viz., an initial formation of monomethylamino- and then production of dimethylaminotetracyclines. The culture of *S. aureofaciens* BC 41 containing ethionine was found to contain 4-methylamino-anhydrochlortetracycline (27) while *S. aureofaciens* ED 3636 on a synthetic medium with ethionine was found to contain 4-methylamino-6-demethylanhydrochlortetracycline (25) and 4-methylamino-6-demethylanhydrotetracycline (24). The cell-free preparation of *S. aureofaciens* S 2242 in the presence of *S*-adenosylmethionine was then found to promote the conversion of 4-amino-anhydrotetracycline (22) to anhydrotetracycline (31) via 4-methylamino-anhydrotetracycline (26) (Miller et al. 1964).

Experiments with blocked mutants failed to prove that anhydrotetracyclines are intermediates of the biosynthetic pathway. Both anhydrochlortetracycline and anhydrotetracycline are toxic for the producing organism (Goodman et al. 1955), and the biochemical block in C6 hydroxylation is probably a lethal mutation. Only the blocked mutant *S. aureofaciens* 1E 6113 was found to contain 6-demethylanhydrochlortetracycline (30) produced together with small amounts of 6-demethylchlortetracycline (39) (McCormick and Jensen 1969). The high toxicity of anhydrotetracyclines is probably due to their inhibitory action on RNA accumulation. Silverman and Atherly (1978) showed that in *Escherichia coli* this process is suppressed by anhydrotetracycline concentrations tenfold lower than those of other tetracycline compounds.

McCormick et al. (1962) demonstrated the conversion of anhydrochlortetracycline (32) in a culture of *S. aureofaciens* BC 41 to chlortetracycline (41), anhydrotetracycline (31) to tetracycline (40), or anhydrochlortetracycline (32) to dehydrochlortetracycline (36) in the blocked mutant *S. aureofaciens* S 1308, 6-demethylanhydrotetracycline (29) to 6-demethyltetracycline (38) in the blocked mutant *S. aureofaciens* S 2242, and 6-demethylanhydrochlortetracycline (30) to 6-demethylchlortetracycline (39) in the blocked mutant *S. aureofaciens* S 2311.

C4 methylation of the tetracycline nucleus is catalyzed by tetracycline methyltransferase (*S*-adenosylmethionine : dedimethylamino-4-aminoanhydrotetracycline *N*-methyltransferase). The enzyme was described by Miller and Hash (1975a) and found in *S. aureofaciens* and *S. rimosus*. The authors assume that the enzyme introduces both the methyl groups. The determination of the enzyme activity in a cell-free preparation is based on the measurement of incorporation of label from [^{14}C]*S*-adenosylmethionine into the reaction product – anhydrotetracycline. Aminoanhydrotetracycline was used as substrate. Study of the substrate specificity also showed the methylation of 7-chloro-, 6-demethyl-, 2-carboxamido-2-nitrile-, and 4-methylaminoderivatives of 4-amino-anhydrotetracycline.

j) C6 Hydroxylation

Hydroxylation of anhydrotetracyclines yields corresponding dehydrotetracyclines. Enzyme hydroxylation in position-C6 is probably a highly nonspecific process since it yields a large number of metabolites. When C6 methylation is blocked, after the cyclization of ring A, *S. aureofaciens* ED 1369 and V 828 directly yield protetrone (1) by C6 hydroxylation and subsequent reduction (McCormick 1966; McCormick and Jensen 1968). Reduction and lactonization of this compound gives ekatetrone (2) (Podojil et al. 1978; Přikrylová et al. 1978).

In the methylated series, a block in cyclization of ring A leads to the direct formation of the oxanthranol derivative "anthron" (3), which was identified by McCormick et al. (1968 b) in a culture of *S. aureofaciens* S 2242.

In the nonmethylated series, the biosynthetic sequence, including the cyclization of ring A, gives the naphthacenequinone derivative (6) from pretetramid (4) as demonstrated in the mutant *S. aureofaciens* K 147 (McCormick 1969) and another shunt product 6-hydroxy-6-methylpretetramid (7) from 6-methylpretetramid (5) in *S. aureofaciens* K 114 (McCormick 1965).

If C4 hydroxylation has taken place 4-hydroxy-6-methylpretetramid (9) probably yields the corresponding C6-hydroxylated derivative aureovocidin (10), which was identified in *S. aureofaciens* 8425 as aglycone of the glucoside aureovocin (Vaněk et al. 1971).

The existence of hypothetical intermediates – 6-demethyl-6-deoxytetramid green in the nonmethylated and 6-deoxytetramid green in the methylated series (Vaněk et al. 1971) – is indicated by the identification of A–C diquinone (11) in *S. aureofaciens* ED 1424 and of tetramid green (12) in *S. aureofaciens* V 655 (McCormick 1969); these substances are probably also formed by a direct hydroxylation of the hypothetical substances.

Blocked mutants of the nonmethylated series were also found to produce other substances arising from the hypothetical 6-demethyl-6-deoxytetramid green. Among these substances are tetramid blue (13) formed in *S. aureofaciens* E 504 probably due to another series of reactions after a block in C4a,12a hydration and C7 chlorination (McCormick 1965) and chloro-A–C-diquinone (14), a product of the mutant *S. aureofaciens* 1E 1407 (McCormick 1969) probably formed by direct C6 hydroxylation of the hypothetical 6-demethyl-6-deoxy-7-chlorotetramide green (Vaněk et al. 1971). The same intermediate gives rise to chlortetramid blue (15) in the mutant *S. aureofaciens* 1E 6113 and E 504, probably after a transfer of the amino group to C4 and double *N*-methylation (McCormick 1969).

In the biosynthetic sequence leading to tetracycline antibiotics, 6-demethyldehydrochlortetracycline (34) described by McCormick (1969) in *S. aureofaciens* E 504 is an intermediate of 6-demethylchlortetracycline (39). This substance, which arises by C6 hydroxylation of 6-demethylanhydrochlortetracycline (30), is highly unstable and is usually degraded to chlortetramid blue (15). In the methylated series a nonchlorinated dehydrotetracycline (35) is a biosynthetic intermediate formed by C6 hydroxylation. Its formation was documented by Miller et al. (1965) during the conversion of anhydrotetracycline (31) in a cell-free preparation from *S. aureofaciens* E 504. Dehydrochlortetracycline (36) was described as the product of the biochemical mutant *S. aureofaciens* S 1308 blocked in the final reduction (McCormick et al. 1958 a).

C6 hydroxylation of anhydrotetracyclines is catalyzed by anhydrotetracycline oxygenase. Běhal et al. (1979 a) identified this enzyme in *S. aureofaciens* and

S. rimosus. The enzyme assay is based on the measurement of absorbance at 345 nm (maximum of absorption of anhydrotetracyclines, different from the maximum for dehydrotetracyclines and tetracyclines). The cell-free extract is incubated with anhydrotetracycline in the presence of NADPH and O_2. The decrease in absorption at 440 nm is directly proportional to the amount of anhydrotetracycline transformed to dehydrotetracycline.

k) Final Reduction

The final reduction of the 5a,11a double bond, described by McCormick et al. (1958b), completes the transformation of appropriate 5a,11a-dehydrotetracyclines to antibiotically active final products. Thus 6-demethyltetracycline (38), a product of the biochemical mutant *S. aureofaciens* S 604, was described by McCormick et al. (1957) similar to its chlorinated analogue 6-demethylchlortetracycline (39). Tetracycline (40) was described as a product of the biochemical mutants *S. aureofaciens* with a low chlorination ability (Doerschuk et al. 1959).

The formation of chlortetracycline (41), a standard metabolite in the species *S. aureofaciens*, by the final reduction of the 5a,11a double bond was proved by McCormick et al. (1958b) through a biological reduction of dehydrochlortetracycline (36) in a culture of *S. aureofaciens* BC 41 and V 138.

The final reduction of the 5a,11a double bond is catalyzed by NADP: tetracycline 5a(11a) dehydrogenase (Miller and Hash 1975b). The enzyme was detected in *S. aureofaciens* and its determination is based on the investigation of the antibiotic activity in a cell-free extract containing antibiotically inactive 7-chloro-5a(11a)-dehydrotetracycline and NADPH. The antibiotic activity of the resulting chlortetracycline corresponds to the activity of the enzyme.

The reaction in a cell-free extract does not require the presence of the so-called cosynthetic factor I which is assumed to participate in hydrogen transfer during the reduction (Miller et al. 1960). An addition of the cosynthetic factor I to the culture of the mutant *S. aureofaciens* S 1308 blocked in the final reduction brings about chlortetracycline production. The factor is produced by wild strains; however, the mutant *S. aureofaciens* W 5 produces large amounts of this substance, which is presumably of a flavine or pteridine character.

2. *Streptomyces rimosus*

Miller et al. (1964, 1965) found in their study of biosynthesis of tetracycline substances in a culture of *S. rimosus* inhibited by ethionine, and in the conversion of biosynthetic intermediates in cell-free preparations, that the biosynthetic pathway of oxytetracycline is identical with the pathway of chlortetracycline in *S. aureofaciens* up to the formation of dehydrotetracycline (35).

Besides 4-amino-6-demethylanhydrotetracycline (20) and 4-amino-anhydrotetracycline (22), a culture of *S. rimosus* T 1686B on a synthetic medium with ethionine was found also to contain 4-methylamino-6-demethylanhydrotetracycline (24) and 4-methylamino-anhydrotetracycline (26). In contrast to *S. aureofaciens* ethionine does not block C6 methylation (Miller et al. 1964). Dulaney et al. (1962) found 4-methylethyloxytetracycline (28) in a culture of *S. rimosus* on a semisynthetic medium containing ethionine.

Dehydrotetracycline (35) is probably transformed to dehydrooxytetracycline (37) by C6 hydroxylation. This substance was not isolated and evidence of its existence was obtained during bioconversions of dehydrotetracycline (35) to oxytetracycline (43) in an *S. rimosus* American Type Culture Collection (ATCC) 13224 cell-free extract (MILLER et al. 1965). The authors found that NADPH and O_2 are necessary for C5 hydroxylation. The small amount of tetracycline (40) synthesized from dehydrotetracycline (35) in the absence of O_2 (MILLER et al. 1965) is in keeping with the finding of PERLMAN et al. (1960) that *S. rimosus* is capable of producing tetracycline (40). The transformation of dehydrooxytetracycline (37) to oxytetracycline (43) is assumed to involve a final reduction of the 5a,11a double bond under the participation of NADPH (MILLER et al. 1965).

In contrast to *S. aureofaciens, S. rimosus* is incapable of C7 chlorination of the tetracycline nucleus; on the other hand, it performs its C5 hydroxylation. In addition, it does not produce 6-demethyloxytetracycline even in the presence of ethionine (ZYGMUNT 1962). However, in the presence of ethionine it is capable of producing 6-demethyl intermediates 4-amino-6-demethylanhydrotetracycline (20) and 4-methylamino-6-demethylanhydrotetracycline (24) (MILLER et al. 1964). MCCORMICK et al. (1962) showed that *S. rimosus* T 1686B does not metabolize 6-demethylanhydrochlortetracycline (30) or anhydrochlortetracycline (32); only anhydrotetracycline (31) is transformed to oxytetracycline (43). This points to the substrate specificity of one of the two terminal reactions.

MILLER (1967) assumes that this specific site is C6 hydroxylation. Anhydrotetracycline oxygenase of *S. rimosus* is thus a strictly specific enzyme unlike the enzyme from *S. aureofaciens*, which catalyzes C6 hydroxylation of substrates with hydrogen or halogen on C7 and hydrogen or methyl on C6 and even with the hydroxyl group on C5 (MCCORMICK et al. 1962).

The terminal dehydrogenase does not possess such strict specificity as documented by the formation of 5-hydroxychlortetracycline (44) from dehydrochlortetracycline (36) in cell-free preparations of *S. rimosus* BE 541 (MITSCHER et al. 1966) or in the culture of *S. rimosus* ATCC 13224 (MARTIN et al. 1967). The reaction requires NADPH and O_2 (MILLER 1967).

III. Transformation of the Tricyclic Decaketide

The transformation of the tricyclic decaketide is assumed to involve the same biosynthetic reactions as the transformation of the nonaketide. The only intermediate of this pathway leading to 2-acetyl-2-decarboxamidotetracyclines was described by MCCORMICK et al. (1962). In a culture of *S. aureofaciens* F 2242, 2-acetyl-2-decarboxamido-anhydrotetracycline (45) was transformed to 2-acetyl-2-decarboxamidotetracycline (46). This indicates that the presence of the carboxamide group on C2 is not a necessary condition for the reaction and that the formation of 2-acetyl-2-decarboxamidotetracyclines is catalyzed by an identical synthetase complex as the transformation of carboxamide derivatives. This is further confirmed by the formation of 2-acetyl-2-decarboxamidotetracycline (46) in the culture of *S. aureofaciens* S 6422, i.e., in a blocked mutant incapable of malonamyl CoA formation (MCCORMICK 1966). The formation of 2-acetyl-2-decarboxamidotetracycline (46) and 2-acetyl-2-decarboxamidochlortetracycline (47) as minor components accompanying tetracycline (40) and chlortetracycline (41) was described by MILLER and HOCHSTEIN (1962). Likewise LANCINI and SENSI (1964) identified 2-acetyl-2-decarboxamidotetracycline (46) in a culture of *S. psammoticus*.

Streptomyces rimosus also produces, apart from oxytetracycline (43), a minor substance: 2-acetyl-2-decarboxamidooxytetracycline (48) (HOCHSTEIN et al. 1960). Biochemical mutants isolated in some laboratories are characterized by a predominant production of decarboxamido compounds (FROLOVA et al. 1971; HOCHSTEIN et al. 1960; MCCORMICK 1966).

IV. Genetic Loci Responsible for the Biosynthesis of Tetracyclines

VANĚK et al. (1971) assume that the genetic loci controlling the synthesis of enzymes participating in the final biosynthetic reactions of chlortetracycline (transformation of the hypothetical tricyclic nonaketide) are grouped into the so-called *ctc* operon. Metabolic blocks – mutations of these genes – lead to the formation of corresponding mutant metabolites.

This idea is supported by the results of genetic analysis of oxytetracycline production in *S. rimosus*. BORONIN and MINDLIN (1971) subjected to genetic analysis blocked mutants of *S. rimosus* and found two groups of loci responsible for the biosynthesis of oxytetracycline; the groups were localized near the loci for streptomycin resistance. Likewise, ALAČEVIĆ (1976) described on a linkage map of *S. rimosus* R 7 four clustered *otc* loci corresponding to four complementary groups of nonproducing mutants.

Oxytetracycline biosynthesis is also controlled by extrachromosomal DNA (BORONIN and SADOVNIKOVA 1972). These genetic determinants seem to be responsible for the synthesis of a factor protecting the protein-synthesizing system of *S. rimosus* against its own antibiotic (BORISOGLEBSKAYA et al. 1979).

E. Regulation of the Biosynthesis of Tetracyclines

I. Saccharide Metabolism

The first data on the regulation of biosynthesis of tetracycline antibiotics were provided by classical studies concerned with the effect of phosphate ions (BIFFI et al. 1954). Addition of orthophosphate to cultivation medium of *S. aureofaciens* caused a sharp drop in chlortetracycline yield, increased consumption of sucrose, and an accumulation of pyruvic acid in the medium.

To reveal the relationship of the producer's metabolism to the biosynthesis of chlortetracycline, DI MARCO et al. (1956) added metabolic inhibitors into the medium. If the direct oxidative pathway was blocked by arsenite so that glycolysis became the main pathway, the production of the antibiotic was substantially decreased, consumption of sucrose was enhanced, and pyruvic acid was formed in increased amounts. Addition of orthophosphate potentiated this effect while iodoacetic acid suppressed the inhibition. Iodoacetate and fluoride, two inhibitors of glycolysis, caused an increased antibiotic production in a low-production strain of *S. aureofaciens*; on the other hand, 2,4-dinitrophenol and sodium azide decreased the production appreciably (Vaněk 1958). These results have to be evaluated with caution since none of the inhibitors has a completely specific effect; however, they indicate that increased yields were achieved by blockage of the glycolytic pathway.

These studies pointed indirectly to the importance of an equilibrium between the glycolytic and oxidative metabolism of saccharides. Direct proof of the presence of the hexosemonophosphate oxidative pathway in *S. aureofaciens* was provided by Boretti et al. (1956), who concluded that phosphate ion inhibits the formation of heptoses and hexoses during direct oxidation, thereby stimulating glycolysis. The two alternative pathways of sugar metabolism – glycolysis and the pentose cycle – were proved in *S. aureofaciens* by Shen et al. (1959), who also proposed, independently of the above authors, a hypothesis of the shift in sugar metabolism from the hexosemonophosphate pathway to glycolysis under the action of orthophosphate. According to this hypothesis, however, orthophosphate has no effect on transketolase and transaldolase, which catalyze further metabolism of ribose-5-phosphate in the pentose cycle (Boretti et al. 1956), but inhibits rather glucose-6-phosphate dehydrogenase, with an attendant accumulation of pyruvate, and shifts thus the reaction in favor of glycolysis. Rokos and Procházka (1957) proposed that the ratio between oxidative and glycolytic sugar degradation, and thus chlortetracycline yield, may be changed depending on the carbon source used in the medium.

Attempts to affect the sugar metabolism and the chlortetracycline production by inhibitors were successful only when these substances were added to the medium in the first 24 h of cultivation. Analogously, the stimulatory effect of benzyl thiocyanate on chlortetracycline biosynthesis was perceptible only in the initial stages of cultivation (Pecák et al. 1958). The increased sensitivity of cultures to external interventions was confirmed by Matelová et al. (1955), who found an adverse effect of lowered oxygen supply at the beginning of cultivation on chlortetracycline production. Hošťálek (1964a), using specifically labeled glucose molecules, found that the intensity of the pentose cycle in intermittently aerated culture is significantly lower than in control culture.

The intimate relationship between sugar metabolism and oxytetracycline biosynthesis in *S. rimosus* was documented by Horváth and Szentirmai (1962), who found a higher activity of glycolytic enzymes in low-production strains that in production variants.

Further data on the relationship between glycolysis and the pentose cycle and its significance in chlortetracycline yields were provided by the study of the stimulatory effect of benzyl thiocyanate. A follow-up study of oxidation of glucose labeled on C1 or C6 showed (Hošťálek 1964b) that an increasing concentration of the agent reduces the relative proportion of glycolysis in the metabolism of glucose by washed mycelium. The site of effect of the agent is apparently the transport of sugars into the cells (Hošťálek 1964c). This is corroborated by the fact that the stimulating effect of benzylthiocyanate is the most marked in media with rapidly assimilated glucose while in media with slowly utilized fructose the agent has almost no effect (Hošťálek et al. 1958).

The type of carbon source used has a significant effect on the producer's metabolism and thus also on antibiotic yield. If *S. aureofaciens* is grown on a medium containing a rapidly assimilated saccharide (glucose), the submerged culture resembles in its characteristics a culture growing on a medium with sucrose and an excess of orthophosphate. Typical features of such a culture are increased rate of sugar consumption and a growth in the form of thick basophile hyphae with a large content of nuclear elements and nucleic acids (BORETTI et al. 1955; PROKOFIEVA-BELGOVSKAYA and POPOVA 1959). The same effect was observed by KAC (1960) in submerged culture of *S. aureofaciens* growing on a medium with glucose.

The negative effect of rapidly assimilated sources of carbon or phosphate ions on the production of tetracycline antibiotics can be interpreted as a carbon catabolite regulation of biosynthesis (HOŠŤÁLEK 1980). BĚHAL et al. (1982) described the repression of anhydrotetracycline oxygenase synthesis in a *S. aureofaciens* culture due to an increased orthophosphate concentration in the medium. ERBAN et al. (1983) found a low activity of this enzyme in a culture growing on a glucose-containing medium. The mechanism of the inhibitory effect is not known but the mediator of the catabolite regulation is likely to be a phosphorylated compound accumulated in the cell owing to a rapid saccharide metabolism. This phenomenon, which was described in the catabolite regulation of bacterial endospore formation (FREESE et al. 1972), was also observed by MADRY et al. (1979) during the inhibition of tylosine biosynthesis by orthophosphate. These conclusions are confirmed by recent results of BĚHAL et al. (1982), who found that orthophosphate added to the culture in the growth phase inhibits the synthesis of anhydrotetracycline oxygenase until it disappears from the medium. About 1 h after phosphate ion exhaustion the synthesis of the enzyme is restored.

The basic building unit of the tetracyclines is malonyl CoA; this fact indirectly indicates the significance of the glycolytic pathway, which yields two molecules of malonyl CoA from one glucose molecule. The negative effect of intensive glycolysis can therefore be attributed to an increased accumulation of phosphorylated intermediates in the cell, which can repress the formation of the enzyme system synthesizing the antibiotic.

II. Formation of Malonyl CoA

High chlortetracycline production is best accomplished in biochemical variants in which pathways leading to malonyl CoA are potentiated while reactions tapping this intermediate from the tetracycline biosynthetic pathway are suppressed. This assumption was confirmed in experiments comparing the activity of the tricarboxylic acid cycle in the low-production strain of *S. aureofaciens* related to the wild strain, and in a high-production variant. In a stationary phase the low-production strain was characterized by a high activity of tricarboxylic acid cycle enzymes whereas in the high-production variant its activity in the period of intensive chlortetracycline synthesis dropped considerably (HOŠŤÁLEK et al. 1969a). The activity of the tricarboxylic acid cycle was paralleled by the ATP level in the mycelium; in high-production variants the ATP content in the production phase was tenfold higher than in the wild strain (JANGLOVÁ et al. 1969).

Lipogenesis, whose activity is connected only with the vegetative phase, does not represent a competitive pathway of malonyl CoA utilization in *S. aureofaciens* (BĚHAL et al. 1969 a, b). Lipogenesis activity, measured by the incorporation of labeled acetate into lipids, corresponds to the activity of acetyl CoA carboxylase during cultivation (BĚHAL and VANĚK 1970) and to the maximum activity of NADPH-generating systems – malate dehydrogenase (decarboxylating) and the pentose cycle (JECHOVÁ et al. 1969).

In the intensive chlortetracycline biosynthesis period, acetyl CoA carboxylase activity is low. BĚHAL et al. (1977) proved that in this period the activity of the whole enzyme sequence catalyzing the formation of malonyl CoA via acetyl CoA carboxylation, i.e., pyruvate kinase and the pyruvate dehydrogenase complex, decreases. A characteristic feature of the high-production variant is a rise in the activity of phosphoenolpyruvate carboxylase, which yields oxalacetate. Gas chromatography was used to prove the formation of malonate from oxalacetate-4-[^{14}C] in a cell-free extract. The reaction required the presence of HSCoA and NAD^+.

The formation of malonyl CoA in an alternative pathway was confirmed by the incorporation of labeled substrates into the antibiotic molecule. The ratio of pyruvate and acetate incorporation indicates that the pyruvate dehydrogenase complex is not a limiting enzyme system in the biosynthesis of the tetracycline skeleton, since acetate incorporation does not appreciably exceed the incorporation of pyruvate. Also, the radioactivity of the carbamoyl group (determined after Hofman's degradation) is about the same after incorporation of acetate-2-[^{14}C], pyruvate-3-[^{14}C], and malonate-2-[^{14}C], amounting to about 2.8% (BĚHAL et al. 1977). This attests to the high randomization of acetate units described by CATLIN et al. (1969) in the incorporation of acetate-2-[^{14}C] into the oxytetracycline molecule. The carbamoyl group is originally a carboxyl group of malonate and should thus not be radioactive if the malonyl CoA were formed by the classical carboxylation of acetyl CoA. If other carbon atoms arriving from the carboxyl group of acetate (malonate) have the same radioactivity, the molecule of the antibiotic is seen to be formed from malonyl CoA formed in an alternative metabolic pathway.

This result, indicating that the building blocks of secondary metabolites are formed in metabolic pathways different from those giving rise to identical intermediates utilized in primary metabolism, is still unique. The formation of malonyl CoA utilized both for the biosynthesis of lipids and oligoketide secondary metabolites is usually assumed to proceed by an identical mechanism catalyzed by the same enzymes.

III. Energy Metabolism

Intact function of the tricarboxylic acid cycle under nonproduction conditions, when the producer's metabolism is not limited by phosphate ions, brings about a high level of ATP in the cells (ČURDOVÁ et al. 1976). The regulatory mechanism controlling the activity of the tricarboxylic acid cycle in *S. aureofaciens* is the allosteric inhibition of citrate synthase (HOŠŤÁLEK et al. 1969 b) and phosphoenolpyruvate carboxylase (Voříšek et al. 1969, 1970) by ATP. Both enzymes are inhibited in concentrations ten times higher than the concentrations of ATP in the mycelium of a wild strain. It is therefore improbable that this mechanism would play a role in the control of tetracycline biosynthesis.

Striking differences in ATP level under production and nonproduction conditions induced Čurdová et al. (1976) to determine the energy charge of the culture, i.e., the ratio [(ATP) + 1/2 (ADP)]/[(ATP) + (ADP) + (AMP)]. The determination of actual ATP level in cells is not a sufficient indicator of intensity of energy metabolism since it does not include the rate of its turnover – synthesis and degradation.

During the cultivation of *S. aureofaciens* the authors recorded a drop in energy charge. A particularly striking drop was found in the low-production strain, viz., from a value of 0.7 in the vegetative phase to a transient value below 0.2. This fluctuations was not due to changes in the degree of phosphorylation of adenylates present in the system but to a sharp increase in ADP and AMP levels, probably a consequence of RNA degradation. *S. aureofaciens* polynucleotide phosphorylase degrades RNA to nucleotide diphosphates (Šimúth et al. 1975) which are further cleaved by ATP diphosphohydrolase to monophosphates (Hošťálek et al. 1981). These results confirmed the substantially lower ATP level in a high-production variant compared with the low-production strain. However, the energy charge level during cultivation is almost identical in the two strains. In the production variant the total adenylate synthesis is apparently suppressed and the possibility of formation of high-energy bonds at the ATP level is reduced.

Another important group of high-energy phosphate compounds in *S. aureofaciens* are inorganic polyphosphates (Kulaev 1979). The low level of polyphosphate fractions (low-polymer and high-polymer) in the high-production strain (Kulaev et al. 1976) also confirms the low activity of its energy metabolism. The low-production strain synthesizes polyphosphates mostly at the expense of ATP with the aid of ATP: polyphosphate phosphotransferase, in both the vegetative and the stationary phase. Another enzyme of polyphosphate synthesis, 1,3-diphosphoglycerate polyphosphate phosphotransferase, was active in this strain in the vegetative phase. While its participation in polyphosphate synthesis in the low-production strain in the stationary phase was negligible, in the high-production variant its activity increased significantly in the period of intensive antibiotic formation. The strain is characterized by low activity of the tricarboxylic acid cycle and the terminal oxidation in the production phase; the formation of polyphosphate high-energy bonds takes place as early as during glycolysis, at the 1,3-diphosphoglycerate level.

The resulting polyphosphates are utilized in *S. aureofaciens* for sugar phosphorylation. Hošťálek et al. (1976b) also identified, apart from hexokinase catalyzing the formation of glucose-6-phosphate from ATP, polyphosphate glucokinase. A conspicuous maximum of ATP glucokinase activity was observed in the vegetative phase, followed by a slight drop at the 48th h and then a slight increase in its activity in both strains. Polyphosphate glucokinase was identified in the mycelium only after 20 h of cultivation; its activity increased sharply (especially in the high-production variant) and reached a maximum in the 48th h, in the period of an intensive antibiotic synthesis.

It is not yet clear which polyphosphate fraction participates in sugar phosphorylation. Studies of ^{32}P incorporation into polyphosphate fractions of mycelium pointed to the rise in the rate of synthesis of high-polymer polyphosphates after 36 h of cultivation. The level of this fraction was also the highest throughout the cultivation. The participation of high-polymer polyphosphates is also confirmed by the rise of activity of high-polymer polyphosphatase in the high-production strain associated with the rise in activity of 1,3-diphosphoglycerate polyphosphate phosphotransferase (Kulaev et al. 1976).

F. Biosynthesis of Macromolecules and the Production of Tetracyclines

I. Nucleic Acid Metabolism

The significance of nucleic acid metabolism in the synthesis of tetracycline antibiotics was stressed by Boretti et al. (1955). The authors found that the level of proteins and nucleic acids in the mycelium decreased more rapidly under the conditions of high chlortetracycline yields. These findings were confirmed cytologically by Scotti and Zocchi (1955), who described thick basophile hyphae with high RNA content in a culture of *S. aureofaciens* in the vegetative phase of cultivation. The production phase was characterized by a low content of RNA in thin hyphae. Similar results were obtained by Prokofieva-Belgovskaya and Orlova (1956). Doskočil et al. (1958, 1959) described a conspicuous maximum in RNA level in about the 10th h of cultivation in *S. rimosus* and *S. aureofaciens*, whereas the DNA content in the culture was almost stable. Zelinka and Schnittová (1966) also found that the rapid drop in RNA level was a characteristic feature of high-yield chlortetracycline fermentations. The lowering of content of nucleic acid in the mycelium was reflected in an increased level of their degradation products. Šimúth and Zelinka (1970) found hypoxanthine, guanosine, and cytosine in the fermentation medium; their levels increased with proceeding chlortetracycline biosynthesis. Addition of exogenous chlortetracycline to the culture in the 20th h was reflected chiefly in an increased level of hypoxanthine and cytosine. Degradation products of nucleic acids, i.e., nucleotides (AMP, CMP), nucleosides, and hypoxanthine were also found in acid-soluble mycelial fraction.

These findings stimulated further research into the relationship between chlortetracycline production and the activity of nucleolytic enzymes, e.g., extracellular ribonuclease and acid phosphatase. The level of ribonuclease increased with proceeding cultivation while phosphodiesterase and acid phosphatase exhibited a maximum at the end of the vegetative phase. No alkaline phosphatase activity could be detected in the cultivation medium (Zelinková and Zelinka 1969). The intracellular levels of ribonuclease and phosphodiesterase had a different time course. The high-production strains showed two maxima of activity of the two enzymes, the first one at the end of the exponential phase and the second one after the 45th h of cultivation (Jeloková et al. 1974). Extracellular ribonuclease was purified (Bačová et al. 1971) and was proved to be a guanyl specific ribonuclease (Zelinková et al. 1971). An identical enzyme was found in mycelial homogenate of *S. aureofaciens*. It is probably bound to the cell wall or to the plasma membrane (TIMKO et al. 1976a).

The rate of RNA synthesis in *S. aureofaciens* reaches a maximum in about the 12th h of cultivation. This was confirmed by the time course of RNA polymerase (nucleoside triphosphate-RNA-nucleotidyltransferase – DNA dependent). MALÍKOVÁ et al. (1972) determined the activity of the enzyme during cultivation, using DNA isolated from *S. aureofaciens* as a matrix. Activity was found to rise up to the 12th h, then drop sharply; no detectable activity was found after the 30th h. ŠIMÚTH et al. (to be published) isolated RNA polymerase from *S. aureofaciens* mycelium in the initial phases of growth when tetracycline is not yet produced. The enzyme has properties similar to those of other bacterial RNA polymerase and is inhibited by rifampicin and chlortetracycline. The study of kinetics of RNA synthesis by [^{14}C] uracil or [^{14}C] uridine pulse labeling (ŠIMÚTH et al. 1979a; MIKULÍK and VANĚK 1979) revealed a maximum incorporation in *S. aureofaciens* after about 10 h of cultivation.

An integral part of the multienzyme system participating in the nucleic acid metabolism in *S. aureofaciens* is polynucleotide phosphorylase. The enzyme catalyzes both the polymerization of ribonucleoside diphosphates and the reverse reaction – in the presence of phosphate ion it phosphorylates polynucleotides, giving rise to nucleoside diphosphates. It takes part in the elimination of messenger RNA after translation and a regeneration of building blocks for new RNA synthesis. The activity of the enzyme culminates in the 20th h, i.e., at the time of active protein synthesis; it decreases in the production phase but persists until the end of cultivation (ŠIMÚTH and ZELINKA 1971). ŠIMÚTH et al. (1975) found that a purified preparation of polynucleotide phosphorylase is competitively inhibited by chlortetracycline. The enzyme attacks the 16S and 23S molecules of rRNA, the substrate structure being the factor limiting the rate of phosphorolytic degradation (PARAJKOVÁ et al. 1977).

II. Interaction of Tetracycline Antibiotics with Ribosomes

The finding that bacterial protein synthesis is inhibited by tetracycline antibiotics promoted the study of interaction of these substances with the protein-synthesizing apparatus of the producer. *S. aureofaciens* produces amounts of chlortetracycline 100 times greater than the concentration which totally inhibits the growth of sensitive bacterial cells. The first experiments showed that chlortetracycline at 1-m*M* concentration altered the sedimentation profile of 70S ribosomes, causing their sedimentation (VANĚK et al. 1969; ZELINKA and SABO 1969). Chlortetracycline is probably bound to the ribosomes via Mg^{2+} ions (MIKULÍK et al. 1971a; ZELINKA and SABO 1969). Ribosome aggregation produced by tetracycline was proved in the study of the ultrastructure of *S. aureofaciens* during cultivation. LUDVÍK et al. (1971) found ribosomal aggregates in the cyctoplasm of a production variant after 48 h of cultivation. Ultrastructural changes corresponded to changes in the ribosome sedimentation profile (MIKULÍK et al. 1971b).

Application of [^{3}H]tetracycline showed that the antibiotic was bound to 70S and 100S ribosomal dimers; the major part of radioactivity was associated with 30S subunits while a smaller proportion was associated with 50S subunits. A quantity of 320 molecules was found to be bound reversibly to one ribosome, one tetracycline molecule per one ribosome being bound irreversibly (Mikulík et al. 1971 c). Spectral studies of tetracycline binding to ribosomes showed that the antibiotic was bound to both the ribosomal RNA and ribosomal proteins (Mikulík et al. 1971 a).

Timko et al. (1976 b) studied the content of ribosomes and RNA in *S. aureofaciens* during cultivation. The largest number of ribosomes in the cytoplasm was found after 12 h; the content decreased until the 36th h and then remained constant until the end of cultivation. A similar time course was obtained when the content of 16S and 23S RNA was determined in the mycelium (ribosomes make up 80% of the total RNA content).

A certain proportion of the RNA is probably degraded after ribosome aggregation owing to the action of the chlortetracycline produced by the cell. Jeloková et al. (1976) showed that the degradation of rRNA by enzymes bound to ribosomes of *S. aureofaciens* increased in the presence of chlortetracycline. The increase in chlortetracycline production found in the presence of cadaverine (0.1%) added to medium at the beginning of cultivation (Zelinka 1968) is probably associated with stabilization of ribosomes in the production phase. The presence of cadaverine stabilizes the RNA level after the 36th h of cultivation; it probably protects ribosomal structure so that RNA is degraded more slowly by ribonuclease. This makes it possible to extend the period of active formation of specific synthetases paricipating in the synthesis of the antibiotic (Zelinka and Sedláček 1968).

This is apparently also connected with the increase in tetracycline production in the biochemical mutant of *S. aureofaciens* obtained by Colombo et al. (1981). The strain, which was resistant to higher orthophosphate concentrations in the medium and attained higher antibiotic yields as compared with the parent strain even at higher growth rates, exhibited, during cultivation, a higher RNA level which did not decrease during the production phase.

III. Protein Synthesis

Mikulík et al. (1971 c) found that exogenous tetracycline penetrated through the *S. aureofaciens* cell wall and accumulated in the cells; however, the penetration into the mycelium of the production variant was lower than that into low-production strain mycelium under identical conditions. Addition of 500 μg/ml tetracycline in the 4th h of cultivation caused a 37% inhibition of protein synthesis in the production variant and completely inhibited tetracycline production. The same addition brought about a complete inhibition of leucine incorporation in a low-production strain. The same dose of the antibiotic, added to a 16-h-old culture of the high-production variant, had no effect on the final tetracycline yield. The added tetracycline was neither modified nor inactivated by the growing culture. The same differences in the sensitivity of low-production and high-production strains were found by Šimúth et al. (1979 a), who studied the effect of chlortetracycline on the rate of RNA synthesis.

Ribosomal 30S fraction prepared from a 10-h-old culture of *S. aureofaciens* and containing endogenous mRNA was used to study the effect of tetracycline on in vitro protein synthesis; added to the system at a concentration of 40 μg/ml, the antibiotic caused a 50% inhibition of the process (MIKULÍK et al. 1971c).

In a medium containing sucrose, soybean flour, corn-steep liquor, and mineral salts, the protein synthesis in a culture of *S. aureofaciens* reaches a maximum around the 20th h of cultivation; this was found by [^{14}C]leucine incorporation (MIKULÍK et al. 1971c; ŠIMÚTH et al. 1979a) and [^{14}C]phenylalanine incorporation (MIKULÍK and VANĚK 1979). With increasing age of the culture the rate of protein synthesis declines, the rate observed at the end of cultivation reaching about one-tenth of the maximum rate observed in the vegetative phase. Nevertheless, throughout the cultivation the RNA and the protein synthesis remain active.

As found by incorporation of [^{14}C]leucine into *S. aureofaciens* cells (BĚHAL et al. 1979b), 75% of the protein synthesized between the 16th and 17th h of growth is degraded by the 48th h of cultivation. This phenomenon is apparently associated with the degradation of cells formed in the vegetative phase and with the formation of thin hyphae typical of the production phase. Protein synthesis continues throughout the cultivation, its rate being 10%–15% of the maximum rate from the first, preparatory phase; it ceases around the 90th h of cultivation when chlortetracycline synthesis also ceases. The activity of transaminases increases in the production phase, probably attendant to the utilization of the carbon moiety of amino acids from degraded proteins for the antibiotic synthesis (BĚHAL et al. 1977).

Attempts at elucidating the molecular basis of gene expression during tetracycline biosynthesis prompted the study of protein synthesis in cell-free systems of *S. aureofaciens*. MIKULÍK and VANĚK (1979) studied the activity of 70S ribosomes during translation initiation, using ApUpG or Qβ RNA as a template. The *S. aureofaciens* ribosomes from a culture producing chlortetracycline were found to have relatively little activity in the formation of the initiation complex. The formation of the complex was stimulated by high concentrations of IF-3 from *Escherichia coli*, although IF-3 was not inactivated by tetracycline. The authors assume that the antibiotic inhibits the binding of IF-3 to RNA by integrating with rRNA at the same binding site. The study of translation of poly(U) in a hybrid system containing 30S and 50S ribosomes also showed that *S. aureofaciens* ribosomes were less active than the reference ribosomes of *E. coli*.

WEISER et al. (1981) purified a polypeptide chain elongation factor Tu from an *S. aureofaciens* mycelium and compared it with the Tu elongation factor from *E. coli*. Despite differences in molecular mass and heat stability, the two factors were found to be structurally similar.

To preclude possible negative effects of high-phosphorylated nucleotides (which are integrated into the protein-synthesizing apparatus and inactivate it) and the chlortetracycline produced, ŠIMÚTH et al. (1979b) isolated basic components of the cell-free protein-synthesizing system prior to the formation of the above substances in the culture. They worked with a mycelium from the second vegetative generation inoculated with the first generation in which RNA synthesis had not yet reached a maximum (as measured by incorporation of [^{14}C]uracil into the acid-insoluble mycelial fraction). In contrast to a culture inoculated with an old inoculum, the cell-free system controlled by poly(U) in this culture (6-h-old second vegetative generation) had activity about 10 times higher. The rate of synthesis of [^{14}C]polyphenylalanine found with poly(U) prepared by polymerization of uridine diphosphate in situ (using production strain polynucleotide phosphorylase) was about double that found with exogenous poly(U). The protein synthesis was not suppressed completely even by very high (200 µg/ml) doses of chlortetracycline. According to the authors this is due to residual chlortetracycline-resistant protein synthesis (ŠIMÚTH et al. 1979a; MIKULÍK and VANĚK 1979). ŠIMÚTH et al. (1979b) recommended the determination of RNA synthesis intensity as a suitable test for evaluating the quality of inoculum for industrial fermentations.

IV. High-Phosphorylated Nucleotides

The research into the regulation of biosynthesis of tetracycline antibiotics has recently centered around the study of the possible role of high-phosphorylated nucleotides. These effectors control the phenotype expression of genomes by regulating the transcription or translation of appropriate operons. MIKULÍK and VANĚK (1979) and ŠIMÚTH et al. (1979a) identified these substances by chromatography on phosphorus excretion index (PEI)-cellulose after pulse labeling of *S. aureofaciens* mycelium with ^{32}P. A drop in the rate of RNA synthesis was accompanied by an increased synthesis of nucleotide phosphates whose level had dropped after the decline in protein synthesis, i.e., in the period of an intensive antibiotic formation. Exogenous chlortetracycline added to the culture suppressed the synthesis of some high-phosphorylated nucleotides, especially guanosine tetraphosphate (ŠIMÚTH et al. 1979a). In *S. rimosus* a drop in guanosine tetraphosphate synthesis is observed on increasing the concentration of produced oxytetracycline in mycelium (ŠŤASTNÁ and MIKULÍK 1981). ŠIMÚTH et al. (1981) studied the transcription activity of RNA polymerase from *S. aureofaciens* in vitro. An addition of guanosine tetraphosphate was found to cause a significant inhibition of the enzyme. Thus high-phosphorylated nucleotides may possibly participate in the control of gene expression during intensive RNA synthesis in the first, preparatory phase of cultivation.

G. Conclusion

Current knowledge of the regulation of biosynthesis of tetracycline antibiotics makes it possible to consider two basic types of mechanisms affecting the production of these substances. The first of these regulates the expression of genes of the tetracycline biosynthetic pathway, i.e., the production of appropriate synthetases, while the other regulates the self-resistance of the protein-synthesizing apparatus to the produced substance.

Expression of tetracycline biosynthesis takes place before the termination of the so-called balanced growth, i.e., under the conditions when the vegetative growth begins to be limited. As in the fermentation of other antibiotics, the biosynthesis of tetracyclines is usually carried out under orthophosphate limitation but with a sufficient level of other nutrients in medium. When the vegetative growth is favored, the formation of the enzyme system of antibiotic biosynthesis is repressed probably by a catabolite repression mechanism reflecting the accumulation of inhibitory catabolites.

Expression of a nonvegetative genome is characterized by metabolic changes, e.g., the suppression or disappearance of enzyme systems typical of vegetative growth (ATP glucokinase, acetyl CoA carboxylase). The level of these enzymes changes gradually, without sudden change. This may be associated with changes in the relative proportion of different metabolic types of mycelium in the population – thick basophile hyphae are replaced by thin long filaments characteristic of the production phase.

It is not yet clear what is the fundamental condition for the high yield in the high-production variant – a sufficient supply of building units (malonyl CoA) ensured through the blockage of competing metabolic pathways, or high activity of synthetases of the tetracycline pathway. This high activity is essential for the biosynthesis of tetracyclines since the drop in the level of anhydrotetracycline oxygenase at the end of cultivation leads to a cessation of chlortetracycline production.

This is closely connected with another condition for high yields – the self-resistance to produced tetracyclines which are potent inhibitors of protein synthesis. During intensive antibiotic production by the high-yielding variant of *S. aureofaciens* a certain proportion of RNA and protein synthesis remains resistant to any level of tetracyclines dissolved in the cell. The enzyme system accomplishing the formation of these essential macromolecules becomes resistant to the effects of its own antibiotic only after the termination of the first, preparatory phase. It can be thus assumed to be protected by a certain, probably inducible, system which nullifies the action of the produced metabolite. Such a system was also proposed by Jones (1979) in the actinomycin producer *Streptomyces antibioticus*. Like tetracycline antibiotics, actinomycin is a potent inhibitor of DNA-dependent RNA synthesis. A highly purified RNA polymerase from *S. antibioticus* has properties similar to those of enzymes from other gram-positive of gram-negative bacteria and, unlike a crude mycelial enzyme preparation, cannot catalyze transcription in the presence of actinomycin.

The presence of such a substance or a protective system is a necessary prerequisite for high yields of tetracycline antibiotics. The proposed protective system is obviously identical with the inducible mechanism of "resistance" of *S. rimosus*, whose synthesis is controlled by extrachromosomal DNA. Borisoglebskaya et al. (1979) assume that the system is a specific protein which, in high-production strains, switches off the inhibitory action of tetracycline antibiotics on protein synthesis. The protected protein-synthesizing system then probably ensures intact production of specific synthetases during the production process in high-production variants.

References

Alačević M (1973) Genetics of tetracycline-producing streptomycetes. In: Vaněk Z, Hošťálek Z, Cudlín J (eds) Genetics of industrial microorganisms. Actinomycetes and fungi. Academia, Prague, pp 59–70

Alačević M (1976) Recent advances in *Streptomyces rimosus* genetics. In: Macdonald KD (ed) Second international symposium on the genetics of industrial microorganisms. Academic, London, pp 513–519
Backus EJ, Duggar BM, Campbell TH (1954) Variation in *Streptomyces aureofaciens*. Ann NY Acad Sci 60:86–101
Bačová M, Zelinková E, Zelinka J (1971) Exocellular ribonuclease from *Streptomyces aureofaciens*. I. Isolation and purification. Biochim Biophys Acta 235:335–342
Běhal V, Vaněk Z (1970) Regulation of biosynthesis of secondary metabolites. XII. Acetyl-CoA carboxylase in *Streptomyces aureofaciens*. Folia Microbiol (Prague) 15:354–357
Běhal V, Procházková V, Vaněk Z (1969a) Regulation of biosynthesis of secondary metabolites. II. Fatty acids and chlortetracycline in *Streptomyces aureofaciens*. Folia Microbiol (Prague) 14:112–116
Běhal V, Cudlín J, Vaněk Z (1969b) Regulation of biosynthesis of secondary metabolites. III. Incorporation of 1-^{14}C-acetic acid into fatty acids and chlortetracycline in *Streptomyces aureofaciens*. Folia Microbiol (Prague) 14:117–120
Běhal V, Podojil M, Hošťálek Z, Vaněk Z, Lynen F (1974) Regulation of biosynthesis of excessive metabolites. XVI. Origin of the terminal group of tetracyclines. Folia Microbiol (Prague) 19:146–150
Běhal V, Jechová V, Vaněk Z, Hošťálek Z (1977) Alternate pathways of malonylCoA formation in *Streptomyces aureofaciens*. Phytochemistry 16:347–350
Běhal V, Hošťálek Z, Vaněk Z (1979a) Anhydrotetracycline oxygenase activity and biosynthesis of tetracyclines in *Streptomyces aureofaciens*. Biotechnol Lett 1:177–182
Běhal V, Vaněk Z, Hošťálek Z, Ramadan A (1979b) Synthesis and degradation of proteins and DNA in *Streptomyces aureofaciens*. Folia Microbiol (Prague) 24:211–216
Běhal V, Grégrová-Prušáková J, Hošťálek Z (1982) Effect of inorganic phosphate and benzyl thiocyanate on the activity of anhydrotetracycline oxygenase in *Streptomyces aureofaciens*. Folia Microbiol (Prague) 27:102–106
Biffi G, Boretti G, Di Marco A, Pennella P (1954) Metabolic behaviour and chlortetracycline production by *Streptomyces aureofaciens* in liquid culture. Appl Microbiol 2:288–293
Birch AJ (1957) Biosynthetic relations of some natural phenolic and enolic compounds. Fortschr Chem Org Naturst 14:186–216
Birch AJ, Snell JF, Thomson PJ (1962) Studies in relation to biosynthesis. Part XXVIII. Oxytetracycline (Terramycin). J Chem Soc 425–429
Blumauerová M, Mraček M, Vondráčková J, Podojil M, Hošťálek Z, Vaněk Z (1969a) Regulation of biosynthesis of secondary metabolites. IX. The biosynthetic activity of blocked mutants of *Streptomyces aureofaciens*. Folia Microbiol (Prague) 14:215–225
Blumauerová M, Hošťálek Z, Mraček M, Podojil M, Vaněk Z (1969b) Regulation of biosynthesis of secondary metabolites. X. Metabolic complementation of blocked mutants of *Streptomyces aureofaciens*. Folia Microbiol (Prague) 14:226–231
Blumauerová M, Hošťálek Z, Vaněk Z (1972) Biosynthesis of tetracyclines: Problems and perspectives of genetic analysis. In: Terui G (ed) Fermentation technology today. Society of Fermentation Technology, Osaka, pp 223–232
Boretti G, Di Marco A, Scotti T, Zocchi P (1955) Variazioni morfologiche e biochimiche dello *Streptomyces aureofaciens* in relazione alla produzione di clorotetraciclina. G Microbiol 1:97–105
Boretti G, Di Marco A, Julita P, Raggi F, Bardi U (1956) Presenza degli enzimi della via esosomonofosfato ossidativa nello *Streptomyces aureofaciens*. G Microbiol 1:406–416
Borisoglebskaya AN, Perebityuk AN, Boronin AM (1979) Study on resistance of *Actinomyces rimosus* to oxytetracycline (in Russian). Antibiotiki 24:883–889
Boronin AM, Mindlin SZ (1971) Genetical analysis of *Actinomyces rimosus* mutants with the impaired synthesis of the antibiotic (in Russian). Genetika (Moscow) 7:125–131
Boronin AM, Sadovnikova LG (1972) The elimination of oxytetracycline resistance in *Actinomyces rimosus* by acridine dyes (in Russian). Genetika (Moscow) 8:174–176
Catlin ER, Hassal CH, Parry DR (1969) The biosynthesis of phenols. Part XVIII. Carbon-14 labelling in rings C and D of oxytetracycline incorporating (2-^{14}C)-acetic acid. J Chem Soc C Org Chem 1363–1366

Colombo AL, Crespi-Perellino N, Grein A, Minghetti A, Spalla C (1981) Metabolic and genetic aspects of the relationship between growth and tetracycline production in *Streptomyces aureofaciens*. Biotechnol Lett 3:71–76

Čurdová E, Křemen A, Vaněk Z, Hošťálek Z (1976) Regulation of biosynthesis of secondary metabolites. XVIII. Adenylate level and chlortetracycline production in *Streptomyces aureofaciens*. Folia Microbiol (Prague) 21:481–487

Darken MA, Berenson H, Shirk RJ, Sjolander NO (1960) Production of tetracycline by *Streptomyces aureofaciens* in synthetic media. Appl Microbiol 8:46–51

Delić V, Pigac J, Sermonti G (1969) Detection and study of cosynthesis of tetracycline antibiotics by an agar method. J Gen Microbiol 55:103–108

Di Marco A, Pennella P (1959) The fermentation of the tetracyclines. In: Hockenhull DJD (ed) Progress in industrial microbiology, vol I. Heywood, London, pp 45–92

Di Marco A, Boretti G, Julita P, Pennella P (1956) Researches on carbohydrate metabolism in *Streptomyces aureofaciens* in connection with chlortetracycline production. Rev Ferment Ind Aliment 11:140–146

Dimroth P, Walter H, Lynen F (1970) Biosynthese von 6-Methylsalicylsäure. Eur J Biochem 13:98–110

Doerschuk AP, McCormick JRD, Goodman JJ, Szumski SA, Growich JA, Miller PA, Bitler BA, Jensen ER, Matrishin M, Petty MA, Phelps AS (1959) Biosynthesis of tetracyclines. I. The halide metabolism of *Streptomyces aureofaciens* mutants. The preparation and characterization of tetracycline, 7-chloro^{36}-tetracycline and 7-bromotetracycline. J Am Chem Soc 81:3069–3075

Doskočil J, Sikyta B, Kašparová J, Doskočilová D, Zajíček J (1958) Development of the culture of *Streptomyces rimosus* in submerged fermentation. J Gen Microbiol 18:302–314

Doskočil J, Hošťálek Z, Kašparová J, Zajíček J, Herold M (1959) Development of *Streptomyces aureofaciens* in submerged culture. J Biochem Microbiol Technol Eng 1:261–271

Duggar BM (1948) Aureomycin: a product of the continuing search for new antibiotics. Ann NY Acad Sci 51:177–181

Dulaney EL, Putter I, Drescher D, Chaiet L, Miller WJ, Wolf FJ, Hendlin D (1962) Transethylation in antibiotic biosynthesis. I. An ethyl homolog of oxytetracycline. Biochim Biophys Acta 60:447–449

Erban V, Novotná J, Běhal V, Hošťálek Z (1983) Growth rate, sugar consumption and the expression of anhydrotetracycline oxygenase in *Streptomyces aureofaciens*. Folia Microbiol (Prague) 28:262–267

Finlay AC, Hobby GL, P'an SY, Regna PP, Routien JB, Seeley DB, Shull GM, Sobin BA, Solomons IA, Vinson JW, Kane JH (1950) Terramycin, a new antibiotic. Science 111:85

Freese E, Oh KY, Freese EB, Diesterhaft MD, Prasad C (1972) Suppression of sporulation of *Bacillus subtilis*. In: Halvorson HO, Hanson R, Campbell LL (eds) Spores, vol V. American Society for Microbiology, Washington, pp 212–221

Friend EJ, Hopwood DA (1971) The linkage map of *Streptomyces rimosus*. J Gen Microbiol 68:187–197

Frolova VI, Rosenfeld GS, Listvinova SN (1971) A study on biosynthetic products of *Actinomyces rimosus* mutants. Isolation and identification of 2-acetyl-2-decarboxamide-oxytetracycline (ADOT) (in Russian). Antibiotiki (Moscow) 16:687–691

Gatenbeck S (1961) The biosynthesis of oxytetracycline. Biochem Biophys Res Commun 6:422–426

Goodman JJ, Matrishin M (1961) Effect of sulfadiazine on the synthesis of demethylchlortetracycline by *Streptomyces aureofaciens*. J Bacteriol 82:615

Goodman JJ, Matrishin M (1964) Effect of norleucine on the synthesis of demethylchlortetracycline by *Streptomyces aureofaciens*. Nature 201:190

Goodman JJ, Miller PA (1962) The effect of antimetabolites on the biosynthesis of tetracyclines. Biotechnol Bioeng 4:391–402

Goodman JJ, Matrishin M, Backus EJ (1955) The effect of anhydrochlortetracycline on the growth of actinomycetes. J Bacteriol 69:70–72

Goodman JJ, Matrishin M, Young RW, McCormick JRD (1959) Inhibition of the incorporation of chloride into the tetracycline molecule. J Bacteriol 78:492–499

Goodman JJ, Matrishin M, McCormick JRD (1963) Reversal of chlorination inhibitors in *Streptomyces aureofaciens*. Nature 198:1093–1094

Gourevitch A, Misiek M, Lein J (1955) Competitive inhibition by bromide of incorporation of chloride into the tetracycline molecule. Antibiot Chemother 5:448–452

Hendlin D, Dulaney EL, Drescher D, Cook T, Chaiet L (1962) Methionine dependence and the biosynthesis of 6-demethylchlortetracycline. Biochim Biophys Acta 58:635–636

Hlavka JJ, Boothe JH (1973) The tetracyclines. Fortschr Arzneimittelforsch 17:210–240

Hochstein FA, Stephens CR, Conover LH, Regna PP, Pasternack R, Gordon PN, Pilgrim FJ, Brunings KJ, Woodward RB (1953) The structure of Terramycin. J Am Chem Soc 75:5455–5475

Hochstein FA, Schach von Wittenau M, Tanner FW Jr, Murai K (1960) 2-Acetyl-2-decarboxamidoöxytetracycline. J Am Chem Soc 82:5934–5937

Hopwood DA (1967) Genetic analysis and genome structure in *Streptomyces coelicolor*. Bacteriol Rev 31:373–403

Horváth I, Szentirmai A (1962) Glucose catabolism of *Streptomyces rimosus*. Acta Microbiol Acad Sci Hung 9:105–116

Hošt'álek Z (1964a) Relationship between the carbohydrate metabolism of *Streptomyces aureofaciens* and the biosynthesis of chlortetracycline. I. The effect of interrupted aeration, inorganic phosphate and benzyl thiocyanate on chlortetracycline biosynthesis. Folia Microbiol (Prague) 9:78–88

Hošt'álek Z (1964b) Relationship between the carbohydrate metabolism of *Streptomyces aureofaciens* and the biosynthesis of chlortetracycline. II. The effect of benzyl thiocyanate on the respiration of washed mycelium of *Streptomyces aureofaciens*. Folia Microbiol (Prague) 9:89–95

Hošt'álek Z (1964c) Relationship between the carbohydrate metabolism of *Streptomyces aureofaciens* and the biosynthesis of chlortetracycline. III. The effect of benzyl thiocyanate on carbohydrate metabolism of *Streptomyces aureofaciens*. Folia Microbiol (Prague) 9:96–102

Hošt'álek Z (1980) Catabolite regulation of antibiotic biosynthesis. Folia Microbiol (Prague) 25:445–450

Hošt'álek Z, Herold M, Nečásek J (1958) Die Beeinflussung der Chlortetracyclinproduktion und des Kohlenhydratverbrauches durch Benzylrhodanid. Naturwissenschaften 45:543–544

Hošt'álek Z, Tintěrová M, Jechová V, Blumauerová M, Suchý J, Vaněk Z (1969a) Regulation of biosynthesis of secondary metabolites. I. Biosynthesis of chlortetracycline and tricarboxylic acid cycle activity. Biotechnol Bioeng 11:539–548

Hošt'álek Z, Ryabushko TA, Cudlín J, Vaněk Z (1969b) Regulation of biosynthesis of secondary metabolites. IV. Inhibition of citrate synthase in *Streptomyces aureofaciens* by adenosine triphosphate. Folia Microbiol (Prague) 14:121–127

Hošt'álek Z, Blumauerová M, Vaněk Z (1974) Genetic problems of the biosynthesis of tetracycline antibiotics. In: Ghose TK, Fiechter A, Blakebrough N (eds) Advances in biochemical engineering, vol 3. Springer, Berlin Heidelberg New York, pp 13–67

Hošt'álek Z, Blumauerová M, Ludvík J, Jechová V, Běhal V, Čáslavská J, Čurdová E (1976a) The role of the genome in secondary biosynthesis in *Streptomyces aureofaciens*. In: Macdonald KD Second international symposium on the genetics of industrial microorganisms. Academic, London, pp 155–177

Hošt'álek Z, Tobek I, Bobyk AM, Kulaev IS (1976b) Role of ATP-glucokinase and polyphosphate glucokinase in *Streptomyces aureofaciens*. Folia Microbiol (Prague) 21:131–138

Hošt'álek Z, Blumauerová M, Vaněk Z (1979) Tetracycline antibiotics. In: Rose AH (ed) Economic microbiology, vol 3. Secondary products of metabolism. Academic, London, pp 293–353

Hošt'álek Z, Jechová V, Čurdová E, Vořišek J (1981) Phosphatase activity in glycocalyx of *Streptomyces aureofaciens*. In: Schaal KP, Pulverer G (eds) Actinomycetes. Fischer, Stuttgart, pp 281–286

Hutchinson CR (1981) The biosynthesis of tetracycline and anthracycline antibiotics. In: Corcoran JW (ed) Antibiotics, vol IV, Biosynthesis. Springer, Berlin Heidelberg New York, pp 1–11

Hütter R (1967) Systematik der Streptomyceten unter besonderer Berücksichtigung der von ihnen gebildeten Antibiotika. Karger, Basel

Janglová Z, Suchý J, Vaněk Z (1969) Regulation of biosynthesis of secondary metabolites. VII. Intracellular adenosine-5'-triphosphate concentration in *Streptomyces aureofaciens*. Folia Microbiol (Prague) 14:208–210

Járai M (1965) Biochemical chlorination inheritance in *Streptomyces aureofaciens*. Acta Microbiol Acad Sci Hung (Budapest) 11:409–416

Járai M, Kollár J (1962) Biochemical studies on *Streptomyces aureofaciens*. II. Ionic influences on the formation of chlortetracycline. Acta Microbiol Acad Sci Hung 9:145–148

Jechová V, Hošt'álek Z, Vaněk Z (1969) Regulation of biosynthesis of secondary metabolites. V. Malate dehydrogenase (decarboxylating) in *Streptomyces aureofaciens*. Folia Microbiol (Prague) 14:128–134

Jeloková J, Zelinková E, Zelinka J (1974) Activity of nucleolytic enzymes in mycelium of *Streptomyces aureofaciens* during fermentation. Biológia (Bratislava) 29:207–212

Jeloková J, Zelinková E, Mucha J, Zelinka J (1976) Intracellular nucleolytic enzymes in *Streptomyces aureofaciens* II. In: Zelinka J, Balan J (eds) Proceedings of the second international symposium on ribosomes and ribonucleic acid metabolism. Slovak Academy of Sciences, Bratislava, pp 147–154

Jones GH (1979) Purification of RNA polymerase from actinomycin producing and non-producing cells of *Streptomyces antibioticus*. Arch Biochem Biophys 198:195–204

Kabuto C, Silverton JV, Akiyama T, Sankawa V, Hutchison RD, Steyn PS, Vleggaar R (1976) X-Ray structure of viridicatumtoxin: a new class of mycotoxin from *Penicillium viridicatum* Westling. J Chem Soc Chem Commun 728–729

Kac LN (1960) Cytological investigation of the development of a chlortetracycline producer on media containing different carbon sources (in Russian). Antibiotiki 5:29–32

Koike J, Tazawa I, Arai T (1967) Genetic relatedness among streptomycetes producing tetracycline antibiotics, studied by means of deoxyribonucleic acid association. Int J Syst Bacteriol 27:58–60

Kulaev IS (1979) The biochemistry of inorganic polyphosphates. Wiley, Chichester

Kulaev IS, Bobyk AM, Tobek I, Hošt'álek Z (1976) Possible role of high-molecular weight polyphosphates in the biosynthesis of chlortetracycline in *Streptomyces aureofaciens* (in Russian). Biokhimiya 41:343–348

Lancini GC, Sensi P (1964) Isolation of 2-acetyl-2-decarboxamidotetracycline from cultures of *Streptomyces psammoticus*. Experientia 20:83–84

Lein J, Sawmiller LF, Cheney LC (1959) Chlorination inhibitors affecting the biosynthesis of tetracycline. Appl Microbiol 7:149–151

Ludvík J, Mikulík K, Vaněk Z (1971) Fine structure of *Streptomyces aureofaciens* producing tetracycline. Folia Microbiol (Prague) 16:479–480

Lynen F, Tada M (1961) Die biochemischen Grundlagen der „Polyacetat-Regel". Angew Chem 73:513–519

Madry N, Sprinkmeyer R, Pape H (1979) Regulation of tylosin synthesis in *Streptomyces*. Effects of glucose analogs and inorganic phosphate. Eur J Appl Microbiol Biotechnol 7:365–370

Makarevich VG, Laznikova TN (1963) Some data on the comparative study of chlortetracycline-producing strains of *Actinomyces aureofaciens* LSB-2201 and LSB-16 (in Russian). Antibioliki 8:195–201

Makarevich VG, Slugina MD, Upiter GD, Zaslavskaya PL, Gerasimova TM (1976) Regulation of tetracycline biosynthesis by control of antibiotic-producing organism growth (in Russian). Antibiotiki 21:205–210

Malíková S, Šimúth J, Zelinka J (1972) Activity of DNA-dependent RNA-polymerase in metabolism of *Streptomyces aureofaciens*. Biológia (Bratislava) 27:449–453
Martin JH, Mitscher LA, Miller PA, Shu P, Bohonos N (1967) 5-Hydroxy-7-chlortetracycline. I. Preparation, isolation and physicochemical properties. Antibiot Agents Chemother 1966:563–567
Matelová V, Musílková M, Nečásek J, Šmejkal F (1955) The influence of interrupted aeration on chlortetracycline production (in Czech). Preslia (Prague) 27:27–34
McCormick JRD (1965) Biosynthesis of the tetracyclines. In: Vaněk Z, Hošt'álek Z (eds) Biogenesis of antibiotic substances. Publishing House Czechoslovak Academy Science, Prague, pp 73–91
McCormick JRD (1966) Biosynthesis of the tetracyclines: an integrated biosynthetic scheme (Part I and II). In: Herold M, Gabriel Z (eds) Antibiotics. Advances in research, production and clinical use. Butterworths, London, pp 556–574
McCormick JRD (1967) Tetracyclines. In: Gottlieb D, Shaw PD (eds) Antibiotics, vol II. Biosynthesis. Springer, Berlin Heidelberg New York, pp 113–122
McCormick JRD (1969) Point-blocked mutants and the biogenesis of tetracyclines. In: Sermonti G, Alačević M (eds) Genetics and breeding of *Streptomyces*. Yugoslavian Academy Science & Arts, Zagreb, pp 163–176
McCormick JRD, Jensen ER (1965) Biosynthesis of the tetracyclines. VIII. Characterization of 4-hydroxy-6-methylpretetramid. J Am Chem Soc 87:1794–1795
McCormick JRD, Jensen ER (1968) Biosynthesis of tetracyclines. X. Protetrone. J Am Chem Soc 90:7126–7127
McCormick JRD, Jensen ER (1969) Biosynthetis of the tetracyclines. XII. Anhydrodemethylchlortetracycline from a mutant of *Streptomyces aureofaciens*. J Am Chem Soc 91:206
McCormick JRD, Sjolander NO, Hirsch U, Jensen ER, Doerschuk AP (1957) A new family of antibiotics: the demethyltetracyclines. J Am Chem Sec 79:4561–4562
McCormick JRD, Miller PA, Growich JA, Sjolander NO, Doerschuk AP (1958a) Two new tetracycline-related compounds: 7-chloro-5a-(11a)-dehydrotetracycline and 5a-epi-tetracycline. A new route to tetracycline. J Am Chem Soc 80:5572
McCormick JRD, Sjolander NO, Miller PA, Hirsch U, Arnold NH, Doerschuk AP (1958b) The biological reduction of 7-chloro-5a(11a)-dehydrotetracycline to 7-chlorotetracycline by *Streptomyces aureofaciens*. J Am Chem Soc 80:6460–6461
McCormick JRD, Hirsch U, Sjolander NO, Doerschuk AP (1960) Cosynthesis of tetracyclines by pairs of *Streptomyces aureofaciens* mutants. J Am Chem Soc 82:5006–5007
McCormick JRD, Miller PA, Johnson S, Arnold N, Sjolander NO (1962) Biosynthesis of the tetracyclines. IV. Biological rehydration of the 5a,6-anhydrotetracyclines. J Am Chem Soc 84:3023–3025
McCormick JRD, Johnson S, Sjolander NO (1963a) Biosynthesis of the tetracyclines. V. Naphthacenic precursors. J Am Chem Soc 85:1692–1693
McCormick JRD, Reichenthal J, Johnson S, Sjolander NO (1963b) Biosynthesis of the tetracyclines. VI. Total synthesis of a naphthacenic precursor: 1,3,10,11,12-pentahydroxynaphthacene-2-carboxamide. J Am Chem Soc 85:1694
McCormick JRD, Joachim UH, Jensen ER, Johnson S, Sjolander NO (1965) Biosynthesis of the tetracyclines. VII. 4-Hydroxy-6-methylpretetramid, an intermediate accumulated by a blocked mutant of *Streptomyces aureofaciens*. J Am Chem Soc 87:1793–1794
McCormick JRD, Jensen ER, Johnson S, Sjolander NO (1968a) Biosynthesis of the tetracyclines. IX. 4-Amino-dedimethylaminoanhydrodemethylchlortetracycline from a mutant of *Streptomyces aureofaciens*. J Am Chem Soc 90:2201–2202
McCormick JRD, Jensen ER, Arnold NH, Corey HS, Joachim UH, Johnson S, Miller PA, Sjolander NO (1968b) Biosynthesis of the tetracyclines. XI. The methylanthrone analog of protetrone. J Am Chem Soc 90:7127–7129
Mikulík K, Vaněk Z (1979) Interrelationship between primary and secondary metabolism in actinomycetes. In: Luckner M, Schreiber K (eds) Regulation of secondary product and plant hormone metabolism. Pergamon, Oxford, pp 199–208

Mikulík K, Karnetová J, Křemen A, Tax J, Vaněk Z (1971 a) Protein synthesis and production of tetracycline in *Streptomyces aureofaciens*. In: Ericson A (ed) Radiation and radioisotopes for industrial microorganisms. International atomic energy agency, Vienna, pp 201–222

Mikulík K, Blumauerová M, Vaněk Z, Ludvík J (1971 b) Characterization of ribosomes of a strain of *Streptomyces aureofaciens* producing chlortetracycline. Folia Microbiol (Prague) 16:24–30

Mikulík K, Karnetová J, Quyen N, Blumauerová M, Komersová I, Vaněk Z (1971 c) Interaction of tetracycline with protein synthesizing system of *Streptomyces aureofaciens*. J Antibiot 24:801–809

Miller MW, Hochstein FA (1962) Isolation and characterization of two new tetracycline antibiotics. J Org Chem 27:2525–2528

Miller PA (1967) Cell-free studies on the biosynthesis of the tetracyclines. Dev Ind Microbiol 8:96–108

Miller PA, Hash JH (1975 a) *S*-Adenosylmethionine-dedimethylamino-4-aminoanhydrotetracycline *N*-methyltransferase. In: Hash JH (ed) Methods in enzymology, vol XLIII. Antibiotics. Academic, New York, pp 603–606

Miller PA, Hash JH (1975 b) NADP-Tetracycline 5a(11a)dehydrogenase. In: Hash JH (ed) Methods in enzymology, vol XLIII. Antibiotics. Academic, New York, pp 606–607

Miller PA, McCormick JRD, Doerschuk AP (1956) Studies of chlortetracycline biosynthesis and the preparation of chlortetracycline-C^{14}. Science 123:1030–1031

Miller PA, Sjolander NO, Nalesnyk S, Arnold N, Johnson S, Doerschuk AP, McCormick JRD (1960) Cosynthetic factor I, a factor involved in hydrogen-transfer in *Streptomyces aureofaciens*. J Am Chem Soc 82:5002–5003

Miller PA, Saturnelli A, Martin JH, Mitscher LA, Bohonos N (1964) A new family of tetracycline precursors: *N*-demethylanhydrotetracyclines. Biochem Biophys Res Commun 16:285–291

Miller PA, Hash JH, Lincks M, Bohonos N (1965) Biosynthesis of 5-hydroxytetracycline. Biochem Biophys Res Commun 18:325–331

Minieri PP, Firman MC, Mistretta AG, Abbey A, Bricker CE, Rigler NE, Sokol H (1954) A new broad spectrum antibiotic product of the tetracycline group. Antibiot Annu 1953–1954:81–87

Mitscher LA (1968) Biosynthesis of the tetracycline antibiotics. J Pharm Sci 57:1033–1049

Mitscher LA, Martin JH, Miller PA, Shu P, Bohonos N (1966) 5-Hydroxy-7-chlorotetracycline. J Am Chem Soc 88:3647–3648

Orlova NV, Pushkina ZT (1972) Oxytetracycline production by *Actinomyces rimosus* under conditions of addition of nutrients during biosynthesis (in Russian) Antibiotiki 17:108–114

Parajková M, Šimúth J, Zelinka J (1977) Characterization of products of phosphorolysis of *Streptomyces aureofaciens* ribonucleic acid. Collect Czech Chem Commun 42:2718–2722

Pecák V, Čížek S, Musil J, Čerkes L, Herold M, Bělík E, Hoffman J (1958) Stimulation of chlortetracycline production by benzyl thiocyanate. J Hyg Epidemiol Microbiol Immunol 2:111–115

Perlman D, Heuser LJ, Dutcher JD, Barrett JH, Boska JA (1960) Biosynthesis of tetracycline by 5-hydroxytetracycline-producing cultures of *Streptomyces rimosus*. J Bacteriol 80:419–421

Perlman D, Heuser J, Semar JB, Frazier WR, Boska JA (1961) Process for biosynthesis of 7-chloro-6-demethyltetracycline. J Am Chem Soc 83:4481

Podojil M, Vaněk Z, Běhal V, Blumauerová M (1973) Regulation of biosynthesis of excessive metabolites. XIV. Incorporation of (U-^{14}C) asparagine into the molecule of tetracycline. Folia Microbiol (Prague) 7:415–417

Podojil M, Vaněk Z, Přikrylová V, Blumauerová M (1978) Isolation of ekatetrone, a new metabolite of producing variants of *Streptomyces aureofaciens*. J Antibiot 31:850–854

Podojil M, Blumauerová M, Vaněk Z, Čulík K (1984) The tetracyclines: properties, biosynthesis and fermentation. In: Vandamme EJ (ed) Biotechnology of industrial antibiotics. Dekker, New York, pp 259–279

Pridham TG (1977) Physiological characteristics and the species concept in Actinomycetales. Dev Ind Microbiol 18:287–297

Přikrylová V, Podojil M, Sedmera P, Vokoun J, Vaněk Z, Hassall CH (1978) The structure of ekatetrone, a metabolite of strains of *Streptomyces aureofaciens*. J Antibiot 31:855–862

Prokofieva-Belgovskaya AA, Orlova NV (1956) Growth and development characteristics of actinomycetes producing streptomycin, chlortetracycline and oxytetracycline during submerged biosynthesis of the antibiotic (in Russian). Izv Akad Nauk SSSR, Ser Biol 5:59–66

Prokofieva-Belgovskaya AA, Popova LA (1959) The influence of phosphorus on the development of *Actinomyces aureofaciens* and on its ability to produce chlortetracycline (in Russian). Mikrobiologiya (Moscow) 28:7–13

Prokofieva-Belgovskaya AA, Pestereva GD, Rudaya SM (1956) Growth and development characteristics of *Actinomyces rimosus* during submerged formation of the antibiotic (in Russian). Mikrobiologiya (Moscow) 25:666–674

Rokos J, Procházka P (1957) Relation of the metabolism of various carbohydrates to the production of chlortetracycline in *Streptomyces aureofaciens* (in Czech). Česk Mikrobiol (Prague) 2:251–253

Scotti T, Zocchi P (1955) Studio della struttura del micelio di *Streptomyces aureofaciens* in coltura sommersa. G Microbiol 1:35–43

Sekizawa Y (1955) A biochemical chlorination in *Streptomyces*. J Biochem (Tokyo) 42:217–219

Sensi P, DeFerrari GA, Gallo GG, Rolland G (1955) Bromotetracycline, a new antibiotic. I. Isolation and physical and chemical characteristics. Farmaco [Sci] 10:337–345

Shen S-C, Chen J-P, Koo T-A (1959) Pentose metabolism and the influence of orthophosphate on the paths of sugar degradation of *Streptomyces aureofaciens*. Sci Sin 8:733–745

Shirling EB, Gottlieb D (1968) Cooperative description of type cultures of *Streptomyces*. III. Additional species descriptions from first and second studies. Int J Syst Bacteriol 18:279–392

Shirling EB, Gottlieb D (1969) Cooperative description of type cultures of *Streptomyces*. IV. Species descriptions from the second, third and fourth studies. Int J Syst Bacteriol 19:391–512

Shirling EB, Gottlieb D (1972) Cooperative description of type strains of *Streptomyces*. V. Additional descriptions. Int J Syst Bacteriol 22:265–394

Silverman RH, Atherly AG (1978) Unusual effect of 5a,6-anhydrotetracycline and other tetracyclines. Inhibition of guanosine 5′-diphosphate 3′-diphosphate metabolism, RNA accumulation and other growth-related processes in *Escherichia coli*. Biochim Biophys Acta 518:267–276

Šimúth J, Zelinka J (1970) Nucleic acid degradation products of *Streptomyces aureofaciens*. J Antibiot 23:242–249

Šimúth J, Zelinka J (1971) The activity of polynucleotide phosphorylase in *Streptomyces aureofaciens* (in Slovak). Biologia (Bratislava) 26:239–243

Šimúth J, Zelinka J, Polek B (1975) Polynucleotide phosphorylase from *Streptomyces aureofaciens*: purification and properties. Biochim Biophys Acta 379:397–407

Šimúth J, Hudec J, Chau HT, Dányi O, Zelinka J (1979a) The synthesis of highly phosphorylated nucleotides, RNA and protein by *Streptomyces aureofaciens*. J Antibiot 32:53–58

Šimúth J, Trnovský J, Dányi O, Zelinka J (1979b) A cell free proteosynthetic system of *Streptomyces aureofaciens*. I. Translation of poly(U) prepared in situ by polynucleotide phosphorylase from *Streptomyces aureofaciens* in the presence of inhibitors. Biologia (Bratislava) 34:963–970

Snell JF, Wagner RL, Hochstein FA (1956) Radioactive oxytetracycline (Terramycin). I. Mode of synthesis and properties of the radioactive compound. In: Proceedings of the international conference on peaceful uses of atomic energy, vol 12, Radioactive isotopes and ionizing radiation in agriculture, physiology and biochemistry. Unites Nations, Geneva, pp 431–434

Snell JF, Birch AJ, Thomson PL (1960) The biosynthesis of tetracycline antibiotics. J Am Chem Soc 82:2402

Šťastná J, Mikulík K (1981) Role of highly phosphorylated nucleotides and antibiotics in the development of streptomycetes. In: Schaal KP, Pulverer G (eds) Actinomycetes. Fischer, Stuttgart, pp 481–486

Stephens CR, Conover LH, Pasternack R, Hochstein FA, Moreland WT, Regna PP, Pilgrim FJ, Brunings KJ, Woodward RB (1954) The structure of aureomycin. J Am Chem Soc 76:3568–3575

Timko J, Zelinková E, Halás Š, Zelinka J (1976a) A ribonuclease in the cell debris of *Streptomyces aureofaciens*. Biologia (Bratislava) 31:665–673

Timko J, Sabo B, Zelinka J (1976b) Nucleic acids and ribosomes from mycelium of *Streptomyces aureofaciens* during fermentation. Biologia (Bratislava) 31:703–708

Turley RH, Snell JF (1966) Biosynthesis of tetracycline antibiotics. In: Snell JF (ed) Biosynthesis of antibiotics, vol 1. Academic, New York, pp 94–120

Vaněk Z (1958) Stimulatory substances for the synthesis of chlortetracycline by *Streptomyces aureofaciens*. Folia Biol (Prague) 4:100–106

Vaněk Z, Cudlín J, Mikulík K (1969) Biogenesis and genetical regulations of synthesis of secondary metabolites. In: Sermonti G, Alačević M (eds) Genetics and breeding of *Streptomyces*. Yugoslavian Academy Science & Arts, Zagreb, pp 180–186

Vaněk Z, Cudlín J, Blumauerová M, Hošt'álek Z (1971) How many genes are required for the synthesis of chlortetracycline. Folia Microbiol (Prague) 16:225–240

Vaněk Z, Tax J, Komersová I, Sedmera P, Vokoun J (1977) Anthracyclines. Folia Microbiol (Prague) 22:139–159

Villax I (1962) *Streptomyces lusitanus* and the problem of classification of the various tetracycline-producing *Streptomyces*. Antimicrob Agents Chemother 661–668

Voříšek J, Powell AJ, Vaněk Z (1969) Regulation of biosynthesis of secondary metabolites. IV. Purification and properties of phosphoenolpyruvate carboxylase in *Streptomyces aureofaciens*. Folia Microbiol (Prague) 14:398–405

Voříšek J, Powell AJ, Vaněk Z (1970) Regulation of biosynthesis of secondary metabolites. XIII. Specific allosteric properties of phosphoenolpyruvate carboxylase in *Streptomyces aureofaciens*. Folia Microbiol (Prague) 15:153–159

Weindling R, Tresner HD, Backus EJ (1961) The host-range of a *Streptomyces aureofaciens* actinophage. Nature 189:603

Weiser J, Mikulík K, Bosch L (1981) Studies on the elongation factor Tu from *Streptomyces aureofaciens* producing tetracycline. Biochem Biophys Res Commun 99:16–22

Zaitseva ZM, Mindlin SZ (1965) Properties of *Actinomyces aureofaciens* mutants producing 6-demethylchlortetracycline (in Russian). Mikrobiologiya (Moscow) 34:91–100

Zelinka J (1968) Regulatory aspects of chlortetracycline fermentation. Biologia (Bratislava) 23:169–174

Zelinka J, Sabo B (1969) The effect of chlortetracycline on ribosome properties of the strain *Streptomyces aureofaciens* (in Slovak). Biologia (Bratislava) 24:462–467

Zelinka J, Schnittová D (1966) Nucleic acids level in the mycelium of *Streptomyces aureofaciens* during fermentation (in Slovak). Biologia (Bratislava) 21:536–539

Zelinka J, Sedláček J (1968) Effect of cadaverine on the level of ribonucleic acids in *Streptomyces aureofaciens*. Biologia (Bratislava) 23:913–916

Zelinková E, Zelinka J (1969) Biosynthesis of the exocellular ribonuclease and non-specific phosphodiesterase by *Streptomyces aureofaciens* (in Slovak). Biologia (Bratislava) 24:456–461

Zelinková E, Bačová M, Zelinka J (1971) Exocellular ribonuclease from *Streptomyces aureofaciens*. II. Properties and specificity. Biochim Biophys Acta 235:343–352

Zygmunt WA (1962) Selective inhibition in *Streptomyces rimosus*. J Bacteriol 84:1126–1127

Note Added in Proof

Since the submission of the manuscript several studies of tetracycline biosynthesis have appeared, some of which bring important new data.

Thomas and Williams (1983a) used incorporation of [1-^{13}C] and [1,2-$^{13}C_2$] acetate into the molecule of oxytetracycline with subsequent NMR spectroscopy to exactly prove the exclusive oligoketide origin of the tetracycline nucleus and the direction of folding of a hypothetical linear intermediate. These results can be compared with those obtained by de Jesus et al. (1983) in their study of incorporation of specific labelled [^{13}C] and [^{18}O] acetate into the molecule of viridicatumtoxin. They found acetate folding opposite to that found in oxytetracycline biosynthesis. The origin of C2 and the carboxamide carbon from an intact acetate unit along with the nonacetate origin of C3 signify that viridicatumtoxin is biosynthetically different from streptomycete tetracycline antibiotics.

The polyacetate theory of formation of a linear precursor of oxytetracycline was confirmed also by incorporation of [1-^{13}C,$^{2}H_3$] acetate; the deuterium labelling was found only at C7 and C9 (Thomas and Williams 1984). Labelling studies with [1,2,3-$^{13}C_3$] malonate provided evidence for the origin of the carboxamide substituent directly from an intact malonate unit (Thomas and Williams 1983b). An open question is still the stage at which the formation of the amide bond takes place.

In the field of genetic regulation of the biosynthetic process the study of Rhodes et al. (1981) aimed at a biochemical and genetic characterization of *S. rimosus* mutants blocked in oxytetracycline biosynthesis. Genetic analysis showed the existence of two chromosomal clusters responsible for individual steps of the biosynthetic pathway. The genes for the reactions to 4-aminoanhydrotetracycline were mapped in a position between *cys*D3 and *rib*B1, genes for further metabolic steps (transformation of anhydrotetracycline) in a diametrically opposite region between *pro*A3 and *ade*A2.

References

de Jesus AE, Hull WE, Steyn PS, van Heerden FR, Vleggaar R (1982) Biosynthesis of viridicatumtoxin, a mycotoxin from *Penicillium expansum*. J Chem Soc Chem Commun 902–904

Rhodes PM, Winskill N, Friend EJ, Warren M (1981) Biochemical and genetic characterization of *Streptomyces rimosus* mutants impaired in oxytetracycline biosynthesis. J Gen Microbiol 124:329–338

Thomas R, Williams DJ (1983a) Oxytetracycline biosynthesis: mode of incorporation of [1-^{13}C]- and [1,2-$^{13}C_2$]-acetate. J Chem Soc Chem Commun 128–130

Thomas R, Williams DJ (1983b) Oxytetracycline biosynthesis: origin of the carboxamide substituent. J Chem Soc Chem Commun 677–679

Thomas R, Williams DJ (1984) Oxytetracycline biosynthesis: mode of incorporation of [1-^{13}C,$^{2}H_3$] acetate. J Chem Soc Chem Commun 443–444

CHAPTER 5

Chemical Modification of the Tetracyclines

W. Rogalski

A. Introduction

The tetracyclines are a group of broad-spectrum antibiotics which, even 30 years after their discovery, have retained a prominent position in the treatment of infectious diseases.

A wealth of literature has accumulated on the subject of tetracyclines. In the 16-year period from 1965 to 1980 alone more than 10,000 publications appeared dealing with chemical, pharmacological, and medical aspects, serving to indicate the intense interest and activity surrounding this series of antibiotics.

Chemical research during recent decades in the field of tetracyclines can be divided into the following four groups:

1. Isolation and structure determination of tetracyclines (Chaps. 2 and 3, this volume)
2. Synthesis of degradation and transformation products of natural tetracyclines with the aim of obtaining compounds with better chemotherapeutic properties (Sect. B, this chapter)
3. Experiments for total synthesis of natural tetracyclines or their immediate biologically active derivatives
4. Total synthesis of unnatural tetracyclines with new structures which can be achieved neither by fermentation nor by semisynthesis (Sect. C, this chapter).

Over the past decade or two, however, the widespread use of tetracyclines has led to an alarming rise in the number of resistant organisms, so that their usefulness is beginning to become somewhat limited. Further factors affecting their use and effectiveness are toxicity, poor absorption, and molecular instability.

In the past 3 decades enormous effort has been directed toward modifying the structure of tetracyclines in an attempt to improve their properties and, above all, their antibacterial activity. A threefold approach has been adopted:

1. Genetic manipulation of tetracycline-producing microorganisms (Hošťálek et al. 1974) in the hope that mutants might produce tetracyclines having different characteristics
2. Structural modification of existing tetracyclines by partial synthesis
3. Preparation of totally synthetic tetracyclines having a structure not capable of being copied by semisynthetic or fermentation methods.

There follows a summary of work performed using approaches 2 and 3. The resultant products are classified as: (1) semisynthetic tetracyclines and (2) totally synthetic unnatural tetracyclines.

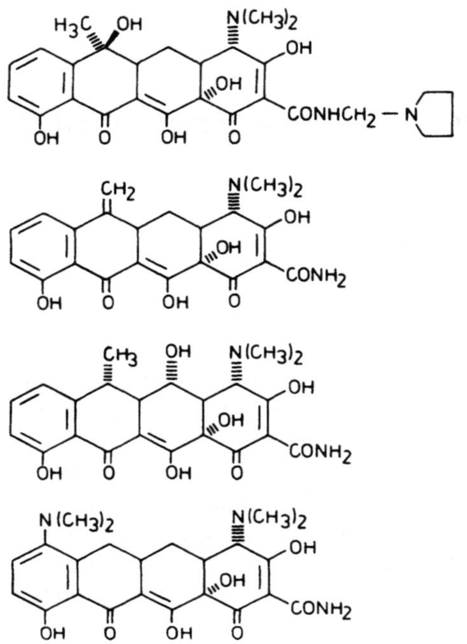

Rolitetracycline 1

Methacycline 2

Doxycycline 3

Minocycline 4

Fig. 1. The four medicinally important semisynthetic tetracyclines

Semisynthesis is a term used to denote chemical modification of a tetracycline obtained by fermentation procedures. The process uses the natural product as starting material for the modification. Although more than 1,000 tetracycline derivatives have been prepared by this means (Dürckheimer 1975), only tetracyclines (1)–(4) (Fig. 1) have attained any significance in the treatment of infectious diseases.

The total synthesis of complex organic natural products such as tetracyclines was a tremendous challenge to many chemists. Chapter 3 deals with the total synthesis of natural products, so that the present chapter sets out merely to discuss the total synthesis of unnatural tetracyclines which can be prepared neither by fermentation methods nor by semisynthetic means.

In the past 2 decades innumerable review articles have been written about tetracyclines, reflecting research trends in this field. Many review articles have dealt specifically with studies into semisynthetic tetracyclines and their structure-activity relationships (Barrett 1963; Money and Scott 1968; Clive 1968; Blackwood and English 1970; Hlavka and Boothe 1973; Dürckheimer 1975; Mitscher 1978; Brown and Ireland 1978; Boothe and Hlavka 1978).

In more recent years there has been an increased appreciation of the structural features necessary for achieving the desired biological activity and this in turn has led to a better understanding of the interrelationships between structure, configuration, conformation, and biological activity.

Since the discovery of tetracyclines there have been many reactions aimed at modifying the tetracycline molecules. The following survey singles out from the

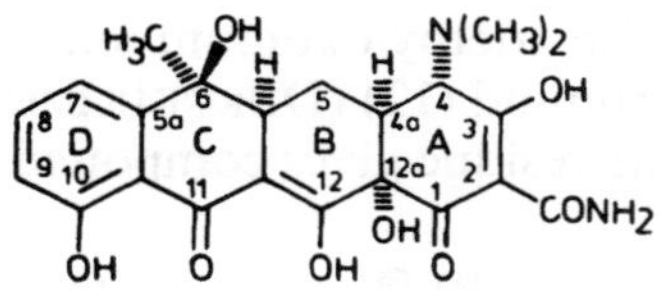

Tetracycline 5

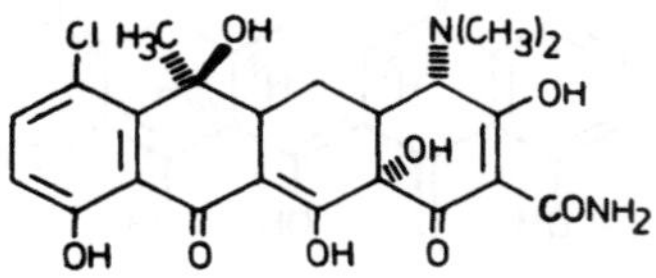

Chlortetracycline 6

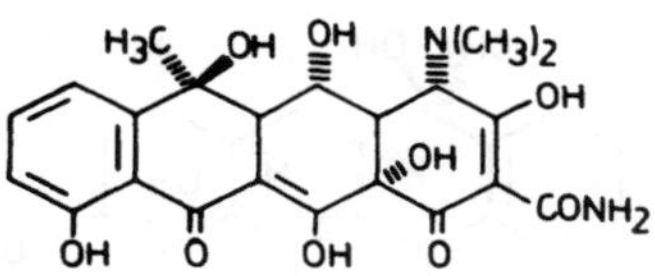

Oxytetracycline 7

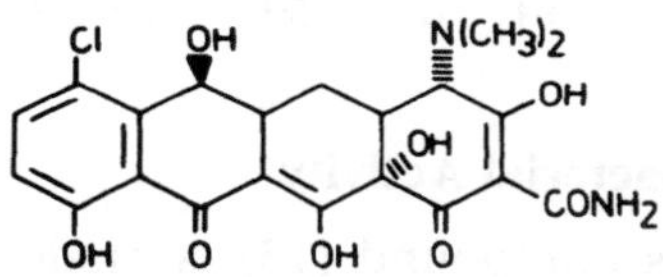

Demethylchloro-tetracycline 8

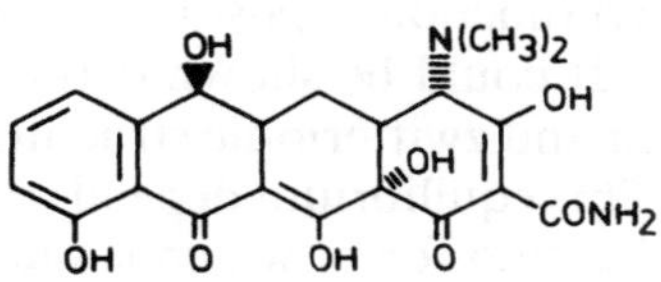

Demethyl-tetracycline 9

Fig. 2. Structure of the relevant tetracyclines used as starting material for modification

wide range of material available only those typical structural variations which have provided a better knowledge of structure-activity relationships and of structural features essential for the biological activity. The text is arranged so as to deal separately with modifications at each position of the molecule. Formula (5) shows the absolute stereochemistry of tetracycline, the way in which the rings are denoted, and the numbering given to C atoms in the tetracyclic ring system. Starting material for all semisynthetic modifications consisted of tetracyclines which were made accessible by fermentation reactions. Their structures are shown in Fig. 2.

B. Semisynthetic Tetracyclines

I. Modifications at the C1 and C3 Positions

1. Chemistry

There is virtually no mention in the literature of modifications at positions 1 and 3. The keto-enol system between carbon atoms 1 and 3 is highly delocalized, extremely slow to react, and present in an equilibrium of two enol forms, as evident in compounds (10) and (11). Alkylation with triethyloxonium tetrafluoroborate with base catalysis leads to the alkoxy compound (12) (DÜRCKHEIMER 1975). Exchanging the 1-ethoxy group for the glycine residue gives compound (13).

10 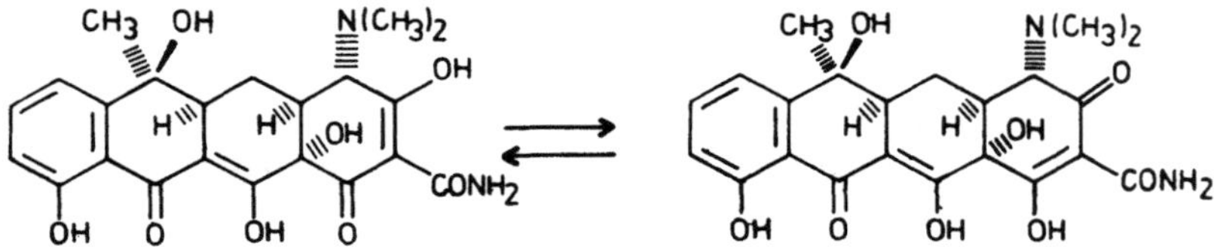 11

12 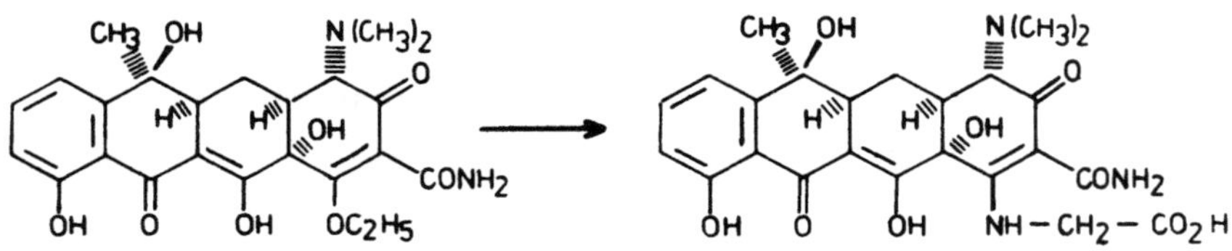 13

2. Effect of Structural Variation on Antibacterial Activity

Compound (12) has no activity whereas compound (13) is moderately active (DÜRCKHEIMER 1975). Apparently a carbonyl function in positions 1 and 3 is essential for providing full tetracycline activity. It could be shown (STEZOWSKI 1976) that an equilibrium between the nonionized and zwitterionic structure of tetracyclines is important for biological activity. This equilibrium depends on the nature of the solvent, and water tends to favor the keto form, which is the form of the zwitterion. This keto-enol tautomerism of ring A is a feature common to all biologically active tetracyclines. Blocking this system by forming derivatives at C1 and C3 should therefore result in loss of antibacterial activity.

II. Modifications at the C2 Position

1. Chemistry

Normally, all tetracyclines have a carboxamide group at the 2 position. When oxytetracycline (7) is being prepared by fermentation, however, a by-product occurs bearing an acetyl group at the 2 position instead of the usual carboxamide group (HOCHSTEIN et al. 1960; MILLER and HOCHSTEIN 1962).

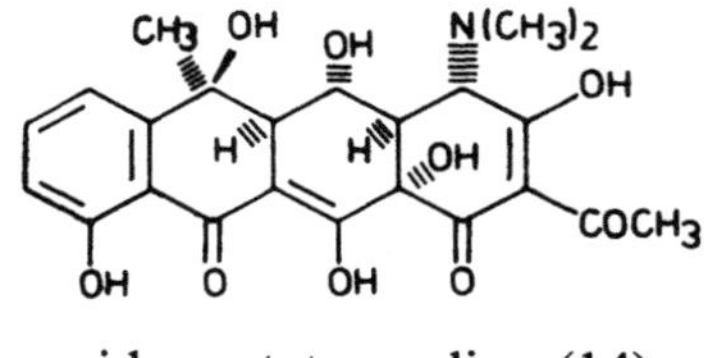 14

2-Acetyl-2-decarboxamidooxytetracycline (14) possesses only about 10% of the normal tetracycline antibacterial activity, thus illustrating that alterations made to the carboxamide group can produce changes in the properties of the molecule.

The carboxamide group in position C2 withstands many reactions even under harsh conditions. Certain types of reaction, however, are capable of modifying this group. One of these reactions is the Mannich reaction, which takes tetracycline as a basis for producing new tetracycline derivatives. The reactivity of the carboxamido group in tetracyclines and the interesting properties exhibited by their condensation products have evoked considerable interest in products of this type and have given rise to a wealth of literature and hundreds of patents concerning the amino alkylation of tetracyclines (BARRETT 1963; BRUNZELL 1962; CHENEY et al. 1958; HÜTTENRAUCH and KEINER 1966). The compounds which can be produced by these means are so numerous as to preclude a mention of all of them in this review, though three substances which are repeatedly quoted in the literature shall be singled out for special mention.

Treatment of tetracycline with morpholine and formaldehyde gives the very readily water-soluble derivative *N*-morpholinomethyltetracycline (15) (GOTTSTEIN et al. 1959).

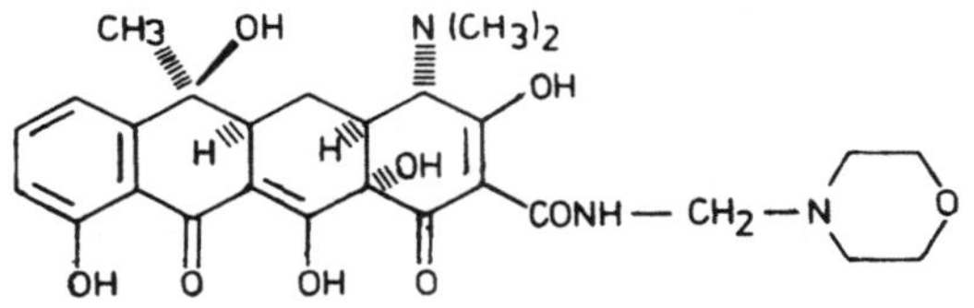

15

Hydrogenolysis over Raney nickel or treatment with aqueous sodium hydrogen sulfite solution reconverts compound (15) into tetracycline (5).

Similarly, *N*-pyrrolidinomethyltetracycline (1) can be prepared from tetracycline (5), pyrrolidine, and formaldehyde (SIEDEL et al. 1958).

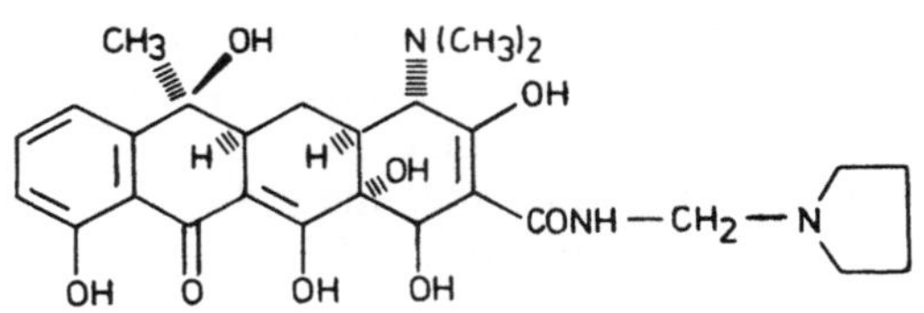

1

This base is more than 2,500 times more water-soluble than tetracycline in the physiological pH range. This property has made it particularly suitable for parenteral use in infectious diseases. Rolitetracycline hydrolyzes in solution to produce an equilibrium consisting of rolitetracycline and tetracycline (HUGHES et al. 1974).

Reacting tetracycline with formaldehyde and lysine gives *N*-lysinomethyltetracycline (16) (DE CARNERI et al. 1961). Here again, the only slightly soluble tetracycline base is transformed into a freely soluble compound.

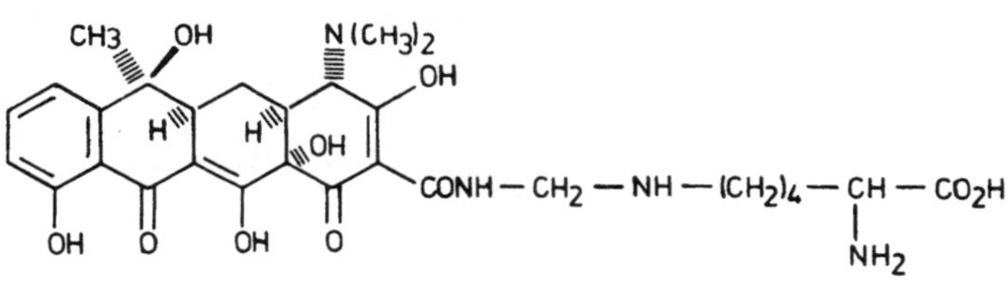

16

When reacted with α-amino acids, tetracyclines give rise to compounds which readily break down in solution, while amino acids where the amino group is in the γ or ε position as well as diamino acids form consistent and relatively more stable condensation products (BERNARDELLI et al. 1967).

Recently the Mannich base prepared by condensation of tetracycline with formaldehyde and glucosamine was described (CHANDRA et al. 1980). It is reported that the glucosamine derivative is more effective in vitro than tetracycline in gram-negative bacterial strains.

Mannich bases of the types described are as a rule freely water-soluble. A number of them are widely used in medicine owing to their excellent pharmacological properties. These Mannich bases are extremely labile, however, in aqueous solutions, hydrolyzing back into the starting materials. This reversion to the original tetracycline is probably responsible for their antibacterial activity.

The methylol compound (17) was isolated by reacting chlortetracycline with formaldehyde alone (TUBARO and BANCI 1964).

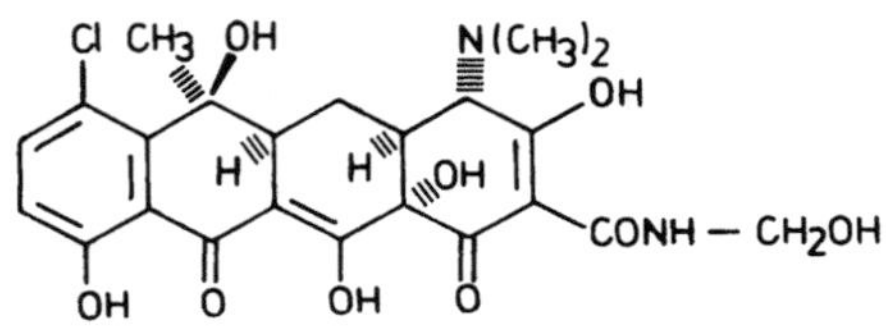

17

Like the Mannich bases, this compound is water-soluble and combines the advantages of being less toxic and better tolerated.

A further class of carboxamide-substituted compounds, namely the alkoxyalkyltetracyclines, is obtained by condensing a tetracycline with an aldehyde in alcohol (TAMORRIA and ESSE 1965; MARTELL et al. 1967b). The simplest member of this group is *N*-(2-methoxy)methyltetracycline (18), which is obtained by refluxing tetracycline (5) in methanol with formaldehyde.

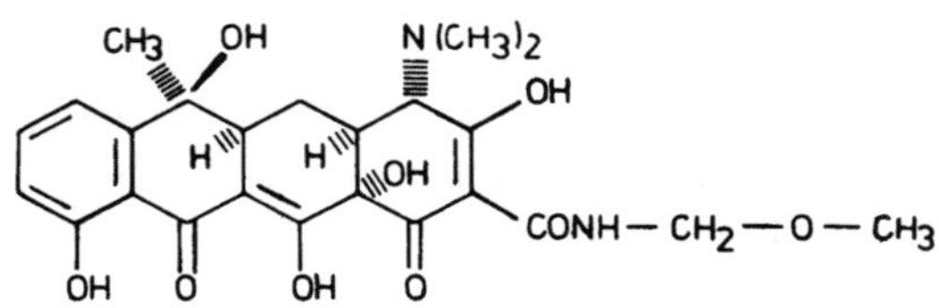

18

The alkoxylalkyltetracyclines exhibit considerably reduced in vitro activity. The larger the residue, the more quickly the product hydrolyzes to tetracycline, the actual antibacterially active substance. The alkoxyalkyl group could if desired be used as a protective group for the carboxamido group, should it be necessary to treat tetracycline or one of its derivatives with dehydrating agents in the event that nitrile formation might occur under such conditions but should be prevented.

Compound (19), *N*-(3-phthalidyl)tetracycline, precipitates out when tetracycline (5) is heated with phthalaldehyde.

The derivative is very freely water-soluble at above pH 9, though it is insoluble in acids (GRANATEK et al. 1963).

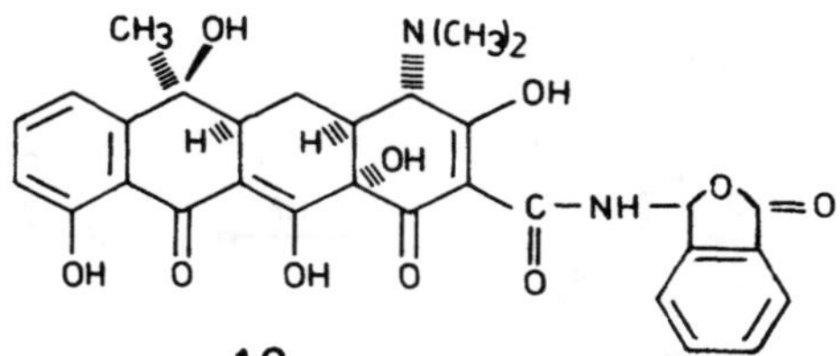

19

Treatment of tetracyclines in pyridine with arylsulfonyl chlorides causes the amide function in the 2 position to be dehydrated to give the nitrile (20) (STEPHENS et al. 1955, 1963). Tetracyclines (21) and (22) can be prepared in this way too. Under certain circumstances the C10 sulfonate ester may also be formed.

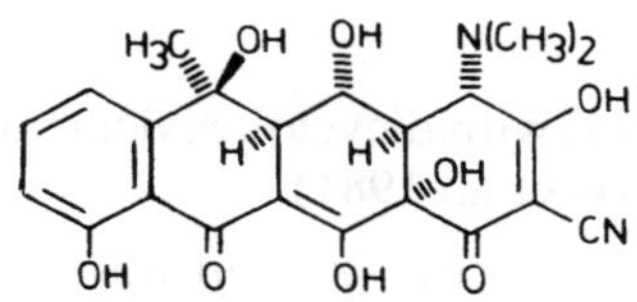

20

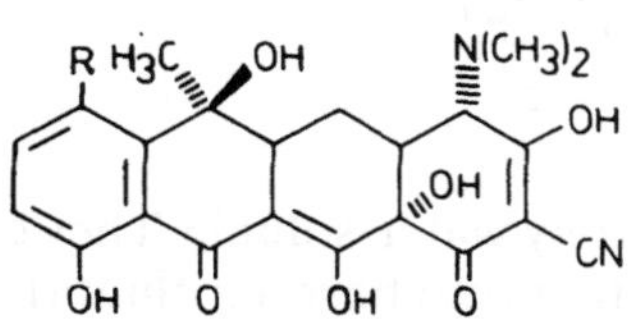

21 a : R = H
21 b : R = Cl

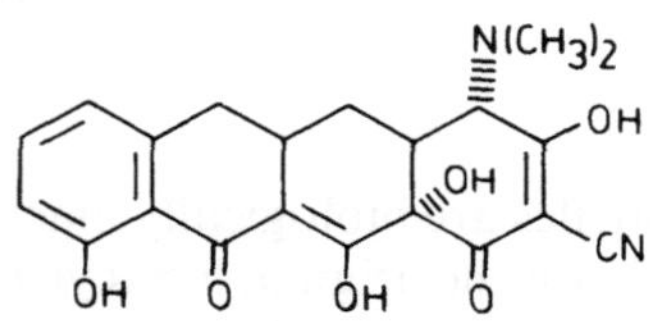

22

The mechanism in Fig. 3 seems to be the most probable for the course of the reaction from amide to nitrile:

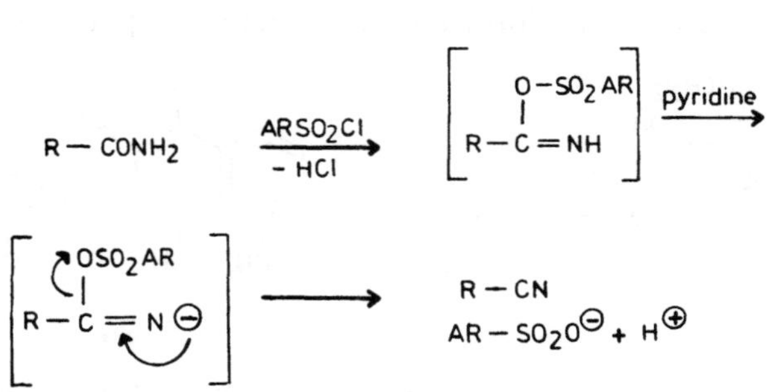

Fig. 3. Mechanism for the modification of amide to nitrile

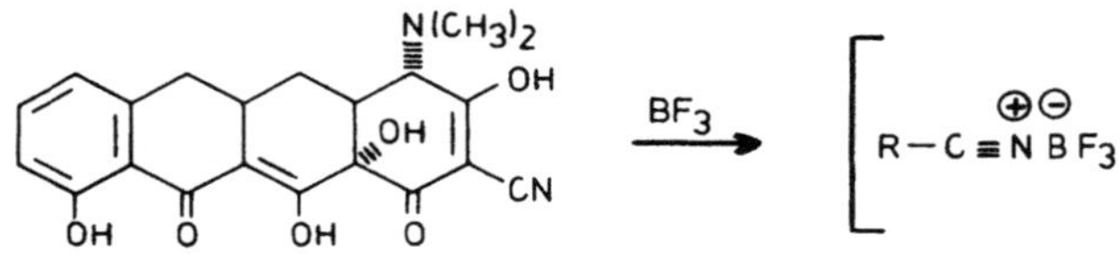

22

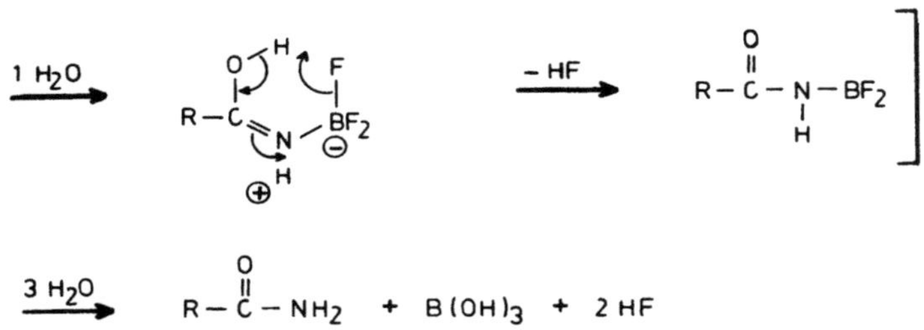

Fig. 4. Proposal for the mechanism of nitrile hydrolyzation (see also MITSCHER 1978)

Treatment of doxycycline (3) with dicyclohexylcarbodiimide in methanol provided the nitrile (22a) (VALCAVI et al. 1981).

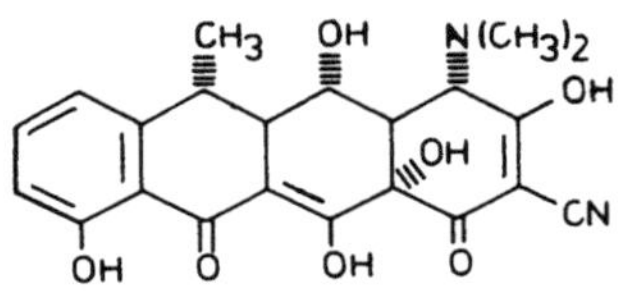

22a

The nitriles are biologically inactive and barely water-soluble. They can be reconverted into the original tetracycline by reacting with boron trifluoride in acetic acid with subsequent hydrolysis (Fig. 4) (BEEREBOOM and BUTLER 1962; MITSCHER 1978).

The corresponding alkylated amides can be obtained by applying the Ritter reaction to the nitriles (STEPHENS et al. 1963). Treatment of 6-demethyl-6-deoxytetracycline nitrile (22) with isobutylene in sulfuric and acetic acids gives rise to the *N*-alkylated amide (23). In the presence of the 6-hydroxy group the corresponding anhydro amides are formed in this reaction step, e.g., compound (24).

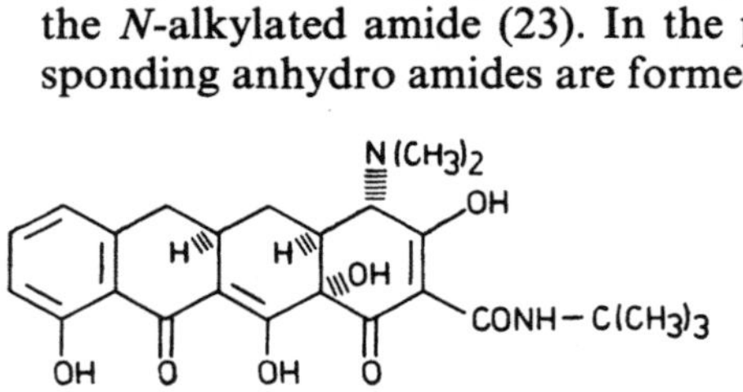

23

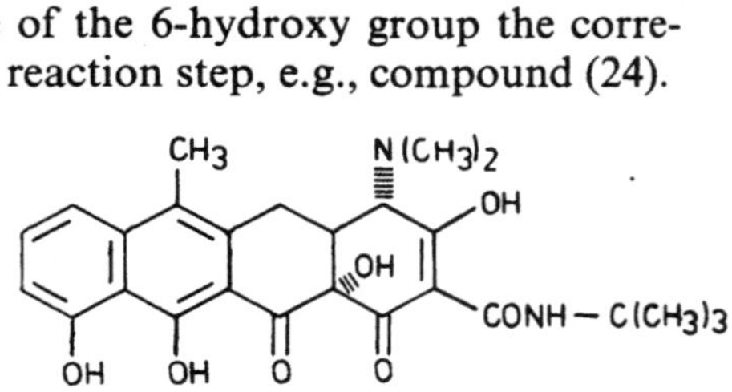

24

N-tert-Butyl-6-demethyl-6-deoxytetracycline (23) exhibits only moderate in vitro activity against gram-positive bacteria. By contrast, the substance is devoid of all gram-negative and in vivo activity. Compound (23) has more significant lipophilic properties than compound (98) with the unsubstituted amide group (BLACKWOOD and ENGLISH 1970). This may explain why such compounds do not exhibit the same activity against gram-negative bacteria as the tetracyclines themselves and why their effect is exercised predominantly against gram-positive bacteria.

Based on these considerations it was hoped that it might be possible to modify the antibacterial spectrum of the tetracyclines to a lesser extent by forming a mono-*N*-methyl compound and thus to produce useful antibiotics. This aim was pursued along semisynthetic and also totally synthetic lines.

Treatment of minocycline (4) with chloromethylmethyl sulfide in a strong acid produces the correspondingly substituted amide (25), which gives the desulfurized product (26) with Raney nickel in boiling ethanol (BERNARDI et al. 1975a).

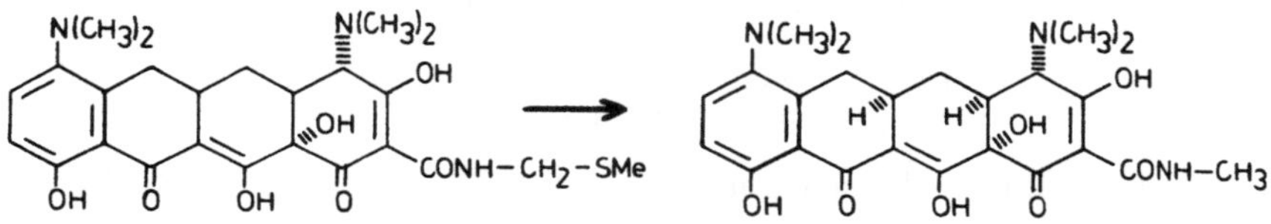

25 26

While having a somewhat less pronounced antibacterial activity, the *N*-methyl compound (26) has a similar spectrum to that of minocycline.

Treatment of tetracycline nitriles with, for instance, hydroxymethylenephthalimide in strong acids (Einhorn reaction) produces a condensation product similar to the Mannich products, e.g., compound (27), this being without any antibacterial activity (MARTELL 1967b). Compound (27) treated with boiling methanol in the presence of *n*-butylamine gives the amine (28), which is highly unstable and is degraded to 6-demethyl-6-deoxytetracycline.

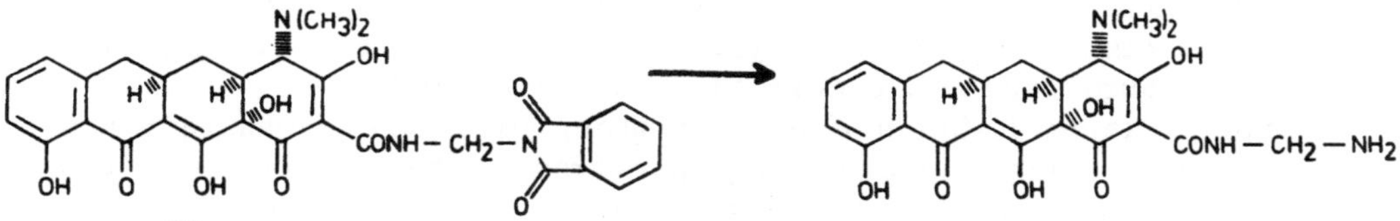

27 28

N-Cycloheptatrienyltetracyclines (29) have properties similar to those of the tetracycline Mannich bases and are also similar in their behavior (DÜRCKHEIMER 1975). Acids cause them to revert to tetracycline, e.g., compounds (29) and (30).

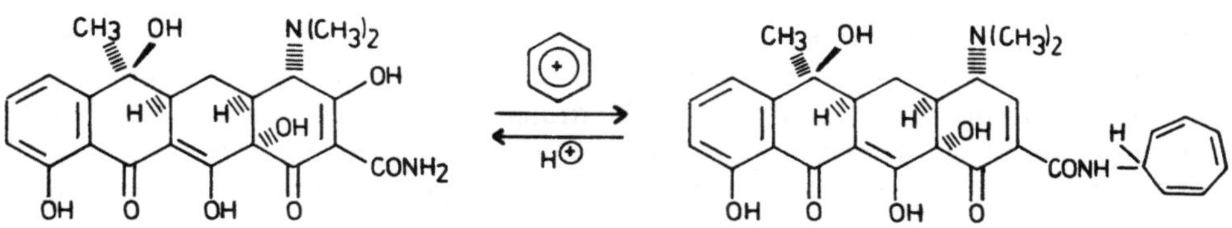

30 29

Further reactions at the C2 atom have been carried out (VALCAVI et al. 1981). The nitrile (22a) was converted with hydrogen cloride in ethanol to the 2-ethoxy-carbonyl compound (22 b).

To obtain the 2-thioamide (22 c), doxycycline hydrochloride (3) was treated with P_2S_5 in dioxane. Reduction of (22 c) over Raney nickel gave the 2-amino-methyl derivative (22 d), a highly unstable compound.

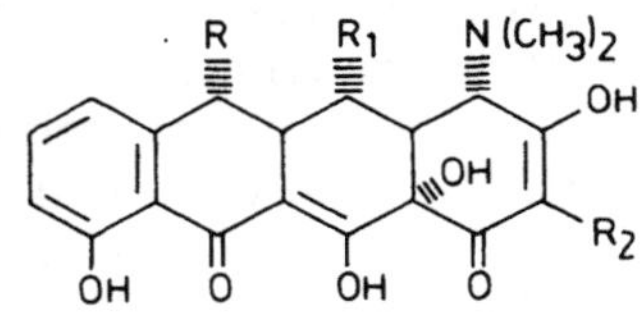

3 : R = CH_3 ; R_1 = OH ; R_2 = $CONH_2$ (doxycycline)
22 a : R = CH_3 ; R_1 = OH; R_2 = CN
22 b : R = CH_3 ; R_1 = OH; R_2 = $COOC_2H_5$
22 c : R = CH_3 ; R_1 = OH; R_2 = $CSNH_2$
22 d : R = CH_3 ; R_1 = OH; R_2 = CH_2NH_2

For modification of chelocardin (211) at the C2 atom, see Sect. C.II.1.

2. Effect of Structural Variation on Antibacterial Activity

The structure-activity relationships at the C2 position can be summed up as follows:

Replacement of the C2 carboxamido group by an aldehyde (KORST 1972 a), aldimine (KORST 1972 b), or acetyl group leads to a loss of activity. Tetracycline nitriles are totally inactive. Substitution of a methyl group for a hydrogen at the amidonitrogen does not exert any considerable influence on the in vitro activity. Large residues, such as those of *tert*-butyl and cycloheptyl, are disadvantageous (Table 1).

Owing to the degree of instability of the substituted tetracyclines in aqueous, acidic, or alkaline solutions, derivatives are re-cleaved to give the starting materials, this determining the extent of their antibacterial activity.

Mannich aminoalkylation of the amide group gives rise to derivatives which are freely water-soluble in the physiological pH range, which hydrolyze slowly in vitro and in vivo, and which thus possess the same spectrum of activity as the starting materials. It is thanks to these properties that *N*-pyrrolidinomethyltetracycline (1) and lysinomethyltetracycline (16), in particular, have become medicinally important antibiotics.

Regarding the influence of the *N*-*tert*-butyl group on the properties of the molecule it was proposed (BLACKWOOD and ENGLISH 1970) that the remarkable reduced in vitro and in vivo antibacterial activity of the *N*-*tert*-butyl-6-demethyl-6-deoxytetracycline (23) in comparison to 6-demethyl-6-deoxytetracycline is the result of the highly lipophilic nature of the molecule. X-ray crystal structure analysis of *N*-*tert*-butyl-8-methoxy-6-demethyl-6-deoxytetracycline (GLATZ et al. 1979) shows that there is a striking difference between the *N*-*tert*-butyl-8-methoxy compound and 5-oxytetracycline concerning the hydrogen bonding in the A-ring chromophore. The reason is more likely to be the electron-donating character of

Table 1. Antibacterial activity of natural tetracyclines and tetracyclines modified at the C2 Position

Structure	Name	Minimum inhibitory concentrations (μg/ml)		
		Staphylococcus aureas 5	*Streptococcus pyogenes*	*Escherichia coli*
(6)	Chlortetracycline	0.19	0.04	1.56
(7)	Oxytetracycline [a]	0.55	0.07	1.09
(5)	Tetracycline [a]	0.21	0.06	0.73
(8)	Demethylchlortetracycline	0.11	0.04	0.33
(1)	Rolitetracycline [b]	Equivalent to tetracycline		
(21 b)	Chlortetracyclinonitrile [c]	>100	>100	>100
(21 a)	Tetracyclinonitrile [d]	>100	>100	>100
(14)	2-Acetyl-2-decarboxamido-oxytetracycline [e]	3	3	50
–	2-Acetyl-2-decarboxamidotetracycline [f]	3	0.7	50
(23)	6-Demethyl-6-deoxy-N^2-*t*-butyltetracycline [a]	0.7	1.0	>100

[a] Blackwood and English (1970)
[b] Siedel et al. (1958)
[c] Stephens et al. (1954)
[d] Stephens (1962)
[e] Hochstein et al. (1960)
[f] Miller and Hochstein (1962)

the *tert*-butyl group on the amide nitrogen. This causes an increase of the partial negative charge on the amide oxygen and it is believed that this higher degree of protonation displayed by *N-tert*-butyl-8-methoxy-6-demethyl-6-deoxytetracycline than by 5-oxytetracycline may be indicative of stabilization of the nonionized form with respect to the zwitterionic two molecular species which are important for biological activity. Stabilization of the nonionized form in the equilibrium of the nonionized and zwitterionic structure would result in increased lipophilicity. Although these are the results of the investigation of *N-tert*-butyl-8-methoxy-6-demethyl-6-deoxytetracycline it is highly probable that in the case of the simpler analogue (23) the same effects must be involved.

It has been reported (Gulbis and Everett 1976; Williamson and Everett 1975) that tetracycline nitrile (21) is not found to adopt the conformation of the nonionized structure. Tetracycline nitrile lacks the amide carbonyl group, which is important as the proton acceptor in the formation of the hydrogen bond present in all crystal structure analyses in which conformation of the nonionized structure has been observed (Prewo and Stezowski 1977). It is characteristic for the conformation of the nonionized structure that this form is stabilized by a strong hydrogen bond in the enolic A-ring chromophore. But the nonionized form contributes to the biological activity of the tetracyclines by adopting this structure in the hydrophobic regions of biological systems (Stezowski 1976). The lack of this structure means therefore loss of activity.

To summarize, the amide carbonyl appears to be essential for tetracycline activity but not the amide nitrogen.

III. Modifications at the C4 Position

1. Chemistry

Considerable effort has been devoted to modifying the substituents at the C4 position in the tetracyclines by chemical means, whereby the configuration of the substituents has been exceedingly important.

The C4 β-epimers differ considerably in their properties from those with a normal configuration. The most important difference is the antibacterial in vitro activity. It has been found that β-epimers account for about 5% of the activity of normal tetracyclines (DOERSCHUK et al. 1955). Accounts have been given of conditions which promote or hinder epimerization (MCCORMICK et al. 1957; HUSSAR et al. 1968). Epimerization is reported to occur in various solvent systems within a pH range of about 2–6. The degree of epimerization is increased by several buffers such as phosphates, citrates, or acetates. The kinetics of C4 epimerization in tetracyclines have also been investigated (REMMERS et al. 1963).

The process of epimerization in an acid solution has been described (RIGLER et al. 1965) and is shown in Fig. 5.

Tetracycline (5) epimerizes more readily than oxytetracycline (7) (JAROWSKI 1963). It is assumed that the hydroxy group in the 5 position of oxytetracycline forms a hydrogen bridge with the dimethylamino group, thus stabilizing the configuration of the dimethylamino group in the 4 position [see formula (31)] (HUSSAR et al. 1968). Moreover, it was observed that the nature of the substitution at the C2 atom (Mannich compounds) has some influence on the epimerization in oxytetracycline derivatives. Results of the investigations are not unequivocal, however, and in fact are partially contradictory (HUSSAR et al. 1968; HÜTTENRAUCH and KEINER 1966). No explanation has as yet been found for these contradictory results. Under alkaline conditions 4-epitetracyclines are converted almost completely back to the bioactive α-isomer in the presence of chelating metals (KORST et al. 1968).

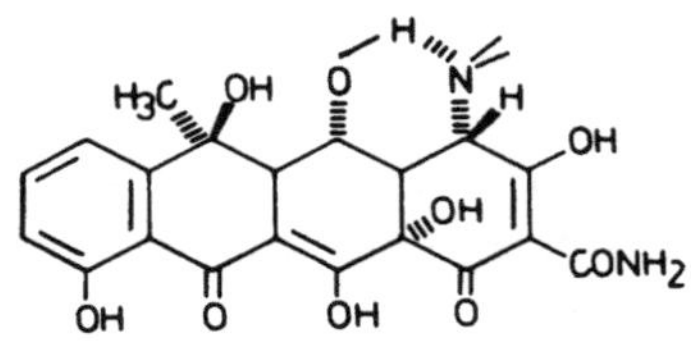

31

In strong-acid solutions the tetracyclines are dehydrated to anhydrotetracyclines. In 1*N* HCl, for instance, 4-epianhydrotetracycline (33) is obtained from

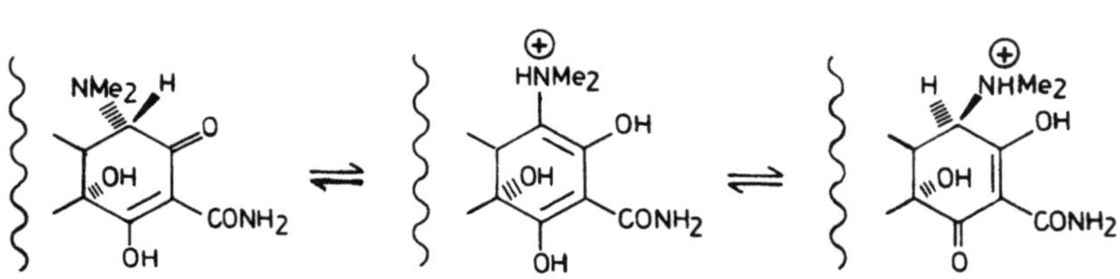

Fig. 5. Epimerization process at the C4 position

4-epitetracycline (32) with no appreciable isomerization (McCormick et al. 1956; Kelly 1964).

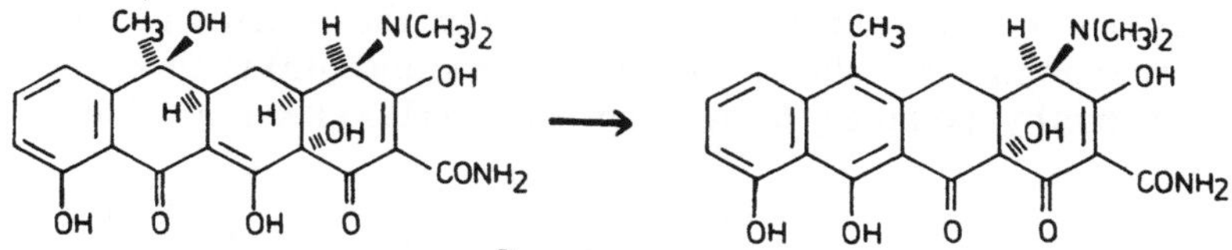

32 33

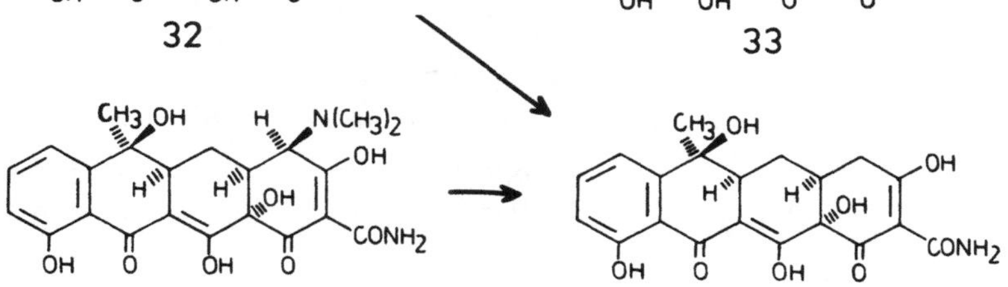

34 35

Treating both C4 epimers (32) and (34) with zinc in glacial acetic acid for 6 h at 30 °C gives dedimethylaminotetracycline (35) (McCormick et al. 1956).

In the preparation of quaternary ammonium compounds with methyl iodide, the quaternary ammonium salts (36) are formed only from tetracycline (5) and chlorotetracycline (6) at room temperature over a period of 1 week. Oxytetracycline (7) is degraded under these conditions (Boothe et al. 1958).

Treatment of salt (36) with zinc in glacial acetic acid gives 4-dedimethylaminotetracycline (37) (Boothe et al. 1958). Deamination can also be achieved by photolysis of tetracycline (5) (Hlavka and Bitha 1966). 4-Epitetracycline (34) undergoes no photoelimination under these conditions.

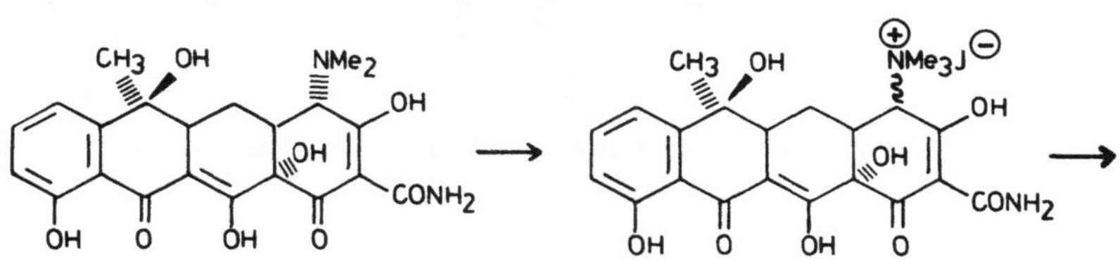

5 36

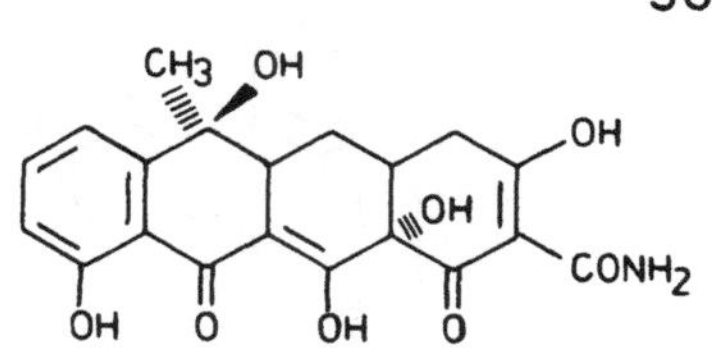

37

The quaternary ammonium compounds tend to form various reaction products all according to the conditions under which they react (Fig. 6). Refluxing tetracycline methyl betaine (36) in acetonitrile leads to the formation of 4a,12a-anhydro-4-dedimethylamino-4-hydroxytetracycline (39) or (40) (Boothe et al. 1958). If betaine (36) or (38) is refluxed in methanol, ring B opens forming esters (41) or (42) and the γ-lactam (43) or (44) (Hlavka et al. 1968). Acid treatment of betaine (36) yields anhydrobetaine (45), which can be transformed by boiling in acetonitrile into 4-hydroxy-6-methylpretetramide (46). Treating compounds (46) and (47) with hydrogen iodide in phenol gives the 6-methylpretetramide (48). As the formulae in Fig. 6 show, however, compound (46) is also produced from tetracycline methyl betaine (36) by other routes (HLAVKA et al. 1968).

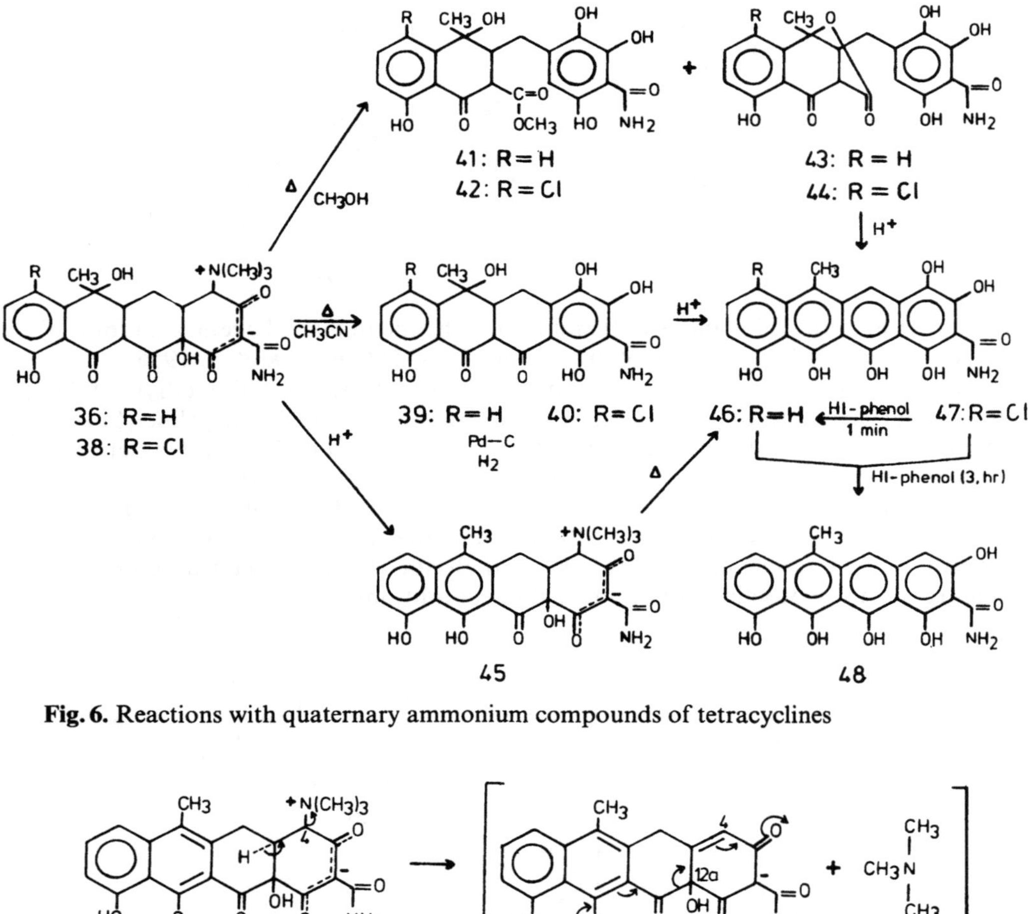

Fig. 6. Reactions with quaternary ammonium compounds of tetracyclines

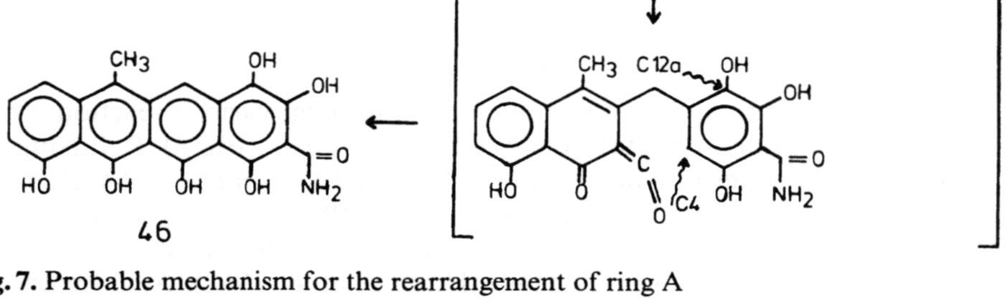

Fig. 7. Probable mechanism for the rearrangement of ring A

There are various mechanisms for transforming (45) into (46); the most probable reaction is that shown in Fig. 7. Opening of ring B between C atoms 12 and 12a and rotation of ring A are followed by ring closure between C atoms 12 and 4 to give 4-hydroxy-6-methylpretetramide (46) (HLAVKA et al. 1968).

A further unusual reaction sequence proceeds from tetracyclines (5) and (9) via the stable hemiketals (57) and (58), which in turn form the starting material for various substituted amino compounds of type (59) and (60). These tetracyclines, which are substituted differently at the 4 position, were particularly interesting because it was apparent that it might thus be possible to modify the properties of tetracyclines.

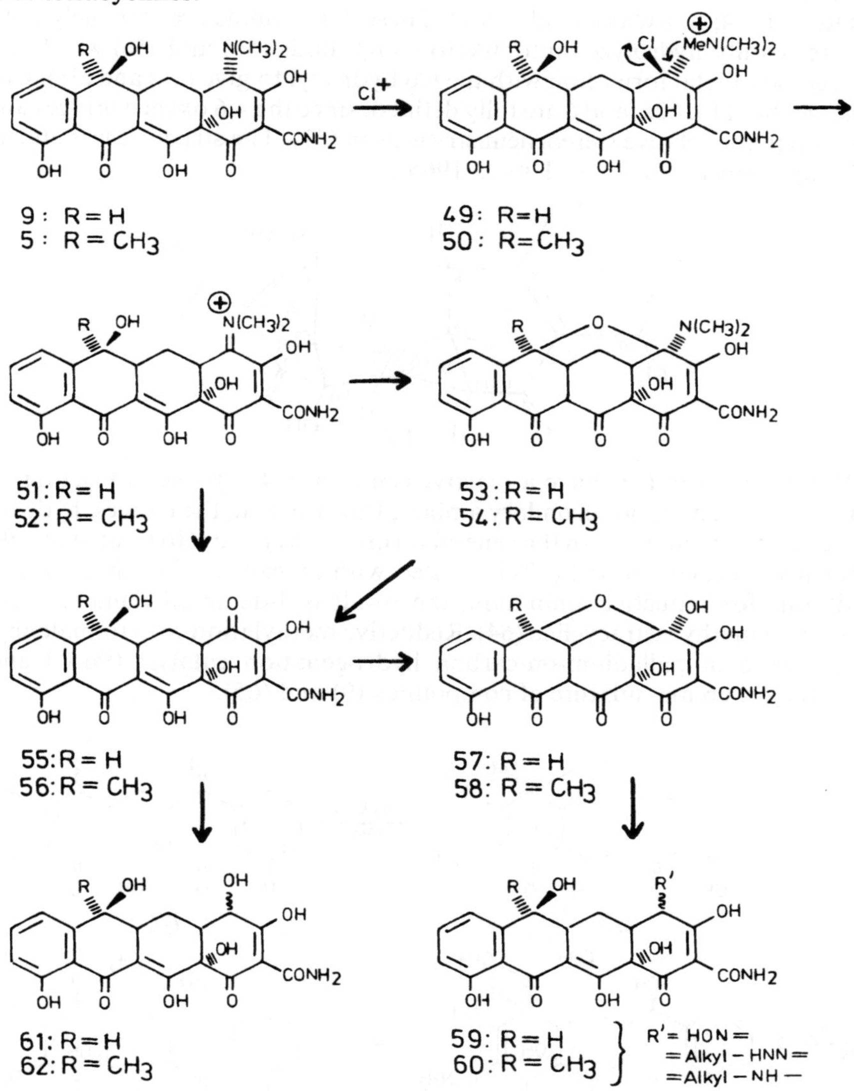

Fig. 8. Reactions leading to the 4,6-hemiketals

Treating (5) and (9) with positive chlorine, copper acetate, or mercury acetate leads via compounds (49) and (50) to the imino compounds (51) and (52), which are transformed in the presence of water to the 4-keto compounds (55) and (56). These easily react through a nucleophilic reaction of the 6-hydroxy group with the 4-keto group to form the 4,6-hemiketals (57) and (58).

For the conversion of the 4-amino compound to the 4-keto intermediate the following reactive mechanism has been proposed (Fig. 8) (BLACKWOOD and STEPHENS 1965; ESSE et al. 1964a; HLAVKA and BOOTHE 1973). Under anhydrous conditions the C6 hydroxy group of compound (51) or (52) reacts with the 4-imino group to produce compounds (53) and (54) (ESSE et al. 1964a; BLACKWOOD and STEPHENS 1964; SCHWARZ et al. 1967). These compounds are extremely unstable and are readily hydrolyzed into 4-keto compounds (55) and (56) which in turn undergo hemiketal formation with the C6 hydroxyl to give (57) and (58). Carbon atoms 4a, 5a, 11a, 12a, and 6 are fully defined, since the 4,6 oxygen bridge can only occur when the relative stereochemistry is as in (57). The structure was elucidated by X-ray analysis (VAN DEN HENDE 1965).

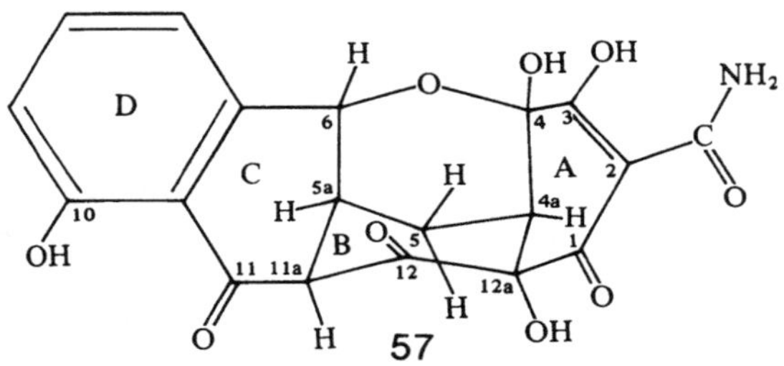

57

Ketals (57) and (58) have a reactive center at C4 capable of reacting with a number of primary and secondary amines, thus forming the oximes, hydrazones, and substituted amines with the general formulae (59) and (60) (ESSE et al. 1964b). If, for instance, compound (57) is treated with an excess of methylamine under conditions for reductive amination, the result is 4-dedimethylamino-4-methylamino-6-demethyl-tetracycline (64). Reductive methylation with formaldehyde in the presence of palladium-on-carbon hydrogenation catalyst (Pd-C) and H_2 yields the C4 epimer mixture of compounds (9) and (65).

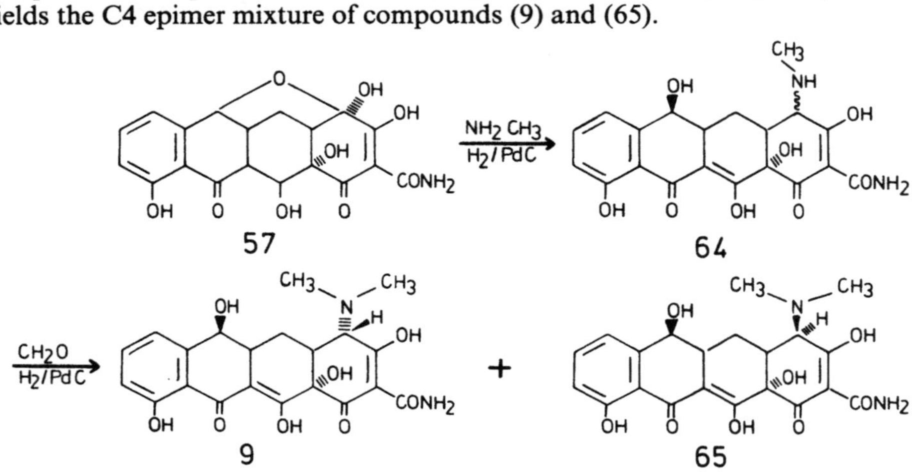

57 64 9 65

Since fermentation produces only tetracyclines with a dimethylamino group (except for ethylmethylaminotetracycline when ethionine is used in the fermentation), the 4,6-hemiketals (57) and (58) represent a useful starting material for the preparation of various substituted C4 amino compounds. Unfortunately, however, the end products often turn out to have the main product in the undesired 4-epi configuration, since by reduction of the double bond of the intermediates the catalyst can more readily gain access to the compounds from the open α-side, leading to a β-configuration of the amino group. This procedure was used to prepare a whole series of amines variously alkyl-substituted at the C4 position. Although many of these derivatives with the "natural" configuration at the C4 atom are antibacterially active, they all prove to be less active than the tetracyclines themselves.

Unsubstituted C4 amino compound (67) can be prepared by various means, in each case taking the 4,6-hemiketal of (58), for instance, as starting material. Reacting (58) with hydrazine gives the hydrazone (66), which is reduced with zinc dust in aqueous acetic acid or with sodium hydrogen sulfite to give the 4-epi-4-amino-4-dedimethylaminotetracycline (67). Compound (67) can also be obtained, however, by treating the oxime (68) with zinc dust or by direct reductive amination of (68) with hydrogen, PtO_2, and an excess of hydroxylamine in dimethylformamide (BLACKWOOD and STEPHENS 1964).

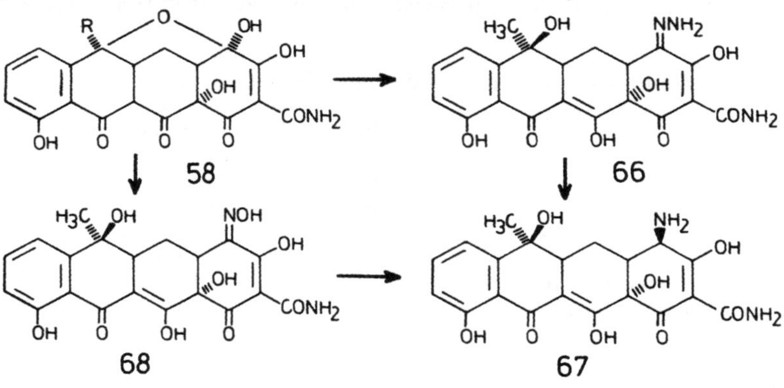

4-Dedimethylamino-4β-aminotetracycline (67) can be transformed in hot aqueous bicarbonate solution to the lactam (69). Dehydrating (69) results in the anhydro derivative (70) (BLACKWOOD and STEPHENS 1965).

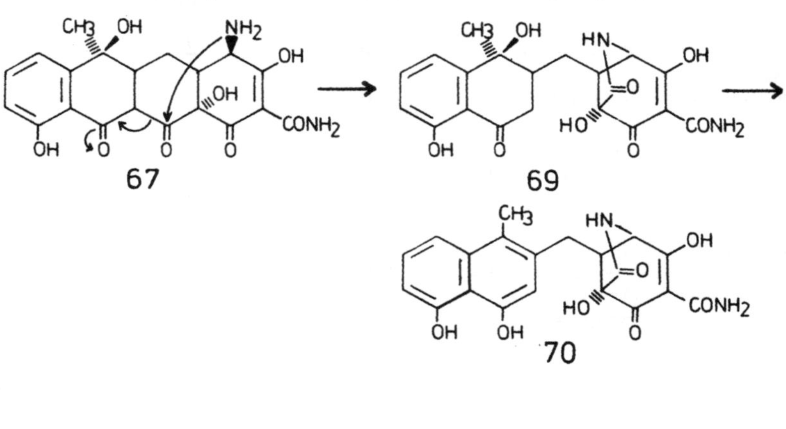

Reduction of hemiketal (58) with hydrogen and a catalyst, sodium hydrogen sulfite, or with zinc dust leads to the α,β-epimer mixture of the 4-hydroxy compound (71). Acid treatment of (71) yields the corresponding 5a,6.-anhydro derivative (72) (BLACKWOOD and STEPHENS 1964).

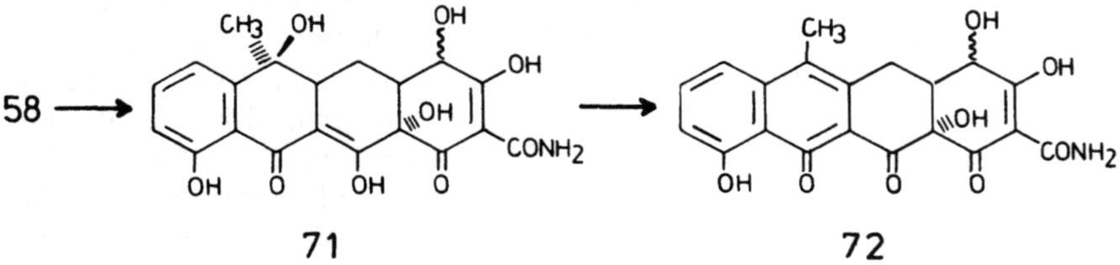

2. Effect of Structural Variation on Antibacterial Activity

The antibacterial activity of tetracyclines modified at the C4 position can be summarized as follows (Tables 2 and 3).

The amino group at the C4 position is not crucial to the antibacterial in vitro activity (BLACKWOOD and ENGLISH 1970). While 4-dedimethylamino-6-demethyl-6-deoxytetracycline (73), 4-dedimethylaminotetracycline (74), and 4-dedimethylaminooxytetracycline (75) do still possess antimicrobial activity against gram-

Table 2. Antibacterial activity of tetracyclines modified at the C4 position[a]

Name	Minimum inhibitory concentrations (μg/ml)		
	Staphylococcus aureus 5	*Streptococcus pyogenes*	*Escherichia coli*
Tetracycline[a]	0.21	0.06	0.73
4-Dedimethylaminooxytetracycline[b]	25	12	50
4-Dedimethylaminotetracycline[c]	12	6	100
4-Dedimethylamino-6-demethyl-6-deoxytetracycline[d]	0.8	1.5	25
4-Epitetracycline[e]	6	3	12
6-Methylenetetracycline methiodide[f]	12	3	>100
4-Oxo-4-dedimethylaminotetracycline-4,6-hemiketal	>100	>100	>100
4-Oximino-4-dedimethylamino-tetracycline[g]	>100	>100	>100
4-Hydrazone-4-dedimethylamino-tetracycline[g]	50	25	>100
4-Hydroxy-4-dedimethylamino-tetracycline[g]	> 10	5	>100

[a] BLACKWOOD and ENGLISH (1970)
[b] HOCHSTEIN et al. (1953)
[c] BOOTHE et al. (1958)
[d] STEPHENS et al. (1963)
[e] STEPHENS et al. (1956); DOERSCHUK et al. (1955)
[f] BLACKWOOD et al. (1963)
[g] BLACKWOOD and STEPHENS (1965)

Table 3. In vitro activity of various N4 analogues of 6-demethyltetracycline against *Staphylococcus aureus* relative to tetracycline. (Esse et al. 1964b)

NRR[1]		Activity relative to tetracycline
—R	R′	100%
CH_3	CH_3	96%
CH_3	C_2H_5	75%
CH_3	C_3H_7	50%
C_2H_5	C_2H_5	25%
CH_3	C_2H_4OH	12%

positive bacteria, they are virtually ineffective against gram-negative organisms. In vivo they are completely devoid of activity.

The dimethylamino group in the 4 position is thus essential for maintaining full in vitro and in vivo activity in tetracyclines (McCormick et al. 1957, 1960).

The lack of the dimethylamino group prevents the formation of the zwitterion and strongly favors the enolic structure of the A-ring. It has been shown that an equilibrium between the nonionized and zwitterionic structure is necessary for the antibacterial activity. From this it is understandable why the dimethylamino group is so important for the full in vitro and in vivo activity.

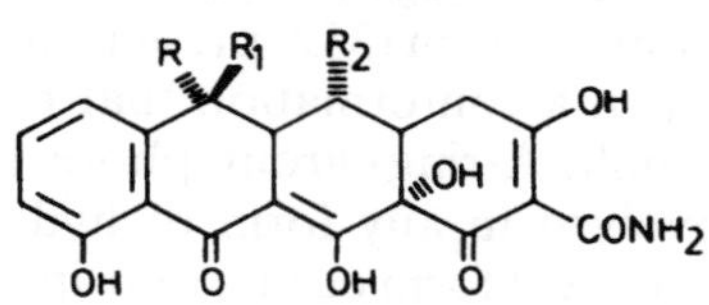

73: $R = R_1 = R_2 = H$
74: $R = CH_3$; $R_1 = OH$ $R = H$
75: $R = CH_3$; $R_1 = R_2 = OH$

The natural α-configuration at position 4 is also essential, as the corresponding C4 epimeric compounds exhibit mostly reduced antibacterial activity (Kende et al. 1961). Because of the relatively short distances between the C4 atom and C6 and O6 atoms in the conformation of the nonionized structure, it is sterically impossible for the 4-epitetracyclines to adopt this conformation. The interaction directly influences the equilibrium between the nonionized and zwitterionic structure necessary for the in vitro activity. This may explain the biological inactivity of the 4-epitetracyclines (Stezowski 1976). Replacement of the dimethylamino group with a primary amino group does not alter the in vitro activity (Martin et al. 1973; Urbach et al. 1973). A methylamino group, on the other hand, causes a slight drop in activity, while a diethylamino group and longer-chained alkylamino groups lead to more pronounced loss of activity as the chain length increases, as shown in Table 3 (Esse et al. 1964b).

Removal of the amino group or loss of its basic character through quaternization, acylation (Dürckheimer 1975), or conversion into an oxime, hydrazone, or tetracycloxide considerably reduce the activity or nullify it altogether.

For the tetracycline methiodide (36) it was shown (GULBIS and EVERETT 1976) that the molecule cannot adopt the conformation of the nonionized form because it lacks the hydrogen atom at the C3 oxygen necessary for the formation of the enolic A-ring chromophore (PREWO and STEZOWSKI 1977). This is significant since the tetracyclines are thought to act via an equilibrium between a nonionized and zwitterionic structure. Any substitution on or adjacent to ring A that interferes with the equilibrium may serve to decrease the antibacterial activity as it is the case with the tetracycline methiodide.

One prerequisite for good in vivo activity is optimum distribution in the body. It was discovered in earlier investigations that at a physiological pH the tetracyclines occur in zwitterionic form, simultaneously forming the lipophilic tetracycline species. This was explained in terms of the formation of an inner salt of the zwitterionic form, consisting of a dimethylammonium cation and a tricarbonylmethyl anion, whereby a neutralization effect is supposed to result (COLAIZZI and KLINK 1969; TUTE 1975). In more recent X-ray testing of tetracyclines, it was shown that there are no interactions between positive and negative charge (STEZOWSKI 1976).

It is assumed, in fact, that two tetracycline forms are in solvent-dependent equilibrium, namely a zwitterionic and a nonionized form. The chemical structure of the zwitterion (351) has two charge centers which are associated at the protonated dimethylamino group, whereas the negative charge is distributed over the tricarbonylmethane system. Thus the dimethylamino group of zwitterionic form is both inter- and intramolecular hydrogen bonded and therefore a highly polar species. In contrast, the nonionized form (352) presents a molecular structure of considerable reduced polarity in a conformation that has extensive intramolecular hydrogen bonding in the enolic A-ring chromophore. In this structure the dimethylamino group is not involved in any form of hydrogen bonding (STEZOWSKI 1976). Even when the nonionized form occurs only in very low concentrations (indeed, under physiological conditions the zwitterionic form appears to be the predominant form of the natural tetracyclines), it is nevertheless the nonionized form which is responsible for distribution in the body, since it is by far the more lipophilic of the two component forms (PURICH et al. 1973; TERADA and INAGI 1975; PREWO and STEZOWSKI 1977).

To summarize, these investigations show quite plainly that the dimethylamino group is the most favorable substituent for achieving optimum in vitro and in vivo activity and that the α-configuration is essential.

IV. Modifications at the C5 Position

1. Chemistry

Oxytetracycline (6) is the only compound in the tetracycline series bearing a hydroxy group at the C5 atom.

Transformations at C5 have been restricted to esterification of the 5-hydroxy group as described below, and direct introductions. One characteristic of this series is that it is readily esterified. Under the conditions for acylation the 12a-hydroxy group is esterified at the same time, so that two equivalents of acylating agent give the C12a, C5 diacetate (76) (HOCHSTEIN et al. 1953; BARRETT 1963).

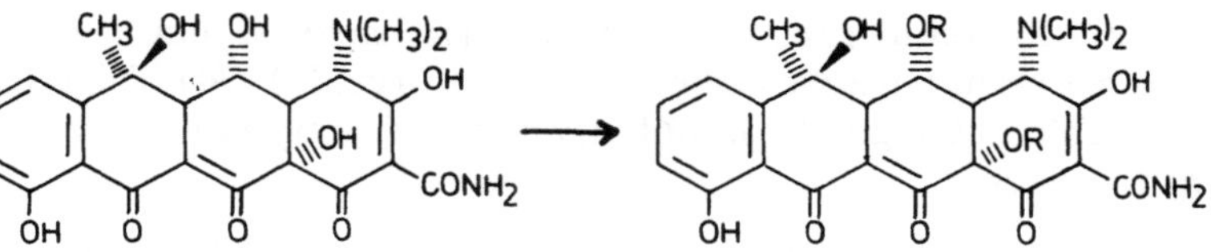

6 76

Esterification reactions using strong acids (HF, CH_3SO_3H) produce exclusively the C5 esters. This is the method which was used for the 6-deoxytetracyclines, deoxycycline (3), and methacycline (2) (BERNARDI et al. 1974). One chemical method for introducing the oxygen function to the C5 atom takes as a basis 5a,11a-dehydrotetracycline (77) (SCHACH VON WITTENAU et al. 1963). The reaction yields compound (78) via an SN2′ mechanism when a strong acid and the corresponding alcohol are used, with simultaneous aromatization of ring C. A β-configuration is assumed for the introduced substituents. Unlike their corresponding hydroxy compounds, C5 alkoxy compounds are relatively stable.

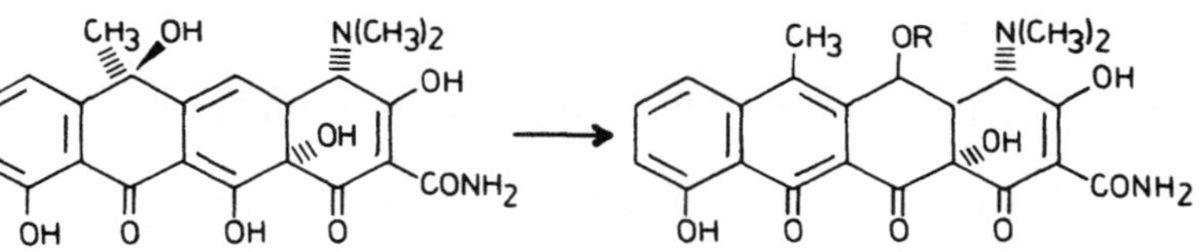

77 78

2. Effect of Structural Variation on Antibacterial Activity

The 5-hydroxy group itself has no influence on antibacterial activity (BARRETT 1963), but only on stability, absorption, and pharmacokinetics. Esterification of the 5-hydroxy group generally leads to a loss of activity. While certain of the 5-hydroxy esters (Table 4), e.g., compounds (79) and (80), show notable in vitro ac-

Table 4. In vitro antibacterial activity of 5-hydroxyesters of compounds (79) and (80). (BERNARDI et al. 1974)

Compounds	Minimum inhibitory concentrations (μg/ml)			
	Staphylococcus aureus 209	*Staph. aureus* ATCC 12715	*Escherichia coli*	*Klebsiella pneumoniae*
Methacycline	0.07	>20	0.31	0.31
(79a) $R=CH_3CO$	0.15	5	0.62	0.62
(79b) $R=(C_2H_5)_2CHCO$	0.62	0.62	>2.5	>2.5
(79c) $R=C_6H_5CH_2CO$	0.31	0.62	>2.5	>2.5
Doxycycline	0.15	>20	0.31	0.31
(80a) $R=CH_3CO$	0.31	>20	1.25	1.25
(80b) $R=(C_2H_5)_2CHCO$	>2.5	>20	>2.5	>2.5
(80c) $R=p\text{-}CH_3C_6H_4CO$	0.62	0.62	>2.5	>2.5

tivity against tetracycline-resistant gram-positive bacteria, they have only limited activity against gram-negative bacteria (BERNARDI et al. 1974). This effect is probably attributable to the greater lipophility of these compounds through the alkyl residue of the ester.

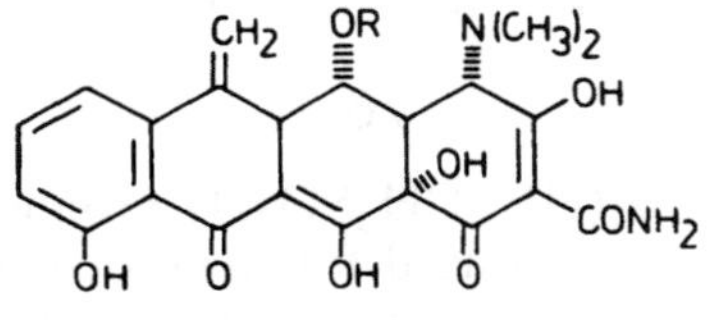

79

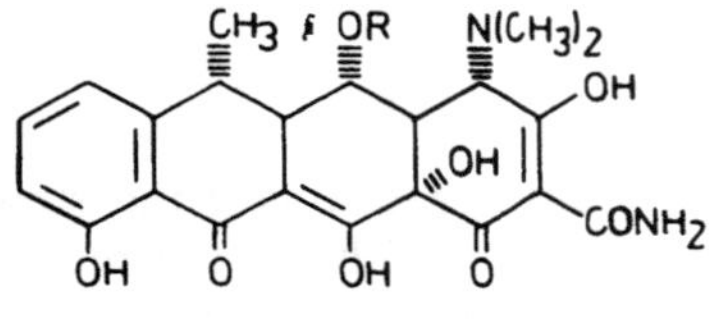

80

The 5-formyl derivative of doxycycline and methacycline has proven to have superior therapeutic activity to that of the corresponding 5-hydroxy compound. This is explained in terms of better absorption following oral administration (BERNARDI et al. 1974). None of the modifications performed at C5 has been able to change decisively the biological activity of the molecule for the better. Generally speaking, the 5 position does not appear to be particularly crucial to tetracycline activity.

There is only one exception, which was published quite recently (VALCAVI et al. 1981).

Reaction of doxycycline (3) and methacycline (2) with Ac_2O in dimethylsulfoxide provided the products (80a) and (79a) respectively. Both compounds proved to be practically inactive.

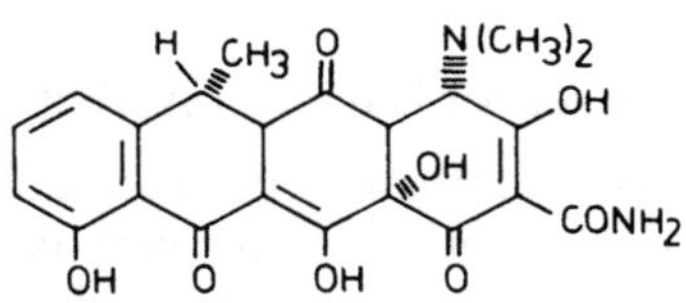

80 a

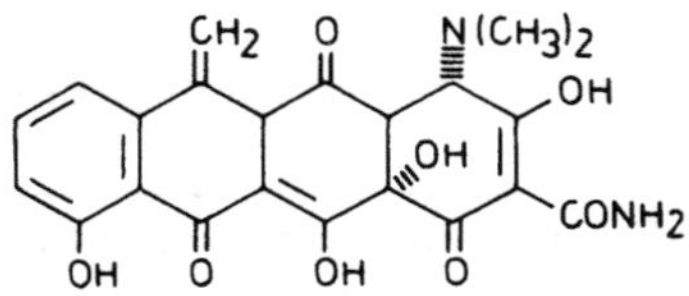

79 a

V. Modifications at the C5a Position

1. Chemistry

The normal stereochemistry at the tetracycline C5a position is the α-configuration. 5a,11a-Dehydro-7-chlorotetracycline (82) is the intermediate product in the biosynthesis of tetracyclines (MCCORMICK et al. 1958). The 5a,11a-dehydro compound (82) is also obtained by treating 7,11a-dichlorotetracycline (81) with te-

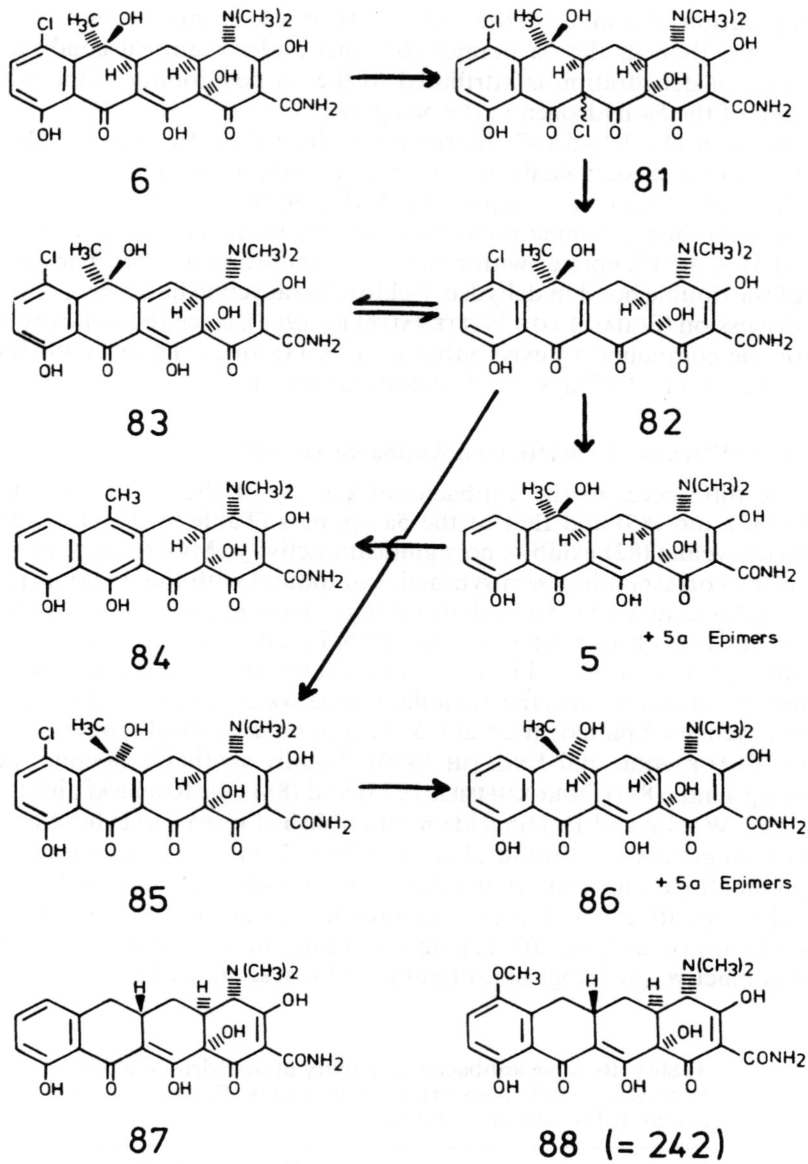

Fig. 9. Reactions affecting position 5a

traethylammonium chloride (Fig. 9) (McCormick et al. 1965). Compound (81) can again be prepared from 7-chlorotetracycline (6). Catalytic hydrogenation of compound (82) results not only in tetracycline (5) with a natural α-configuration of the hydrogen at the C5a atom but also the corresponding 5a epimer (McCormick et al. 1958; Martell et al. 1967c).

Dehydration to anhydrotetracycline (84) proceeds more rapidly in tetracycline (1 min) than in the 5a epimer (67 min) under identical conditions. The slower rate of dehydration is attributed to the *cis* positioning of the 6-hydroxy group and of the 5a-hydrogen in the 5a epimer.

Treating 5a,11a-dehydro-7-chlorotetracycline (82) with hydrogen fluoride in the presence of two equivalents of water results, with reversal of the configuration at the C6 atom, in the 6-epi compound (85) (Fig. 9) (MARTELL et al. 1967c). Catalytic reduction of the double bond again results in the two C5a epimers. Compound (86) is the C6 epimer with natural configuration at C5a. The precise position of the double bond in dehydro-7-chlorotetracycline has been a point of frequent discussion (SCHACH VON WITTENAU et al. 1963), since theoretically it is possible for the compound to exist either as a 5a,11a or as a 5,5a tautomer [compounds (82) and (83)] (PREWO and STEZOWSKI 1980).

2. Effect of Structural Variation on Antibacterial Activity

There are differences in the antibacterial activity of the 5a,11a-dehydro compounds (82) and (85) and that of the 5a epimers (Table 5). 5a,11a-Dehydro-7-chlorotetracycline (82) exhibits no significant activity (McCORMICK et al. 1958), whereas the corresponding semisynthetic compound with the unnatural configuration at C6 [compound (85)] exhibits both in vitro and in vivo activity (MARTELL et al. 1967c). It has been postulated that the 5,5a-tautomer (83) is the actual active compound (BLACKWOOD and ENGLISH 1970; SCHACH VON WITTENAU et al. 1963), since this structure contains the phenoldiketone system of the medicinally important tetracyclines. Epimerization at C5a is supposed generally to result in loss of activity (BLACKWOOD and ENGLISH 1970). Totally synthetic 5a-epitetracyclines [e.g., compounds (87) (DÜRCKHEIMER 1975) and (88) (W. Rogalski and R. Kirchlechner; H. Wahlig and E. Dingeldein, unpublished research] exhibit an in vitro activity similar to that of natural tetracycline. Totally synthetic 6-demethyl-6-deoxy-5a-methyltetracycline (89) exhibits a high level of activity both against tetracycline-sensitive and tetracycline-resistant gram-positive organisms. The compound has virtually no effect against gram-negative organisms. The 5a epimer of (89) is inactive (W. Rogalski, unpublished research, see Sect. C.V).

Table 5. Relative antibacterial activity of dehydro-7-chlorotetracyclines and 5a-epitetracyclines against *Staphylococcus aureus*. (MARTELL et al. 1967c)

Name	Relative activity	
	In vitro	In vivo
Tetracycline	1.0	1.0
6-Epitetracycline	0.6	–
5a-Epi-6-epitetracycline	0.4	–
5a-Epitetracycline	Inactive	
5a(11a)-Dehydrochlortetracycline	Inactive	
6-Epi-dehydrochlortetracycline	1.5	0.5

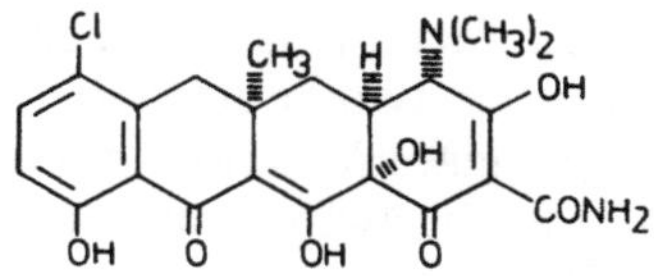

89 (= 273)

The activity of 7-chlorotetracycline (in vitro and in vivo), the antibacterial activity of 5a-epi-7-chlorotetracycline (in vitro), and the total absence of activity in dehydro-7-chlorotetracycline, as compared with the surprising presence of activity (in vitro and in vivo) in dehydro-7-chloro-6-epitetracycline, give grounds for supposing that various structural changes in the BCD chromophore and thus in conformation result from reversing the configuration at C5a, from dehydrating the BC-ring system, or from reversing the configuration at C6, and that these changes are responsible for the varying degrees of inactivation of the individual molecules (PREWO and STEZOWSKI 1980).

Following analysis of the molecular structures it was postulated that two types of tetracycline base, a zwitterionic and a nonionized form, are important for biological activity to exist. These two forms are in a solvent-dependent equilibrium (HUGHES et al. 1979). Furthermore, both forms have characteristic conformations. It was discovered that the conformation of the 5a-epi-7-chlorotetracycline cation differed considerably from that of the zwitterionic form of the tetracycline base and the cation and is very similar to the conformation of nonionized oxytetracycline (PREWO and STEZOWSKI 1980). It was inferred from this that the equilibrium between the zwitterionic and nonionized form of the 5a-epi-7-chlorotetracycline cation differs from the equilibrium of other medicinally important tetracyclines.

This result correlates with the finding that 5a-epi-7-chlorotetracycline is active in vitro though not in vivo. Further findings would also suggest that the zwitterion of the 5a-epi-7-chlorotetracycline base, if indeed it is formed at all, assumes the conformation of the nonionized form as opposed to the conformation assumed by the tetracyclines which have in vivo activity (PREWO and STEZOWSKI 1980). In the tetracyclines showing in vivo activity there are always equilibria between nonionized and zwitterionic forms with different conformation. In vivo activity is dependent on the presence of the zwitterionic conformation. Investigation of the conformation of 5a-epi-7-chlorotetracycline shows that there are only slight steric interactions between rings A and C, whereas most tetracyclines having the natural configuration at C5a exhibit considerable interactions between rings A and C. These interactions probably have a direct influence on the equilibrium between zwitterionic and nonionized free bases of tetracyclines possessing in vivo activity.

Determining the chemical structure of dehydro-7-chlorotetracycline is hampered by the possibility of tautomerization in the BCD-ring system. Two tautomers have been found to crystallize from water and organic solvents (SCHACH VON WITTENAU et al. 1963). More recent investigations (PREWO and STEZOWSKI 1980) suggest that the tautomer from chloroform must have the structure of 5a,11a-dehydrochlortetracycline (82), whereby the compound is supposed to occur in the nonionized form. It is regarded as probable that the dehydro-7-chlorotetracycline undergoes two tautomeric structural transformations upon passing from the aqueous phase into a nonaqueous environment. In the one case ring A is involved insofar as the zwitterionic form passes to the nonionized form; in the other case the BCD-ring system is involved.

The 5a,11a double bond causes the β-hydroxyketone structure of the BCD chromophore to break down, this structure being a feature of all medicinally important tetracyclines. The dehydro-7-chlorotetracyclines are antibacterially inactive (BLACKWOOD and ENGLISH 1970; MCCORMICK et al. 1958).

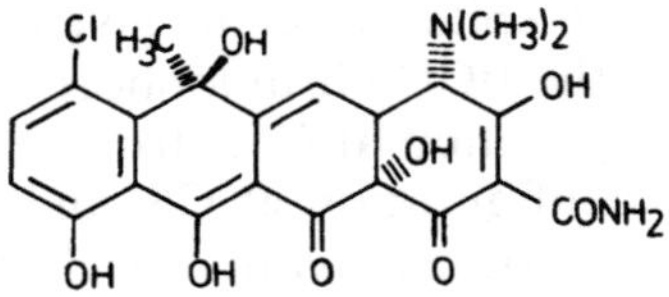

90

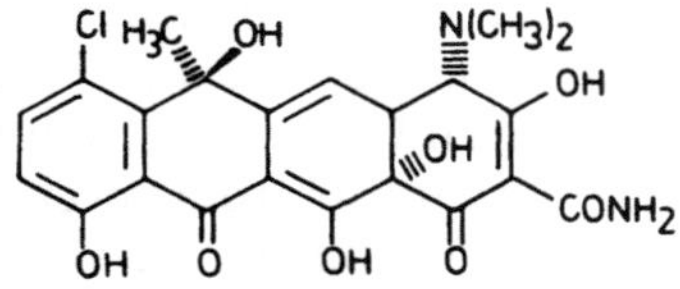

91

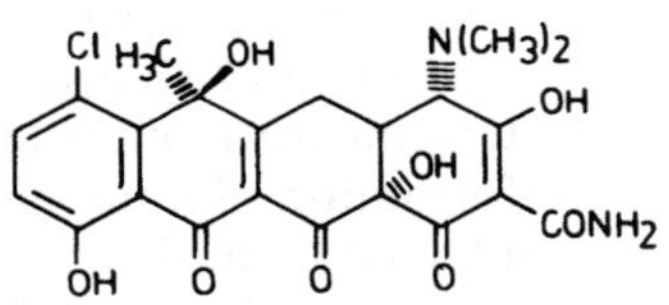

82

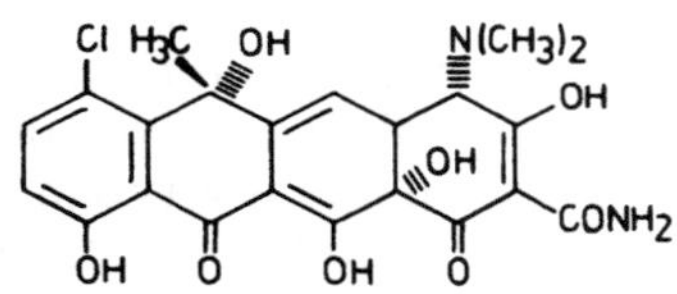

93

It is assumed that a number of tautomeric forms occur, giving rise, by crystallization from aqueous solution, to the mixture of two tautomers (90) and (91). They are assumed to be zwitterionic forms.

Unlike the dehydro-7-chlorotetracyclines, the corresponding 6-epi compound possesses significant in vitro and in vivo antibacterial activity (Table 5) (MARTELL et al. 1967c; BLACKWOOD and ENGLISH 1970). Structure (93) is probably the tautomeric form of 6-epi-dehydro-7-chlorotetracycline, this form being responsible for antibacterial efficacy, since the β-hydroxyketone structure important for ensuring antimicrobial activity is present in the BCD-ring system. The presence of a second double bond in ring B is probably of relatively little significance as far as the conformation of the molecule is concerned. The fact that the 6-epimer exhibits significant in vitro and in vivo activity, while compound (91) with normal configuration at C6 is ineffectual, indicates that different conformations are favored in the two C6 isomer equilibria. The reason for this is probably to be found in the difference in steric interactions of the β-substituents at C6, methyl instead of hydroxy, and hydrogen at C4 (PREWO and STEZOWSKI 1980).

These investigations plainly show that modifications in the structure or in the stereochemistry of the tetracycline BCD chromophore produce changes in the chemical and biological behavior of these compounds; these changes can be interpreted in terms of molecular conformational characteristics.

VI. Modifications at the C6 Position

1. Chemistry

Modifications at the C6 atom have produced by far the greatest success in evolving highly active tetracyclines.

The hydroxy group at C6 makes the molecule unstable to both acids and bases. Treatment of tetracycline (5) with acids gives anhydrotetracycline (24) while treatment of the same starting material with bases gives isotetracycline (94).

Numerous attempts have been made to reconvert anhydrotetracycline into tetracycline. This has been found to be possible (Fig. 10) through the action of oxygen on a benzene solution of anhydrotetracycline (24) when irradiated with a fluorescent lamp for 6 days (SCOTT and BEDFORD 1962). The hydroperoxide (95) was obtained as intermediate product, which was transformed by catalytic reduction to 5a,11a-dehydrotetracycline (96), this being identical with the natural product. Further catalytic reduction of the 5a,11a-double bond gives tetracycline (5) and the corresponding 5a epimer (97). The substances were obtained in poor yield. Better results were achieved with N^2-*t*-butyl compounds since the lipophilic nature of the latter makes them more soluble in organic solvents.

The two 6-demethyltetracyclines (8) and (9), prepared by fermentation, also serve as starting material for modifications at C6 (Fig. 10). Catalytic hydrogenolysis (MCCORMICK et al. 1960; STEPHENS et al. 1963) of these fermentation products in dimethylformamide (DMF)/water and palladium/carbon catalyst gives the 6-demethyl-6-deoxytetracyclines (98). The tetracyclic compound (98) is the simplest of all tetracyclines having full antibacterial activity. It is extremely stable to the action of both acids and bases. It was these properties which permitted a number of hitherto impossible electrophilic substitution reactions to be performed. The chemistry of these reactions is summarized in Sect. 7 (Figs. 14–16).

Catalytic hydrogenolysis with a noble metal (MCCORMICK et al. 1960; SCHACH VON WITTENAU et al. 1962; STEPHENS et al. 1963) also made it possible to transform tetracycline (5) and oxytetracycline (7) into the corresponding 6-β-methyl-6-deoxytetracyclines (99) and (100). The yields of (99), for example, are rather unsatisfactory since under the reaction conditions not only is anhydrotetracycline (24) formed but there is also an over-reduction of the starting material to compound (101). Tetracyclines (99) and (100) are extremely acid-stable and are eminently suitable for aromatic substitution, which will be dealt with in the next section.

Whenever tetracyclines are reacted with *N*-chlorosuccinimide (NCS), it is the structure of the tetracycline which predetermines what reaction product will be obtained. Treatment of tetracyclines (5) and (7) with NCS in 1,2-dimethoxyethane produces the 11a-chlorotetracycline-6,12-hemiketals (102) (Fig. 11) (BLACKWOOD et al. 1963). Reduction with hydrogen sulfite gives the starting tetracycline (5). Treatment of (102) with anhydrous HF under mild conditions, however, leads to the formation of the 11a-chloro-6-methylenetetracyclines (104), which may be transformed with sodium hydrogen sulfite into the 6-methylenetetracycline (106). Blocking the 11a position with chlorine prevents a C11, C11a enolization. This means that endocyclic dehydration is suppressed in favor of exo-

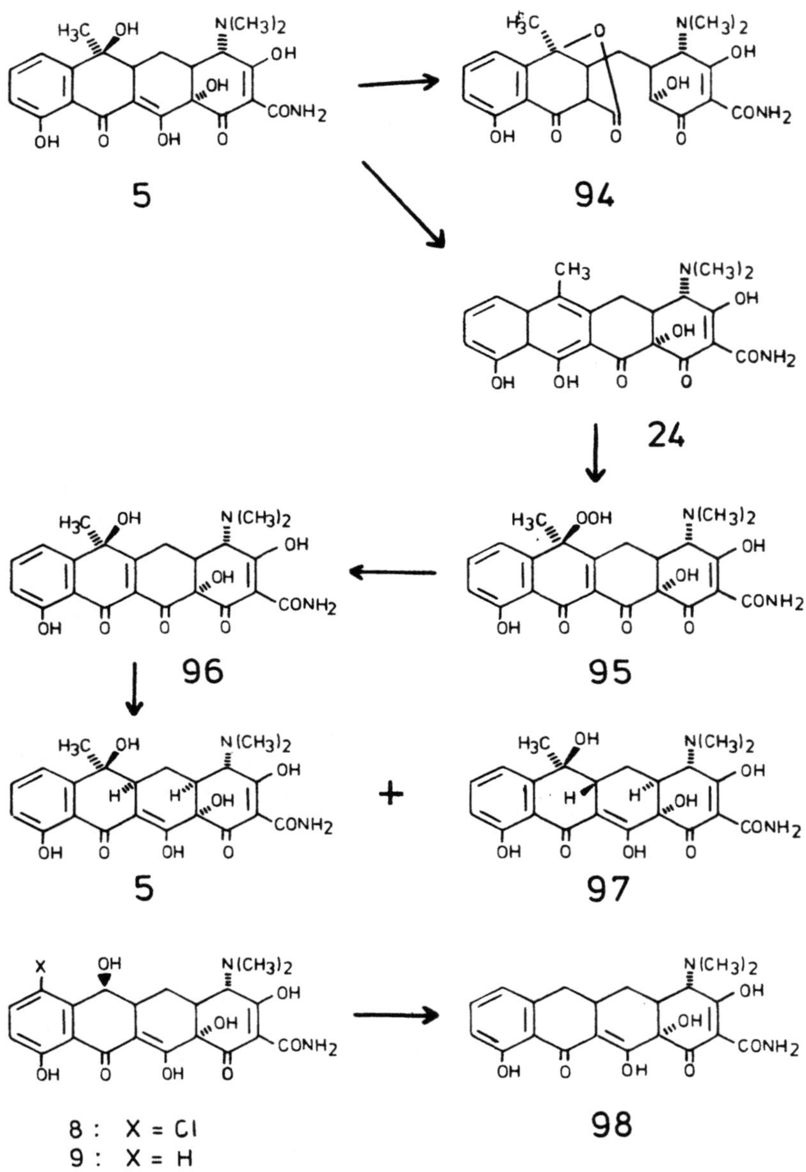

Fig. 10. Variations at the C6 position

cyclic dehydration, whereby the C6 methyl group has three hydrogens available for the reaction in comparison with one at C5a.

Although the 11a-chloro compound (102) has a decreased in vitro activity the reduction of (102) occurs also in vivo to the fully biologically active 6-methylene-tetracycline (106).

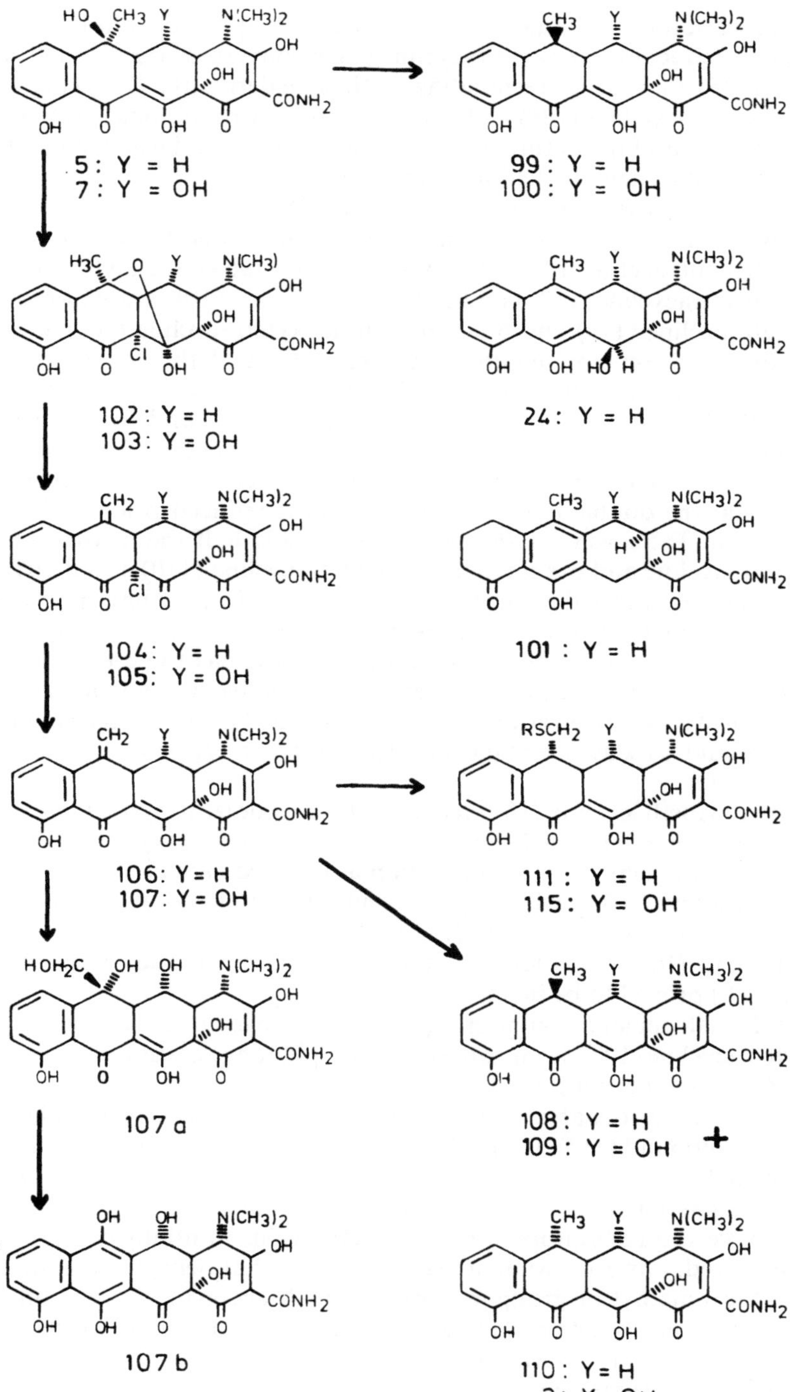

Fig. 11. Synthesis of methacycline and doxycycline

By application of the same three-step reaction sequence (chlorination, dehydration, and reduction), 5-oxytetracycline (7) is converted, via the intermediates (103) and (105), into the corresponding methylene derivative (107) (Fig. 11).

The new tetracyclines (106) and (107) possess in vitro biological activity which is higher than that of the natural tetracyclines. In practice the activity largely corresponds to that of demethylchlorotetracycline.

The 6-methylenetetracyclines (106) and (107) have themselves been used as starting material for a number of new tetracyclines substituted at the C6 atom (Fig. 11) (Stephens et al. 1963; Blackwood et al. 1963). Catalytic reduction of 6-methylenetetracyclines (106) and (107) produces a 1:1 mixture of 6-α-methyl-6-deoxytetracycline (110) and 6-β-methyl-6-deoxytetracycline (108) as well as a 1:1 mixture of 6-α-methyl-6-deoxytetracycline (3) and the corresponding 6-β-epimer (109). Catalytic reduction with 11a-chloro compounds (104) or (105) leads largely to the formation of 6-β-methyltetracyclines (108) and (109), since the absorption of the molecule on the surface of the catalyst occurs from the α-side on account of the molecular conformation. This reductive process presupposes, however, that the double bond at the C6 atom is reduced prior to the halogen atom at C11a. Tetracycline (108) possesses roughly half the in vitro activity of natural tetracycline and 6-α-methyl-6-deoxytetracycline (110) about 70% of this activity. The α-epimer is therefore somewhat more effective than the β-epimer.

Within the 5-oxytetracycline series, the 6-β-compound (109) possesses only about 30% of the activity of 5-oxytetracycline, whereas the α-epimer (3) is 1.4 times as active. Moreover, the α-epimer is highly active in vivo and has a longer half-life. 6-α-Methyloxytetracycline (3) was launched onto the market in 1967 as doxycycline and is today one of the most frequently prescribed tetracyclines in the world.

5-Hydroxymethacycline (107) reacts with the oxidizing system $OsO_4/KClO_3$ in methanol/water giving the 6-demethyl-6-hydroxymethyloxytetracycline (107a) probably with the unnatural configuration at C6 (Valcavi et al. 1981).

When reacting (107a) with periodic acid under mild conditions 6-demethyl-6-hydroxyanhydrooxytetracycline (107b) was obtained.

Compound (107a) was less active than the parent tetracycline, while compound (107b) proved to be inactive.

The 11a-halogenated compound (105), the halogenated version of 6-methyleneoxytetracycline (107), is unstable in certain pH ranges, resulting in an opening of ring B to produce compound (112). Under more acidic conditions, however, compound (105) is so stable that treatment with *N*-chlorosuccinimide in liquid HF yields compound (113), from which the 7-chloro compound (114) can be obtained through dechlorination with hydrogen sulfite. The latter derivative is more than six times as active as 6-methyleneoxytetracycline (107).

The preparation of uniform 6-α-methyltetracyclines initially posed a problem. This was solved, however, when it was discovered that benzylmercaptans can be added to the 6-methylene group in a sort of anti-Markownikov reaction and that 6-α-benzylthiomethylenetetracyclines of the general formula (115) result. Compounds (116)–(125) are typical examples of this category of substances (Fig. 12). Raney nickel desulfuration of compound (120) led to 6-α-methyl-6-deoxytetracycline (3) in good yield. Upon reaction with peroxides or peroxy acids, the mer-

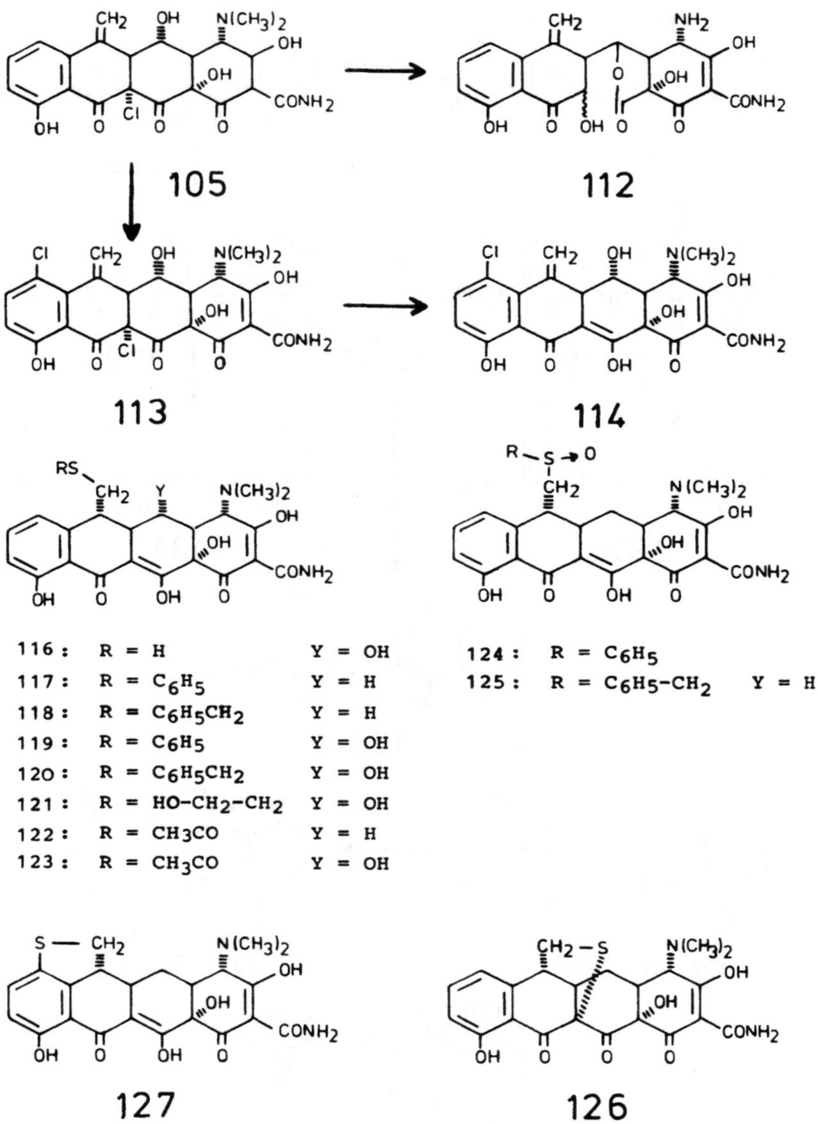

Fig. 12. Reaction products of methacycline

capto compounds (117) and (118) are transformed into the corresponding sulfoxides (124) and (125).

The lipophilic phenyl and benzylmercaptan adducts of 6-methylenetetracyclines show a considerable drop in activity, especially against gram-negative bacteria. Antibacterial activity is increased if the compounds are transformed into the more polar sulfoxides. The thiolacetic acid derivatives such as (122) and (123) are more active by virtue of their polar properties. The same is true of the phenyl-

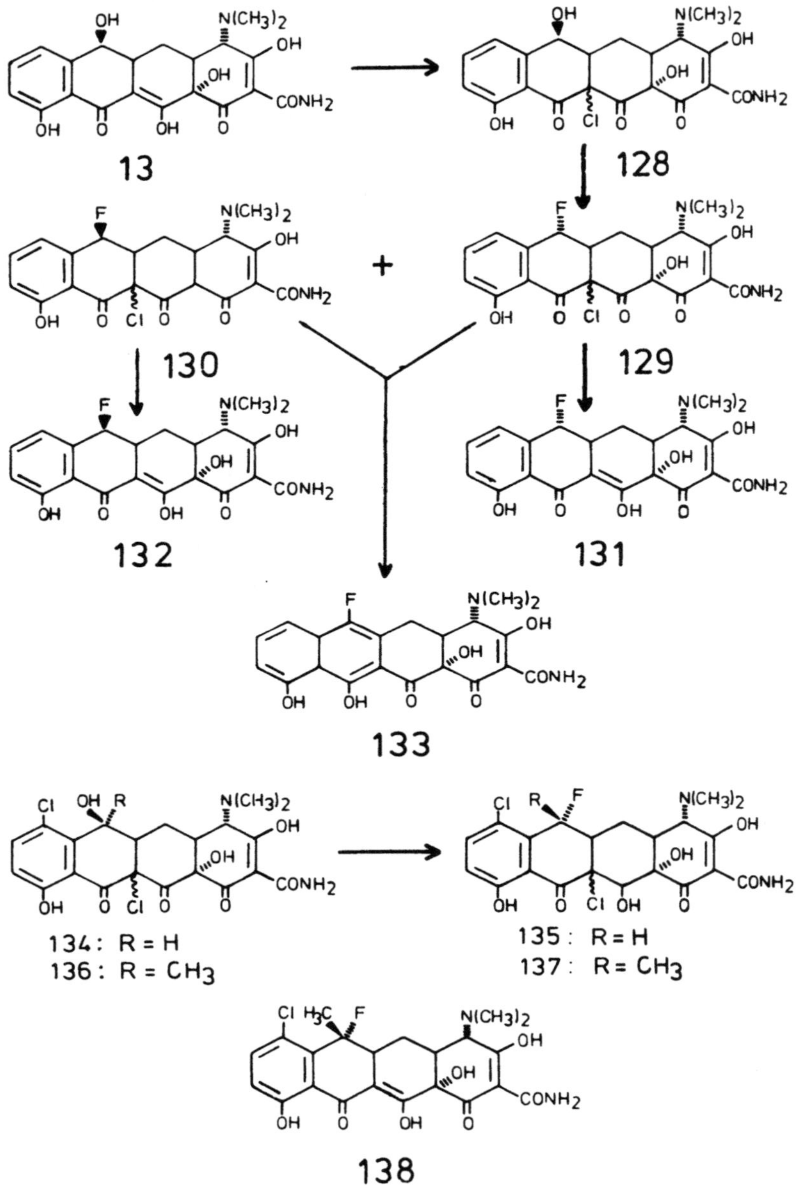

Fig. 13. Synthesis of 6-fluoro compounds

and benzylmercapto compounds of the more polar oxytetracycline, e.g., (119)–(121), and (123) (Blackwood et al. 1963).

A product of particular interest was the cyclic sulfur derivative (126), since this manifests in vivo activity in spite of the fact that in vitro activity is totally lacking. When used in vivo, a metabolic reaction occurs, loosening the bond between sulfur and the C11a atom, causing a derivative to be formed which is antibacterially active. As a direct contrast, compound (127) shows excellent in vitro activity although it is totally devoid of activity in vivo (BLACKWOOD et al. 1963).

Reaction of liquid HF with 11a-chloro-6-demethyltetracycline (128) produces a mixture of two 6-fluorostereo isomers, namely compounds (129) and (130) (Fig. 13). Mild catalytic reduction of both compounds gives 6-α-fluoro-6-demethyl-6-deoxytetracycline (131) and 6-β-fluoro-6-demethyl-6-deoxytetracycline (132) (BITHA et al. 1970). Dehydrochlorination of (129) and (130) with tetraethylammonium bromide in both cases yields the anhydro compound (133).

Compounds (129) and (130) differ in their stability. Whereas the 6-β-fluoro compound (130) forms the anhydro compound (133) at room temperature with elimination of HF, this occurs only under harsher conditions under the action of base in the case of compound (129).

When liquid HF is allowed to act on 7,11a-dichloro-6-demethyltetracyclines (134) and (136), only the more stable 6-α-fluorides (135) and (137) are obtained (Fig. 13). Tetracyclic compounds (134) and (136) experience a reversal of their configuration when allowed to react with hydrogen fluoride, with fluorine being introduced instead of the hydroxy group. Compound (136), for instance, was converted into 7,11a-dichloro-6-α-fluoro-6-β-methyl-6-deoxytetracycline (137), which gives compound (138) upon careful catalytic hydrogenation.

Treatment of (139) with hydrobromic acid in acetic acid causes esterification of the C6 hydroxy group to occur (BITHA et al. 1970). The resulting compound is reduced catalytically to 6-acetoxy-6-demethylchlortetracycline (140). Subsequent catalytic hydrogenation leads to the formation of the 7-dechloro compound (141), which was also obtained by catalytic reduction of the 11a-blocking group of 11a-chloro-6-acetoxy-6-demethyltetracycline.

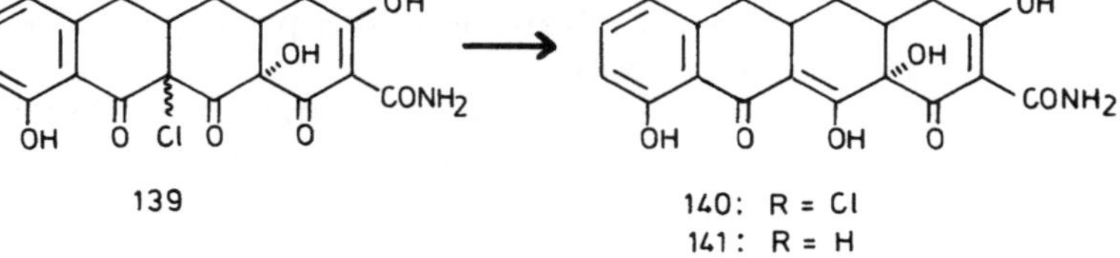

139

140: R = Cl
141: R = H

The result of esterifying the 6-β-hydroxy group in (139) is that the corresponding 7-chloro compound (140) is twice as active and the 7-dechloro analogue (141) only 0.63 times as active as tetracycline against *Staphylococcus aureus*.

2. Effect of Structural Variation on Antibacterial Activity

Modifications at C6 of the tetracyclic ring structure were extremely fruitful in the development of new, more active tetracyclines. Neither the 6-methyl group nor the 6-hydroxy group turned out to contribute appreciably to the antibacterial effect. Elimination of the 6-hydroxy group produces tetracyclines which are both more lipophilic and more stable to acids. Doxycycline (3) is the most important member of this group and has found widespread use in the treatment of infectious diseases. In its spectrum and intensity of activity and in its mode of action, doxy-

Table 6. Antibacterial in vitro activity of 6-fluoro-substituted and 6-acetoxy-substituted tetracyclines. (BITHA et al. 1970)

Name	Percentage activity[a]
Tetracycline	100
6-α-Fluoro-6-demethyl-6-deoxytetracycline	200
6-β-Fluoro-6-demethyl-6-deoxytetracycline	12
6-α-Fluoro-7-chloro-6-deoxytetracycline	400
6-α-Fluoro-7-chloro-6-demethyl-6-deoxytetracycline	13
6-α-Fluoro-6-deoxytetracycline	30
6-β-Acetoxy-7-chloro-6-demethyl-tetracycline	200
6-β-Acetoxy-6-demethyltetracycline	63

[a] Approximate activity against *Staphylococcus aureus*; activity of tetracycline = 100%

cycline is comparable with the other tetracyclines. Differences are to be found, however, in the pharmacokinetics of doxycycline, this product being absorbed more swiftly following oral administration and to a greater extent than other tetracyclines. It has a considerably longer half-life and undergoes roughly 20% tubular resorption in the kidney. Consequently, doses can be kept considerably lower, this in turn causing fewer side effects in the intestinal tract. These favorable properties represent a considerable advancement in the field of tetracyclines, although it must be added that the advancement is in the kinetics of doxycycline rather than in its activity.

Doxycycline has a methyl group in the α-position; 6-epidoxycycline with a methyl group in the β-position is less effective. Indeed, the C6 monosubstituted tetracyclines are more active when substitution takes place at the α-position than compounds substituted at the β-position.

This is the case too for the 6-fluoro-substituted tetracyclines. As it is seen from Table 6, the α-fluoro-substituted analogues are more potent than the β-epimers. Chlorine in the 7 position, an electronic-attracting group, further increases the activity.

Methacycline is another therapeutically useful development. This is a 6-methyleneoxytetracycline having excellent antibacterial activity and at the same time being of high stability. In fact, this applies to all tetracyclines of the 6-methylene series. The primary cause of this is a certain electronic effect of the methylene group in the 6 position, similar to that of a chlorine atom in the C7 position (BLACKWOOD and ENGLISH 1970). The most active compound of all in the 6-demethyl series is 6-demethylchlortetracycline.

Table 7 sets out the antibacterial activities of tetracyclines modified at the C6 position (BLACKWOOD and ENGLISH 1970).

Among the sulfur tetracyclines, lipophilicity of the molecule would appear to play a critical role in determining activity variation; however, steric, conformational, and/or electronic effects are not to be wholly excluded. Larger lipophilic residues in the 6 position like phenyl and benzyl mercaptan adducts of 6-methylene-

Table 7. Antibacterial activity of tetracyclines modified at the C6 Position

Name	Minimum inhibitory concentrations[a] (μg/ml)				
	Klebsiella pneumoniae	*Staphylococcus aureus* 5	*Staphylococcus aureus* (tetracycline resistant)	*Streptococcus pyogenes*	*Escherichia coli*
6-Demethyl-6-deoxytetracycline[b]	0.9	0.2	1.5	0.2	1.5
β-6-Deoxytetracycline[b]	0.5	0.8	9	0.4	6
β-6-Deoxyoxytetracycline[b]	0.4	0.8	200	0.1	12
6-Methyleneoxytetracycline[c]	2.3	0.13	50	0.03	0.43
6-Methylenetetracycline[c]	1.2	0.2	6	0.2	3
6-Methylene-7-chlorooxytetracycline[c]	6.3	0.15	100	0.01	0.8
α-6-Deoxyoxytetracycline[b]	1.4	0.19	8.8	0.04	1.74
α-6-Deoxytetracycline[b]	0.7	0.6	3	0.1	6
13-Mercapto-α-6-deoxyoxytetracycline[c]	0.06	3	>100	1.5	>100
13-Phenylmercapto-α-6-deoxytetracycline[c]	0.01	0.8	0.8	0.2	>100
13-Benzylmercapto-α-6-deoxytetracycline[c]	0.01	0.2	0.4	0.1	>100
13-Phenylmercapto-α-6-deoxyoxytetracycline[c]	0.2	0.2	1.5	0.2	>100
13-Benzylmercapto-α-6-deoxyoxytetracycline[c]	0.26	0.04	1.5	0.04	100
13-(2-Hydroxymethylmercapto)-α-6-deoxyoxytetracycline[c]	0.06	6	>100	0.4	>100
13-Acetylmercapto-α-6-deoxytetracycline[b]	0.6	0.4	12	0.4	50
13-Acetylmercapto-α-6-deoxyoxytetracycline[c]	0.4	0.2	12	0.2	12
13-Phenylmercapto-α-6-deoxytetracycline *S*-oxide[c]	0.4	12.5	100	0.2	50
13-Benzylmercapto-α-6-deoxytetracycline *S*-oxide[c]	0.24	3	>100	0.2	>100
7,13-Epithio-α-6-deoxytetracycline[c]	1.3	0.4	3	0.2	3
11a,13-Epithio-α-6-deoxyoxytetracycline[c]	>0.01	100	>100	50	>100

[a] Bioassay relative to tetracycline (BLACKWOOD and ENGLISH 1970)
[b] Stephens et al. (1963)
[c] Blackwood et al. (1963)

tetracycline lead to a decrease in antibacterial activity, especially against gram-negative bacteria. More polar residues such as sulfoxides or thiolacetic acid residues increase activity. In line with these results, the corresponding sulfide derivatives in the more polar 5-hydroxytetracycline series show much less depression in activity (BLACKWOOD et al. 1963).

In conclusion, the following trend in structure-activity relationships in tetracyclines modified at C6 can be noted. The 6-methylenetetracyclines exhibit superior activity to that of the normal tetracyclines. Furthermore, α-6-deoxytetracyclines are more active than the corresponding β-6-deoxytetracyclines. Finally, the introduction of larger substituents at C6 causes the compounds to be more lipophilic and thus lessens their activity against gram-negative organisms. The more pronounced lipophilic properties of the 6-deoxytetracyclines results in more favorable pharmacokinetics.

VII. Modifications at the C7 and C9 Positions

1. Chemistry

The greater chemical stability of 6-deoxytetracyclines toward acids makes possible a number of electrophilic substitutions in the aromatic D-ring of the tetracyclic ring system under highly acidic conditions.

Positions 7, 8, and 9 are free for substitution to take place. Position 8 is not available, however, for electrophilic substitution owing to the fact that the carbonyl function at the C11 atom exercises an electron-attracting influence on the 8 position, leading to its deactivation. Positions 7 and 9, on the other hand, are activated by the *para-* or *ortho-*positioned hydroxy group at C10. This explains why up to now substitutions are only known in the 7 and 9 positions.

Treating 6-deoxy-6-demethyltetracycline (98) with electrophilic reagents such as nitrate ions, bromine ions (*N*-bromosuccinimide), or methylphthalimide in a strong acid gives the 7-substituted tetracyclines (HLAVKA et al. 1962a; HLAVKA and KRAZINSKI 1963; BOOTHE et al. 1960; PETISI et al. 1962; SPENCER et al. 1963; BEEREBOOM et al. 1960; MARTELL et al. 1967a; MARTELL and BOOTHE 1967). Only nitration leads both to the 7-nitro compound (142) and the 9-nitro isomer (143) (Fig. 14) (BOOTHE et al. 1960). Both compounds are easily distinguished by their characteristic UV spectra. The yield is dependent on the type of substitution at C6. 6-Demethyl-6-deoxytetracycline gives virtually identical yields of 7- and 9-substituted products upon nitration. Using the 6-deoxytetracycline, i.e., in the presence of a methyl group at C6, the yield of the 9-nitro compound is four times as great as that of the 7-nitro compound. The low yield of the latter is attributed to the steric influence of the 6-methyl group on the 7 position, so that the 9 position is more highly favored for electrophilic attack.

Compound (143) has only weak antibacterial activity, whereas the 7-nitro compound (142) is six times more active than tetracycline.

Reduction of the 7-nitro group of 6-demethyl-6-deoxytetracycline gives the corresponding 7-amino compound (144), which shows less activity than tetracycline itself. Reduction of the 9-nitro derivative (143) to the amino group yields compound (145), this being more effective than tetracycline against *S. aureus* and more active than the 9-nitro derivative (BOOTHE et al. 1960; PETISI et al. 1962). The structures of both nitro compounds have been proven (BOOTHE et al. 1960; HLAVKA et al. 1962a; ANDRE and ULLBERG 1957). The most elegant way in which this was achieved was by using tetracycline labeled at the 7 position with tritium for the electrophilic reaction, causing tritium to be replaced by the substituents (BOOTHE et al. 1960).

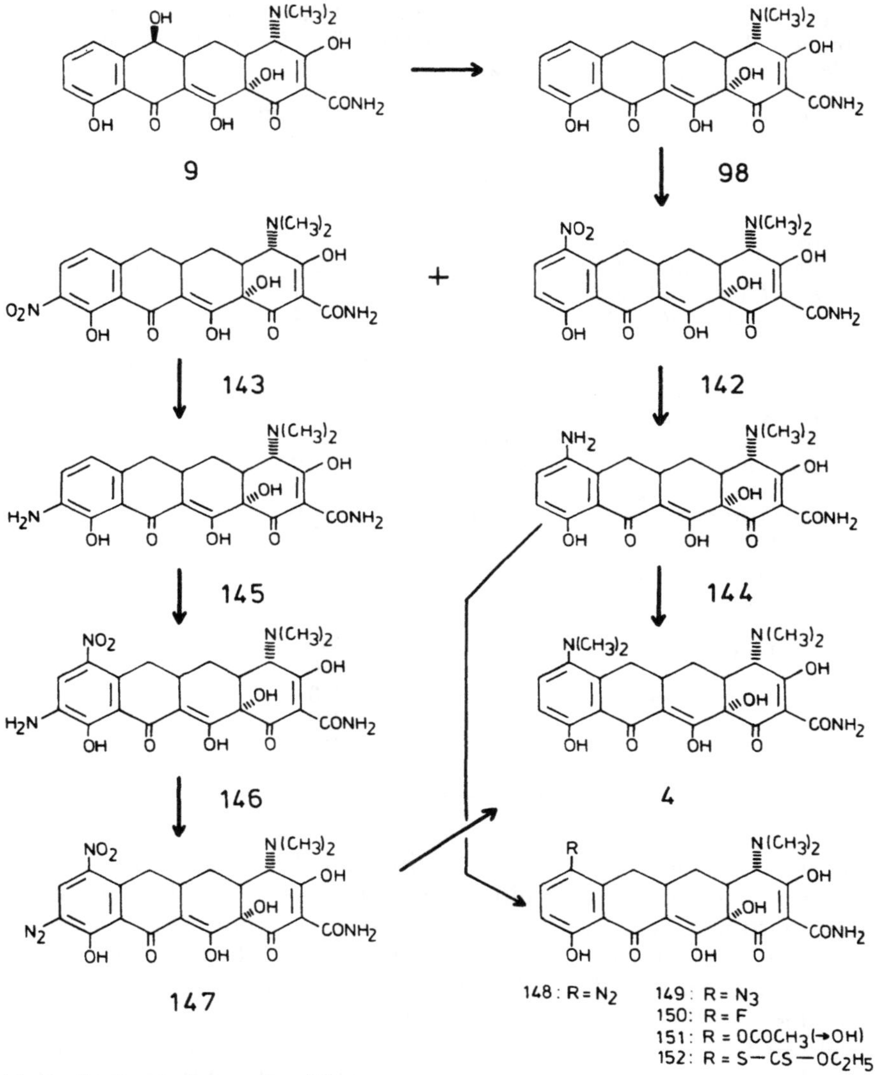

Fig. 14. Synthesis of minocycline (4)

When the 7-amino compound (144) undergoes reductive alkylation, the result is 7-dimethylamino-6-demethyl-6-deoxytetracycline (4), otherwise known as minocycline (Fig. 14) (MARTELL and BOOTHE 1967).

Minocycline possesses the same antibacterial spectrum as natural tetracyclines and furthermore is active against tetracycline-resistant *S. aureus* strains (Table 8). Altering the substituent at the 7-amino group (e.g., lengthening of the alkyl chains) produces a drop in activity as also in the case of the C4 amino group. Conversion of the 9-amino group into a dimethylamino group likewise causes activity to be lost.

Table 8. In vitro activity of 7-dimethylamino-6-demethyl-6-deoxytetracycline (minocycline) compared with that of tetracycline. (MARTELL and BOOTHE 1967)

Organism	Minimum inhibitory concentration (μg/ml)	
	Tetracycline	Minocycline
Tetracycline sensitive		
Bacillus cereus ATCC 10702	0.5	0.25
B. subtilis ATCC 6633	1.0	0.25
Escherichia coli ATCC 9637	15.0	8.0
Myobacterium ranae	2.0	0.5
M. smegmatis ATCC 607	2.0	0.5
Proteus vulgaris ATCC 9484	15.0	2.0
Pseudomonas aeruginosa ATCC 10145	31.0	31.0
Salmonella galinarium Lederle 604	15.0	15.0
Streptococcus faecalis ATCC 8043	2.0	1.0
S. pyogenes C 203	0.5	0.5
Staphylococcus aureus ATCC 6538P	2.0	1.0
S. aureus strain Smith	1.0	0.5
Tetracycline resistant		
Staphylococcus aureus		
strain Rose ATCC 14154	250	4
strain No. 3	250	8
5	250	4
9	>250	4
15	>250	8
20	>250	4
23	>250	8

The yield of 7-nitro compound upon nitration of 6-demethyl-6-deoxytetracycline is poor since the 7- and 9-nitro compounds (142) and (143) are formed in equal proportions, these then having to be separated laboriously. As a result the manufacturing costs for the clinically important product minocycline were high. However, a way was found of utilizing the 9-nitro compound (143) for preparing minocycline. For this the 9-nitro derivative was converted to the amine (145) and again nitrated, giving a good yield of 7-nitro-9-amino-6-demethyl-6-deoxytetracycline (146). Diazotization of (146) gives compound (147). When compound (147) is subjected to catalytic reduction with palladium catalyst, the diazonium group is hydrogenated, the nitro group is reduced to the amine, and, in the presence of formaldehyde, the amino group undergoes reductive alkylation giving minocycline (4) as end product.

Exploitation of the 9-nitro group for minocycline synthesis thus gave a superior total yield of this compound (CHURCH et al. 1971). Considerably improved minocycline yields can be attained, however, by a different reaction sequence. If 6-demethyl-6-deoxytetracycline (98) is treated with *tert*-butanol in methanesulfonic acid, then almost exclusively the 9-*tert*-butyl-substituted compound is obtained (CHURCH et al. 1971; BERNARDI et al. 1975b). The *tert*-butyl group in the 9 position is an excellent protecting group which can be easily removed in anhydrous HF. Nitration of (98) in *tert*-butanol, methanesulfonic acid, and sodium nitrate (i.e., introduction of the protective group in the 9 position with subsequent nitration in one step) gives compound (153) in good yield. Reduction of the nitro group with platinum catalyst in the presence of formaldehyde gives the 7-dimethylamino compound (154). Subsequent removal of the protective group in the 9 position with trifluoromethanesulfonic acid gives 7-dimethylamino-6-demethyl-6-deoxytetracycline (minocycline) (4) in a very good overall yield.

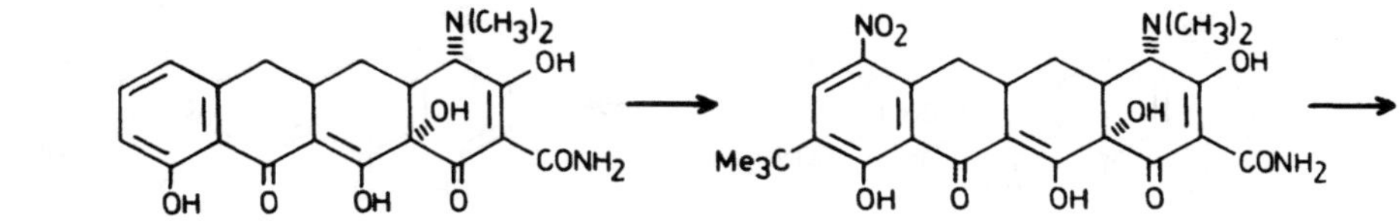

98 153

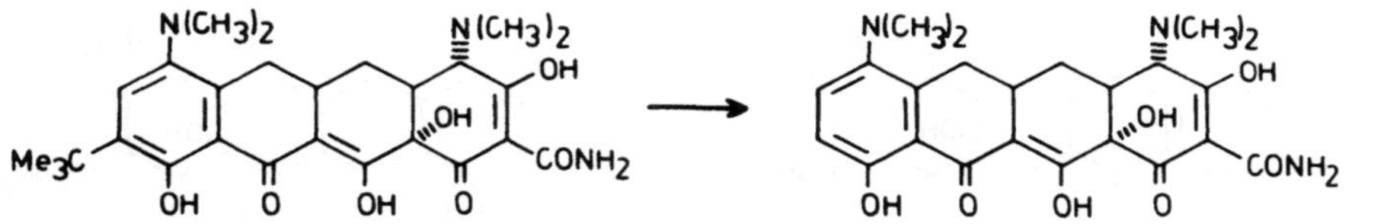

154 4

The 7-amino compound (144) is also the starting compound for a number of further modifications at the C7 atom. Conversion into the 7-diazonium compound (148) with butyl nitrite and transformation of the diazonium group with azide, fluoride, acetic acid, and xanthate gives the corresponding 7-azide (149), 7-fluoride (150), 7-acyloxy (151), and 7-xanthate (152) (Beereboom et al. 1960; Boothe et al. 1960; Hlavka et al. 1962a, b).

Attempts at directly introducing oxygen in the 7 position have been unsuccessful. In fact, this only succeeds by hydrolyzing the 7-acetoxy compound (151), which in turn can only be prepared by photolysis of the tetracyclic 7-diazonium compound (148) in the presence of acetic acid (Hlavka et al. 1962b). The 7-hydroxy-6-demethyl-6-deoxytetracycline (155) thus prepared has considerably poorer antibacterial activity than tetracycline.

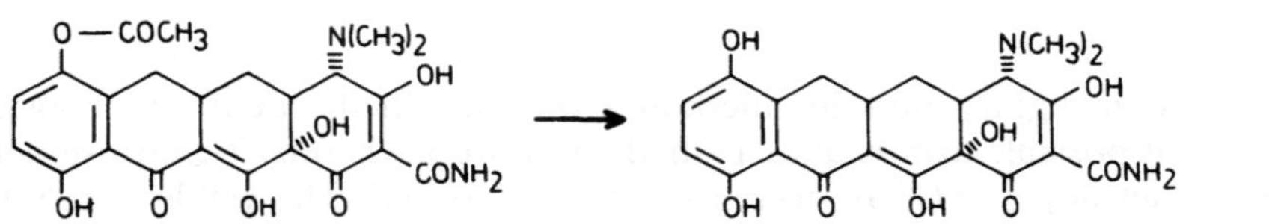

151 155

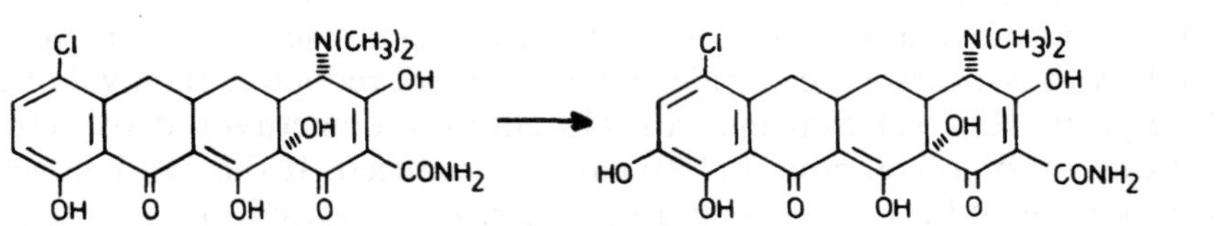

156 157

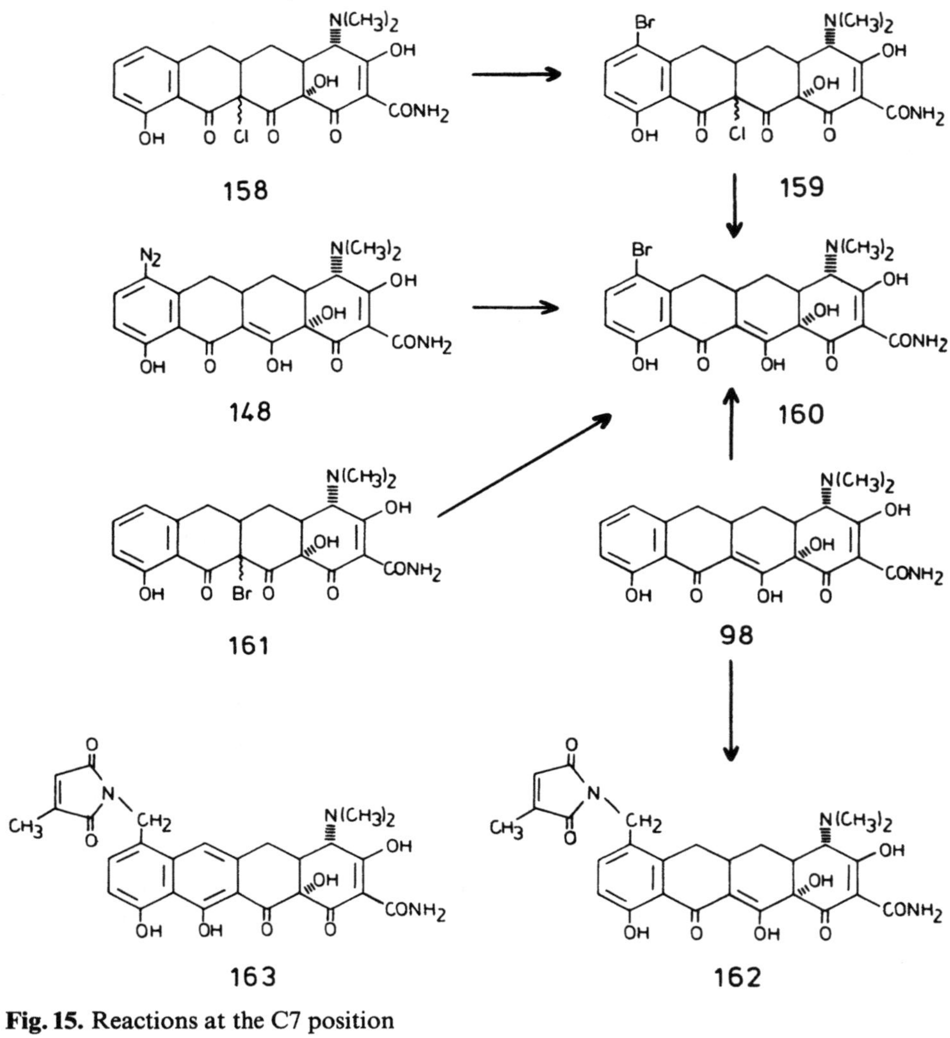

Fig. 15. Reactions at the C7 position

Using a slightly modified method with a modified Udenfriend reagent (SHU 1966) it is possible to introduce a 9-hydroxy group, whereby 7-chloro-6-demethyl-6-deoxytetracycline (156) serves as starting material. The yields of (157) are totally unsatisfactory, however. Even though the antibacterial activity of (157) was adequate this compound has never achieved any significance.

The 7-bromo analogues can be synthesized via a reaction of 11a-chloro compounds with *N*-bromosuccinimide and subsequent reductive removal of the 11a-chloro group (Fig. 15). Starting with 11a-chloro-6-demethyl-6-deoxytetracycline (158) the 7-bromo compound (160) can be produced. If the 11a-halogen group is bromine or iodine, then these groups can be relocated in concentrated acid (HLAVKA et al. 1962a) or by photolysis (HLAVKA and KRAZINSKI 1963) to give the corresponding 7-halogen-substituted tetracyclines. Compound (160) is thus produced from compound (161). The 7-bromo compound (160) is also directly accessible through bromination of (98) in trifluoroacetic acid (BEEREBOOM et al. 1960).

Treatment of 7-diazonium-6-demethyl-6-deoxytetracycline (148) with halides such as NaBr or NaI gives the corresponding 7-halogen compound, e.g., compound (160).

Radioactive 7-iodo-6-demethyl-6-deoxytetracycline was of some interest in tumor diagnosis. Trials in dogs with mammary tumors showed that certain organs such as the liver and kidneys exhibited the highest radioactivity levels, but that the tumor contained twice as much radioactivity as healthy tissues (HLAVKA and BUYSKE 1960).

A further type of 7-substituted tetracycline can be produced by the Tscherniac-Einhorn reaction (MARTELL et al. 1967a). Treating 6-demethyl-6-deoxytetracycline (98) in strong acid with *N*-hydroxyphthalimide gives the corresponding 7-substituted compound (162). All attempts at cleaving the imide group were unsuccessful. The compounds prepared in this way showed a partially better in vitro activity than tetracycline on account of their greater lipophilicity, although they were disappointing in vivo. The same reaction can be used in 6-demethylanhydrotetracycline and the product is compound (163). The in vitro activity is insignificant.

Recently, the synthesis of 7- and 9-methyltetracyclines has been reported. The biotesting of these derivatives showed that antibacterial activity was retained. The 9-methyl compounds, however, exhibit depressed activity relative to the corresponding 7-analogues (BERNARDI et al. 1975c).

The compound 6-α-benzylsulfoxymethylene-6-demethyl-6-deoxytetracycline (125) has been mentioned in connection with modifications at the C6 atom and with substitution at the 6-methylene group. Treatment of this compound with hydrochloric acid (BLACKWOOD et al. 1963) causes alkylation in the 7 position, leading to formation of the pentacyclic dihydrothiophene product (127), the following reaction mechanism (protonation, electrophilic attack, solvolysis, and tautomerization) being assumed (Fig. 16). Compound (127) exhibits broad-spectrum tetracycline-like activity, indicating changes along the upper periphery of the molecule.

The conditions for the electrophilic reaction in the 6-demethyl-6-deoxytetracycline series were not applicable for the 6-deoxyoxytetracycline and 6-methyleneoxytetracycline series. Only two compounds from this group deserve mention, namely 7-chloro-6-methyleneoxytetracycline (164) (BLACKWOOD et al. 1963) and 9-nitro-6-deoxy-6-epioxytetracycline (165) (BEEREBOOM et al. 1960). While the 7-chloro compound was shown to be active, the 9-nitro compound was inactive.

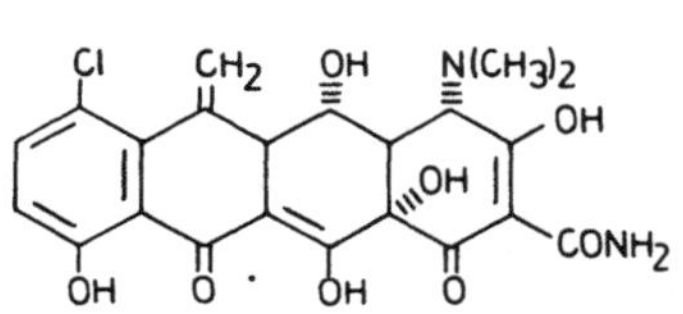

164

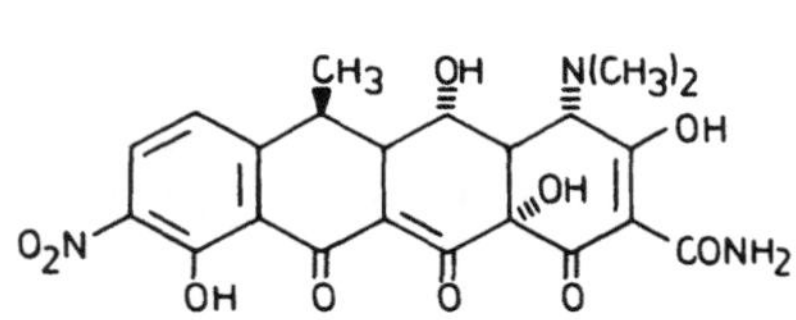

165

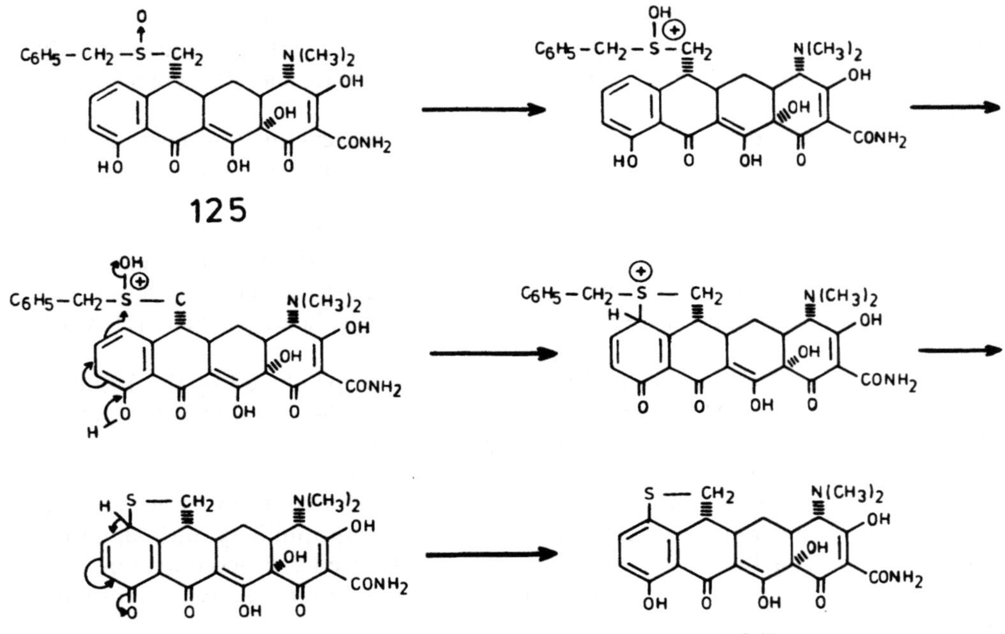

Fig. 16. Reaction mechanism for preparation of the pentacyclic dihydrothiophene product (127)

Using 7-nitro-6-demethyl-6-deoxytetracycline (142) in the nitration reaction leads to formation of the 7,9-dinitro derivative (166), whereas if 9-nitro-6-demethyl-6-deoxytetracycline (167) is used there is no nitration at the 7 position.

The same also applies to the 7-halogen-substituted 6-demethyl-6-deoxytetracyclines. The 7-chloro and 7-bromo compounds (168) and (169) give the 7-halogen-9-nitro derivatives (170) and (171) upon nitration. By carefully reducing the nitro group it was possible to produce in this way the corresponding 9-amino-7-chloro-6-demethyl-6-deoxytetracyclines (172) and 9-amino-7-bromo-6-demethyl-6-deoxytetracyclines (173) (SPENCER et al. 1963).

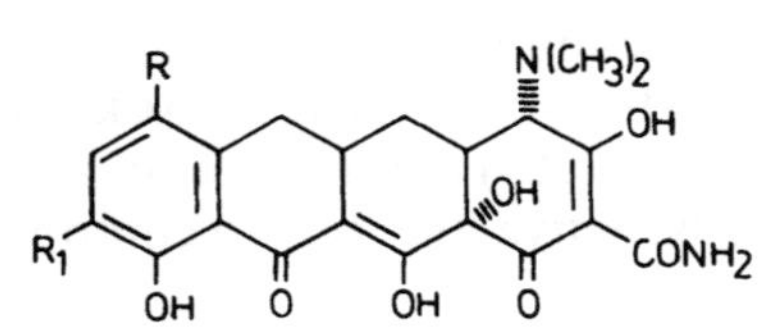

142: R = NO_2	; R_1 = H	170: R = Cl	; R_1 = NO_2
166: R = NO_2	; R_1 = NO_2	171: R = Br	; R_1 = NO_2
167: R = H	; R_1 = NO_2	172: R = Cl	; R_1 = NH_2
168: R = Cl	; R_1 = H	173: R = Br	; R_1 = NH_2
169: R = Br	; R_1 = H	174: R = H	; R_1 = NH_2
		175: R = NO_2	; R_1 = NH_2

Normally an amino group deactivates the ring under highly acidic conditions. Upon nitration of 9-amino-6-demethyl-6-deoxytetracycline (174), however, the 9-amino-6-demethyl-6-deoxy-7-nitrotetracycline (175) is obtained in good yield. Likewise, 9-amino-6-deoxytetracycline can be brominated to give a 9-amino-7-bromo-6-deoxytetracycline analogous to compound (173).

It should also be mentioned that dedimethylaminoanhydrotetracycline can be transformed with *N*-bromosuccinimide into a monobromo compound. It proved impossible to reduce out the bromine from this latter compound with zinc in glacial acetic acid and to exchange the bromine for a dimethylamino group. It is assumed that bromination has resulted in the corresponding 9-bromo derivative. Reacting dedimethylamino-12a-deoxyanhydrotetracycline-10-monomethyl ether with *N*-bromosuccinimide leads to formation of the corresponding 12a-bromo derivative (MUXFELDT and KREUTZER 1961).

2. Effect of Structural Variation on Antibacterial Activity

The acid stability of 6-deoxytetracyclines permitted the use of reactions for ring D substitution which would otherwise have been unthinkable in the presence of the 6-hydroxy group. Many of these new tetracyclines have good in vitro and in vivo activity. Only a very small number, however, showed any significant improvement on the medicinally important tetracyclines. The most important of these compounds is 7-dimethylamino-6-demethyl-6-deoxytetracycline (4), known otherwise as minocycline. It possesses superb activity against tetracycline-sensitive organisms and is also active against tetracycline-resistant gram-positive bacteria, especially against *S. aureus* strains (Table 8) (MARTELL and BOOTHE 1967; REDIN 1966; STEIGBIGEL et al. 1968).

In comparing the activities of various 7-substituted 6-demethyl-6-deoxytetracyclines it is seen (Table 9) that a bromine atom in the 7 position produces a rise in activity, that the 7-chloro compound is more active than the bromo compound, and that an iodine atom in the 7 position has virtually no effect on activity. As a result of this observation it has been assumed that there is a direct connection between the electron activity of the halogen atoms in the 7 position and the biological activity of the compound (HLAVKA et al. 1962a).

An attempt has been made to correlate the antibacterial activity with substitution in ring D through a Free-Wilson approach (FREE and WILSON 1964; PURCELL et al. 1973) or with physicochemical parameters (COLLETT et al. 1970). This attempt was unsuccessful. No direct connection could be discovered between antibacterial activity in vitro and the π value, which can be taken as a measure for the lipophilic nature of the molecule. Chelation is required both for effect on the ribosomes and for transport into the bacterial cells. It is this active process which explains the absence of any correlation between the hydrophobic nature of the molecule and the in vitro antibacterial activity (COLLETT et al. 1970). A connection could only be expected if the tetracyclines were to gain access to the bacterial cell by passive diffusion.

A correlation could be established between the electronic structure and antibacterial activity of the substituents in ring D of the tetracyclines via the use of the square of the Hammet substituents index (CAMARATA et al. 1970) or pertur-

Table 9. In vitro activity of tetracyclines modified at positions C7 and C9. (BLACKWOOD and ENGLISH 1970)

Name	Minimum inhibitory concentration[a] (μg/ml)			
	Staphylococcus aureus 5	*Staphylococcus aureus* (tetracycline resistant)	*Streptococcus pyogenes*	*Escherichia coli*
6-Demethyl-6-deoxytetracycline	0.2	1.5	0.2	1.5
7-Nitro-6-demethyl-6-deoxytetracycline	0.2	12.5	0.04	0.15
7-Amino-6-demethyl-6-deoxytetracycline	1.5	100	0.2	0.8
7-Dimethylamino-6-demethyl-6-deoxytetracycline	0.1	0.8	0.02	3
7-Chloro-6-demethyl-6-deoxytetracycline	0.03	0.8	0.1	1.5
7-Bromo-6-demethyl-6-deoxytetracycline	0.3	0.8	0.2	3
9-Nitro-6-demethyl-6-deoxytetracycline	1.5	25	0.8	1.5
9-Amino-6-demethyl-6-deoxytetracycline	1.5	25	0.1	1.5
9-Dimethylamino-6-demethyl-6-deoxytetracycline	6	50	3	12
9-Chloro-6-demethyl-6-deoxytetracycline	1.5	12	0.8	12

[a] Bioassay relative to tetracycline

bation energy (PERADEJORDI et al. 1971). The predicted activities are of the same order as observed in vitro activities with some exception; i.e., 7-amino-6-demethyl-6-deoxytetracycline appears as one of more active tetracyclines in these calculations but it is one of the less active. Further it is not possible to carry over the calculation to the in vivo activity.

Nevertheless, the results described in this section show clearly that as a rule the introduction of strong electron-withdrawing groups at the C7 atom increases in vitro activity, whereas electron-donating groups cause a decrease in activity. Amine functions can either be of the strongly attracting type or of the type which concedes electrons, the important difference being whether the amine is protonated or not. pH measurements have shown that under test conditions the amine at C7 should not be protonated. An effect should therefore be anticipated which is opposed to that of a substituent which is attractive toward electrons, i.e., the in vitro activity should be lessened. This is not the case, however, as is shown particularly clearly by 7-dimethylamino-6-demethyl-6-deoxytetracycline (4), minocycline. There is a possible explanation for this (BLACKWOOD and ENGLISH 1970). In the vicinity of the surface of a bacterium there is a microregion of low pH. 7-Dimethylamino-6-demethyl-6-deoxytetracycline was thus protonated and rendered highly attractive to electrons, resulting in heightened in vitro activity. The

7-amino compound on the other hand is a weaker base and thus protonizable to a lesser extent under identical conditions. It thus possesses a less pronounced in vitro activity. Minocycline, on the other hand, is a more lipophilic tetracycline, and its superior activity can be explained also in terms of improved uptake into the bacterial cell via routes not available to the other tetracyclines (McMurry et al. 1982).

The 9-nitro and 9-chloro-6-demethyl-6-deoxytetracyclines have less activity than the corresponding 7-substituted compounds (Hlavka and Boothe 1973), as illustrated in a comparison of activities in Table 9. The reason for this may be a possible hydrogen bridge with the phenolic hydroxy group at C10, which may interfere with the active site in the tetracycline molecule. The 9-amino-6-demethyl-6-deoxytetracyclines are somewhat more active than their 7-analogues, while the 9-dimethylamino compounds exhibit notably reduced activity. Steric factors may play a role here. Nevertheless, in spite of its poorer in vitro activity 9-dimethylamino-6-demethyl-6-deoxytetracycline is surprisingly active in vivo. This makes it possible to conclude that there is a similarly favorable interaction of electron and lipophilic factors in vivo as in minocycline.

In summary it can be stated that the 7-substituents are more favorable for antibacterial activity than those in the 9 position. Compounds with strong electron-withdrawing groups are also the more active. Hence a nitro or dimethylamino group in the 7 position improves the activity most. The most important compound is minocycline, which exhibits superior activity against many bacteria and is also active against a number of tetracycline-resistant organisms (Table 8).

The correlations observed in vitro do not appear to be transferable to in vivo activity.

VIII. Modifications at the C11 and C12 Positions

1. Chemistry

Very little is known about modifications at carbon atoms C11 and C12. When oxytetracycline is heated in dioxane with triethylamine, allooxytetracycline (176) is produced (Schwarz and Applegate 1967). Treating tetracycline with hydrazine gives the pyrazoletetracycline (177), in which the oxygen atoms at C11 and C12 are replaced by nitrogen (Valcavi et al. 1963).

2. Effect of Structural Variation on Antibacterial Activity

Both tetracycline derivatives are inactive. This is not surprising since every modification at this β-dicarbonyl system results in loss of antibacterial activity.

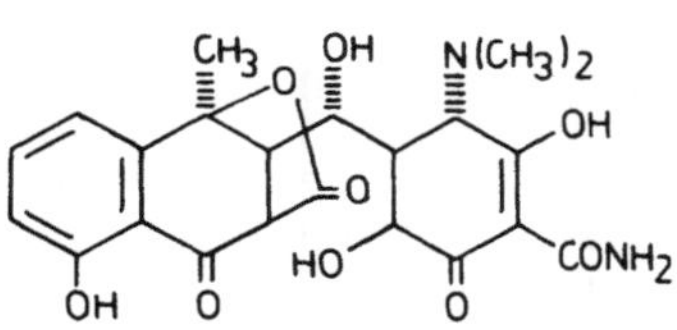

176

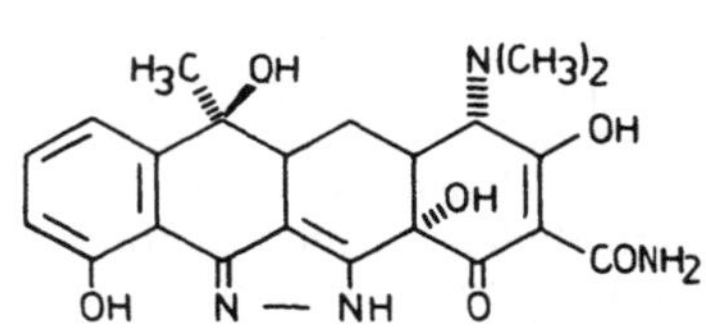

177

IX. Modifications at the C11a Position

1. Chemistry

Modifications at C11a basically comprise halogenation of tetracyclines at this position. This made it possible to block position 11a for reactions which are of importance in 6-methylene chemistry. The 11a-fluoro compound especially was used as an intermediate product on account of its stability and simple catalytic removal for further reactions at C6. The iodine and bromine analogues are less stable than the corresponding chlorine and fluorine compounds (Blackwood et al. 1961, 1963; Rennhard et al. 1961). Both compounds are thus easily transformed in concentrated acid (Hlavka et al. 1962a) or by photolysis (Hlavka and Krazinski 1963) into the corresponding 7-halogenated compounds. Compound (161) thus yields the 7-bromo derivative (160). Transformation by photolysis is solvent dependent. When acetonitrile is used, HBr is split off and anhydrotetracycline (178) is formed.

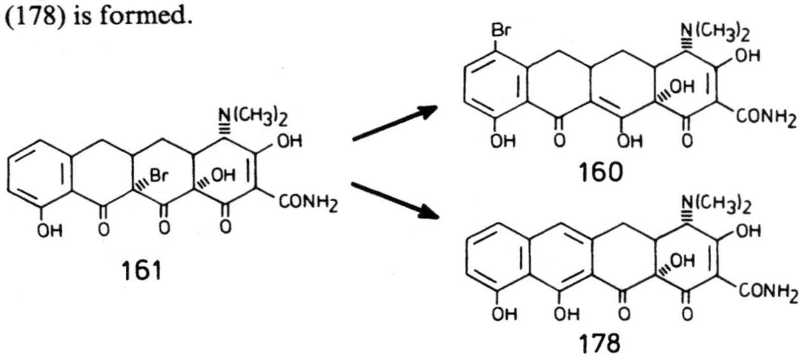

2. Effect of Structural Variation on Antibacterial Activity

Substitution at C11a leads to loss of antibacterial activity (Table 10). The 11,12 β-diketone system is disturbed, which, owing to its chelating properties with mag-

Table 10. In vitro activity of tetracyclines modified at position C11a. (Blackwood and English 1970)

Name	Minimum inhibitory concentration (μg/ml)		
	Staphylococcus aureus 5	*Streptococcus pyogenes*	*Escherichia coli*
11a-Bromo-6-demethyl-6-deoxytetracycline	3	1.5	6
11a-Chloro-6-demethyl-6-deoxytetracycline	6	3	12
11a-Fluoro-6-demethyl-6-deoxytetracycline	100	50	>100
7,11a-Dichloro-6-demethyl-6-deoxytetracycline	12	6	50
11a-Chloro-6-methylenetetracycline	50	12	>100
11a-Chloro-6-methyleneoxytetracycline	100	100	>100
11a-Chlorotetracycline 6,12-hemiketal	100	50	>100
11a-Fluorotetracycline 6,12-hemiketal	50	25	>100

nesium, plays an important role in the active mechanism within the bacterium. By this structural variation the conformation of the zwitterionic and nonionized forms, if they exist, should be very different from that of the antibacterially active tetracyclines. Therefore it is not surprising that the 11a-halogenated compounds are inactive.

X. Modifications at the C12a Position

1. Chemistry

Modifications at C12a have been limited to removal of the 12a-hydroxy group, its reintroduction, and its esterification (Fig. 17).

Removal of the 12a-hydroxy group occurs under reductive conditions and leads to compound (180) (HOCHSTEIN et al. 1960; GREEN and BOOTHE 1960). Treatment of tetracycline (5) with formic anhydride in acetic acid gives the C12a-formyl ester (179) (BLACKWOOD et al. 1960b). Catalytic reduction of the 12a ester leads to the corresponding 12a-deoxytetracycline (180). This method is an alternative to direct reduction of the hydroxy group with zinc/acetic acid. Heating the ester gives the 4a,12a anhydro compound (181). In neutral or basic solutions the formyl ester is unstable. In methanolic solution the ester (179) is split within a few minutes and tetracycline (5) is released again. The tetracycline-C10,12a-diacetates behave similarly. 12a-deoxytetracycline (180) is, under certain conditions, halogenated both in the C11a and in the C12a position (GREEN et al. 1960).

Introduction of the 12a-hydroxy group into the tetracyclic ring system by chemical means was a decisive step forward in the total synthesis of tetracyclines (HOLMLUND et al. 1959; MUXFELDT and KREUTZER 1961; WOODWARD 1963; MUXFELDT et al. 1968). Hydroxylation of the C12a position with the aid of microorganisms has been described (HOLMLUND et al. 1959).

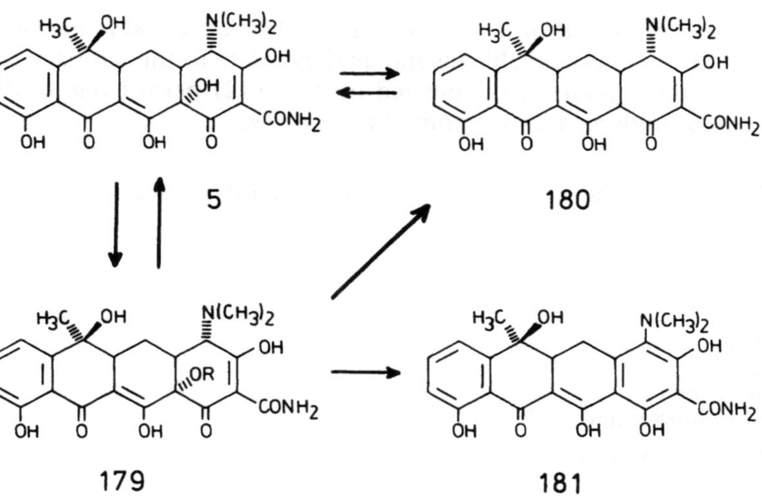

Fig. 17. Reactions affecting position 12a

The C12a hydroxy group divides the tetracyclic ring system into two chromophores, that of ring A and that of rings BCD. There is a characteristic UV spectrum. Upon removal of the C12a hydroxy group the ring system can conjugate completely, this being noticeable in alkaline solutions in a displacement to longer wavelengths.

2. Effect of Structural Variation on Antibacterial Activity

The hydroxy group and the stereochemistry at C12a is important for the activity of the molecule. The 12a epimer is notably less active than the natural tetracycline (Schach von Wittenau et al. 1965). 12a-Deoxytetracycline possesses only about 2% of the in vitro activity of tetracycline (Table 11).

Table 11. In vitro activity of tetracyclines modified at position C12a. (Blackwood and English 1970)

Name	Minimum inhibitory concentration (μg/ml)		
	Staphylococcus aureus 5	*Streptococcus pyogenes*	*Escherichia coli*
12a-Formyltetracycline	0.2	0.2	1.5
12a-Acetyloxytetracycline	3	3	25
12a-Propionyloxytetracycline	3	0.8	100
5,12a-Diacetyloxytetracycline	3	3	25
10,12a-Diacetyloxytetracycline	3	0.8	25

XI. Structure-Activity Relationships

The chemical modifications of fermentation-derived tetracyclines already discussed and the results available insofar as they relate to the antibacterial activity of modified tetracyclines (summarized in Table 12) permit one to deduce the requirements fundamental to tetracycline activity.

Table 12. Relative in vitro activity of tetracyclines modified at positions Cl, C2, C4, C5a, C7, C9, C6, C11a, C12a, and C5

Name	Percentage[a] activity
Tetracycline	100
Chlortetracycline[b]	110
Oxytetracycline[b]	40
6-Demethylchlortetracycline[b]	190
5a,6-Anhydrotetracycline[b]	30
4a,12a-Anhydrotetracycline[b]	0.4
Isotetracycline[b]	Inactive

Table 12 (continued)

Name	Percentage[a] activity
1-Ethoxytetracycline[c]	Inactive
2-Nitrile-2-decarboxamidotetracycline[b]	Inactive
2-Nitrile-2-decarboxamidochlortetracycline[b]	Inactive
Rolitetracycline	100
2-Acetyl-2-decarboxamidotetracycline[b]	7
2-Acetyl-2-decarboxamidooxytetracycline[b]	7
N^2-*t*-Butyl-6-demethyl-6-deoxytetracycline[b]	30
4-Dedimethylaminooxytetracycline[b]	0.8
4-Dedimethylaminotetracycline[b]	2
4-Dedimethylamino-6-demethyl-6-deoxytetracycline[b]	26
4-Epitetracycline[b]	4
4-Epioxytetracycline[b]	4
4-Epi-α-6-deoxyoxytetracycline[b]	7
6-Methylenetetracycline methiodide[b]	2
4-Oxo-4-dedimethylaminotetracycline-4,6-hemiketal[b]	Inactive
4-Oximino-4-dedimethylaminotetracycline[b]	Inactive
4-Hydrazono-4-dedimethylaminotetracycline[b]	0.4
4-Hydroxy-4-dedimethylaminotetracycline[b]	2
Demethyltetracycline[d]	96
4-Ethyl-methylamino-6-demethyltetracycline[d]	75
4-Methyl-propylamino-6-demethyltetracycline[d]	50
4-Diethylamino-6-demethyltetracycline[d]	25
4-Hydroxyethyl-methylamino-6-demethyltetracycline[d]	12
5a,11a-Dehydrochlortetracycline[e]	Inactive
5a-Epitetracycline[e]	Inactive
5a,11a-Dehydro-6-epichlortetracycline[e]	150
5a-Epi-6-epitetracycline[e]	40
6-Demethyl-6-deoxytetracycline[f,g]	160
6-Deoxytetracycline[g]	70
7-Chloro-6-demethyl-6-deoxytetracycline[h]	300
7-Bromo-6-demethyl-6-deoxytetracycline[h]	200
7-Iodo-6-demethyl-6-deoxytetracycline[h]	120
7-Bromo-6-deoxytetracycline[f]	140
7-Iodo-6-deoxytetracycline[f]	60
7-Fluoro-6-demethyl-6-deoxytetracycline[h]	220
7-Nitro-6-demethyl-6-deoxytetracycline[g]	640
7-Amino-6-demethyl-6-deoxytetracycline[g]	40
7-Formamido-6-demethyl-6-deoxytetracycline[g]	35
7-Dimethylamino-6-demethyl-6-deoxytetracycline[i]	200
7-Isopropylamino-6-demethyl-6-deoxytetracycline[j]	100
7-Azido-6-demethyl-6-deoxytetracycline[f]	150
6-Demethyl-6-deoxytetracycline-7-diazonium sulfate[f]	20
7-Acetoxy-6-demethyl-6-deoxytetracycline[h]	120
7-Hydroxy-6-demethyl-6-deoxytetracycline[h]	23
7-Formyloxy-6-demethyl-6-deoxytetracycline[h]	32
7-Ethoxythiocarbonylthio-6-demethyl-6-deoxytetracycline[f]	50
9-Chloro-6-demethyl-6-deoxytetracycline[b]	14
9-Nitro-6-demethyl-6-deoxytetracycline[g]	12
9-Amino-6-demethyl-6-deoxytetracycline[g]	160
9-Dimethylamino-6-demethyl-6-deoxytetracycline[b]	4

Table 12 (continued)

Name	Percentage[a] activity
9-Formamido-6-demethyl-6-deoxytetracycline[g]	225
9-Azido-6-demethyl-6-deoxytetracycline[f]	90
9-Azido-6-deoxytetracycline[f]	10
9-Acetamido-6-deoxytetracycline[g]	24
9-Amino-6-deoxytetracycline[g]	60
9-Nitro-6-deoxytetracycline[g]	1
6-Deoxytetracycline-9-diazonium disulfate[f]	10
6-Demethyl-6-deoxytetracycline-9-diazonium disulfate[f]	17
9-Ethoxythiocarbonylthio-6-demethyl-6-deoxytetracycline[f]	10
7-Chloro-9-nitro-6-demethyl-6-deoxytetracycline[k]	21
7-Bromo-9-nitro-6-demethyl-6-deoxytetracycline[k]	15
7,9-Dinitro-6-demethyl-6-deoxytetracycline[k]	60
9-Amino-7-chloro-6-demethyl-6-deoxytetracycline[k]	525
9-Amino-7-bromo-6-demethyl-6-deoxytetracycline[k]	320
9-Amino-7-nitro-6-demethyl-6-deoxytetracycline[k]	275
9-Amino-7-nitro-6-deoxytetracycline[k]	160
9-Amino-7-bromo-6-deoxytetracycline[k]	140
9-Acetamido-7-nitro-6-deoxytetracycline[k]	15
9-Acetamido-7-bromo-6-deoxytetracycline[k]	75
6-Demethyl-6-deoxytetracycline[g]	160
6-Methylenetetracycline[b]	105
6-Methyleneoxytetracycline[b]	160
6-Methylene-7-chlorooxytetracycline[b]	140
α-6-Deoxyoxytetracycline[b]	110
α-6-Deoxytetracycline[b]	35
β-6-Deoxyoxytetracycline[b]	26
β-6-Deoxytetracycline[b]	26
13-Mercapto-α-6-deoxyoxytetracycline[b]	7
13-Benzylmercapto-α-6-deoxyoxytetracycline[b]	105
13-Benzylmercapto-α-6-deoxytetracycline *S*-oxide[b]	7
13-Benzylmercapto-α-6-deoxytetracycline[b]	105
13-Acetylmercapto-α-6-deoxyoxytetracycline[b]	105
13-Phenylmercapto-α-6-deoxyoxytetracycline[b]	105
13-Phenylmercapto-α-6-deoxytetracycline *S*-oxide[b]	2
13-(2-Hydroxymethylmercapto)-α-6-deoxyoxytetracycline[b]	4
7,13-Epithio-α-6-deoxytetracycline[b]	53
11a,13-Epithio-α-6-deoxyoxytetracycline[b]	Inactive
6-α-Fluoro-6-demethyl-6-deoxytetracycline[l]	200
6-β-Fluoro-6-demethyl-6-deoxytetracycline[l]	12
6-α-Fluoro-6-demethyl-6-deoxychlortetracycline[l]	13
6-α-Fluoro-6-deoxychlortetracycline[l]	400
6-α-Fluoro-6-deoxytetracycline[l]	30
6-β-Acetoxy-6-demethylchlortetracycline[l]	200
6-β-Acetoxy-6-demethyltetracycline[l]	63
11a-Chloro-6-demethyl-6-deoxytetracycline[b]	3
7,11a-Dichloro-6-demethyl-6-deoxytetracycline[b]	2
11a-Chloro-6-methylenetetracycline[b]	0.4
11a-Fluorotetracycline 6,12-hemiketal[b]	0.4
12a-Deoxy-6-demethyl-6-deoxytetracycline[b]	7
12a-Formyltetracycline[b]	105

Table 12 (continued)

Name	Percentage[a] activity
12a-Acetyloxytetracycline[b]	7
5,12a-Diacetyloxytetracycline[b]	7
10,12a-Diacetyloxytetracycline[b]	7
12a-Epi-4-dedimethylaminooxytetracycline[b]	Inactive
α-6-Deoxyoxytetracycline[m, n]	100
5-Formyloxy-α-6-deoxytetracycline[m]	100
5-Acetyloxy-α-6-deoxytetracycline[m]	50
5-Chloropropyloxy-α-6-deoxytetracycline[m]	25
6-Methyleneoxytetracycline[m]	200
5-Formyloxy-6-methylenetetracycline[m]	200
5-Acetyloxy-6-methylenetetracycline[m]	100
5-Chloropropyloxy-6-methylenetetracycline[m]	100

[a] Activities were measured turbidimetrically against *Staphylococcus aureus* by the method of PELCAK and DORNBUSH (1948); activity of tetracycline = 100%
[b] BLACKWOOD and ENGLISH (1970)
[c] DÜRCKHEIMER (1975)
[d] ESSE et al (1964)
[e] MARTELL et al (1967)
[f] HLAVKA et al (1962a)
[g] PETISI et al (1962)
[h] HLAVKA et al (1962b)
[i] MARTELL and BOOTHE (1967)
[j] HLAVKA and BOOTHE (1973)
[k] SPENCER et al (1963)
[l] BITHA et al (1970)
[m] BERNARDI et al (1974)
[n] Approximate activity against *Staphylococcus aureus* 209 P; activity of α-6-deoxyoxytetracycline = 100%

1. Structure

Structurally the most simple tetracycline having complete biological activity is partially synthetic 6-demethyl-6-deoxytetracycline.

The fundamental prerequisites for its antibacterial activity are the linear arrangement of the four rings, the phenoldiketone system of rings BCD, and the tricarbonylmethane system of ring A with its basic function at the C4 atom. Any change sustained by the ring system as a result of cleavage of a ring (e.g., iso-tetracycline), or aromatization of one or more additional rings, causes a marked decrease in activity in vitro and complete loss of activity in vivo. Any change in the two chromophore systems, made up of rings BCD and ring A, either by removal of the 12a-hydroxy group or by introduction of a substituent in the 11a position to form longer or shorter chromophores, causes the activity to drop sharply.

Any change made to the oxygens at the C11,C12-β-ketone system reduces biological activity. This is hardly surprising when one considers that the phenoldiketone system possesses considerable chelatization ability (MITSCHER et al. 1968, 1969; WILLIAMSON and EVERETT 1975; GULBIS and EVERETT 1975; JOGUN and STEZOWSKI 1976), which constitutes an important aspect of the active mechanism on the receptor side of the ribosomes and is a prerequisite for transport into the bacterial cell.

The amide hydrogen at C2 can be replaced by methyl without loss of activity. Larger groups tend to cause the activity to deteriorate unless they are cleavable in water.

The 4-dimethylamino group can be replaced by a primary or monomethyl-substituted amino group with no appreciable loss of in vitro activity. All other modifications to substituents at the nitrogen, e.g., longer alkyl chains or acyl residues, bring about a decrease in activity.

Indeed, the upper periphery of the molecule, the hydrophobic portion, can be varied in many possible ways from C atoms 5–9. This may produce an increase in antibiotic activity. Steric interactions or hydrogen bridges formed by substituents at C9 with the oxygen at C10 lead to loss of activity.

The most important structural modifications have taken place at C atoms 6 and 7. This gave rise to the two most important products, doxycycline (3) and minocycline (4). They are both of greater chemical stability, are more antibacterially active, and have more favorable pharmacokinetics.

2. Conformation and Configuration

With the advent of X-ray structural analysis it was possible for the first time to elucidate the conformation of the molecular structure and the stereochemical configurations of tetracyclines (HIROKAWA et al. 1959; TAKEUCHI and BUERGER 1960; DONOHUE et al. 1963; CID-DRESDNER 1965; HUGHES et al. 1971; VON DREELE and HUGHES 1971).

Conformation has also been investigated under physiological conditions using the circular dichroism method (MITSCHER et al. 1968, 1969, 1972). It can be concluded from the results obtained that the BDC-ring system is essentially planar and that the AB-ring system can undergo considerable conformational changes, whereby the conformation at physiological pH values is not necessarily the active conformation.

NMR spectroscopy has been involved in determining the conformation of the molecule (SCHACH VON WITTENAU and BLACKWOOD 1966) and the role of metal binding in the activity of tetracyclines (WILLIAMSON and EVERETT 1975; GULBIS and EVERETT 1975, 1976). Results of the metal binding studies in tetracyclines were interpreted as an indication of a magnesium-ion-induced conformational change of tetracyclines.

In more recent X-ray crystallography studies the conformation and the hydrogen-bonding interactions of nonionized and zwitterionic forms of tetracyclines are discussed (STEZOWSKI 1976, 1977; JOGUN and STEZOWSKI 1976; PREWO and STEZOWSKI 1977, 1980; HUGHES et al. 1979). It was shown that the tetracycline bases in their zwitterionic and nonionized forms can exhibit very differing conformations. The transition between the two conformers involves a twist about the bond C4a–C12a at the juncture of the A- and B-rings. The zwitterionic form seems to be the dominant form even in the presence of only slight concentrations of water. This form is important therefore in determining the activity of tetracyclines in aqueous media. The nonionized form of the molecule is probably that form which is responsible for solubility in the lipid phase.

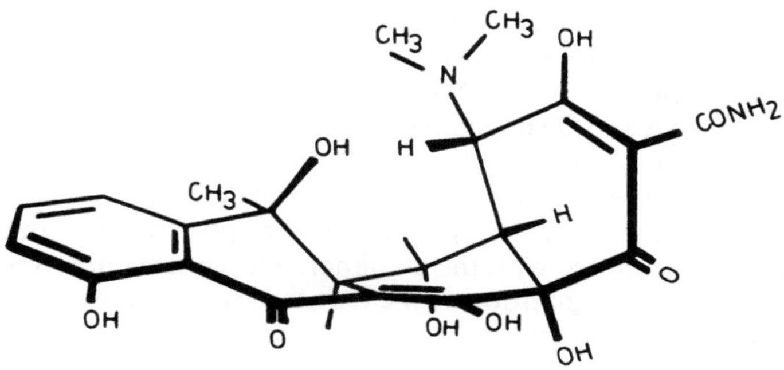

Fig. 18. The conformation of oxytetracycline 7

One of the limitations of the X-ray crystal structure studies is the static nature of the measurements, and a limitation of the circular dichroism studies is the simulated physiological conditions under which the molecules were investigated. Therefore it must be kept in mind that none of the conformations may give a true reflection of the molecule under the condition in the bacteria or under the natural physiological conditions. The range of conformations accessible to the basic four-ring system and the relative stabilities of different conformers are matters of considerable importance for the biological activity. The conformation of the nonionized form of the oxytetracycline base is shown as follows (Fig. 18).

From the evidence assembled in the foregoing it can be seen that the biologically active tetracycline molecule has to fulfill the following conditions: planarity of the two ketone-enol systems C11/C12 and C1/C3 in the BCD- and A-ring chromophore separated by a *cis* arrangement of the 12a-hydroxy group.

The configuration at atoms C4a, C5a, and C12a largely determines the conformation of the molecule. For full activity to be achieved by the molecule it is necessary for it to occur in the natural configuration (CONOVER et al. 1962). For in vivo activity the proton at the C4 atom has to be in the normal, β-configuration. However, activity is not principally dependent on the substituents and their configuration at carbon atoms 5, 5a, and 6.

It is known that of the three tetracyclines oxytetracycline, α-6-deoxyoxytetracycline, and β-6-deoxyoxytetracycline, oxytetracycline is the least lipophilic (BLACKWOOD and ENGLISH 1970). Substitution of a hydrogen atom for the 6-hydroxy group in the conformation of the nonionized oxytetracycline should cause an increase in the lipophilicity of the molecule. Indeed, this is the case. However, the α-6-deoxyoxytetracycline shows a considerably greater increase in lipophilicity than the 6 epimer when the two are compared with oxytetracycline. The greater lipophilicity of the α-6-deoxyoxytetracycline is in agreement with the retention of the observed conformation and a reduction of the polarity of the substituents (STEZOWSKI 1976).

In β-6-deoxyoxytetracycline the methyl group adopts the position otherwise taken by the hydroxy group. This produces greater interactions between the larger methyl group at the C6 atom and the hydrogen at the C4 atom. Consequently the conformation of the molecule is changed in the direction of the zwitterionic form. This causes the intramolecular hydrogen bonds between the hydroxy group at C5 and C12a to be reduced, thus raising the polarity of the molecule (STEZOWSKI 1976). Two opposing effects thus cause a decrease in the lipophilicity of the β-epimer: (1) reduction in polarity of the molecule by removing the C6 hydroxy group and (2) increase in the polarity of the molecule by the conformational modification described.

The sum of these effects determines the property of the molecule. The overall increase in polarity is in agreement with the lower lipophilicity of the β-6-deoxyoxytetracycline as compared with the α-epimer. The conclusions to be drawn are that substitution and configuration at the C6 atom can thus influence conformation and hence tetracycline activity.

3. Electron Structure

Information on structure-activity relationships was gained in experiments in which quantum mechanical calculations were applied to study the influence of centers and substituents on tetracycline activity (CAMMARATA et al. 1970; PERADEJORDI et al. 1971). It was shown that there is a correlation between the in vitro activity and electronic structure.

The results from semisynthesis can be summarized as follows. Generally speaking, there seems to be a correlation between the substituents in positions 7 and 9 and their effect on in vitro activity. But the activities of the tetracyclines analogously substituted at these centers do not parallel. Introduction of electron-withdrawing groups at C7, such as nitro and chloro groups, increase in vitro activity whereas the 9-nitro and 9-chloro compounds show depressed activity relative to the 7-analogous compounds. However, electron-donating substituents at C7, e.g., oxygen and amino, reduce the in vitro activity, with the reverse being true at C9 for the amino derivative.

The heightened activity of 6-methylenetetracyclines can also be explained in terms of an electron effect of this type (BLACKWOOD and ENGLISH 1970).

It must be noted, however, that in actual fact not only substituents which are strong electron donors but also those with a strong acceptor effect raise tetracycline activity. One example of this is 7-dimethylamino-6-demethyl-6-deoxytetracycline, minocycline.

The dimethylamino group is a strong electron donor group and consequently ought to be less active than tetracycline. In reality, however, it is more active. In fact it is two to eight times more active than tetracycline (BLACKWOOD and ENGLISH 1970).

Amine functions may either be strong electron acceptors or electron donors, depending on whether the amine is protonated or not. Under physiological conditions the C7 amino group is not protonated. An effect ought to be expected which is opposite to that of an electron-accepting substituent and which is noticeable in the form of reduced in vitro activity. This is not the case, however, as quite clearly demonstrated by 7-dimethylamino-6-demethyl-6-deoxytetracycline. There is possibly an explanation for this behavior, which was discussed already. On the surface of a bacterium there is a microregion of low pH, which would cause the 7-dimethylaminotetracycline to become protonated and thus become a strong electron acceptor. The result of this would be increased in vitro activity.

The simple 7-amino compound, on the other hand, is a weaker base and is thus less protonatable under identical conditions. The simple compound thus is less active in vitro. Apparently the correlations found in vitro are not valid as regards in vivo activity.

In quantum-mechanical investigations into structure-activity relationships it was shown that the π electron donor character of the phenoldiketone system is important (PERADEJORDI et al. 1971). This is significant insofar as it is assumed that the tetracyclines exercise their activity on ribosomes via chelation of the oxygen functions at the C10, C11, and C12 atoms. It appears at present that magnesium chelation (LAST 1969) is involved and that the tetracyclines are transported into the bacterial cell via a magnesium complex, although the role of magnesium binding in the activity of tetracyclines is not yet well defined (WILLIAMSON and EVERETT 1975) and has recently been questioned (TRITTON 1977).

The influence of substituents on the electron properties of the C6 atom and the phenoldiketone system makes it possible to correlate the biological properties of tetracyclines. Any modification in substituents at carbon atoms 5–9 yields derivatives of quantitatively varying activity.

A general statement can be made, namely that substituents which increase the electron-donating capacity of the phenoldiketone system raise antibacterial activity.

It is difficult, of course, to distinguish between a structural modification which alters the ability of tetracyclines to react on the receptor side of ribosomes and one which alters the ability of tetracyclines to penetrate the bacterial cell wall.

4. Lipophilicity

The active mechanism by which tetracyclines act on ribosomes in the interior of the bacterial cell requires that they enter the organism via an active transport mechanism. It is known that the lipophilicity of tetracyclines exercises an influence on antibacterial activity (BLACKWOOD and ENGLISH 1970). The more lipophilic a tetracycline is, the greater is its activity against gram-positive tetracycline-resistant organisms, while lipophilicity has no bearing on effectiveness against gram-positive tetracycline-sensitive bacteria (Tables 13–15). In vitro and in vivo

Table 13. Lipophilicity and antibacterial activity of four medicinally important tetracyclines

Name	Lipophilicity[a]	Minimum inhibitory concentration (µg/ml)		
		Staphylococcus aureus 5[b]	*S. aureus*[b] tetracycline resistant	*Escherichia coli*[b]
Tetracycline	0.025	0.21	60	0.73
Oxytetracycline	0.036	0.55	>100	1.09
Doxycycline	0.600	0.19	8.75	1.74
Minocycline	1.100	0.1	0.8	3.0

[a] Apparent partition between octanol and pH 7.5 buffer. (COLAIZZI and KLINK 1969)
[b] BLACKWOOD and ENGLISH (1970)

Tab. 14. Correlation between partition coefficient and in vitro and in vivo activity. (FOURTILLAN and LEFÈBVRE 1980)

Structure	Name	Partition coefficient $CHCH_3/H_2O$ (pH = 7)	In vitro activity *MIC* (μg/ml) *Staphylococcus aureus*	In vivo activity *Staphylococcus aureus* ED_{50} (mg/kg) in mice p.o.	s.c.
(6)	Chlorotetracycline	–	0.19	7.6	3
(7)	Oxytetracycline	0.11	0.55	7.2	2.6
(5)	Tetracycline	0.105	0.21	5.81	1.23
(2)	Methacycline	0.117	0.13	4.50	1.19
(8)	Demethylchlorotetracycline	0.148	0.11	6.00	1.63
(3)	Doxycycline	0.63	0.19	2.55	1.00
(4)	Minocycline	39.4	0.1	3.5	–

Table 15. Composite values of pharmacokinetic parameters of some tetracyclines in man. (TOON and ROWLAND 1979)

Structure	Name	Partition coefficient octanol/water (pH 7.5)	Fraction unbound in plasma (fu)	Half-life $T_{1/2}$ (h)	Renal clearance (CL_R) 1/h	Nonrenal clearance (CL_{NR}) 1/h	Volume of distribution (liters)
(7)	Oxytetracycline	0.025	0.690	9.2	5.92	2.54	112.31
(5)	Tetracycline	0.036	0.405	9.0	4.41	2.94	95.45
(8)	Demethylchlorotetracycline	0.050	0.250	14.0	2.12	3.77	118.99
(6)	Chlorotetracycline	0.13	0.300	5.6	1.93	8.79	86.62
(2)	Methacycline	0.43	0.220	11.1	2.73	6.37	145.76
(3)	Doxycycline	0.60	0.125	22.0	1.10	1.40	79.37
(4)	Minocycline	1.10	0.240	16.0	0.90	7.28	188.86

activity against gram-positive tetracycline-resistant staphylococci has already been described for minocycline (MARTELL and BOOTHE 1967).

As distinct from the tetracycline-sensitive gram-positive bacteria, tetracycline-sensitive gram-negative bacteria are highly influenced by lipophilicity. The more lipophilic a tetracycline is, the weaker is its activity against gram-negative tetracycline-sensitive bacteria. It may lose its activity altogether. The reported influence of lipophilicity on activity is connected with the varying lipid contents of the membranes of gram-positive and gram-negative bacteria. Various experts suppose that there is a connection between resistance to antibiotics and the lipid contents of bacterial cell walls (NIKAIDO and NAKAE 1979; NEU 1978). This supposition is given weight by the observation that resistant *Staphylococcus* strains, for instance, have a higher lipid level than strains which are sensitive to antibiotics. By way of contrast, higher lipophilicity shown by tetracyclines is not exactly an advantage as regards the uptake of these compounds in gram-negative bacteria. Also, there is no difference in the lipid content of membranes between tetracycline-sensitive and tetracycline-resistant gram-negative bacteria.

It is important to distinguish clearly between two membranes as present in gram-negative bacteria:

1. The outer membrane, forming a lipid-containing, hydrophobic zone and exercising more a sieve function against substances penetrating the bacterium.
2. The inner, cytoplasmic membrane, which also contains lipids but through which the substances penetrate the cell interior via an active transport mechanism. This membrane represents the main substance barrier. The two membranes are separated by the periplasmic space.

Whether the lipophilic character of the tetracyclines determines if the outer membrane is penetrated and whether it also influences active transport through the cytoplasmic membrane are questions which have hitherto not been answered. It is assumed (HUGHES et al. 1979), however, that the hydrophilic/hydrophobic nature of the tetracycline molecule permits permeation through a series of polar and nonpolar barriers to occur as a result of conformational changes occasioned by a condition of equilibrium between a zwitterionic and nonionized form. The nature and extent of these changes directly affect the hydrophilic/hydrophobic properties of the molecule and ought consequently to be codeterminant in the degree of permeation.

In vivo activity cannot be predicted on the basis of in vitro findings. It correlates very haphazardly with electron and lipophilic properties. Whereas optimum lipophilicity is a prerequisite for in vivo activity, strong electron-accepting substituents in tetracycline would appear to reduce in vivo activity, thus running counter to in vitro findings. Strong electron-donating substituents, on the other hand, increase in vivo activity whereas they reduce in vitro activity.

Minocycline seems to combine favorable electron factors with favorable lipophilic factors. It is assumed that the ion group is transformed into an electron-accepting group through a possible protonation of the 7-dimethylamino group in the biophase of bacteria with low pH. Better activity should be the consequence. This is the case. Minocycline has an increased activity against tetracycline-resistant staphylococci, but the activity against gram-negative bacteria is not decreased (REDIN 1966). Minocycline is so far the most lipophilic compound of the tetracyclines. This makes it fair to assume that a modified form of uptake of this compound into the bacterium exists on account of its greater lipophilicity (McMURRY et al. 1975). This would also explain the apparent but by no means normal rise in activity of compounds having an electron-donating substituent in the 7 position, which ought really to cause activity to be reduced.

Because of the similarity of structures between natural tetracyclines and minocycline it is supposed that all these tetracyclines are transported into the cells by a common tetracycline transport system. There are indications, however, that minocycline, hitherto the most active of the tetracyclines, appears to have more possibilities of entering the bacterial cell than the natural tetracyclines (McMURRY et al. 1982). Hence its increased activity may stem from greater penetration into the cell. Penetration may ensue not only by the common tetracycline transport system but also via a route unique to minocycline. Generally speaking, there appear to be more transport routes open to the cell interior for tetracyclines having special characteristics than for the natural tetracyclines.

Two effects can be explained by this hypothesis.

1. By assuming that two different transport systems exist for minocycline it is possible to understand how there can be a higher concentration of minocycline in what are otherwise tetracycline-resistant organisms and how protein synthesis is either impaired or inhibited.
2. It would also be possible to explain how minocycline appears to be only a weak inducer of tetracycline resistance, attributed to part of the tetracycline entering the cell by the tetracycline-specific route, while that part which enters the organism by the minocycline-specific route apparently induces no resistance.

Results obtained with the 7-hydroxy compound support this hypothesis. The 7-hydroxy group is also an electron-donating substituent. The compound itself is not more lipophilic, however, than the normal tetracycline. The electron and lipophilic properties do not thus coincide favorably, so that the 7-hydroxy derivative exhibits the anticipated drop in activity (HLAVKA and BOOTHE 1973).

5. Pharmacokinetic Activity

Two review articles appeared very recently on the structure-activity relationship of natural and semisynthetic important tetracyclines.

The physicochemical properties, in particular the lipid/water solubility of the tetracyclines, determine their physiological distribution, providing the basis for the structure-activity relationship in vitro and in vivo (FOURTILLAN and LEFÈBVRE 1980). It could be shown that the tetracycline ring structure is specific for antibacterial activity, differences being in the polarity of the substituents on C5, C6, and C7. Partition coefficients between $CHCl_3$ and water vary from 0.105 (tetracycline) to 39.4 (minocycline) and are maximum at pH 5.5.

Tetracyclines with high lipid solubility, in particular minocycline and doxycycline, can cause resistance to tetracyclines of lower partition coefficients.

In mice infected with *Staphylococcus aureus*, the LD_{50} for tetracyclines given p.o. and s.c. was inversely proportional to the partition coefficient. The best correlation between in vivo and in vitro activity was found with doxycycline, supporting the hypothesis that the most effective substances are those with a partition coefficient nearest to 1 in this system. Moreover, tetracycline and minocycline, with in vitro activity equivalent to doxycycline, were both less active than doxycycline in vivo (Table 13 a).

Distribution studies in dogs showed that diffusion of free drug from serum to tissues was proportional to partition coefficient.

The principal pharmacokinetic parameters of seven tetracyclines after per os administration of 100–500 mg were tabulated. The variances of the distribution and half-life show a parallel to those of the partition coefficient from the most water-soluble chlorotetracycline to a maximum with doxycycline and decreasing with minocycline.

Two generations of tetracyclines were distinguished. The first included the natural tetracyclines and the second the semisynthetic tetracyclines minocycline and doxycycline, which was characterized by a persistence of high serum and tissue levels.

In a further investigation quantitative structure pharmacokinetic activity relationships were examined in a series of tetracyclines (TOON and ROWLAND 1979).

As can be seen from Table 13 b, the fraction of drug unbound in plasma (fu) varies within the series, but log 1/fu tends to increase linearly with log PC (partition coefficient, octanol/water, pH 7.5). Elimination half-life ($t_{1/2}$) correlated poorly with degree of plasma binding.

A poor correlation also exists between volume of distribution and either PC or log PC.

The same is the case with the total renal clearance and lipophilicity, but the renal clearance is directly proportional to the fraction unbound in plasma.

No correlation exists between nonrenal clearance and log PC but the values of nonrenal clearance tend to be inversely proportional to the fraction of unbound drug.

However, when correcting the differences in fu, a highly significant positive correlation exists between volume of distribution based on unbound drug and log PC, indicating that, as in plasma, drug binding to tissue components increases with lipophilicity.

The results of this investigation show further that, besides lipophilicity, other factors, possibly steric and ionic, are also largely responsible for differences in efficiency.

The analysis illustrates the need to resolve pharmacokinetic parameters into component parts, before attempting to relate the influence of structural modification on pharmacokinetics.

6. Summary

The first part of this review was devoted to the chemical modifications of the fermentation-derived tetracyclines and to the identification of the structural requirements for biological activity. Important improvements have been achieved by increasing the stability of the molecule due to deletion of the 6-hydroxy group. Furthermore the solubility of the molecule could be increased due to substituents at the C2 carboxamide group, the derivatives of which hydrolyze into the starting materials in aqueous solution. Still further improvements have been achieved by increasing the lipophilic nature of the molecule, resulting mainly in better pharmacokinetic properties of some tetracyclines due to modifications of the center C6 and C7 of the tetracycline ring system. The goal of improved antibacterial activity due to a decrease in the minimum inhibitory concentration and by a marked improvement in the spectrum of activity could not be achieved.

C. Totally Synthetic Unnatural Tetracyclines

Work on the development of new tetracyclines had been centred for a number of years around semisynthetic procedures. In fact, more than 1,000 tetracycline derivatives have been produced by this means. The advantage offered by semisynthesis was the relative speed with which new compounds could be developed. However, the number of reactions available for this type of synthesis is limited. What is more, modifications are only possible at certain positions within the molecule.

The total outcome of this line of research has been three marketable products. The first was methacycline (2), a 6-methylene-oxytetracycline, which was followed by doxycycline (3), being the reduction product of methacycline. The third product referred to is minocycline (4), which has improved in vitro antibacterial activity against staphylococci. One feature all have in common is superiority in their pharmacokinetics over the natural tetracyclines, this making them important antibiotics for treating infectious diseases.

One thing which has not been possible, however, even with these structural modifications is the elimination of the gaps in the spectrum of activity of the tetracyclines.

It was hardly surprising, therefore, that a certain degree of resignation set in: "It has up to now proven impossible to alter the basic bacteriostatic characteristics of tetracycline through chemical modifications. Nor has it been possible to extend the spectrum of activity to any significant extent. The growing number of tetracycline-resistant strains is viewed with concern" (DÜRCKHEIMER 1975).

What pathogenic microorganisms have managed to do is to adapt to the natural antibiotics and their derivatives obtained by slight, partial-synthetic modification in such a way as to become resistant to the antibiotics, so that these are now no longer an adequate means of combatting the bacteria. In view of this problem, the search for new antibiotics has continued unabated. Nature's reserve of therapeutically effective antibiotics appears to be limited. Despite intensive efforts it is only seldom that a new antibiotic which is both effective and toxicologically acceptable is found. It is all the more important, therefore, to modify existing antibiotic types of proven status by means of structural alterations which, it is hoped, will render them effective against resistant organisms and, what is more, offer advantages as regards their pharmacology.

Total synthesis widens the scope for modification, since the number of feasible reactions can be enlarged considerably. Whereas total synthesis was earlier chiefly a means of proving the constitution of complex natural substances, it has nowadays become a means of fulfilling other objectives such as the development of economical synthesis procedures in cases where raw materials have become scare and the synthesis of physiologically interesting derivatives of natural products not accessible by partial synthesis.

Total synthesis of tetracyclines enables modification to take place at positions in the molecule which could be ruledout as being impossible in semisynthesis. The previous paper dealt with structural aspects which are imperative if the necessary antibacterial activity is to be attained. With proper appreciation of these structure-activity relationships it is possible to conceive structures which exceed by far the semisynthetic modifications. It is perfectly feasible, for instance, to aim for structures not possessing the full tetracycline structure but nevertheless fulfilling the criteria imposed in order for tetracycline activity to exist. Total synthesis thus offers a way of widening the bounds of possible tetracyclic compounds, permitting more profound insight to be gained into structure-activity relationships.

One can assume that tetracyclines exercise their effect by complexing with the ribosomes in the bacterial cell. It has also been shown that all tetracyclines inhibit protein synthesis to the same extent in extracellular ribosomes. When, however, the site at which the tetracyclines are to unfold their activity lies within the bacterial cell, the ability of the tetracycline to penetrate the cell is a determinant factor as regards the tetracycline activity. In other words, tetracycline activity is a function of permeability. Permeability is directly affected, however, by the structure of the tetracycline, by the configuration of substituents within the molecule, and by conformation, all of which are instrumental in determining the lipophilicity of the molecule; lipophilicity for its part has a decisive influence on the antibacterial and pharmacological characteristics of the substance in question.

One resistance mechanism which has been developed by microorganisms and which in particular seems to play a role in tetracyclines involves a curtailment of the antibiotic substance's ability to penetrate the cell membrane.

While in tetracycline-sensitive bacteria tetracyclines are able to penetrate the inner cell membrane of bacteria using a specific transport system, resistant organisms such as *Escherichia coli* quickly synthesize a membrane protein upon contact with tetracyclines, this quite clearly affecting the permeability. Be that as it may, minocycline on the other hand manages to attain higher intracellular concentrations than the natural tetracyclines even in a number of tetracycline-resistant pathogens. It is a matter for conjecture as to whether this effect is based on only limited recognition of this structural variant as being a tetracycline or whether minocycline is able to use additional transport routes. At all events, one can conclude that through suitable structural modifications it is possible to produce tetracycline variants which attain adequate intracellular concentrations even in tetracycline-resistant organisms.

I. General Synthetic Pathways

The literature offers two pathways for synthesizing complete, active tetracycline derivatives. The totally synthetic route of Woodward and the Pfizer Company is much more circuitous than the totally synthetic pathway of Muxfeldt and coworkers and gives considerably inferior yields (Conover et al. 1962; Korst et al. 1968; Muxfeldt and Rogalski 1965; Muxfeldt et al. 1979). It is only logical, therefore, that attempts at finding new tetracyclines not producible by semisyn-

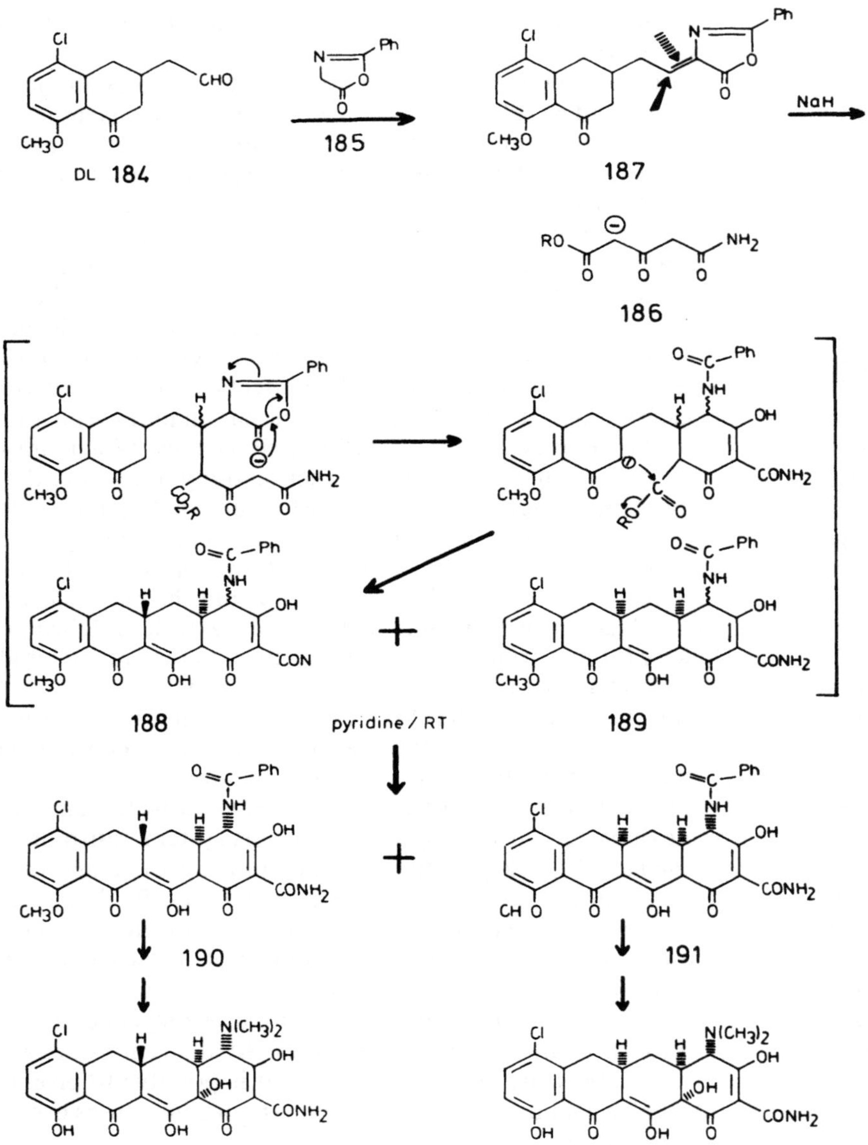

Fig. 19. Synthesis of the tetracycline ring system

thetic means have generally followed the synthetic pathway of Muxfeldt, which is distinguished by a particularly elegant structuring of rings A and B. Three building blocks are required: a tetralonaldehyde (184), an oxazolinone (185) (or thiazolinone), and the amide of monomethyl 3-oxoglutarate (186). These three building blocks are then condensed step by step via the oxazolone (187) to produce the tetracyclic ring system (188) and (189). There follow various other transformations such as epimerization to (190) and (191), as well as hydrolysis, oxidation, and alkylation, leading to the end products (192) and (193) (Fig. 19). The synthetic route as well as the end product can be widely varied by suitable choice of building blocks. Principally, those positions in the molecule can be varied which are indicated with arrows in the general formula (194) (Fig. 20). There are two distinct phases in the synthesis. The first has as its objective a tetralonaldehyde (195) (Fig. 20) and involves the construction of the subsequent CD-rings. The substituents in the subsequent C5–C10 positions of the tetracyclic ring system are already fixed by the tetralonacetaldehyde structure. This means that all structural modifications in a subsequent tetracycline ring system can be deliberately planned into the synthesis of the aldehyde with a view to the desired ultimate structure for the tetracycline. The second phase comprises the formation, already described, of rings A and B by the following, generally applicable procedure.

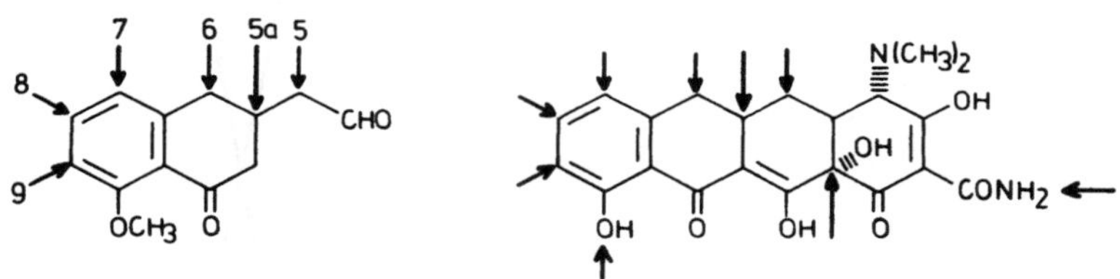

195 194

Fig. 20. Positions indicated with *arrows* can be varied by synthesis

The tetralone-3-acetaldehyde (184) is an important intermediate product in the synthesis of tetracyclic compounds. Condensation of this substance with oxazolone (185) gives the unsaturated azlactone (187), this being an extremely good Michael acceptor. In a subsequent reaction sequence with the amide of monomethyl 3-oxoglutarate it forms the carbon skeleton typical of all the tetracyclines. This "single-pan method" comprises three reaction steps which together permit all the necessary substituents to be introduced in ring A. The procedure is stereo-unspecific.

The first reaction is a reversible Michael addition with acetone dicarboxylic acid ester monoamide, whereby (by virtue of the differences in acidity of the two CH_2 groups next to the carbonyl group, on the one hand when adjacent to an ester group and on the other when adjacent to an amide group) the anion next to the ester function reacts in the presence of NaH with the double bond of (187). This can happen both from the uppermost as well as from the reverse side of the molecule, so that a mixture of two reaction products can be expected differing in their absolute configuration at the C4 atom. The next step is the attack of the second anion on the azlactone, causing ring opening to complete ring A. The next reaction step, a Dieckmann condensation, produces the corresponding tetracyclic compounds. This gives a total of eight possible stereoisomers in various yields. These eight stereoisomers are shown in Fig. 21. Their number can be reduced to four isomers by epimerization using suitable bases. These are grouped in two pairs of antipodes.

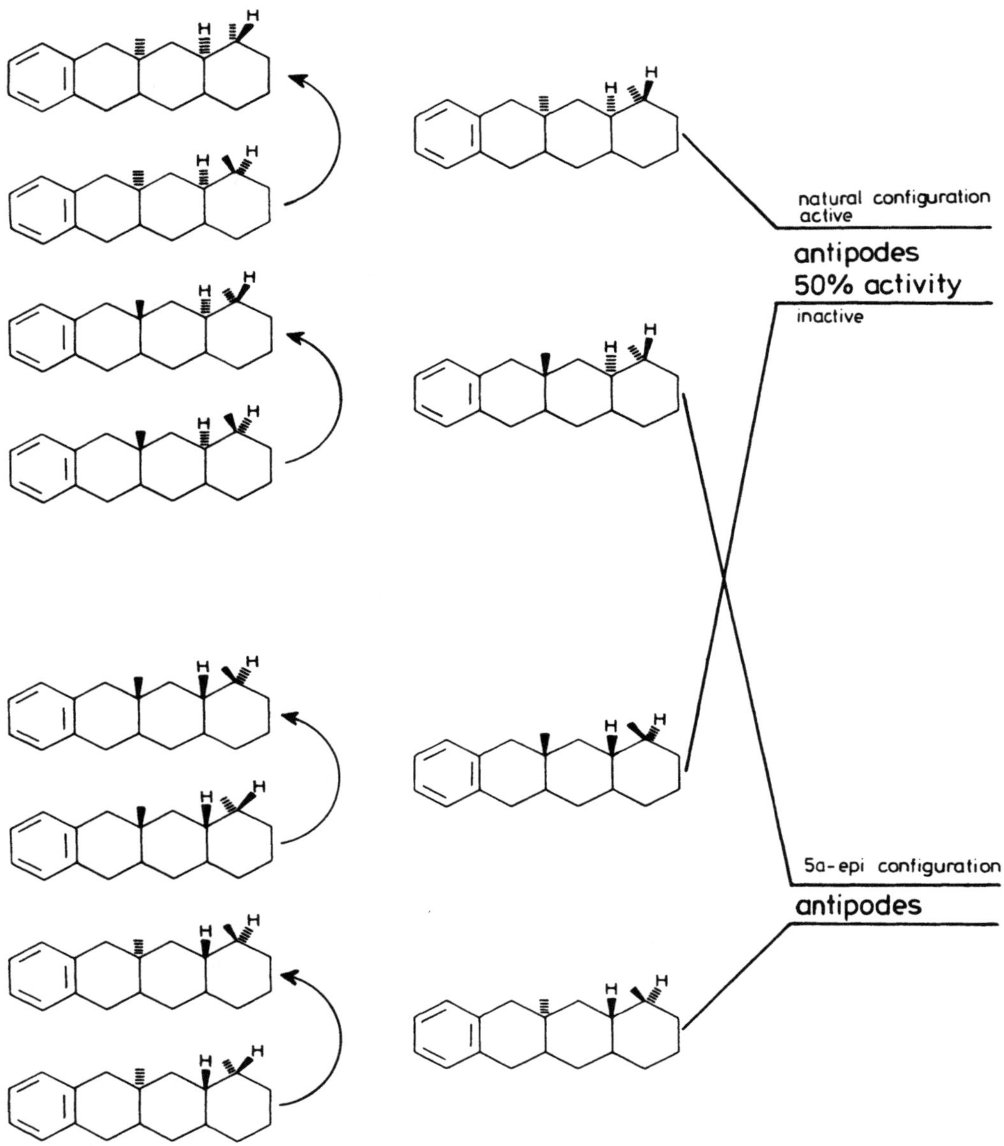

Fig. 21. Stereochemistry at the C4, C4a, and C5a atoms. Cyclization to the tetracycline compounds yields eight possible stereoisomers. Epimerization at the C4 atom with base yields the C4, C4a *trans* hydrogen

In the total synthesis of this simplest racemic tetracyclic compound with *syn* protons at C4a and C5a it is seen that the product is only 50% as effective as the corresponding natural tetracyclines. This seems indicative of the fact that only the antipode with the natural configuration at the asymetrical centers has the full activity whereas the other antipode is apparently devoid of activity.

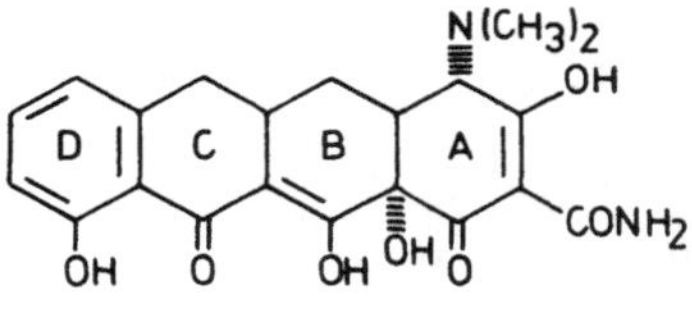

196

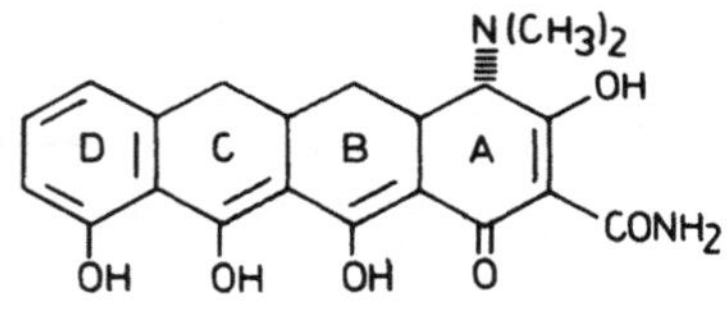

197

Fig. 22. The tetracycline ring system

One characteristic of the tetracyclines is their ring system consisting of four linear-anellated six-membered rings, namely 1,4,4a,5,5a,6,11,12a-octahydronaphthacene, with a characteristic arrangement of the double bonds. A distinction is made between the two chromophore regions A and BCD, which are separated by the 12a-hydroxy group. This ring system (196) has very characteristic UV spectra. The BCD chromophore absorbs at 225, 285, 320, and 360 nm, and the ring A chromophore at 262 nm.

The tetracyclic ring system without the 12a-hydroxy group has a completely different UV spectrum. This is displaced way into the long-wave region and lies between 400 and 500 nm.

Scrutiny of the Dreiding models shows that 12a-deoxytetracyclines with a *cis* configuration of protons at C4a and C5a have a completely enolized, virtually planar, and relatively tension-free ring system conjugated through all four rings [(197), Fig. 22]. In methanolic borate solution complexing leads to a ring system conjugated in this way and absorbing at between 400 and 500 nm.

Observation of 4a,5a-*trans*-12a-deoxytetracycline models suggests that certain torsional stresses must be overcome in order to obtain a system with some degree of planarity. However, since the degree of planarity of the molecule affects the conjugation of the β-tetracarbonyl system, compounds with the *trans* arrangement of protons at C4a and C5a should differ in their absorptivities.

Epimerization at center C4 to C4,C4a-*trans*-arranged hydrogens is performed in pyridine. Dreiding models indicate that compounds with C4a,C4-*trans* protons can assume two conformations. In the one there is an angle of about 90° between the protons at C4a and C4, in the other an angle of 180°. The compound having a *cis* configuration of protons at C4a and C4 can also assume two conformations. In both cases, however, the protons are in the Gauche disposition. This results in a small coupling constant for the two conformations while the large coupling constant in ^{1}H NMR is due to the *trans* configuration of protons at C4a,C4.

II. Anhydrotetracyclines

1. Chemistry

The numerous substituents in the tetracyclic ring system as well as their relative positions to one another make these compounds extremely ready to react with acidic, alkaline, and reductive agents. The effect of acids on tetracyclines has been simply to dehydrate them to anhydrotetracyclines. Thus, for instance, aureomycin (7-chlorotetracycline) (6) is converted in a mild reaction with mineral acids

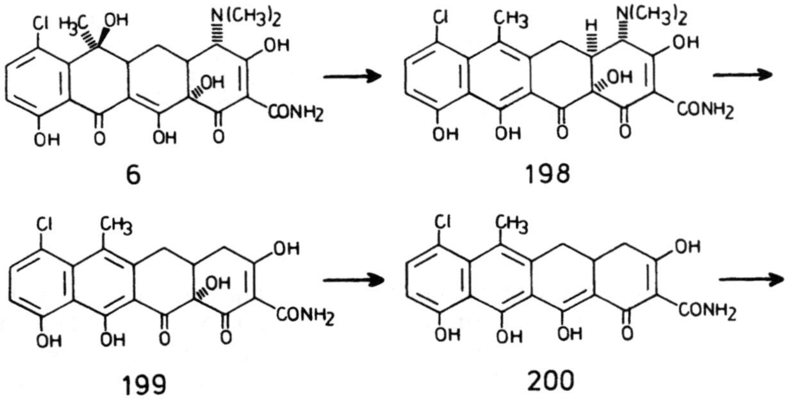

Fig. 23. Degradation of 7-chlorotetracycline to 5a,6-anhydro-7-chlorotetracycline

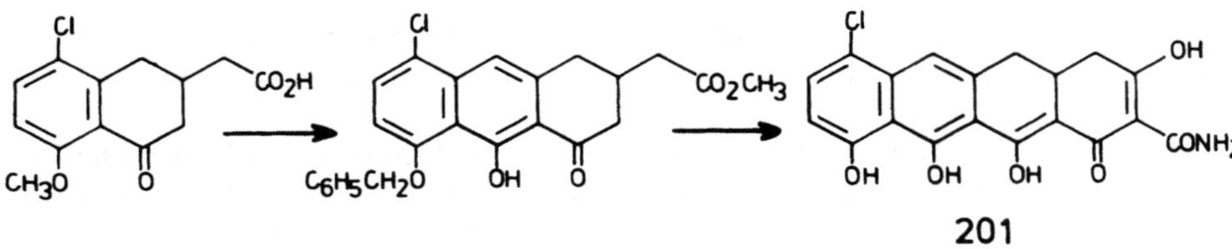

Fig. 24. Synthesis of 6-demethyl-12a-deoxy-7-chloroanhydrotetracycline. (BOOTHE et al. 1959)

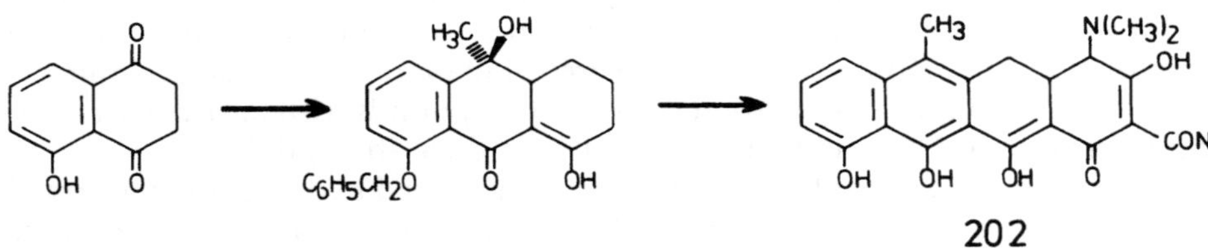

Fig. 25. Synthesis of 12a-deoxyanhydrotetracycline. (GUREVICH et al. 1967)

into anhydroaureomycin (198) (STEPHENS et al. 1954). Further reduction leads to the formation of anhydroaureomycins (199) and (200) (Fig. 23).

Early synthesis work centered round the production of these anhydrotetracyclines. In particular, the research groups of Lederle (Fig. 24) (BOOTHE et al. 1959; KENDE et al. 1961; FIELDS et al. 1960, 1961; WILKINSON and BOOTHE 1961), Shemyakin (Fig. 25) (GUREVICH et al. 1967) and Muxfeldt (Fig. 26) (MUXFELDT 1962) set the synthesis of anhydrotetracyclines as their objective. Synthesis always terminated, however, at a precursor of anhydrotetracycline (198), with compounds (201), (202), and (199) being arrived at. Only when the Muxfeldt synthetic principle had found general applicability was it possible to synthesize anhydrotetracycline (198) (Fig. 27).

Preparation of the condensed azlactone (203) uses the Muxfeldt principle of synthesis (MUXFELDT et al. 1973). The substance can be reacted with monomethyl

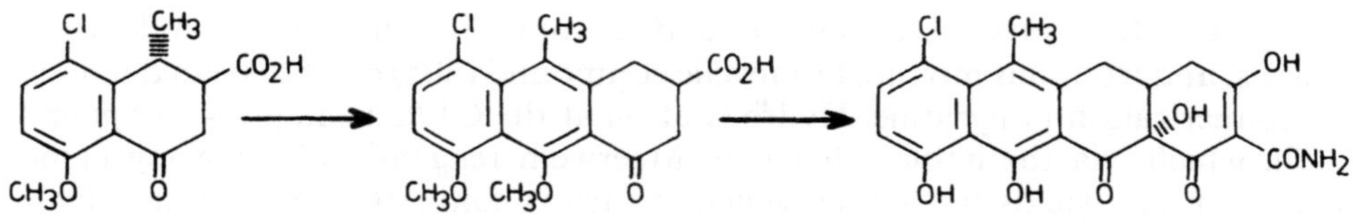

199

Fig. 26. Synthesis of dedimethylaminoanhydrotetracycline. (MUXFELDT 1962)

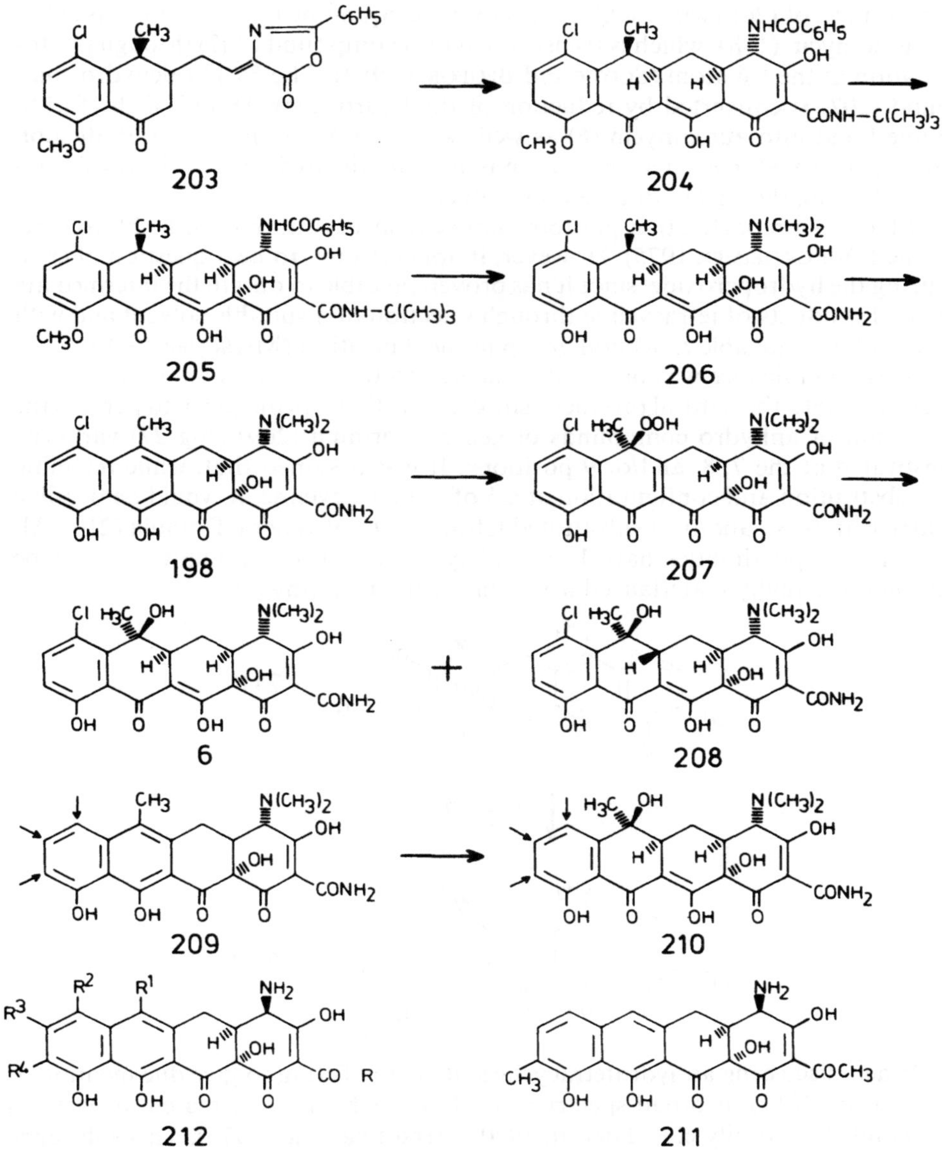

Fig. 27. Synthesis of anhydrotetracyclines

3-oxoglutarate to give a stereoisomer and tautomer mixture of tetracyclic compounds, and from this mixture tetracyclic compound (204) can be isolated following epimerization in pyridine. Hydroxylation at the C12a atom gives compound (205), which, via the imino ether with Meerwein reagent and following imino ether cleavage, yields the amine, which in turn is converted with formaldehyde under reductive conditions into the corresponding 4-dimethylamino compound. Following cleavage of the C10 methoxy group leaving the hydroxy group and after splitting off of the *tert*-butyl group, tetracyclic compound (206) is formed. Dehydration of (206) with dichlorodicyanobenzoquinone in dioxane yields anhydroaureomycin (198), which is transformed into compound (207) through photooxidation at the C6 atom (SCOTT and BEDFORD 1962). The 5a,11a-dehydro compound (207) is converted by reduction of the hydroperoxide and of the 5a,11a double bond into aureomycin (6) as well as into its 5a epimer (208). Reduction can be performed in such a way that initially only the hydroperoxide at C6 is reduced, leaving the 5a,11a double bond intact.

It has been reported that photooxidation is successful only with chlorotetracycline (DÜRCKHEIMER 1975). However, it appears only to be a question of crystallizing the hydroperoxide, since it has proven possible to obtain the intermediate and end products of tetracycline through selection of a suitable solvent and with the aid of a removable *tert*-butyl group in the 9 position (MITSCHER 1978).

Great significance was originally attached to the reconversion of anhydrotetracyclines into the natural products, since the synthetic principle used permits the formation of anhydro compounds of general formula (209) (Fig. 27) variously substituted at the 7, 8, and/or 9 positions. It was assumed that, while retaining the substitution and configuration at C6 of the tetracycline, it would be possible to arrive at 7-, 8-, and/or 9-substituted tetracyclines of general formula (210). Although such possibilities have been widely discussed, compounds of this type have never actually materialized using this synthetic pathway.

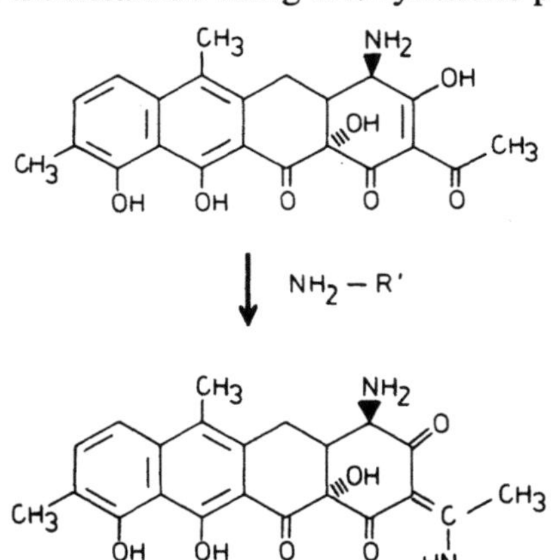

211

211a

When discussing anhydrotetracyclines it is only fitting to give due mention to chelocardin (211), a broad-spectrum antibiotic which was isolated as early as 1956 and structurally elucidated in 1970 (MITSCHER et al. 1970). This substance possesses the ring system of anhydrotetracycline as well as, by contrast, an acetyl group in the 2 position, a primary amino group in the 4 position in β-configuration, and a methyl group in the 9 position. Structural transformations along the lines of general formula (212) via anhydrotetracycline synthesis remain unreported.

However, during the investigation of the chemical modification of chelocardin (211) (CHU and HUCKIN 1980; CHU et al. 1981), it was found that the A-ring β-triketone is the most reactive center in the molecule. It was observed that amines react with β-triketones having an exocyclic carbonyl side-chain to give exclusively β,β′-diketonamines with substitution at the side-chain carbonyl.

Thus the reactions of chelocardin (211) with amines or related compounds lead to products of type (211 a), which possess similar biological activity to that of the parent antibiotic. The possibility of the existence of tautomers and the geometrical isomer at position 2 of the ring system was not excluded.

2. Effect of Structural Variation on Antibacterial Activity

Research into synthesis involving the 5a,6-anhydrotetracyclines has not revealed anything new as regards structure-activity relationships. A residual activity has been described for the 5a,6-anhydrotetracyclines (BLACKWOOD and ENGLISH 1970), which is particularly noticeable against gram-positive bacteria. This activity is thought not to stem, however, from the action principle of the tetracyclines but rather from a different active mechanism (KOSCHEL et al. 1966). Chelocardin (211) has an antibacterial spectrum similar to that of chloramphenicol. It is highly effective in vivo although it exhibits liver toxicity in animals (OLIVER et al. 1962; SINCLAIR et al. 1962), and has thus never been used for therapeutic purposes.

It is conceivable that chelocardine might follow the action principle of 5a,6-anhydrotetracyclines as distinct from the mechanism of the tetracyclines. Although it might have been possible to modify the structure of anhydrotetracyclines using the new synthetic principles, interest shown has been only slight, so that there has since been no deeper involvement in the structure-activity relationships of the anhydrotetracyclines.

III. (±)-B-Nortetracyclines

1. Chemistry

It has already been mentioned that there are possible compounds not possessing the full tetracycline structure and yet fulfilling the criteria fundamental to tetracycline activity. One of these substances is B-nortetracycline (213), in which the B-ring is no longer six but five membered, since the C5 atom has been eliminated from the basic skeleton. This conception was pursued almost simultaneously by the research groups of Hoechst AG (DÜRCKHEIMER 1975) and of E. Merck (W. Rogalski, unpublished research).

In both cases the basic structure is synthesized using the principle developed by Muxfeldt. While Hoechst proceeds from the aldehyde (214) and describes the tetracyclic mixture (215), the E. Merck research group selected the aldehyde (218) (BOOTHE et al. 1959; MUXFELDT and ROGALSKI 1965) to produce the tetracyclic ring system (Fig. 28).

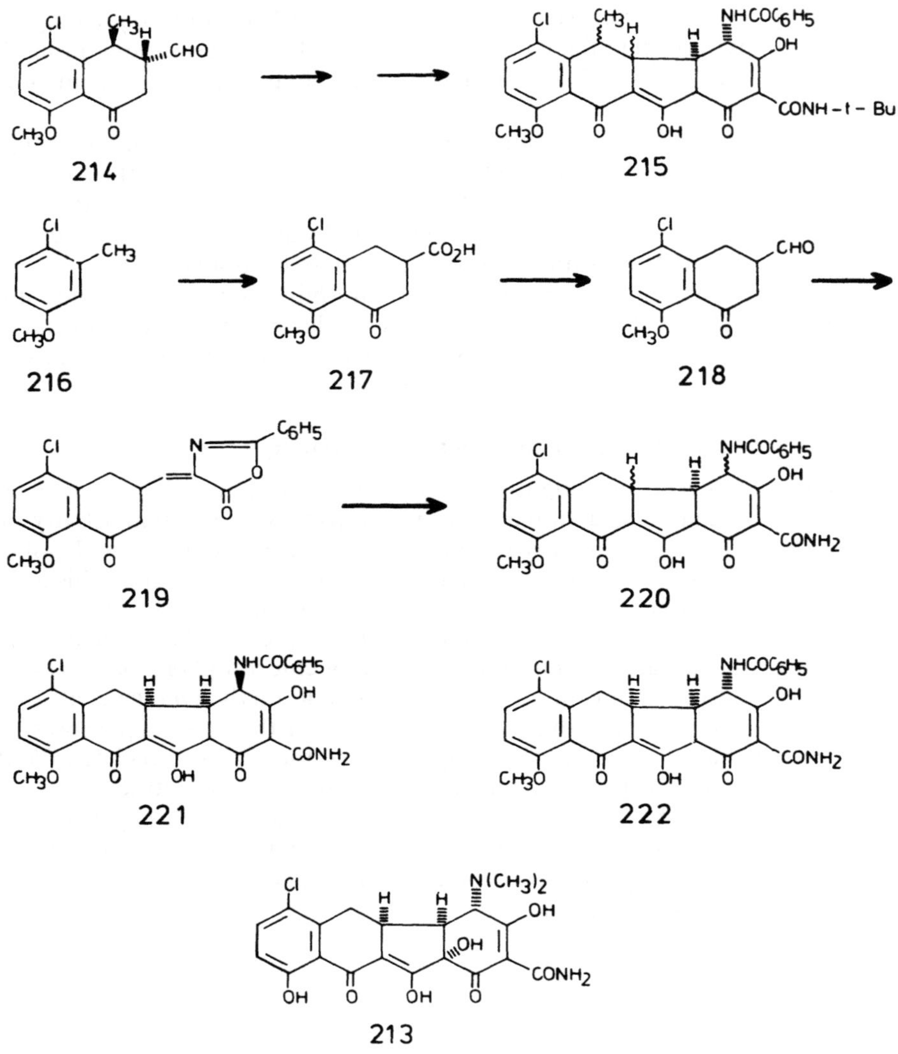

Fig. 28. Synthesis of (±)-B-nortetracyclines

The starting material used by the E. Merck group to synthesize the aldehyde is 1-chloro-2-methyl-4-methoxybenzene (216), which is converted in a three-step process into the tetralonecarboxylic acid (217).

The aldehyde (218) is arrived at in three more steps. When reacted with hippuric acid in acetic anhydride with lead acetate as catalyst, the aldehyde yields the condensed product (219). Reacting (219) with acetonedicarboxylic acid ester monoamide in a mixture of dioxane/dimethyl sulfoxide together with sodium hydride gives the tetracyclic C4, C5a epimer mixture (220) in excellent yield. The two compounds (221) and (222) can be isolated from the isomer mixture. Their UV absorption spectra in $n/10$ molar methanolic borate solution have maxima in the long-wave range at 465 µm, this being characteristic of 12a-deoxytetracyclines.

This would indicate that the tetracyclic ring system is thoroughly conjugated as a result of enolization of the β-dicarbonyl system. The stereochemistry of (221) and (212) can be assigned using nuclear magnetic resonance spectroscopy. The ring system is apparently so stretched by the five-membered ring that all other reactions which are intended to give end product (213) split the ring system. The Hoechst research group similarly describes only compound (215) (DÜRCKHEIMER 1975).

2. Effect of Structural Variation on Antibacterial Activity

There were no new findings regarding structure-activity relationships since the final products sought were never reached. Tests to see whether compound (222) had any antibacterial activity showed only a hint of in vitro activity against a number of gram-positive bacteria, although this is of absolutely no practical significance.

IV. Modification at the C2 Position: (±)-4-Amino-7-chloro-2-*N*-methylcarbonyl-2-decarbonyl-4-dedimethylamino-6-demethyl-6-deoxytetracyclines

1. Chemistry

Total synthesis of (±)-4-amino-7-chloro-2-*N*-methylcarbamyl-2-decarbamyl-4-dedimethylamino-6-demethyl-6-deoxytetracycline (224) involves the deliberate introduction of a methyl group at the carbamyl function in the 2 position.

Synthesis was by the principle of Muxfeldt (URBACH et al. 1973). The racemic aldehyde (184) condenses with hippuric acid in tetrahydrofuran in the presence of basic lead acetate and acetic anhydride to give the oxazolinone (187) (Fig. 29). This is converted with the *N*-methylamide (223) of monomethyl 3-oxoglutarate in tetrahydrofuran in the presence of sodium hydride to give a racemic tetracyclic isomer mixture. Epimerization at the C4 atom with pyridine, oxidation with oxygen in dimethylformamide in the presence of sodium hydride to give the 12a-hydroxy compound, transformation of the C4 benzamido group into an amino group, followed by ether cleavage at the C10 atom lead to the racemic end product (224).

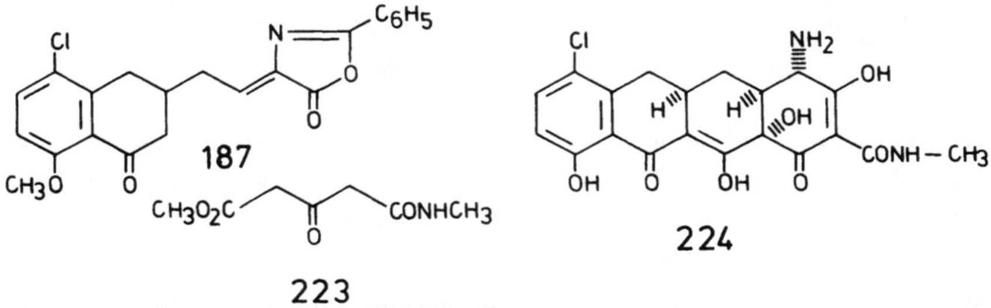

223

Fig. 29. Principle of the synthesis of compound (224)

2. Effect of Structural Variation on Antibacterial Activity

Compound (224) essentially differs from other compounds discovered to date in that it has a primary amino group in the 4 position and a methyl-substituted 2-carbamyl group. It is described as having pronounced bacteriostatic activity. No quantitative data are available. It is known that compounds similar to the one in question fall in line with the general pattern of tetracycline activity. It can be assumed, therefore, that compound (224) represents no particular breakthrough in terms of antibacterial activity.

V. Modifications at the C5a and C6 Positions: (±)-7-Chloro-6-deoxytetracyclines and (±)-7-Chloro-6-demethyl-6-deoxytetracyclines

1. Chemistry

The total synthesis of (±)-7-chloro-6-deoxytetracyclines and (±)-7-chloro-6-demethyl-6-deoxytetracyclines of the natural 6-epi and 5a-epi series essentially involves a deliberate modification of the C6 position, the 5a-epi compound being formed simultaneously as a result of the nonstereospecific composition of the ring system (MARTIN et al. 1973; DÜRCKHEIMER 1975). The ring system is formed using the synthesis principle developed by Muxfeldt. The starting materials used were the two aldehydes (184) and (225) described in the literature as being intermediate products in tetracycline synthesis. These can be converted in a manner analogous to the synthesis described in Sect. B.IV via a number of intermediate steps into the required end products (226)–(232) (Fig. 30).

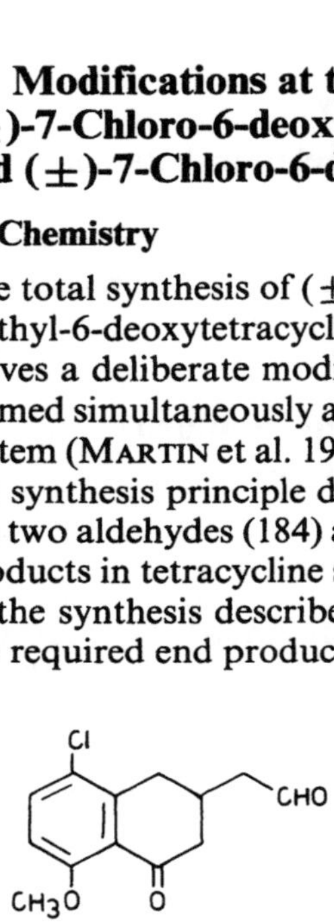

184

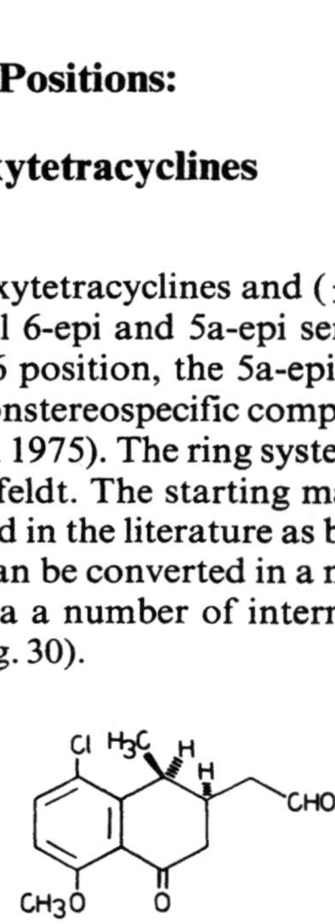

225

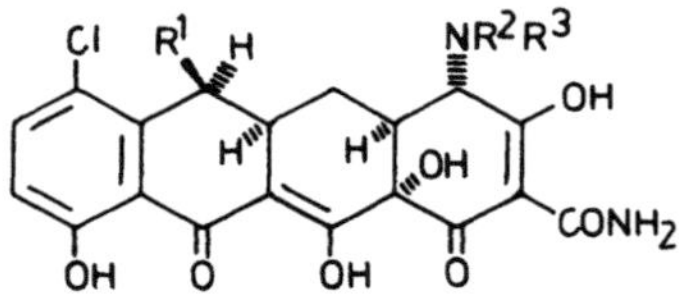

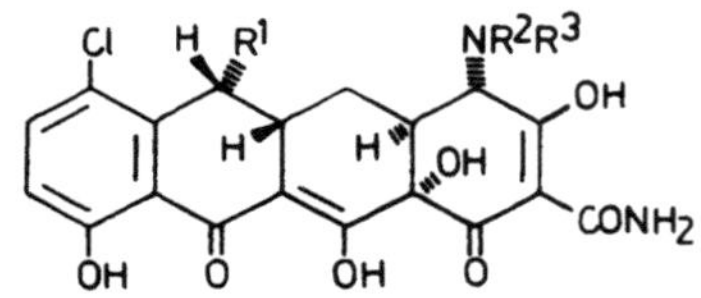

226: R^1 = R^2 = R^3 = H

227: R^1 = CH_3 , R^2 = R^3 = H

228: R^1 = H , R^2 = R^3 = CH_3

229: R^1 = R^2 = R^3 = CH_3

230: R^1 = CH_3 , R^2 = R^3 = H

231: R^1 = R^2 = R^3 = H

232: R^1 = H , R^2 = R^3 = C_2H_5

Fig. 30. Synthesis of (±)-7-chloro-6-deoxytetracyclines and (±)-7-chloro-6-demethyl-6-deoxytetracyclines

2. Effect of Structural Variation on Antibacterial Activity

The tetracyclic compounds (226)–(232) are described as being considerably more lipophilic than the natural tetracyclines (DÜRCKHEIMER 1975). Their antibacterial spectrum is similar in many ways to that of tetracyclines, although a high degree of efficacy against a number of tetracycline-resistant strains is also noted. No quantitative data are available at present. It is known from investigations into other tetracycline series that an increase in the lipophilicity of the tetracyclines is accompanied by an increase in activity against tetracycline-resistant gram-positive organisms, while there is a simultaneous decline in activity against tetracycline-sensitive gram-negative bacteria. The fact that compound (232) is a special case among the above-mentioned totally synthetic tetracyclines comes as no surprise, since enlargement of the substituents at the C4 amino group beyond the methyl group causes the activity to be diminished.

The activity of the tetracyclines described above fell when serum was added and was disappointing in animal trials. The reason for these occurrences is quoted as being a strong, unspecific binding of these antibiotics to serum proteins and tissue components, so that the concentration of free, chemotherapeutically active tetracyclines appears to be no longer adequate to achieve bateriostasis in the organism (DÜRCKHEIMER 1975).

VI. Modification at the C7 Position: (±)-7-Methoxy-6-demethyl-6-deoxytetracyclines

1. Chemistry

The first findings regarding the activity of 5a-epi tetracyclines were contradictory. These substances attracted new interest, however, when they became directly accessible by totally synthetic means.

In order to elucidate the structure-activity relationships, 6-demethyl-6-deoxy-7-methoxytetracyclines and, in particular, their 5a epimers were prepared (W. Rogalski and R. Kirchlechner, unpublished research). The tetracyclic ring system is synthesized by the Muxfeldt principle (Fig. 31). The racemic aldehyde (233) reacts with the thiazolinone in the presence of a base to produce the unsaturated thiazolinone derivative (234), which when reacted with the amide of monomethyl 3-oxoglutarate in tetrahydrafurane (THF) in the presence of sodium hydride produces a mixture of four racemic tetracyclic isomers, from which the two racemic tetracyclines (235) and (236) can be isolated following pyridine-catalyzed epimerization at the C4 atom. Compounds (235) and (236) were then reacted in the manner already described, with end products (240) and (242) being obtained. During synthesis of the end products, compounds (237), (238), and (239) from the natural tetracycline series and compounds (241) and (243) from the 5a-epi series are obtained.

2. Effect of Structural Variation on Antibacterial Activity

In the total synthesis of 6-demethyl-6-deoxy-7-chlorotetracycline, the corresponding racemic 5a epimer (244) was also obtained. Investigation of in vitro ac-

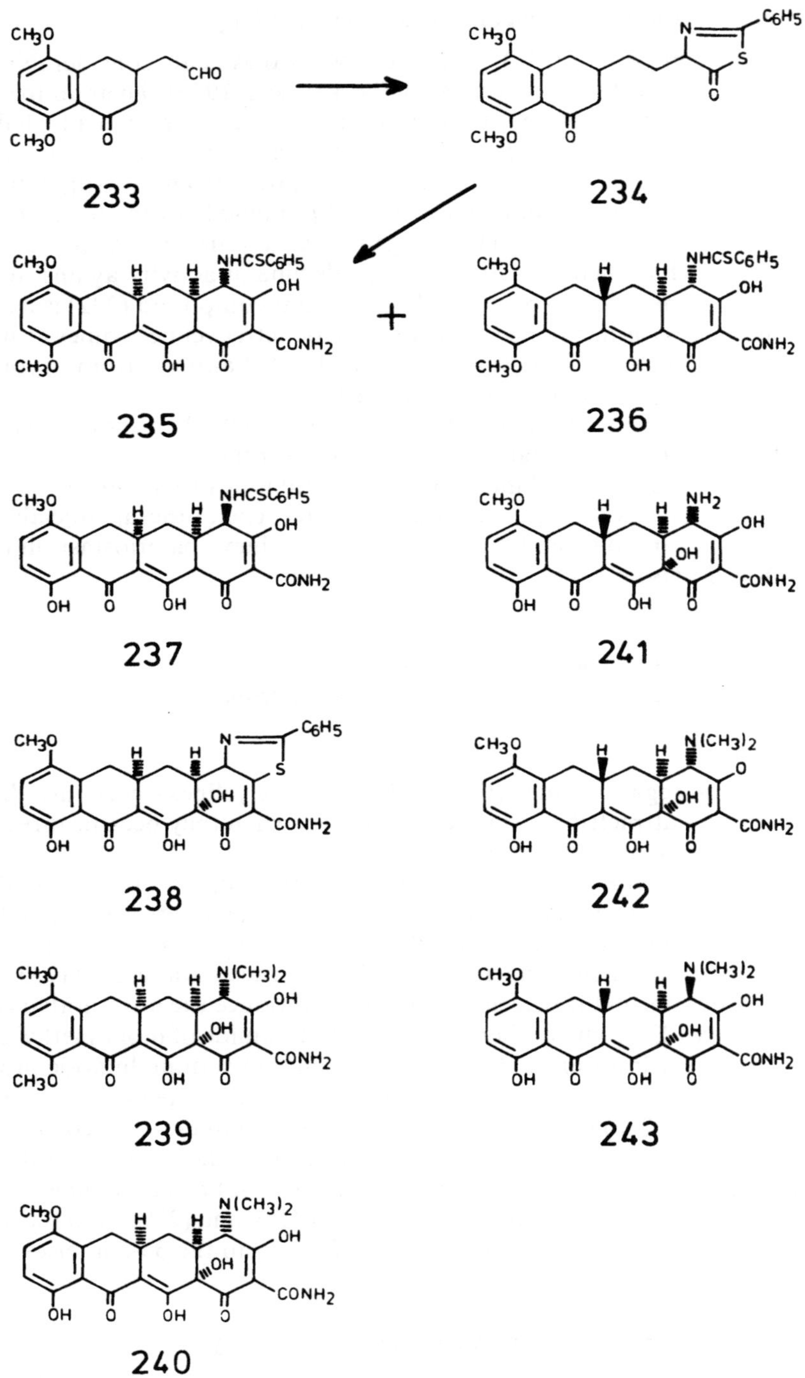

Fig. 31. Synthesis of (±)-6-demethyl-6-deoxy-7-methoxytetracyclines

Table 16. In vitro activity of tetracycline and the racemic 6-demethyl-6-deoxy-5a-epitetracycline. (H. MUXFELDT, unpublished research)

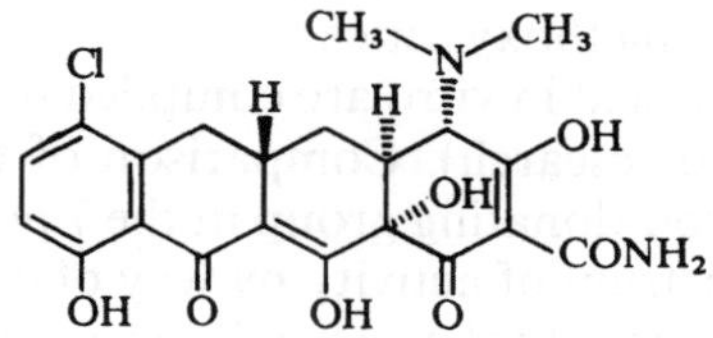

244

Organism	Minimum inhibitory concentrations (μg/ml)	
	Tetracycline	(±)-5a-Epitetracycline
Staphylococcus aureus	50	0.78
Staphylococcus aureus	50	0.04
Streptococcus pyogenes	12.5	0.78
Escherichia coli	100	12.5
Pasturella multocida	6.25	0.19
Salmonella typhosa	100	25

Table 17. In vitro activity of 6-demethyl-6-deoxy-7-methoxytetracyclines modified at positions C4 and C5a. (H. WAHLIG and E. DINGELDEIN, unpublished research)

Organism	Tetracycline	Minimum inhibitory concentrations (μg/ml) Structures					
		5a-α (normal)			5a-β (epi)		
		(237)	(238)	(239)	(241)	(242)	(243)
Escherichia coli C1	0.5	>128	>128	>128	4	4	128
Pseudomonas aeruginosa Ps 1	8	>128	>128	>128	128	>128	>128
Proteus OX19	8	>128	128	>128	4	4	4
Staphylococcus SG 511	0.1	< 0.1	0.5	>128	4	4	4
Streptococcus 3 A	0.1	< 0.1	0.5	>128	4	4	8
E. coli C71	128	>128	>128	>128	16	32	128
E. coli C72	64	>128	>128	>128	16	32	128
E. coli C74	>128	>128	>128	>128	16	32	>128
Aerobacter Ae. 5	64	>128	>128	>128	16	128	>128
A. Ae. 6	128	>128	>128	>128	16	32	>128
P. vulgaris P3	64	>128	>128	>128	16	32	128
P. vulgaris P4	64	>128	>128	>128	16	>128	>128
Staphylococcus aureus Sta 71	64	< 0.1	< 0.1	>128	4	4	4
S. aureus Sta 72	128	< 0.1	0.5	>128	4	4	4
S. aureus Sta 73	64	< 0.1	< 0.1	>128	4	4	4
Streptococcus faecalis 68	64	< 0.1	1	>128	4	8	8
S. faecalis 69	64	< 0.1	1	>128	4	8	8

tivity showed that (244) possesses good in vitro activity against a number of tetracycline-resistant organisms (Table 16) (H. Muxfeldt, unpublished research). The objective was then set of investigating these findings with totally synthetic compounds of the 5a-epi-7-methoxy series.

Results for substances tested in vitro are compiled in Table 17 (H. Wahlig and E. Dingeldein, unpublished research). Comparison of the data obtained shows that, as expected, an electron-donating group in the 7 position generally has a detrimental effect on the spectrum of activity by way of contrast to an electron-accepting group such as chlorine. In the case of compounds (241) and (242) of the 5a-epi series, although a trend is discernible in the expansion of the antibacterial spectrum in the gram-negative and gram-positive regions, the activity attained is of no practical significance and is not of the same itensity as in the 7-chloro series. The 4-epimeric compound (243) has a spectrum of activity which in the gram-positive range is very similar to that of the corresponding compound (242) but which is inferior in the gram-negative range. One striking feature is the in part good efficacy of compounds (237) and (238) against tetracycline-resistant gram-positive organisms. At the same time, however, these compounds are devoid of activity against tetracycline-resistant gram-negative organisms. Clearly, the effect of the greater lipophilicity of these compounds on the antibacterial spectrum makes itself felt. The lipophilicity is due to the lipophilic residues at the C4 atom. Compound (239) is without activity. It possesses all the prerequisites for antibacterial activity except that it has a methoxy group in the 10 position. It is quite clear, then, how crucial the 10-hydroxy group is to the activity.

VII. Modification at the C8 Position: (±)-8-Hydroxy-6-demethoxy-6-deoxytetracyclines

Tetracyclines have undergone innumerable semisynthetic modifications at all conceivable positions except for one which has never been reported, namely at the C8 atom. This position falls strictly within the realms of total synthesis. Position 8 in the tetracyclic ring system has always stirred the imagination, from a structural point of view as well as from the point of view of biosynthetic pathways. It is an astonishing fact that none of the known tetracyclines has an oxygen atom at the C8 atom of the tetracyclic ring system. For biogenetic reasons a hydroxy group should be anticipated in the 8 position (Fig. 32). It has been reported (McCormick and Jensen 1968; Vanek et al. 1974) that for the natural tetracyclines the hypothetical nonaketide (245) is assumed. It has been a source of speculation as to why prior to transformation of (245) to 6-methylpretetramide (246) the 8-keto group is reduced before being cyclized to the hydroxy group and eliminated, since its removal is not essential from a point of view of subsequent reactions (Glatz et al. 1979).

The fact that polyketide precursors can exist where such a reduction of the keto group does not occur is shown by the two antibiotics monardene (247) and chromocycline (248). Monardene (McCapra et al. 1964) is an antibiotic with tranquilizing properties which might stem from a hypothetical tetracycline precursor. Both phenolic hydroxy groups are present in this molecule.

245 246

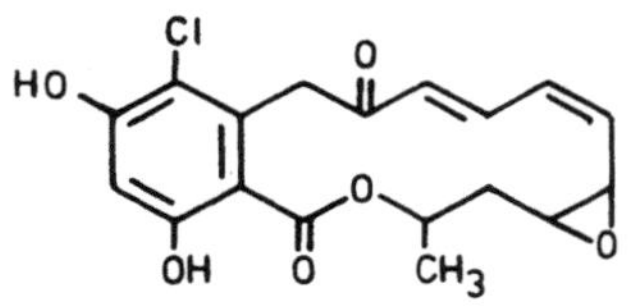

247

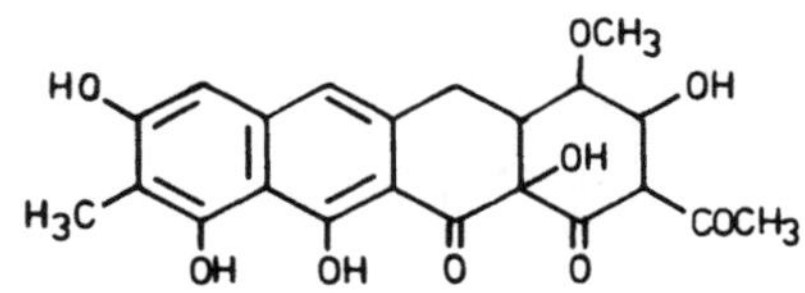

248

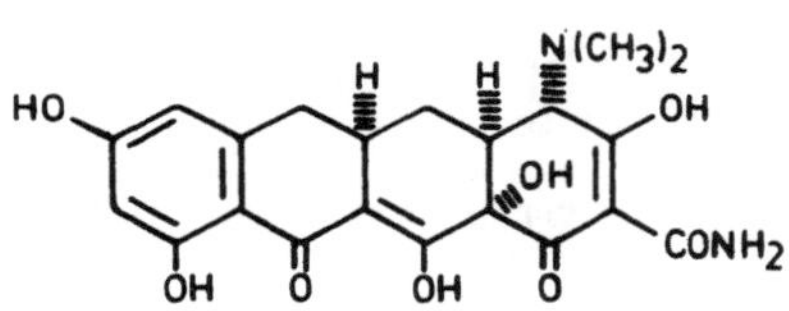

249

Fig. 32. The 8-hydroxy function in the tetracyclic ring system

A hypothetical tetracycline precursor is even more noticeable in the case of chromocycline (248) (BERLIN et al. 1968). This is an antibiotic with a 5a,6-anhydrotetracycline structure, having the discussed hydroxy group in the 8 position.

Moreover, in deviance from the normal tetracyclines it has an acetyl group in the 2 position, a methoxy group in the 4 position and, additionally, a methyl group in the 10 Position.

It has been supposed that the 8-hydroxytetracyclines or their precursors are so toxic for the producing organisms that possibly a mutant incapable of removing this oxygen function at some point in the biosynthesis is destroyed by the product. Whatever conjecture there might be concerning the 8-hydroxy group, it is known that substituents in ring D affect the biological activity of the tetracyclines. The fact that such 8-substituted tetracyclines have never been described makes tetracyclines with an oxygen function in the 8-position an objective very much worth aiming for. As far as is known, only the research group of Muxfeldt and that of E. Merck have made any attempts at synthesizing 8-hydroxytetracycline derivatives.

1. Chemistry

The synthesis of racemic 8-hydroxy-6-demethyl-6-deoxytetracycline (249) (GLATZ et al. 1979) follows the principle of synthesis developed by Muxfeldt (Fig. 33). The starting material used was 3,5-dimethoxybenzoic acid (250). Via

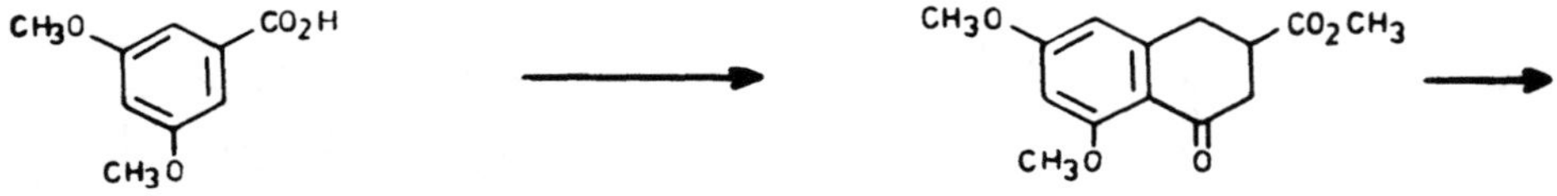

250 251

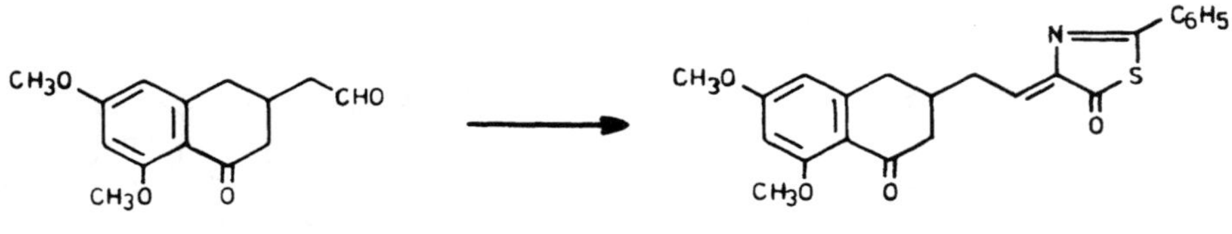

252 253

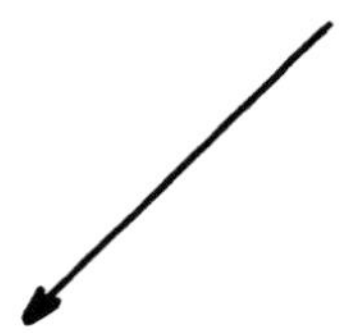

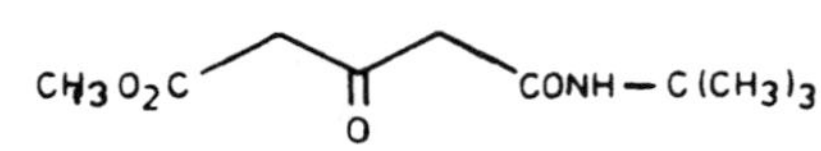

254

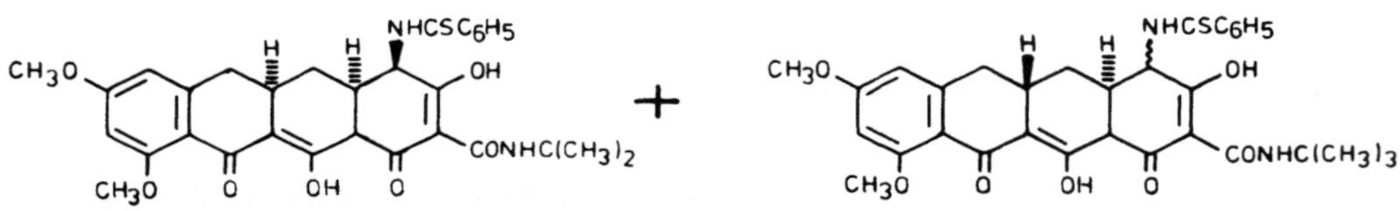

255 256

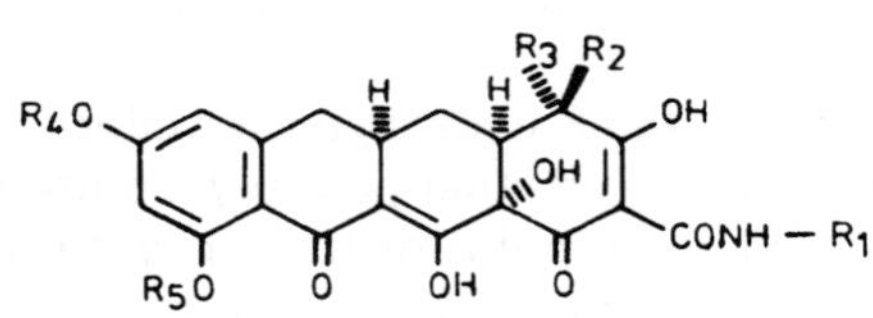

	R^1	R^2	R^3	R^4	R^5
257 :	$C(CH_3)_3$	$NHCSC_6H_5$	H	CH_3	CH_3
258 :	$C(CH_3)_3$	$NH_2 \cdot HCl$	H	CH_3	CH_3
259 :	$C(CH_3)_3$	$N(CH_3)_2$	H	CH_3	CH_3
260 :	$C(CH_3)_3$	H	$N(CH_3)_2$	CH_3	CH_3
261 :	$C(CH_3)_3$	H	$N(CH_3)_2$	CH_3	H
249 :	H	H	$N(CH_3)_2$	H	H

Fig. 33. Synthesis of (±)-8-hydroxy-6-demethyl-6-deoxytetracyclines

several reaction steps the dimethoxytetralonic acid methyl ester (251) was obtained, from which dimethoxytetralonacetaldehyde (252) was produced following several further reactions steps. The aldehyde (252) condensed with hippuric acid and lead acetate in acetic anhydride, producing the azlactone (253). Condensation of (253) with the amide of methyl 3-oxoglutarate (254) produced chiefly the C4 epimer (255) in a 47% yield, while the compound with normal configuration at C4 was only isolated in a 4% yield. The C5a epimer was obtained in a yield of 10% as the 1:1 C4 epimer mixture (256). 12-Hydroxylation of (255) was performed in dimethylformamide with potassium *tert*-butylate in the presence of triethyl phosphite by bubbling in oxygen at −30 °C, leading to compound (257). Transformation of (257) into the amine (258) ensued with triethyloxonium tetrafluoroborate through alkylation of the sulfur atom and subsequent acid hydrolysis of the imino ether. Methylation of the 4-amino group from (258) with formaldehyde under reductive conditions led to compound (259), which readily epimerizes at C4 into a mixture of (259) and (260). The epimerization equilibrium can be displaced, in ethanolic solution for instance, the (260) in a 94% yield, enabling (260) to be produced in pure form by this means. Treatment of (260) with boron tribromide gave the *N-tert*-butyl-8-methoxy-6-demethyl-6-deoxytetracycline (261). Cleaving off all the protective groups from compound (260) with hydriodic acid at 100 °C led to 8-hydroxy-6-demethyl-6-deoxytetracycline (249).

2. Effect of Structural Variation on Antibacterial Activity

It has simply been reported (GLATZ et al. 1979) that tetracyclines (249) and (261) have been tested in vitro for antibacterial activity and in vivo for activity in mice. For both compounds an activity was found which is considerably inferior to that of the normal therapeutically important tetracyclines. Quantitative results have not been published. Thus, any theories regarding the 8-hydroxy group's importance in respect of activity have not been substantiated, at least not in tests performed on pathogens.

The activity found for 8-hydroxy-6-demethyl-6-deoxytetracycline (249) appears to be in agreement with the results found for 7-hydroxy-6-demethyl-6-deoxytetracycline, a compound which has already been discussed in the first section under substitutions at the C7 atom. This also accords with the observation that electron-donating substituents decrease activity unless there is a simultaneous lipophilic effect as in the case of minocycline. Although nothing is known about the lipophilic property of (249), it is certainly fair to assume that it will not differ greatly from that of 7-hydroxy-6-demethyl-6-deoxytetracycline. However, this latter compound is known to be no more lipophilic than the normal tetracyclines. The 7-hydroxy derivative thus exhibited the anticipated decline in activity. The 8-hydroxy derivative (249) apparently behaves in the same manner.

Somewhat more complex, however, is the situation in *N-tert*-butyl-8-methoxy-6-demethyl-6-deoxytetracycline (261), since not only is there the electron-donating methoxy group but also the electron-donating characteristic of the *tert*-butyl substituent at the amide nitrogen, which leads to an increase in the partially negative charge at the amide oxygen. It has been reported on the basis of earlier determinations of crystalline structure that two molecular forms, the zwitterionic form and the nonionized form, are important for the attainment of antibacterial activity (STEZOWSKI 1976; PREWO and STEZOWSKI 1977).

It has been inferred from these findings that lipid-soluble tetracycline is represented through the nonionized conformation of the tetracycline base. The more the equilibrium lies on the side of the nonionized form, the more lipophilic the compound is. The findings from crystalline structure investigations of compound (261) are that the conformation of (261) is similar but not identical with that of the fully associated 5-oxytetracycline base, the difference being mainly in the hydrogen bonding in the A-ring (GLATZ et al. 1979). The reason for the difference in the hydrogen bonding is probably the electron-donating character of the *tert*-butyl substituent on the amide nitrogen causing a higher degree of the negative charge on the amide oxygen and further therefore a relatively high degree of protonization of the amide oxygen in this compound as compared to the natural tetracyclines. It is assumed that the higher degree of protonization may be indicative of the stabilization of the nonionized form of the tetracycline base. Such stabilization would be apparent in the form of an increase in lipophilicity. This would also mean a decrease in antibacterial activity.

In actual fact, compound (261) has a highly lipophilic character and it is considerably less active than the usual medicinal tetracyclines. These statements regarding the activity and lipophilicity of compound (261) are in agreement with reports that the reduced antibacterial activity of *N-tert*-butyl-6-demethyl-6-deoxytetracycline, an analogue of *N-tert*-butyl-8-methoxy-6-demethyl-6-deoxytetracycline (261), is the result of the extremely lipophilic nature of this compound (BLACKWOOD and ENGLISH 1970).

The lipophilicity of compound (261) may partially be caused by a structural effect as discussed above and partially by the hydrophobic nature of the *tert*-butyl group.

Summarizing, it can be stated that tetracyclines having an oxygen function in the 8 position have failed to fulfill the expectations placed in them, namely that they might lead to increased activity. On the contrary, they are considerably less active than the normal tetracyclines.

VIII. Modifications at the C5a Position: (±)-5a-Methyl-6-demethyl-6-deoxytetracyclines

1. Chemistry

In order to afford a better understanding of interrelationships between lipophilicity and the electronic influence of substituents as well of configuration and conformation on the activity of tetracyclines, alkyl substituents were introduced in the 5a position and simultaneously a variety of substitutions was performed in the 7 position (W. Rogalski, R. Kirchlechner, unpublished research). In Fig. 34 the synthesis of (±)-6-demethyl-6-deoxy-7-chloro-5a-methyltetracyclines is described.

Taking 3-methoxybenzyl alcohol as a basis, the benzyl chloride can be produced with thionyl chloride and then, by chlorination, the 2-chloro-5-methoxybenzyl chloride can be prepared in good yield.

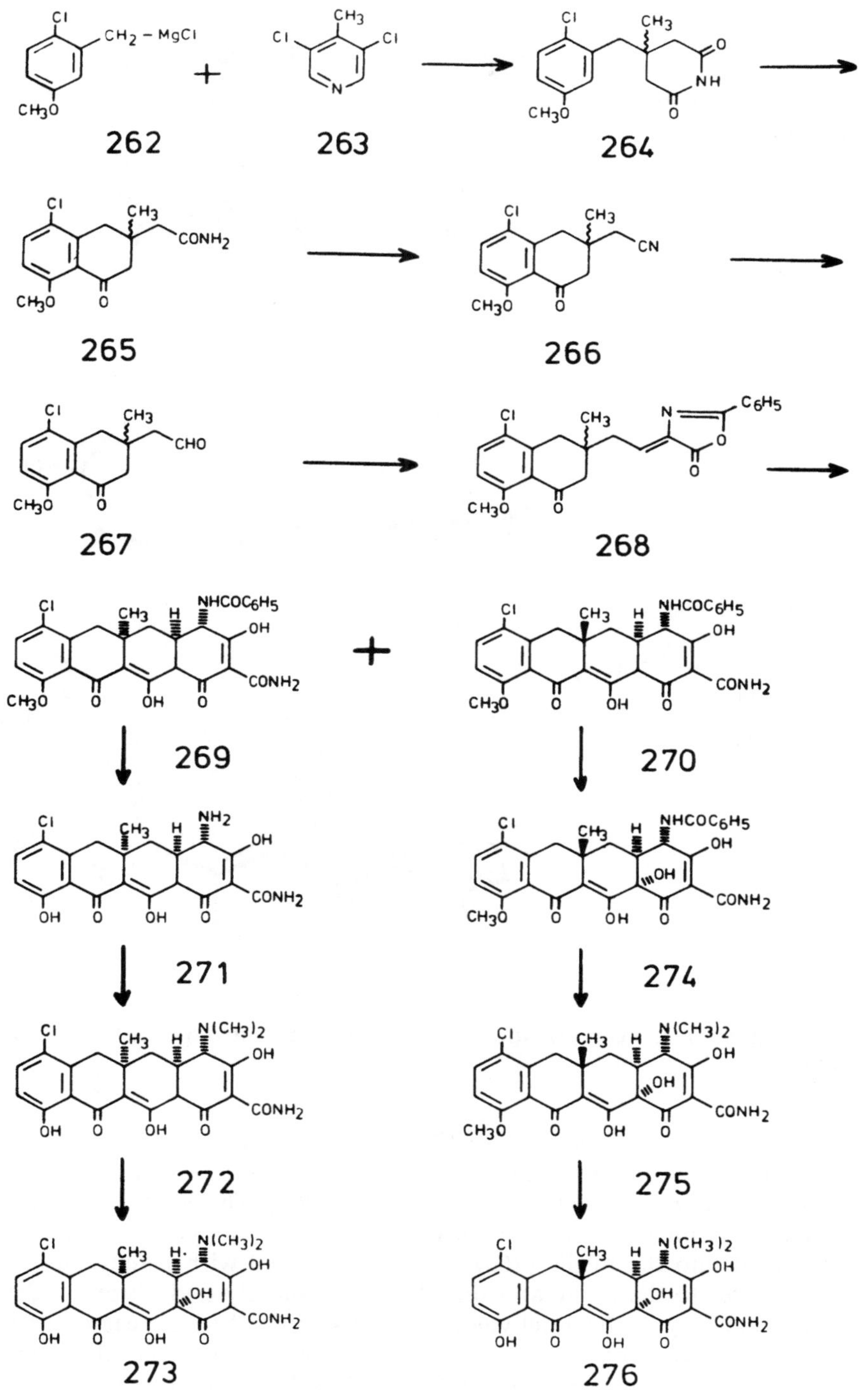

Fig. 34. Synthesis of (±)-6-demethyl-6-deoxy-7-chloro-5a-methyltetracyclines

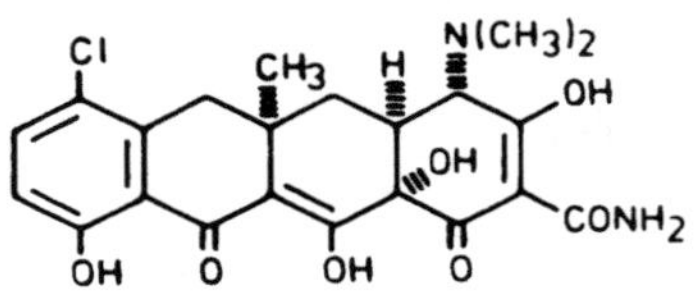

273

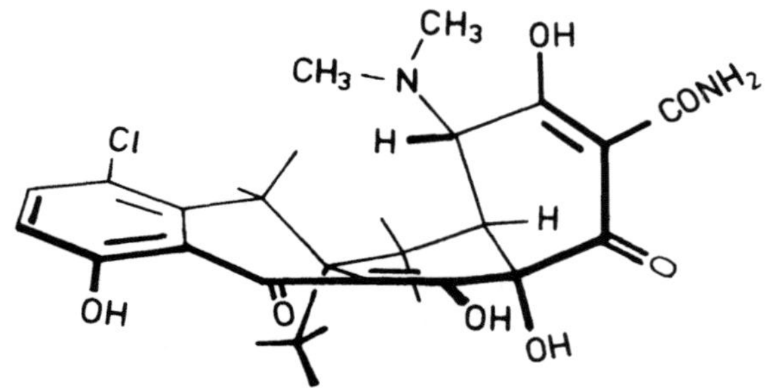

1

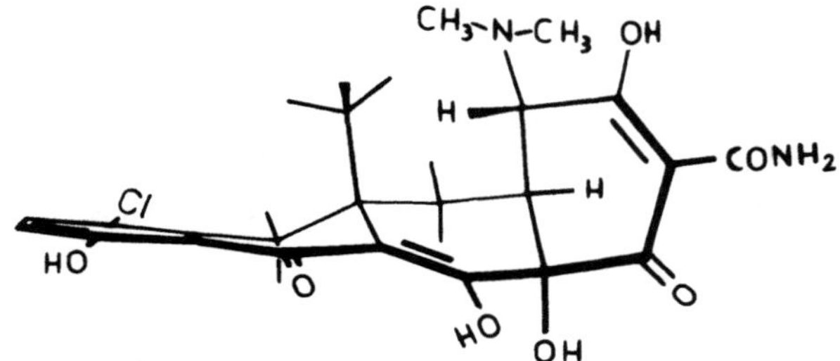

2

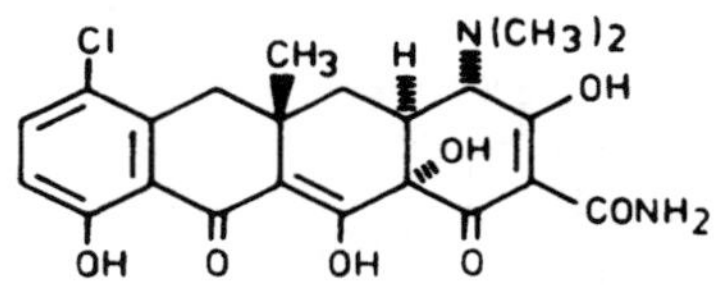

276

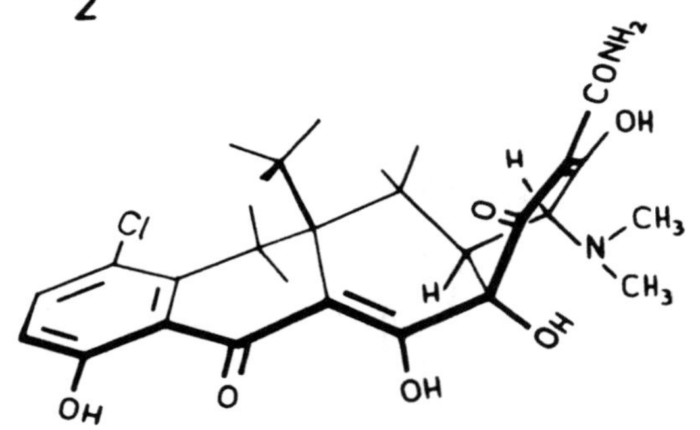

3

Fig. 35. Configuration and conformation of 5a-methyl-substituted 6-demethyl-6-deoxytetracyclines

Applying a Grignard reaction to (262) with 2,6-dichloro-4-methylpyridine (263), the corresponding imide (264) is obtained, which in polyphosphoric acid, for instance, is cyclized to the tetralone derivative (265). The acetamide side chain in the 3 position which is formed thereby is transformed in pyridine with p-toluenesulfonic acid into the nitrile (266), which is reduced with Raney nickel in a phosphate buffer to the imine and this then immediately hydrolyzed under the same conditions to give the aldehyde (267). This could then be reacted with the azlactone, prepared from hippuric acid and, for instance, dicyclohexyl carbodiimide in THF in the presence of $MgSO_4$ and lead acetate to give the azlactone

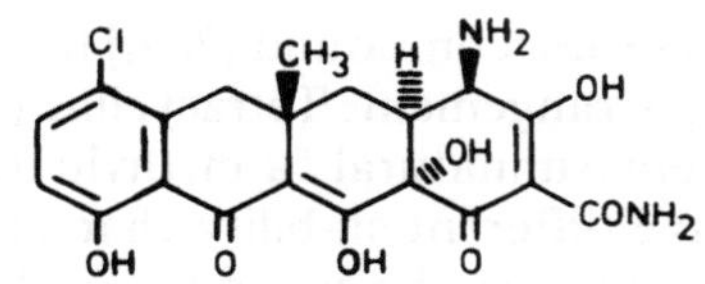

277

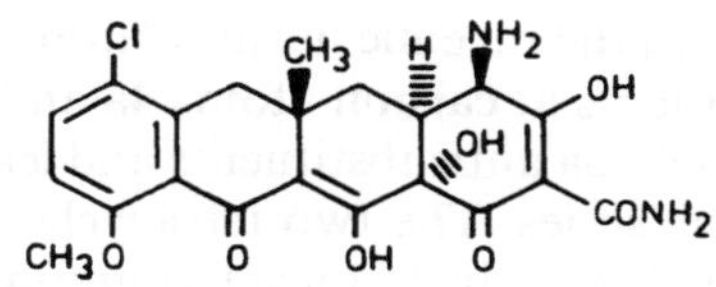

278

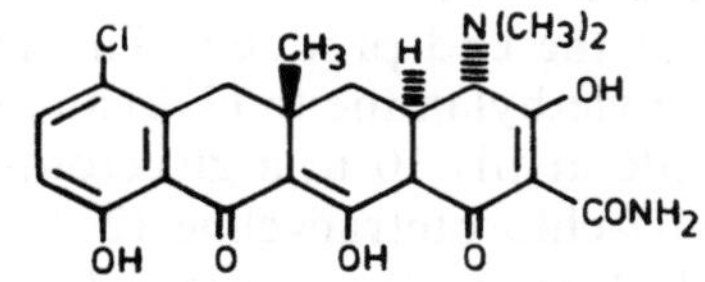

279

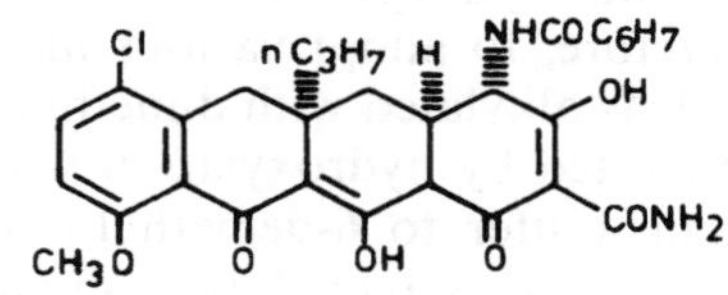

280

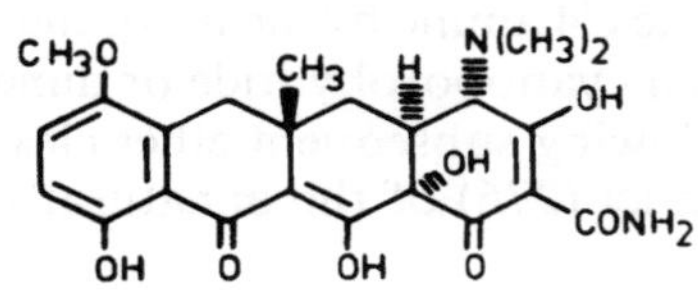

281

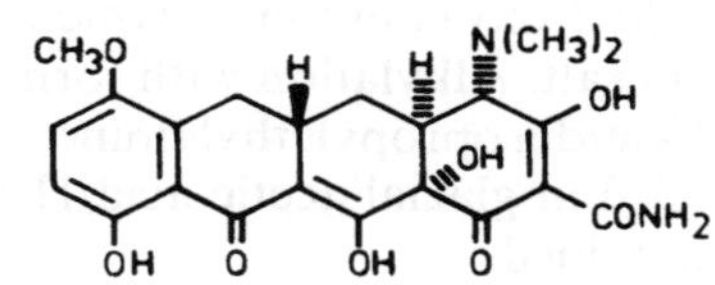

242

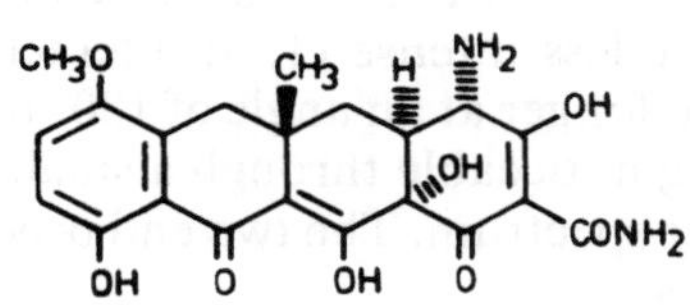

282

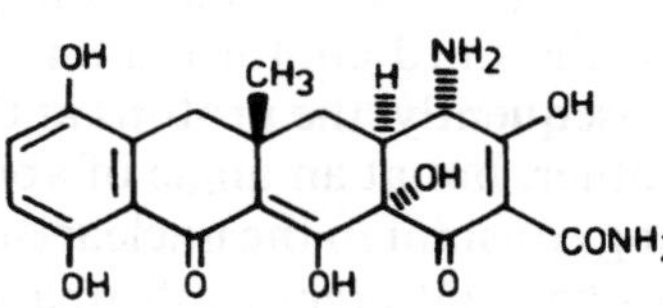

283

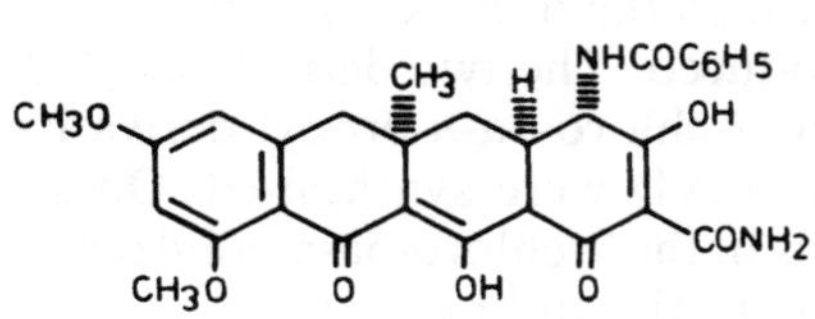

284

Fig. 36. 5a-Substituted 6-demethyl-6-deoxytetracyclines

condensation product (268). This condensation product reacts with the amide of monomethyl 3-oxoglutarate in THF/dimethylsulfoxide (DMSO) with NaH, giving a racemic mixture of tetracyclic compounds. Epimerization of the crude mixture at C4 after working up in pyridine leads essentially to the two racemic tetracyclic compounds (269) and (270), which differ in their stereochemistry at the C5a atom, as already discussed.

In the racemic natural 5a-methyltetracycline series [compound (269)] the substituents at carbon atoms 4a and 5a are in a *syn* arrangement. Tetracycline (270) has 4a,5a antisubstituents and leads into the racemic unnatural 5a-methyltetracycline series. The two tetracyclic compounds have different stability characteristics. While the tetracyclic compound with *syn* protons can be converted in glacial acetic acid/HBr to the ether-cleaved amine (271) in good yield, compound (270) with antihydrogens is destroyed under the same conditions. It was necessary, therefore, to adopt various means of arriving at the end products. The amine (271) is alkylated with dimethyl sulfate/diisopropylethylamine to (272) and then converted by hydroxylation with cerium chloride at pH 10 in a glycerol-phosphate buffer to 6-demethyl-6-deoxy-5a-methyl-7-chlorotetracycline (273). According to analytical data obtained, compound (273) has the configuration and conformation (1) shown in Fig. 35.

In the unnatural series, (270) is first hydroxylated with platinum to give the 12a-hydroxy compound, which is converted to the C4 amine by means of the oxonium salt. Alkylation with formaldehyde/sodium cyanoborohydride or dimethyl sulfate/diisopropylethylamine yields (275). Following subsequent ether cleavage at C10 in glacial acetic acid/HBr, the end product (276) of the unnatural series is obtained.

In the case of final product (276) of the unnatural series all analytical data suggest conformation (3) (Fig. 35). In conformation (2) the interactions between the methyl group at C5a and the proton at C4 are so intense that the molecule slips into the third conformation, in which there are less intense (1, 3) interactions. Consequently, the protons at C4 and C4a are no longer at an angle of 180° to one another, but at an angle of about 45°, this being noticeable through a small coupling constant in the nuclear magnetic resonance spectrum. The two end products thus have different conformations of the A-rings.

Synthesis in the 7-chloro-5a-methyl series produced not only compound (274) but also the 4-epi-5a-epimethyl compounds (277) and (278) (Fig. 36). In order to find out more about structure-activity relationships the 6-demethyl-6-deoxy-5a-epimethyl-7-methoxytetracycline (281) was produced. The two derivatives (282) and (283) could thereby be isolated. Also, the 7-chloro-5a-*n*-propyl derivative (280) and the 8-methoxy-5a-methyl-compound (284) were synthesized. On account of the properties of tetracyclic compounds in the 7-chloro-5a-methyl series, however, the syntheses were not carried through to the end products.

2. Effect of Structural Variation on Antibacterial Activity

Comparison of in vitro screening results (Table 18) for 5a-methyl derivatives in the natural tetracycline series shows clearly that with the increasing progression of substitution in the tetracyclic ring system the antibacterial activity of the molecule also increases. The racemic end product (273) has a spectrum of activity against the test strains which is largely similar to that of tetracycline. Additionally, however, its activity extends to tetracycline-resistant gram-positive organisms. Activity in this region is above that of minocycline. The data obtained seem

Table 18. In vitro activity of tetracyclines modified at positions C5a and C7. (H. WAHLIG and E. DINGELDEIN, unpublished research)

Organism	Minimum inhibitory concentrations (μg/ml)						
	Tetra-cycline	Mino-cycline	5a – nC_3H_7 Structure 280	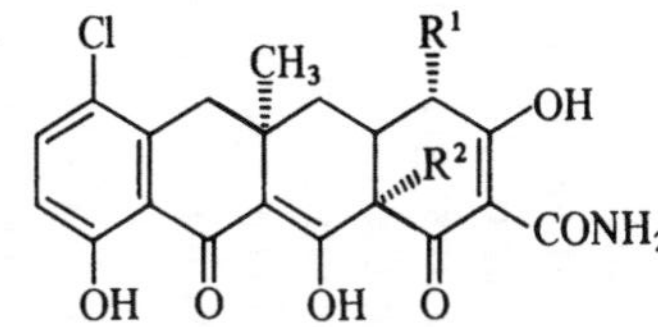			
				$R^1 = NHCOC_6H_5$ $R^2 = H$	$R^1 = NH_2$ $R^2 = H$	$R^1 = N(CH_3)_2$ $R^2 = H$	$R^1 = N(CH_3)_2$ $R^2 = OH$
Escherichia coli C1	0.5	0.5	>128	>128	32	32	8
Pseudomonas aeruginosa Ps1	8	4	>128	>128	> 32	> 32	>128
Proteus OX 21	4	1	>128	>128	4	4	1
Staphylococcus Sg 511	0.1	0.1	8	0.5	0.5	1	0.5
Streptococcus 3A	0.1	0.2	8	1	1	3.2	1
E. coli C71	>128	16	>128	>128	128	> 32	>128
E. coli C72	>128	16	>128	>128	>128	32	>128
E. coli C74	>128	–	>128	>128	>128	32	>128
Aerobacter Ae. 5	>128	–	>128	>128	>128	32	>128
A. Ae. 6	>128	–	>128	>128	>128	32	>128
P. vulgaris P3	>128	64	>128	>128	>128	>128	>128
P. vulgaris P4	>128	–	>128	>128	>128	>128	>128
S. aureus Sta. 71	>128	8	8	–	4	4	1
S. aureus Sta. 72	>128	4	4	–	8	4	0.5
S. aureus Sta. 73	>128	4	8	–	8	4	0.5
Streptococcus faecalis 68	>128	8	32	–	8	4	1
S. faecalis 69	64	8	32	–	8	4	4

to indicate that a simultaneous lessening of activity in the tetracycline-sensitive gram-negative range is to be anticipated.

The 5a-epimethyl derivatives of the unnatural tetracycline series as a whole have poorer activity than compounds in the natural series (Table 19), with 7-methoxy-5a-epimethyl compound (281) being inactive over the entire range, contrasting sharply with the corresponding 7-chloro compounds, in which there is a noticeable extra margin of activity over tetracycline against tetracycline-resistant gram-positive organisms.

What could be the possible explanation for these phenomena? Even during the synthesis the behavior of these compounds, which differs from the behavior of other tetracyclic compounds, became conspicuous. They are so nonpolar that they ran in the solvent front under chromatographic conditions normal for tetracyclines. The increased in vitro activity against gram-positive organisms can thus possibly be the result of an increase in lipophilic character of the 5a-methyltetracyclines. This generally occasions a loss of activity against gram-negative bacteria, as already discussed. Apparently, by introducing the methyl group in the 5a position a splitting of the activity was achieved, in which these compounds have excellent in vitro activity against gram-positive and also against tetracycline-resistant gram-positive organisms. There is no activity, however, against gram-negative bacteria.

The crystallographic elucidations of STEZOWSKI (1976) in tetracyclines showed that two conformations, namely the zwitterionic and the nonionized, are prerequisite for antibacterial activity. Both conformations should be in equilibrium. The chemical structure and conformation of the zwitterionic form is most probably the one playing an essential role in the bloodstream and in the aqueous regions of the bacteria. Analytical data obtained for 7-chloro-5a-methyl-6-demethyl-6-deoxytetracycline (273) suggest that under the conditions obtaining in NMR measurements conformation (1) is present, which is assigned to the nonionized structure (Fig. 35).

Apparently the lack of intramolecular interactions between rings A and C has led to a stabilization of the nonionized form, signaling an increase in lipophilicity. This change may be caused by the structural effect described as well as by the hydrophobic influence of the methyl group. An increase in lipophilicity signifies a reduction in activity, however. This finding is in agreement with earlier findings regarding tetracycline activities (BLACKWOOD and ENGLISH 1970).

In 7-chloro-5a-epimethyl-6-demethyl-6-deoxytetracycline (276) the 5a-methyl group is in the β-configuration. If conformation (2) (Fig. 35) were to be the actual conformation present, there would be strong interactions between the methyl group at C5a and the proton at C4. Sterically, therefore, it is regarded as impossible for the molecule to have this conformation. In NMR the protons C4 and C4a have only a small coupling constant and this implies that under such conditions the molecule must be in conformation (3), which is assigned to the zwitterionic structure. The fact that the molecule is apparently unable to pass into the nonionized conformation may perhaps be a partial explanation for the considerable reduction in activity as compared with the 5a-methyl compound (273), since the nonionized structure and its associated conformation appear to be necessary for the existence of in vitro activity.

Table 19. In vitro activity of tetracyclines modified at positions C5a and C7. (H. WAHLIG and E. DINGELDEIN, unpublished research)

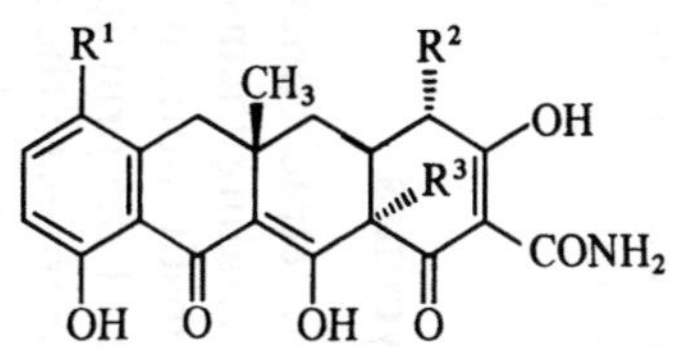

Organism	Minimum inhibitory concentrations (μg/ml)										
	Tetra-cycline	Mino-cycline							4-Epi		
			$R^1=Cl$ $R^2=NH_2$ $R^3=H$	$R^1=Cl$ $R^2=N(CH_3)_2$ $R^3=H$	$R^1=Cl$ $R^2=N(CH_3)_2$ $R^3=OH$	$R^1=OH$ $R^2=NH_2$ $R^3=OH$	$R^1=OCH_3$ $R^2=N(CH_3)_2$ $R^3=OH$	$R^1=OCH_3$ $R^2=N(CH_3)_2$ $R^3=OH$ 5a=H	$R^1=CL$ $R^2=NH_2$ $R^3=OH$	$R^1=CL$ $R^2=NH_2$ $R^3=H$
Escherichia coli C1	0.5	0.5	8	32	8	128	>128	4	32	8
Pseudomonas aeruginosa Ps1	8	4	> 8	>128	128	128	>128	> 8	> 32	> 8
Proteus OX21	4	1	4	4	8	>128	>128	4	4	32
Staphylococcus Sg511	0.1	0.1	4	1	8	1	>128	4	8	1
Streptococcus 3A	0.1	0.2	1	4	8	64	>128	4	4	8
E. coli C71	>128	16	32	128	32	>128	>128	32	>128	>128
E. coli C72	>128	16	32	>128	32	>128	>128	32	>128	>128
E. coli 74	>128	–	128	>128	32	>128	>128	32	>128	>128
Aerobacter Ae. 5	>128	–	128	>128	32	>128	>128	128	>128	>128
A. Ae. 6	>128	–	128	>128	128	>128	>128	32	>128	>128
P. vulgaris P3	>128	64	128	>128	>128	>128	>128	32	>128	>128
P. vulgaris P4	>128	–	128	>128	>128	>128	>128	128	>128	>128
Staphylococcus aureus Sta. 71	>128	8	4	1	32	>128	>128	4	8	4
S. aureus Sta. 72	>128	4	4	4	8	64	>128	4	4	0.5
S. aureus Sta. 73	>128	4	4	1	32	>128	>128	4	8	1
Streptococcus faecalis 68	>128	8	4	4	32	>128	>128	8	8	4
S. faecalis 69	64	8	4	4	32	>128	>128	8	8	4

The situation is different between the 7-chloro-5a-epimethyl compound (276) and the 7-methoxy-5a-epimethyl compound (281). By virtue of their having identical substituents at the C5a atom and in view of the anticipated identical steric interactions, both compounds ought to be in the same conformation. A difference is seen only in the nature of substituents at the C7 atom. While compound (276) has a chlorine substituent, i.e., an electron-accepting atom, compound (281) has the methoxy group in the 7 position, i.e., an electron-donating group. Consequently there ought also to be a difference in antibacterial activity. This is, in fact, the case. Compound (276) exhibits superior activity to (281), even though this is of little practical significance.

A comparison of the activities of 7-methoxy-5a-epi compounds (242) and (281) shows that compound (242) has by far the more favorable antibacterial activity, although the only structural difference is that compound (242) has a proton in the 5a position, whereas compound (281) has a methyl group in β-configuration. In the case of 7-methoxy-5a-epi compound (242) the interactions between the substituent at C5a and the proton at C4 are considerably less intense as a result of the spatially much smaller proton in the 5a position, so that owing to the larger C5a substituent in the 7-methoxy-5a-epimethyl compound (281) greater differences can result between the two molecules also in respect of the interactions between ring A and ring C and thus also of their conformations and their associated zwitterionic and nonionized structures. This may also explain the differences in antibacterial activities (see discussion page 264).

Substitution and configuration at the C5a atom can thus have an influence on conformation and hence on the equilibrium between zwitterionic and nonionized structures. The resultant lipophilicity of the compounds can have a significant effect on tetracycline activity. Electron-accepting or electron-donating substituents in the 7 position exert an additional effect on activity.

IX. Modifications at the C6 Position: 6-Heterotetracyclines

As can be seen from the wealth of publications on semisynthetic tetracyclines, positions 6 and 7 in the tetracyclic ring system are regarded as lending themselves particularly well to modification. Since the scope of possible substitutions at these positions is somewhat limited, a new approach involving use of the principle of isosterism was adopted in order to perform more substantial changes to the tetracycline molecule. Since replacement of a C atom in ring D might possibly occasion too great a change in the aromatic character and thus in the phenol properties of the 10-hydroxy group, the C6 atom was replaced by suitable heteroatoms. The following chemical effects were thus to be expected:

1. Conformational changes as a result of alterations to the 5a-6-6a bond lengths
2. Reversibility of the 5a-6 bond and thus isomerizability at steric center 5a
3. Electron accumulation in the polycarbonyl system through the push effect of the 6-heteroatom.

Of course, from these considerations is could not be foreseen what biological consequences such effects might have. Nevertheless, the effects were such as could not have been achieved by substitution.

1. (±)-6-Oxatetracyclines

a) Chemistry

The fact that up until synthesis of 6-oxatetracyclines the antibacterial activity of a tetracycline with a substituent in the 8 position (Sect. C.VII) had never been described, made tetracyclines with an oxygen function in the 8 position a particularly enticing proposition. The task thus set was the preparation of 8-hydroxy-6-oxatetracycline (295) (W. Rogalski, unpublished research). The ring system is built up according to the principle developed by Muxfeldt.

Starting from phloroglucine (285), compound (286) is obtained by acylation. Etherification of the latter product with dimethyl sulfate gives the dimethyl ether

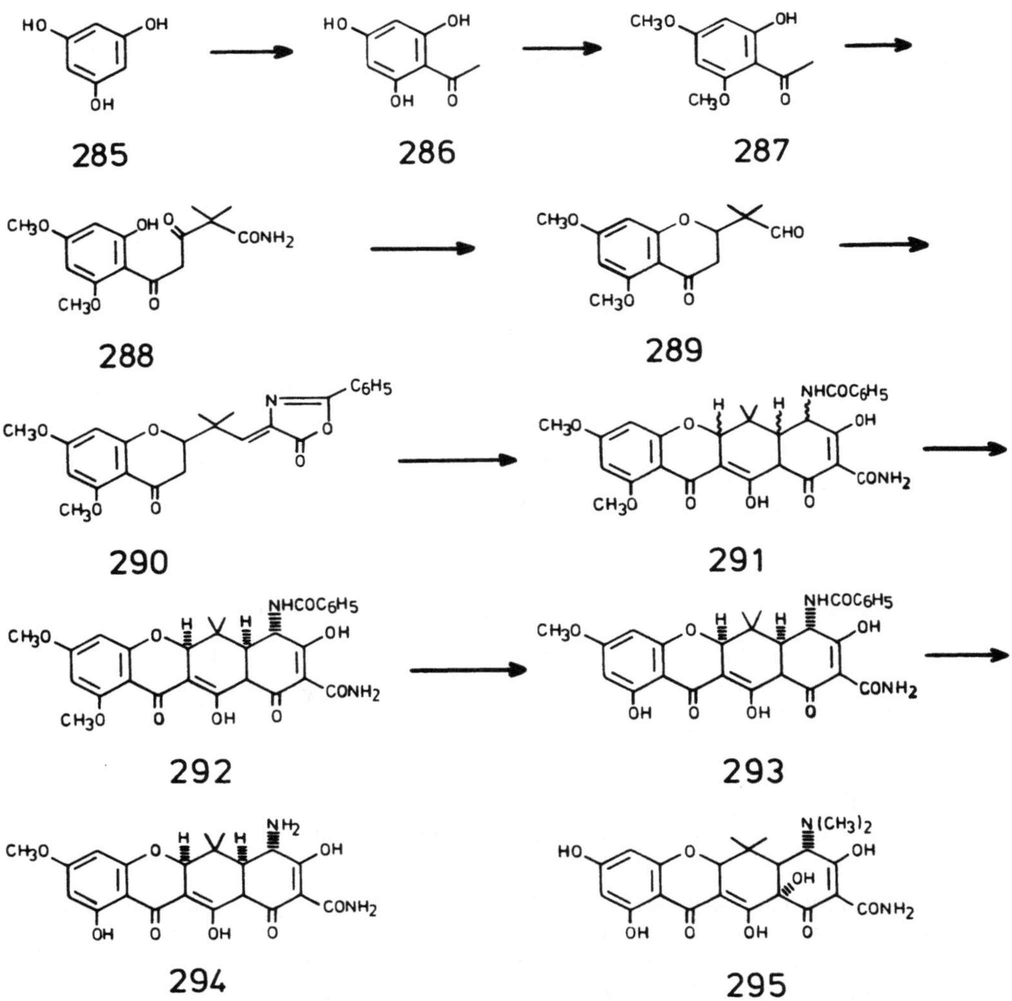

Fig. 37. Synthesis of derivatives of (±)-6-demethyl-6-deoxy-8-hydroxy-6-oxatetracycline

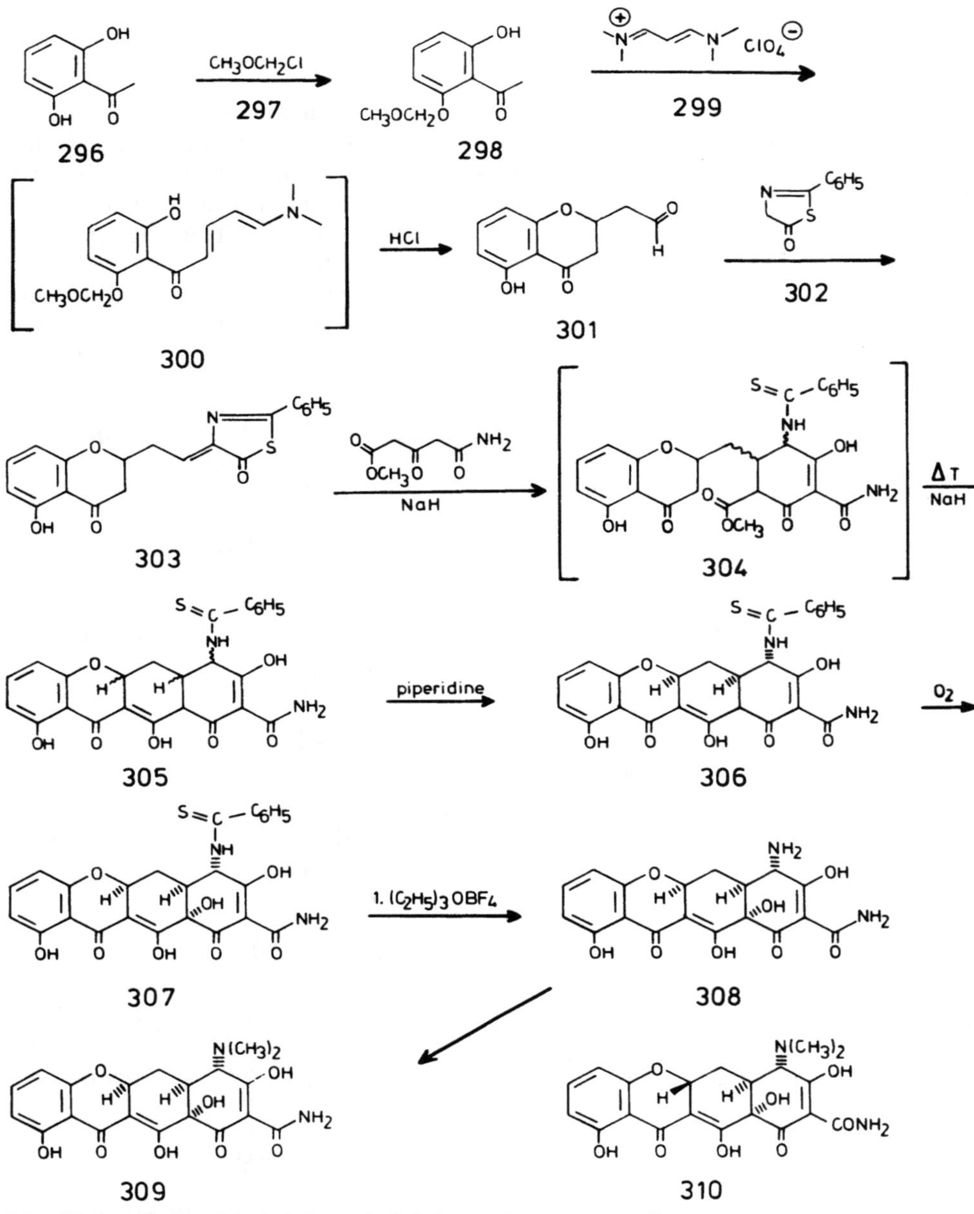

Fig. 38. Synthesis of (±)-6-demethyl-6-deoxy-6-oxatetracycline

(287). Subsequent condensation of (287) with ethyl dimethylcyanoacetic acid in dioxane gives the diketone (288), which is cyclized with sulfuric acid to give 6,8-dimethoxychromanonyl-4-(2)-dimethylacetamide. Following hydration of the double bond the amide is converted via the corresponding nitrile to the 6,8-dimethoxy-chromanonyl-4-(2)-dimethyl-acetaldehyde (289).

The aldehyde is reacted under the conditions already described with the azlactone prepared from hippuric acid to give the unsaturated azlactone derivative (290), this then reacting with the amide of monomethyl 3-oxoglutarate to give a mixture of tetracyclic compounds of general formula (291). Following pyridine-catalyzed epimerization at the C4 atom it was possible to isolate compound (292), which was converted with HBr in glacial acetic acid into the 6-oxa derivative (293). Reaction of the oxonium salt with (293) gives the amine (294) via the imino ether.

The 8-methoxy group in the tetracyclic ring system considerably hampers further reactions. Hence it was not possible to convert the 4-benzamido group into a dimethylamino group, to introduce the *cis*-12a-hydroxy group, and to cleave the 8-methoxy ether with an acceptable amount of effort. Such difficulties were also observed in the synthesis of other 8-methoxy series (W. Rogalski and R. Kirchlechner, unpublished research).

The real aim of preparing a 6-oxatetracycline was attained by a different means. The discovery of a brief and elegant new pathway to the intermediate aldehyde (Fig. 38) enabled the end product to be synthesized in only seven steps (Kirchlechner 1981).

2,6-Dihydroxyacetophenone (296) is alkylated with chloromethyl ether (297) to (298), which is converted with the vinylogous formamidinium salt (299) in pyridine to (300). Following acidic work-up with cleavage of the methoxymethyl ether, compound (300) gives the desired aldehyde (301). This is then reacted with 2-phenyl-3-thiazolin-5-one (302) to give the unsaturated compound (303), which when reacted with the amide of monomethyl 3-oxoglutarate in dioxane with NaH gives a tetracyclic mixture of isomers of general formula (305) via the tricyclic compound (304). In the subsequent treatment of this stereoisomeric mixture with piperidine at 50 °C two different reactions occur. Firstly, there is a $\beta \rightarrow \alpha$-epimerization of the C4 substituent, the result being that the configuration of the normal tetracyclines at C4 is obtained, and secondly the bond O6,C5a opens due to the effect of the base in the 5a-epi compounds, e.g., (311), with formation of the 5a,11a double bond, producing the intermediate product (312), which cannot be isolated, however (Fig. 39). Subsequent ring closure gives compound (306), which

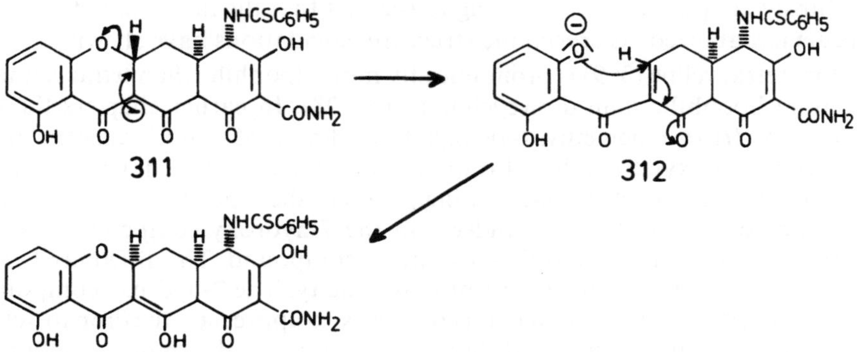

Fig. 39. Mechanism of 5a-epimerization

has the natural configuration in the 5a position. By this means the isomers with 4a,5a anti-hydrogen atoms are converted into the, it seems, thermodynamically more stable isomers with C4a,C5a *syn* hydrogen atoms. Introduction of the *cis*-12a-hydroxy group gives compound (307); conversion of the 4-benzamido function into the amine (308) and alkylation with formaldehyde under reductive conditions gives the 6-demethyl-6-deoxy-6-oxatetracycline (309). Elucidation of the structure of this compound by X-ray analysis could not be performed owing to the fact that no suitable crystals had been obtained. However, such analysis was possible with 5a-epi-6-oxatetracycline (310) (Kollat and Stezowski 1982) isolated from the mother liquors. It was shown that the molecule (310) is in the nonionized form with the associated conformation. The conformation of 5a-epi-6-oxatetracycline nonionized free base is very similar to that of the 5a-epi-6-thiatetracycline analogue and that of the cation of 5a-epi-7-chlorotetracycline in the hydrochloride salt (Prewo et al. 1980; Prewo and Stezowski 1980).

Because of the virtually identical H4,H4a coupling constants in the NMR spectrum of 6-oxatetracycline (309) and 5a-epi-6-oxatetracycline (310) it is assumed that 6-oxatetracycline (309) is likewise in the nonionized form.

b) Effect of Structural Variation on Antibacterial Activity

The 8-methoxy-6-oxatetracycline derivative (294) shows, as has already been observed for these types of compound from other series, how the lipophilic residue at the C4 atom leads to good antibacterial activity against tetracycline-sensitive and tetracycline-resistant gram-positive organisms. Activity against gram-negative bacteria is virtually nil (Table 23). The racemic 6-oxatetracycline (309), on the other hand, is active against the majority of the test strains used and is superior to tetracycline, in fact, in its antibacterial activity. With this class of substances, therefore, it has proved possible to extend the antibacterial spectrum of the tetracyclines.

Three effects, all interrelated, determine the properties of the substance: steric effect, since the space between C5a and C6a is smaller when position 6 is an oxygen atom than the space between C5a and C6a when position 6 is a carbon atom; electronic effect, since electrons are ceded by oxygen to the ring system; and, thirdly, a lipophilic effect, owing to the fact that the nonionized form of the molecule is stabilized, as crystalline structure elucidations have shown.

6-Oxatetracycline (309) is pronouncedly more lipophilic than tetracycline and even more lipophilic than doxycycline (Table 28). In earlier chapters the compounds 7-hydroxy-6-demethyl-6-deoxytetracycline (155) and 7-dimethylamino-6-demethyl-6-deoxytetracycline 4 (minocycline) were described. One thing both have in common is an electron-donating group in the 7 position, which generally causes the activity to decrease. Indeed, in the 7-hydroxy compound this is the case; not so, however, in the 7-dimethylamino compound. The difference between the two lies in their varying degrees of lipophilicity. The 7-hydroxy compound is about as lipophilic as tetracycline. It is thus easy to appreciate the drop in activity. The 7-dimethylamino compound, however, is considerably more lipophilic and has clearly superior in vitro activity. This increase in activity can also be explained in terms of better penetration by the lipophilic compound into the bacterial cell.

Although 6-oxatetracycline has no substituents in the 7 position it does have an electron-donating oxygen function in the 6 position, replacing the C6 atom in ring C. Furthermore, it is more lipophilic than the other tetracyclines, so that the greater activity of 6-oxatetracycline – like that of minocycline – can be interpreted in terms of a higher degree of penetration by the molecule into the organisms.

2. (±)-6-Thiatetracyclines

Results obtained with 6-oxatetracycline show clearly that modifications in the 6 position of the tetracyclic ring system give rise to marked changes in the properties of the molecule. Substitution of a sulfur atom for the oxygen atom in the 6 position should cause an increase in the following effects: electron accumulation in the polycarbonyl system owing to the push effect of the sulfur atom, and changes in the conformation of the molecule through changes made in the bond lengths C5a-S-C6a in the 6-thiatetracyclines so that the space between C5a and C6a is greater when position C is a sulfur atom than the space between C5a and C6a when position 6 is a carbon atom. By performing an additional substitution in the 7 position with electron-accepting and electron-donating groups it ought to be possible to modify the fundamental character of the molecule.

a) Chemistry

Syntheses in the 6-thiatetracycline series were by the Muxfeldt system. The E. Merck research group prepared a total of 22 variously substituted 6-thiatetracyclines by this means (W. Rogalski and R. Kirchlechner, unpublished research; Kirchlechner and Seubert 1982).

There follows a short description of the synthesis of 6-thiatetracycline (327)(Fig. 40), the simplest basic structure in this series, which is also exemplary for all other compounds (Kirchlechner and Rogalski 1980).

The synthesis starts from 2-chloro-4-aminothiophenol (313). It then proved possible to convert the thiophenol (313) smoothly, by reaction with dimethyl glutaconate (314) followed by acid saponification, into the diacid (315), which was cyclized with anhydrous HF to give the thiachromanone (316). Ether cleavage in HBr/glacial acetic acid to form (318) was followed by preparation of the acid chloride and conversion to the aldehyde (319) by means of a Rosenmund reaction.

Reaction of the aldehyde (319) with the azlactone in THF in the presence of lead acetate as a weak base and $MgSO_4$ to take up the water liberated is completed within 15 min at room temperature and gives (320) in good yield.

In the subsequent preparation of the tetracyclic compound by reacting the azlactone with acetone dicarboxylic acid ester monoamide the procedure is as follows. First, the azlactone (320) is dissolved in a mixture of dioxane and DMF, the amide of monomethyl 3-oxoglutarate and NaH are added, and the mixture is then stirred for 30 min at room temperature, the tricyclic ring system (321) being formed. The solution is then refluxed and the reaction mixture is worked up with acidification and dilution of the solution with chloroform, for example. The crude product is a mixture of stereoisomers represented by structure (322).

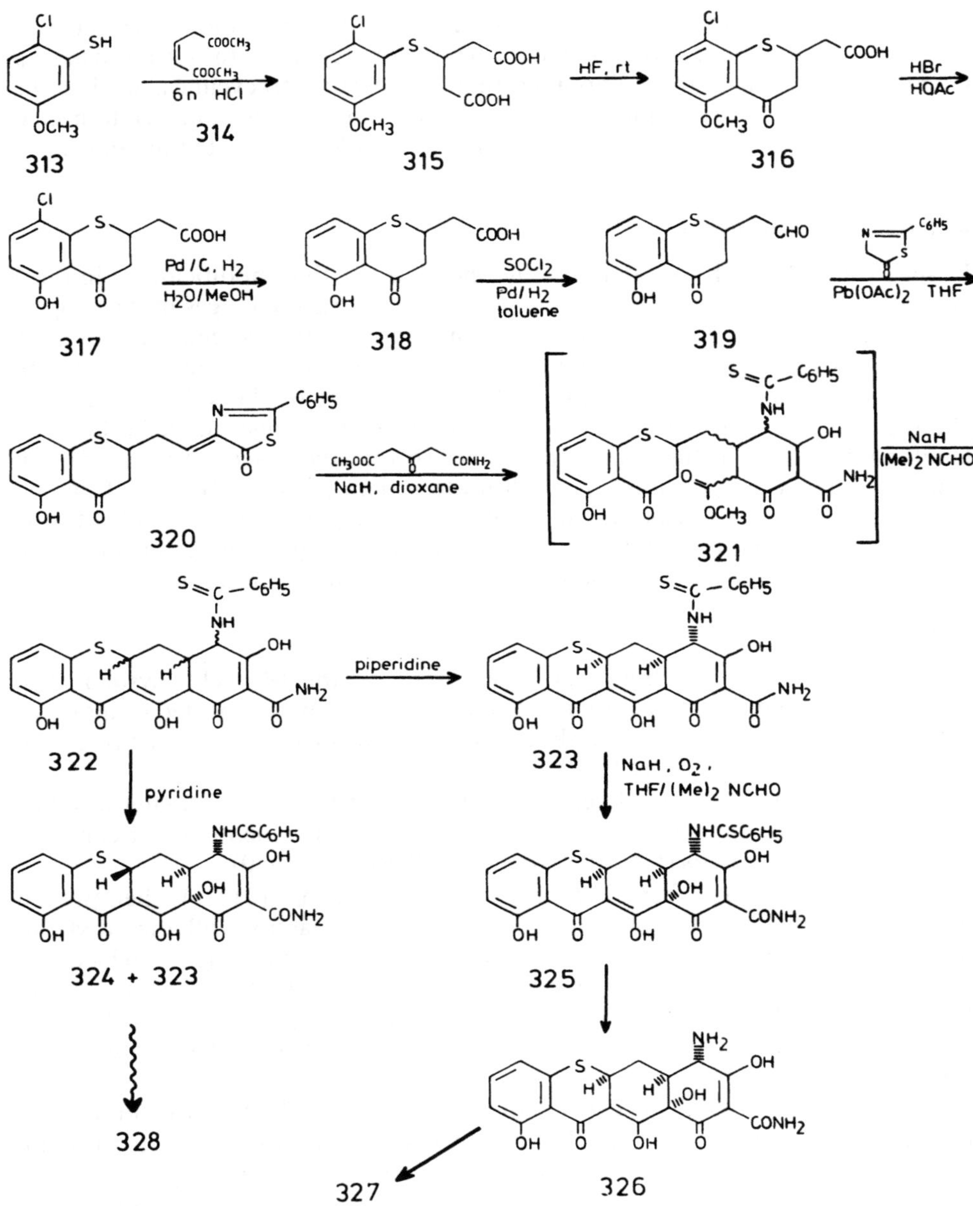

Fig. 40. Synthesis of (±)-6-thiatetracyclines

With the components remaining unseparated, the crude product (322) is dissolved in pyridine and the solution left to stand for 2 days at room temperature, whereupon epimerization at the C4 atom occurs, leaving hydrogens in the *trans*-position on the C4 and C4a atoms. The mixture is then worked up by dilution with a suitable organic solvent and by washing the solution with a dilute acid. The two 5a epimers (324) and (323) can be cleanly separated, as racemic mixtures, by fractional crystallization.

Treatment of the crude product (322) with piperidine at 50 °C for 1 h not only caused C4 epimerization to occur but also epimerization of the C4a,C5a *anti* to its *syn* analogue, as already described for 6-oxatetracycline (Fig. 39). It was thus possible to transform the isomeric mixture (322) quantitatively into the desired isomer (323).

Starting from the pure racemic tetracyclic compound (323) of the natural series, the 12a-hydroxyl group is introduced by treatment with oxygen in a solvent mixture of THF and DMF, in the presence of NaH and triethyl phosphide, to give (325). Hydroxylation takes place largely in the *cis* position, being in accord with the configuration of the natural tetracyclines. Subsequent cleavage of the amide group at the C4 atom under mild conditions using the oxonium salt (Meerwein reagent) gives the imino ether, which on acid work-up of the reaction product is split into benzoic acid ester and the amine compound (326), which is then converted to the end product (327) by a simple method using formaldehyde and sodium cyanoborohydride in methanol. Using the same reaction sequence but starting from the tetracyclic 5a-epi compound (324) and using identical conditions, the end product, 5a-epi-6-thiatetracycline (328) of the unnatural series, is reached.

Allowing H_2O_2 solution to react on (327) and (328) gives the two sulfones (329) and (330). 7-Chloro-6-thiatetracycline 2-dioxide (333) and the 5a epimer (334) were prepared from the thiachromanonic acid (317). Treatment of (317) with 30% H_2O_2 in glacial acetic acid produced the sulfone, which is the analogue of (317), this being converted into the 7-chlorosulfones (333) and (334) in a reaction sequence analogous to (318)–(326) (R. Kirchlechner, unpublished research).

The following substances were also prepared (Fig. 41): the 7-chloro-6-thiatetracyclines (331) and (332), the 7-methoxy-6-thiatetracyclines (335) and (336), the 8-methoxy-6-thiatetracycline (337), the 7-dimethylamino-6-thiatetracyclines (339) and (340), the 10-deoxy-6-thiatetracycline (338), and a number of 6-thiatetracycline derivatives having the general formula (341) (Fig. 42) with variously substituted amino groups at C4.

Surprisingly, the end products in the 6-thiatetracycline series with normal configuration at the C4a and C5a atoms can be converted into the 5a epimers, in the same way as for the 6-oxatetracycline series, using the same mechanism as was described for the 6-oxatetracyclines (Fig. 39). Whereas *before* introduction of the 12a-hydroxy group the compounds with 4a,5a *syn* hydrogen atoms seem to be favored thermodynamically, the 5a-epi compound appears to be thermodynamically favored *following* introduction of the 12a-hydroxy group and *cis* linkage of rings A and B (Kirchlechner 1981).

The 22 end products synthesized are in the form of the racemates. It is known, however, from work performed by the Muxfeldt and Pfizer groups that only one of the enantiomers is biologically active in racemic tetracyclines. It thus seemed appropriate to aim for the preparation of the enantiomeric 6-thiatetracyclines. Indeed, it proved possible in the 7-chloro series to separate the thiachromanone (317) with chinchonine or (+)-1-phenylethylamine into the antipodes. In the further course of the synthesis it also proved possible to obtain the 4a,5a *syn* and the

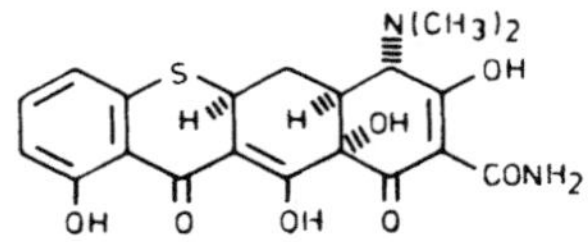

327

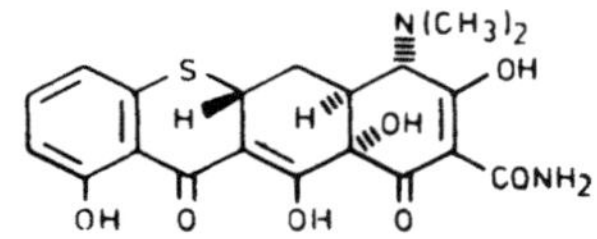

328

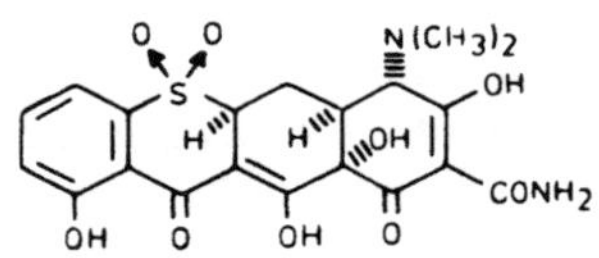

329

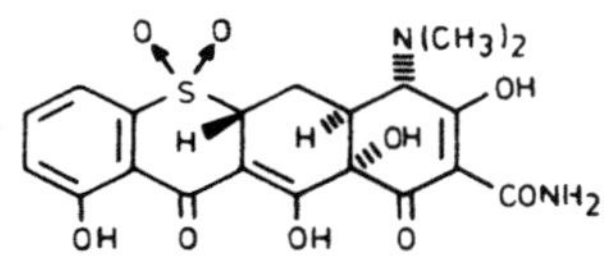

330

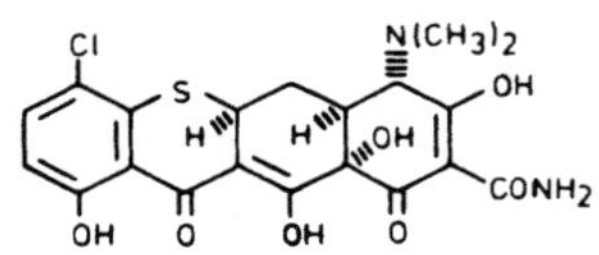

331

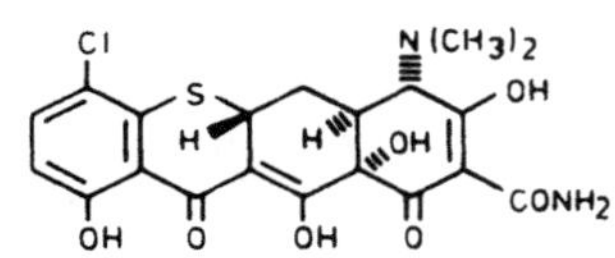

332

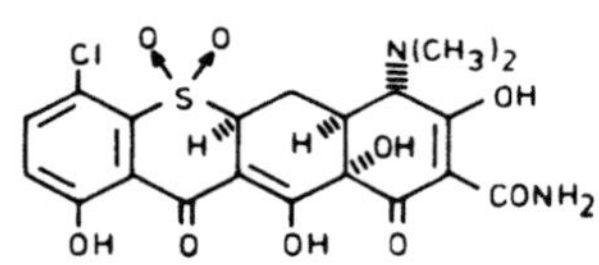

333

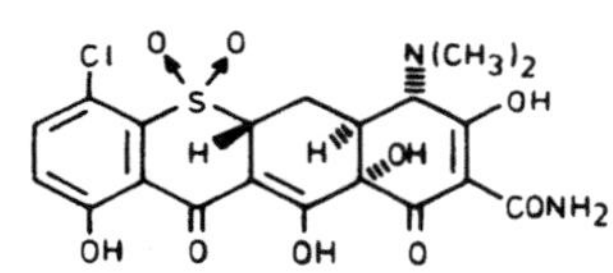

334

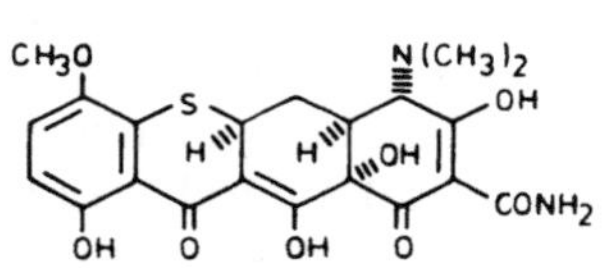

335

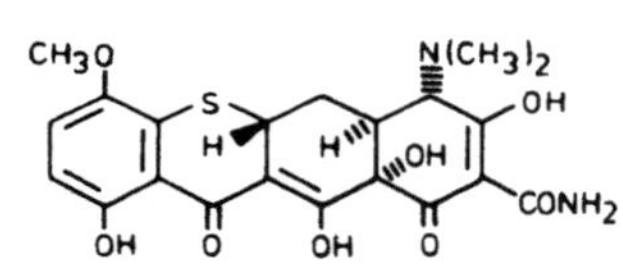

336

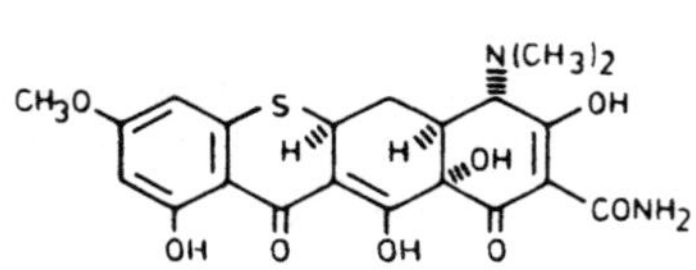

337

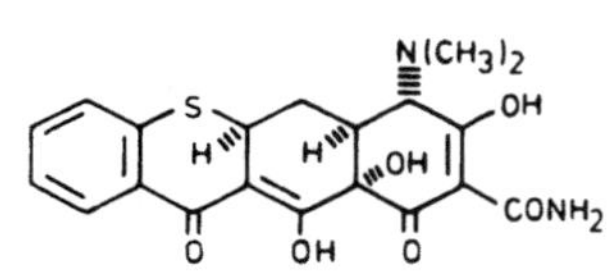

338

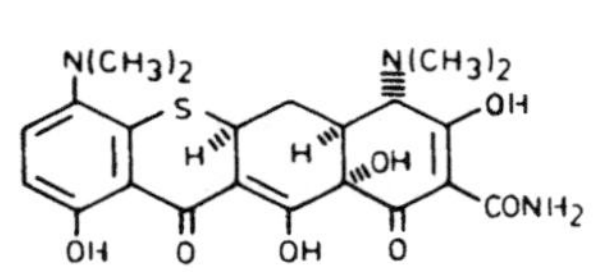

339

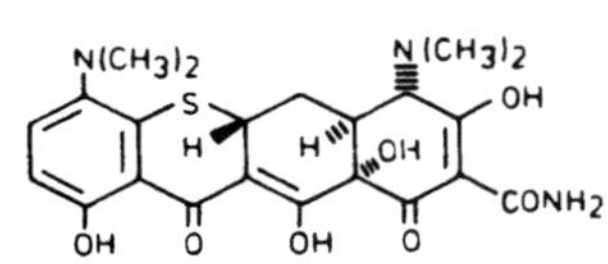

340

Fig. 41. Totally synthetic (±)-6-thiatetracyclines

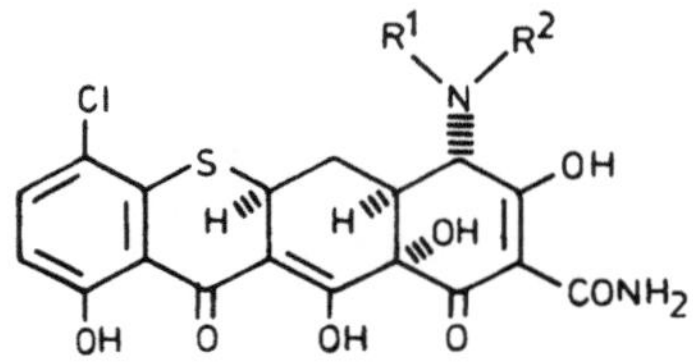

341

342 : $R^1 = R^2 = CH_3$

343 : $R^1 = CH_3$; $R^2 = C_2H_5$

344 : $R^1 = R^2 = C_2H_5$

345 : $R^1 = CH_3$; $R^2 = nC_3H_7$

346 : $R^1 = CH_3$; $R^2 = CH_2 - C_6H_5$

347 : $R^1 = R^2 = n - C_3H_7$

348 : $R^1 = H$; $R^2 = i - C_3H_7$

349 : NR^1R^2 = 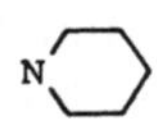

Fig. 42. 7-Chloro-6-thiatetracycline with various substituents at the 4-amino group

4a,5a *anti* products with cyclized ring A, analogues of compound (321) in the 7-dechloro series, in optically active form. Subsequent cyclization to the tetracyclic ring system occurred, however, with complete racemization of center 5a (see mechanism of the 5a epimerization, Fig. 39). The necessary formation of the anion at the C11a atom gives rise, therefore, to a retro Michael addition with removal of the chirality at C5a. Since the reaction is reversible, a situation is created in which although the tetracycline is formed it takes the form merely of a diastereomer mixture, which is separable by chromatography into the optically active components. One of the enantiomeric 7-chloro-6-thiatetracyclines produced in this way showed the anticipated biological activity.

In conclusion, it can be stated that the ease of epimerization of the 6-thiatetracyclines at the C5a atom has a number of consequent effects, as for the 6-oxatetracyclines. While the 5a-epi-6-thiatetracyclines can be used for synthesis in the natural tetracycline series with 4a,5a *syn* hydrogen atoms before 12a hydroxylation, the end products have isomerization characteristics which differ from those of carbocyclic tetracyclines. In the natural tetracyclines epimerization of the 4-dimethylamino group is the preferred isomerization reaction. On the other hand, the 6-thiatetracyclines have a stable substituted 4-amino group, with epimerization at C5a being the preferred reaction.

Superimposition of the Dreiding models of 6-demethyl-6-deoxytetracycline and of 6-thiatetracycline (Fig. 43) shows a certain spatial disagreement between the two molecules, owing to the fact that the distance between atoms C5a and C6a is greater than the distance between these positions in the carbocyclic series. In addition to this structural difference, there is also an electronic one through the sulfur atom in the 6 position, which is so influential as regards the molecule as a whole. The electronic modification can also be influenced by substituents in the

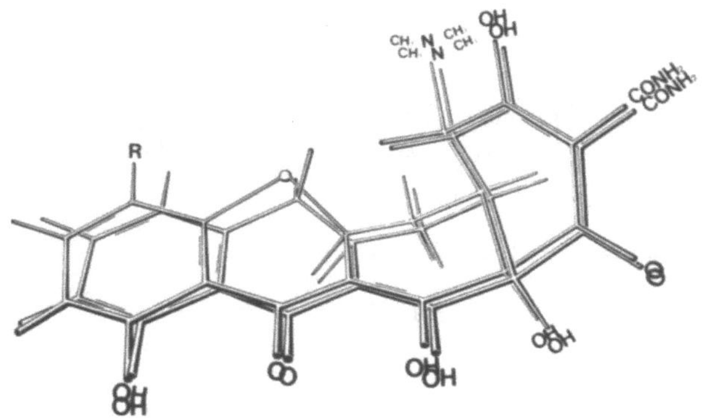

Fig. 43. Superimposition of the Dreiding models of 6-demethyl-6-deoxytetracycline and of 6-demethyl-6-deoxy-6-thiatetracycline

7 position. Crystallographic analyses have been performed (PREWO et al. 1980) both for the 6-thiatetracyclines (327) and (328) and for the 12a-deoxy-11a-hydroxy-6-thiatetracycline. The results are discussed in the next chapter.

b) Effect of Structural Variation on Antibacterial Activity

The end products (327)–(349) of the 6-thiatetracyclines are racemates and we can assume on the grounds of experience gained with other tetracyclines obtained by total synthesis that only one of the enantiomers is biologically active.

α) Activity Against Gram-Positive Bacteria. Taking the simplest compound (Table 20), i.e., one without a substituent at the C7 atom, 6-thiatetracycline (327) has a basic activity far different from that of tetracycline, doxycycline, and minocycline (KIRCHLECHNER et al. 1977; ROGALSKI 1978; TEARE et al. 1981; BAKHTIAR and SELWYN 1982, 1983). Tetracycline-resistant gram-positive bacteria are covered by the active spectrum of 6-thiatetracycline. Chlorine, an electron-attracting group, in the 7 position of the molecule [compound (331)] intensifies the activity somewhat, while a methoxy group [compound (335)] or a dimethylamino group [compound (339)], i.e., electron-donating groups, at the C7 atom reduces the antibacterial activity to a level lower than that in the basic molecule.

β) 5a-Epi Compounds. The third column of Table 21 gives the minimum inhibitory concentrations of two 5a-epi compounds (332) and (336). Comparison with the corresponding 6-thiatetracyclines with natural configuration shows that the different position of the hydrogen at the C5a atom has no effect on the activity of the compounds against either gram-positive or gram-negative bacteria.

γ) Gram-Negative Bacteria. A test of the activity of the 6-thiatetracyclines against gram-negative bacteria gives the following result (Table 21). Looking at the minimum inhibitory concentrations of the base substance (327), we find that it copes with the bacteria usually within the tetracycline spectrum. Furthermore, the tetracycline-resistant bacteria present in the various groups of bacteria also fall within the spectrum of activity. Additionally, however, the spectrum is broadened to include strains of *Proteus mirabilis,* which generally prove resistant

Table 20. In vitro activity (MIC in µg/ml) of 6-thiatetracyclines modified at position C7 in comparison to tetracycline, doxycycline, and minocycline. (ROGALSKI 1978; experimental data by H. WAHLIG and E. DINGELDEIN)

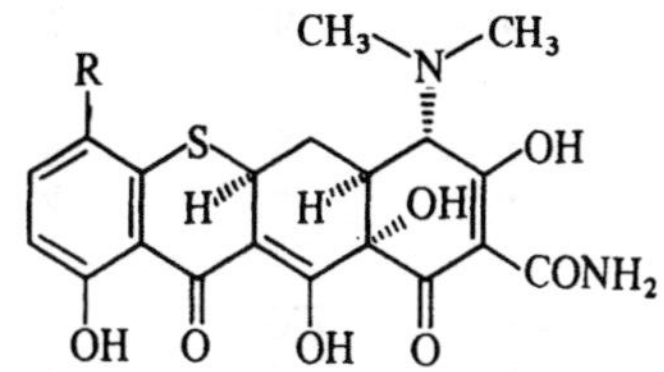

Bacteria	Tetra-cycline	Doxy-cycline	Mino-cycline					5a-Epi	
				R=H Racemate	R=Cl Racemate	R=OCH_3 Racemate	R=$N(CH_3)_2$ Racemate	R=Cl Racemate	R=OCH_3 Racemate
Staphylococcus aureus									
Sta 12	0.1	0.1	< 0.2	0.5	<0.2	0.1	<0.2	<0.2	<0.2
Sta 61	64	2	< 0.2	0.5	<0.2	1	0.5	<0.2	1
Sta 63	0.1	1	< 0.2	0.2	<0.2	0.5	<0.2	<0.2	<0.2
Sta 71	128	16	8	2	<0.2	2	2	0.5	2
Sta 72	>128	16	2	1	<0.2	2	2	0.5	1
Sta 73	128	16	8	0.5	<0.2	2	2	0.5	2
Sta 74	>128	16	4	1	0.2	2	2	<0.2	2
Sta 75	16	4	2	1	<0.2	1	0.5	<0.2	1
Streptococcus pyogenes									
Str 2	0.2	0.05	< 0.2	0.05	<0.2	0.2	0.2	0.2	0.2
Str 8	0.1	0.2	< 0.2	0.5	0.2	0.2	0.2	<0.2	<0.2
Str 26	32	16	8	0.2	<0.2	0.2	–	1	8
Str 27	64	32	16	0.5	1	4	–	1	4
Str 28	64	16	0.5	0.2	<0.2	0.2	–	<0.2	1
Str 30	–	0.05	< 0.2	0.05	<0.2	–	<0.2	0.2	0.2
Str 31	–	0.05	< 0.2	0.05	<0.2	–	0.2	0.2	0.2
Streptococcus faecalis									
Str 68	128	8	16	4	4	4	4	1	2
Str 69	32	16	16	8	8	8	8	1	4
Str 70	64	16	16	8	8	8	16	1	8
Str 75	64	16	16	8	8	8	8	1	8
Str 76	64	16	16	8	8	8	8	2	8

Table 21. In vitro activity (MIC in μg/ml) of 6-thiatetracyclines modified at position C7 in comparison to tetracycline, doxycycline, and minocycline. (ROGALSKI 1978; experimental data by H. WAHLIG and E. DINGELDEIN)

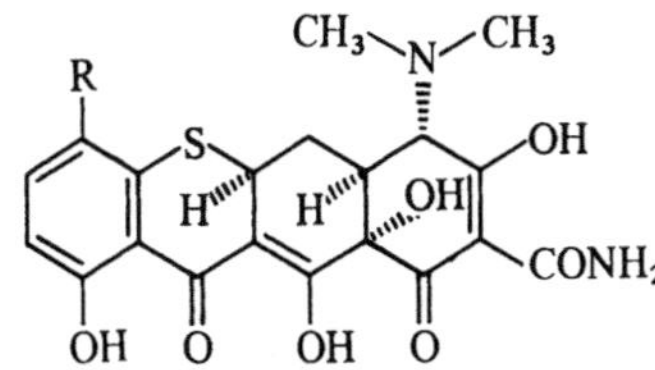

Bacteria	Tetra-cycline	Doxy-cycline	Mino-cycline	R=H Racemate	R=Cl Racemate	R=OCH$_3$ Racemate	R=N(CH$_3$)$_2$ Racemate	5a-Epi R=Cl Racemate	5a-Epi R=OCH$_3$ Racemate
Escherichia coli									
C 1	0.5	0.5	0.5	0.5	0.5	0.5	1	1	0.5
C13	1	2	2	2	2	2	4	2	2
C15	1	0.5	0.2	< 0.2	< 0.2	0.5	0.5	< 0.2	0.5
C41	2	2	4	2	2	4	4	2	4
C65	>128	32	16	4	4	8	–	4	8
C71	>128	32	16	2	4	4	–	4	4
C72	>128	16	8	2	4	8	–	4	8
C73	16	2	1	1	2	2	–	2	2
C75	>128	32	64	–	8	–	–	16	32
Proteus sp.									
P 3	32	32	32	4	2	16	16	4	4
P 4	>128	128	64	2	4	32	32	8	32
P 5	64	64	32	4	2	16	32	2	8
P 6	64	64	32	1	4	16	–	2	8
P 7	64	64	32	4	2	16	–	2	8
P11	32	32	32	4	2	8	16	2	4
P21	2	2	2	0.5	0.2	0.5	–	1	1
Klebsiella enterobius									
Ae5	64	–	16	4	4	4	–	4	4
Ae6	>128	–	64	8	8	8	8	64	32
Pseudomonas aeruginosa									
1	4	1	8	16	16	16	8	16	4
4	16	8	16	8	8	16	–	32	16
5	2	2	2	2	2	4	–	4	4
6	8	8	8	16	8	64	–	8	16
20	16	4	8	8	8	64	32	64	32

Table 22. In vitro activity against tetracycline-resistant bacteria (MIC in μg/ml) of 6-thia-tetracyclines in comparison to tetracycline, doxycycline, and minocycline. (ROGALSKI 1978; experimental data by H. WAHLIG and E. DINGELDEIN)

Bacteria	Tetra-cycline	Doxy-cycline	Mino-cycline	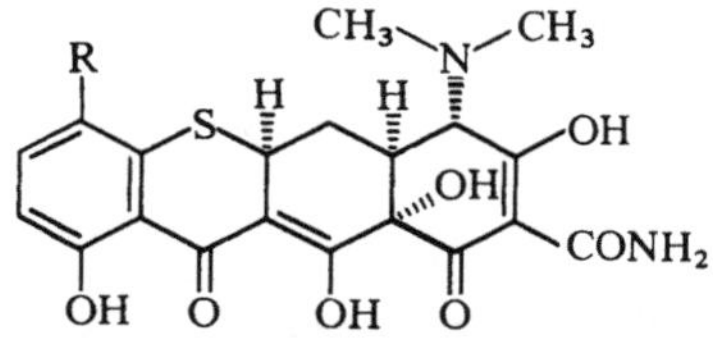		
				$R=H$ Racemate	$R=Cl$ Racemate	$R=OCH_3$ Racemate
Staphylococcus aureus						
7002	128	16	1	1	< 0.2	1
26564	64	8	0.5	1	< 0.2	1
62	32	1	< 0.2	0.5	< 0.2	0.5
64	>128	16	4	2	< 0.2	2
71	128	16	4	1	< 0.2	2
Streptococcus faecalis						
3157	32	16	16	2	4	8
3260	32	8	8	8	4	8
3390	64	16	16	8	4	8
3487	64	16	16	4	4	8
Escherichia coli						
2520	16	4	4	2	4	4
3330	>128	8	4	2	1	4
5910	128	8	4	2	1	1
3407	64	8	1	2	1	2
Proteus sp.						
8412	16	4	2	0.2	0.2	0.5
3547	64	32	16	2	2	4
4073	128	64	32	2	2	8
3638	64	8	16	2	2	16
3015	64	16	8	1	2	8
Klebsiella Enterobius						
1363	4	16	8	8	16	8
1611	128	32	16	8	8	16
4504	32	8	1	2	4	2
4278	>128	32	32	32	16	64
5870	>128	32	64	8	8	32
Pseudomonas aeruginosa						
3068	32	16	8	16	8	16
31312	8	16	4	16	8	16
22068	32	32	32	32	64	64
22351	16	32	16	32	64	32
3157	8	16	8	32	16	16

to tetracycline. Chlorine, an electron-attracting group, in the 7 position [compound (331)] does not alter the activity of the 6-thiatetracycline base molecule (327). If the electron-donating methoxy and dimethylamino groups are present [compound (335) and compound (339)], the spectrum tends to be poorer.

Table 23. Antibacterial activity (MIC in μg/ml) of 6-oxatetracycline, 6-thiatetracycline, and 7-chloro-6-thiatetracycline-*S*-dioxides. (H. WAHLIG and E. DINGELDEIN, unpublished research)

Organism		6-Oxatetra-cycline	6-Thiatetra-cycline	7-Chloro-6-thia-tetracycline-*S*-dioxides	
				5a-α	5a-β
Staphylococcus aureus	102007	–	0.5	>128	128
	102012	1	> 0.1	2	2
	102061	4	0.2	64	64
Streptococcus faecalis	103070	–	2	128	128
	103075	–	2	128	64
β-Hemolytic *Streptococcus*	104030	>16	0.2	0.5	0.2
Bacillus	108012	0.5	–	–	–
Escherichia coli	124001	1	0.2	3	4
	124013	2	–	–	–
	124015	2	0.2	2	4
	124077	2	1	16	16
Salmonella	126022	2	2	8	8
Shigella	127001	0.2	0.2	0.5	0.5
Klebsiella	128001	–	0.5	2	4
Enterobacter	129012	–	4	>128	>128
Serratia	131002	–	4	64	64
Proteus vulgaris	132014	2	0.2	64	64
P. mirabilis	133003	2	2	>128	>128
	133011	4	1	128	128
P. morganii	134018	–	4	>128	>128
P. rettgeri	135016	–	8	>128	>128
P. aeruginosa	120001	16	8	32	32
	120020	4	16	16	32

δ) Tetracycline-Resistant Clinical Strains. Table 22 shows the results of a test in which tetracycline, doxycycline, and minocycline were compared with the 6-thiatetracyclines (327), (331), and (335). In particular, their action on freshly isolated tetracycline-resistant gram-positive and gram-negative bacteria was under scrutiny. Unlike tetracycline, doxycycline, and minocycline, the basic 6-thiatetracycline compound is active in all cases except for the *Pseudomonas* group, with minimum inhibitory concentrations lying within the range of achievable serum concentrations.

Here again, the electron-attracting chlorine group in the 7 position of compound (331) does not change the basic character of the activity of compound (327) in which R is a proton, while the effect of the electron-donating methoxy group of compound (335) manifests itself in a slight reduction of activity.

ε) 6-Thiatetracycline-S-Dioxide. Table 23 sets out the results of in vitro screening performed with the two sulfones (333) and (334). Compared with the corresponding 6-thiatetracyclines (331) and (332), a considerable decrease in activity is observed. The compounds have become devoid of activity against numerous organisms. This applies both to the natural tetracycline series and to the 5a-

Table 24. In vitro activity (MIC in μg/ml) of 6-thiatetracyclines modified at positions C8 and C10 in comparison to tetracycline, doxycycline, and minocycline. (ROGALSKI 1978; experimental data by H. WAHLIG and E. DINGELDEIN)

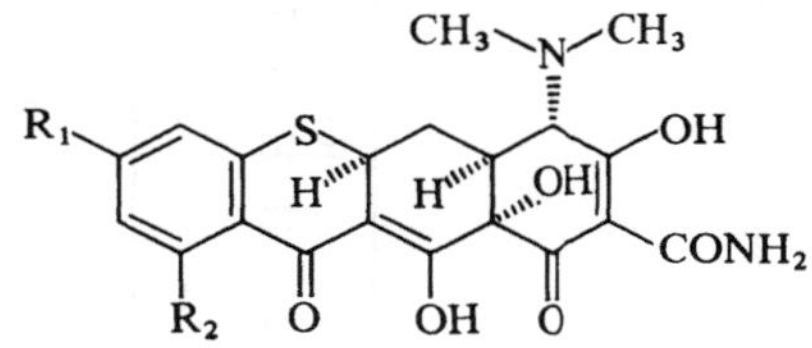

Bacteria	Tetra-cycline	Doxy-cycline	Mino-cycline	$R_1=H$ $R_2=OH$ Racemate	$R_1=OCH_3$ $R_2=OH$ Racemate	$R_1=H$ $R_2=H$ Racemate
Staphylococcus aureus						
Sta 12	0.1	0.1	< 0.2	0.5	0.5	8
Streptococcus pyogenes						
Str 8	0.1	0.2	< 0.2	0.5	1	8
Streptococcus faecalis						
Str 68	128	8	16	4	–	32
Str 69	32	16	16	8	–	64
Escherichia coli						
C 1	0.5	0.5	0.5	0.5	2	32
C 13	1	2	1	2	32	64
C 15	1	0.5	0.2	0.5	1	8
C 41	2	2	1	2	32	–
Proteus sp.						
P 3	32	32	16	4	32	32
P 11	32	64	16	4	64	32
Pseudomonas aeruginosa						
Ps 1	8	1	4	2	128	128

epi series and extends to gram-positive as well as to gram-negative bacteria. The same applies to compounds (329) and (330) as regards their activity. The electron-attracting chlorine group in the 7 position has no influence on the basic character of the molecule.

ζ) 8-Methoxy-6-thiatetracyclines and 10-Deoxy-6-thiatetracyclines. Table 24 shows the activity of two 6-thiatetracyclines (337) and (338). The 8-methoxy group of compound (337) is an electron-donating group and in the case of gram-negative bacteria it causes a decrease in activity as compared with 6-thiatetracycline (327) and even as compared with 7-methoxy-6-thiatetracycline (335). The 10-deoxy compound (338) is even less active against all bacteria, which is not surprising and confirms the assumption that the 10-hydroxy group is absolutely crucial to the activity of the tetracycline molecule.

η) 4-Alkylamino-6-thiatetracyclines. Further modifications of the molecule of 6-thiatetracycline have been performed in order to demonstrate the influence exercised by the alkyl group as it affects lipophilic character. Figure 42 shows the

Table 25. In vitro activity (MIC in μg/ml) of 6-thiatetracyclines with different alkyl substituents at the C4 amino group in comparison to tetracycline, doxycycline, and minocycline. (Rogalski 1978; experimental data by H. Wahlig and E. Dingeldein)

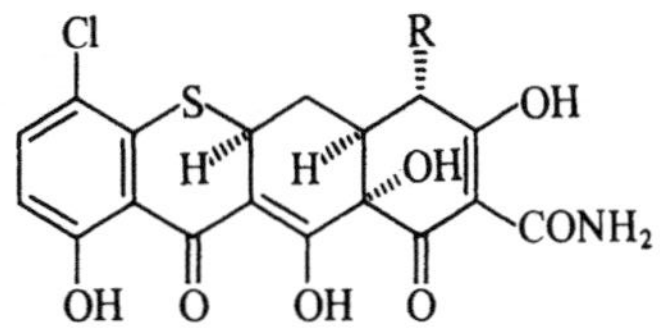

Bacteria	Tetra-cycline	Doxy-cycline	Mino-cycline	R = CH_3 CH_3 N	R = CH_3 C_2H_5 N	R = C_2H_5 C_2H_5 N	R = CH_3 C_3H_7 N	R = CH_3 CH_2-Ph N	R = C_3H_7 C_3H_7 N	R = H i-C_3H_7 N	R = 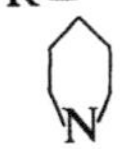
Staphylococcus aureus											
12	0.2	0.1	0.1	<0.2	< 0.1	0.1	0.2	0.1	1	8	0.05
71	64	4	8	–	< 0.1	–	0.2	1	4	16	–
72	>128	4	4	<0.2	< 0.1	–	0.1	0.2	2	16	–
73	>128	8	4	–	< 0.1	–	0.1	0.2	2	16	–
Streptococcus pyogenes 8	0.2	0.2	0.1	0.2	0.2	0.5	0.1	0.1	1	16	0.5
S. faecalis 68	>128	4	16	4	1	–	4	1	4	32	–
S. faecalis 69	32	16	16	8	1	–	4	2	4	32	–
Escherichia coli											
1	0.5	0.5	0.5	0.5	4	16	8	8	>128	128	32
13	1	2	2	2	8	16	16	32	>128	128	128
15	0.5	0.5	0.1	<0.2	0.2	2	8	2	32	64	8
71	>128	16	32	–	8	16	32	64	>128	>128	64
72	128	8	16	–	8		32	64	>128	>128	–
Proteus											
3	64	>64	16	2	8	–	16	64	>128	>128	–
11	32	16	32	2	4	–	8	16	>128	>128	–
21	8	1	1	–	< 0.1	0.1	0.1	0.2	4	16	4
Pseudomonas aeruginosa											
1	16	8	8	2	32	>128	>128	>128	>128	>128	>128

eight 7-chloro-6-thiatetracyclines (342)–(349) with different alkyl substituents on the 4-amino group.

As the alkyl group increases in length, there is an initial slight increase in activity against gram-positive bacteria, while activity against gram-negative bacteria is immediately reduced (Table 25). When the substituent on the amino group reaches a certain size, activity against gram-positive bacteria also diminishes until activity is lost over the entire spectrum. Two effects may be involved.

The increase in lipophilic character resulting from the increase in chain length of the alkyl group causes activity against gram-positive bacteria to increase and activity against gram-negative bacteria to decrease. The steric factor comes into play as the chain length increases, and this has a negative effect on activity.

It is believed that both effects overlap to a greater or lesser degree depending on the size of the alkyl group and lead to the activities mentioned above.

c) Interrelationship Between Structure and Activity of 6-Thiatetracyclines

The introduction of sulfur into the 6 position and the accompanying conformational changes as well as the change in lipophilic and electronic properties are important with regard to the antibacterial activity of the tetracycline. In discussing the relationship between structure and activity in antibacterial substances one must fundamentally distinguish between the ability of the molecule to inhibit protein synthesis by reaction with the ribosomes within the bacterial cell and the ability of the molecule to reach the site of action. The effect of 6-thiatetracyclines on extracellular ribosomes of *Escherichia coli* has been investigated. In these investigations, the compounds inhibited protein synthesis to a degree essentially comparable with the inhibitory effect of the natural tetracyclines.

It may be concluded from the studies performed that the superiority (clearly pronounced in some cases) of the investigated 6-thiatetracyclines in respect of their activity against clinically important groups of bacteria is attributable to a difference in permeability of the cell membrane to the 6-thiatetracyclines. This may be due to the different lipophilic character, different electronic properties, and different conformation of the molecule.

α) Lipophilic Character. There is an interrelationship in the tetracyclines between lipophilic character and biological activity. The tetracyclines which are particularly active against gram-positive bacteria are more lipophilic than those which exhibit a broader activity against gram-negative bacteria. This is interpreted in terms of the different lipid composition of the cell wall of gram-positive and gram-negative bacteria. The introduction of sulfur into the 6 position of the molecule has altered the lipophilic base character of the 6-thiatetracyclines compared with that of the natural tetracyclines. All 6-thiatetracyclines are more lipophilic than tetracyclines, doxycycline, and minocycline. In order to characterize these new tetracyclines by thin-layer chromatography it has been necessary to develop new chromatographic system (Table 26).

An even better means of establishing the lipophilicity of tetracyclines is to study their partition coefficients at various pH values in octanol/phosphate buffer. It is known (COLAIZZI and KLINK 1969) that the tetracyclines are at their most lipophilic in the pH range between 5.0 and 6.5.

Table 26. Thin-layer chromatography of tetracycline derivatives

Structure	Substance	Reference to front value
(3)	Doxycycline	0.1
(309)	6-Oxatetracycline	0.15
(4)	Minocycline	0.3
(327)	6-Thiatetracycline	0.8
(339)	7-Dimethylamino-6-thiatetracycline	0.85

Thin-layer chromatography (TLC) plates were prepared for the separation according to the following procedure (R. Kirchlechner, unpublished research):
Immerse TLC silica gel 60 F-256 plates in a buffer solution of 86 g Na_2HPO_4, 50 g citric acid, and 50 g Titriplex III in 2 liters water plus 2 liters methanol, and dry in air. Then prerun the plates in methyl ethyl ketone saturated with the above buffer, and dry again in air.
The chromatographic separation now ensues: solvent system for the end products was a mixture of dichloromethane, THF, acetone, and water at 48:25/25:2

Table 27. Partition coefficients for tetracyclines at various pH values with *N*-octanol. (R. KIRCHLECHNER, unpublished research)

Drug	Partition coefficient at pH		
	5.5	6.5	7.5
Tetracycline	0.021	0.018	0.014
4-Amino-6-thiatetracycline	0.567	0.697	0.524
Methacycline	0.780	0.720	0.260
Doxycycline	0.790	0.798	0.430
Minocycline	1.170	1.5	1.067
6-Oxatetracycline	1.274	0.575	0.102
7-Methoxy-6-thiatetracycline	9.380	6.530	1.438
7-Chloro-6-thiatetracycline	9.700	6.520	4.710
6-Thiatetracycline	13.650	8.560	2.380

Buffer solutions (phosphate buffer) of pH 5.5; 6.5; 7.5 were used. Five-milliliter portions of buffer solution were extracted with 5 ml octanol; each was placed for 5 min on a Whirl-Mix; absorbance of the starting solution and extracted buffer solutions was measured at 363 nm.

Table 27 gives the lipophilicity of tetracycline, of semisynthetic methacycline, of doxycycline and minocycline, as well as of 6-oxatetracycline and derivatives of 6-thiatetracycline within three different pH ranges (R. Kirchlechner, unpublished research). The figures are in good agreement with data quoted in the literature for natural and semisynthetic tetracyclines (COLAIZZI and KLINK 1969). The table shows in particular the pronounced lipophilicity of several 6-thiatetracycline derivatives. It is seen that 6-thiatetracycline is about 600 times more lipophilic than tetracycline at pH 5.5, 18 times more lipophilic than doxycycline, and 12 times more lipophilic than minocycline.

β) Influence on Gram-Positive Activity. The results of investigations into in vitro activity against gram-positive bacteria permit the conclusion that the altered lipophilic character of the 6-thiatetracyclines based on the introduction of the sulfur atom in position 6 is of no particular importance in respect of the in vitro activity against tetracycline-sensitive gram-positive bacteria.

However, one electronic factor manifests itself inasmuch as the electron-attracting substituent, chlorine, in the 7 position produces an increase in in vitro activity, while in contrast the electron-donating methoxy and dimethylamino substituents weaken the activity.

The influence of the changed lipophilic character is seen most strongly in the case of the tetracycline-resistant gram-positive bacteria. The minimum inhibitory concentrations for the tetracycline-resistant bacteria are of the same order of magnitude as the minimum inhibitory concentrations for tetracycline-sensitive bacteria.

γ) Influence on Gram-Negative Activity. It is known from the natural tetracyclines that activity against tetracycline-sensitive gram-negative bacteria is profoundly influenced by the lipophilic character of these compounds. Experimental results with natural tetracyclines show a general trend toward a decrease in activity against gram-negative bacteria, culminating in total inactivity, as the lipophilic character increases. The influence of the lipophilic character on activity against gram-negative bacteria proves to be quite different in the case of the 6-thiatetracyclines. Unlike in the natural tetracyclines, the activity against tetracycline-sensitive gram-negative bacteria remains preserved in spite of the substantially increased lipophilic character of the 6-thiatetracyclines. Furthermore, activity against tetracycline-resistant gram-negative bacteria increases until it matches the activity against tetracycline-sensitive bacteria. Owing to the fact that activity exists against the otherwise tetracycline-resistant *Proteus* strains, the spectrum is broadened even further. In addition, an electronic effect on in vitro activity manifests itself in the sense that, while the electron-attracting chlorine substituent produces no substantial change in activity, the electron-donating substituents reduce in vitro activity.

δ) Influence of the 7-Dimethylamino Group. The antibacterial activity of 7-dimethylamino-6-thiatetracycline has proved disappointing. This compound in particular was expected to exhibit good in vitro activity compared with minocycline. In fact, the opposite is the case. It may be possible to explain this paradox.

In the vicinity of the surface of bacteria, as already discussed, there is a microregion of low pH. Accordingly, the 7-dimethylamino group of minocycline (4) would, in this region, become protonized and hence strongly electron-attracting. This would result in an increased in vitro activity. By the same token, the 7-dimethylamino group of the 6-thiatetracycline would be more weakly basic and thus less protonizable than minocycline under the same conditions. The group would then be less electron-attracting, manifesting itself in poorer antibacterial activity. To this extent, the relatively poor in vitro activity of this compound, compared with the other three thiatetracyclines and with minocycline, would be understandable.

It is also possible, however, that a steric effect of the 7-dimethylamino group is seen in a structure differing from the natural tetracyclines through the sulfur atom in the 6 position.

ε) Factors Influencing the Electronic Structure. From the quantum chemical approach to structure-activity relationships in tetracyclines (CAMMARATA et al. 1970; PERADEJORDI et al. 1971), it is known that the effect of substituents on the electronic properties of the C6 atom and of the phenoldiketone region of the tetracyclines causes antibacterial properties to be graduated.

Introduction of the hetero atom S in position 6 is supposed to effect a considerable change in the electronic properties of this center.

Also, the sulfur forces electrons into the tetracyclic ring system, resulting in an increase in electron density in the β-polycarbonyl system. Hence the electronic conditions in the phenoldiketone system of the 6-thiatetracyclines should be different from those in the natural tetracyclines and these conditions may modify the properties of the molecule. It is known that the Π-electron donor ability of the phenoldiketone moiety is important to the activity and that the phenoldiketone structure is involved in the magnesium-chelating reaction.

ζ) Influence of the Sulfur Dioxide Group. The 6-thiasulfones have only slight antimicrobial activity. This may be due to the fact that the two oxygen substituents on the sulfur atom give rise to steric interactions between the β-substituents in the 6 position and the hydrogen atom C4, these interactions causing the molecule to assume conformations different from those of medicinally important tetracyclines. Also, changes in the electronic properties of the molecule could be the reason for the marked loss of in vitro activity.

η) Influence of the 11a-Hydroxy Group. It should be mentioned that the structure of the third substance tested, 11a-hydroxy-12a-dioxy-6-thiatetracycline, differs considerably from that of the antibacterially active tetracyclines and that the conformation of the nonionized form of the free base differs widely from that of 6-thiatetracycline (327) and its 5a epimer (328).

d) Conclusion

The synthesis of the 6-thiatetracyclines has permitted, for the first time, modification of the basic bacteriostatic character of the tetracyclines. It has proved possible to broaden the spectrum of activity decisively and to increase the intensity of the activity. The compounds are bactericidally active against many freshly isolated organisms in clinical practice (Table 29, next section).

Replacement of the CH_2 group in the 6 position of the tetracyclic ring system with sulfur results in the introduction of new structural, electronic, and conformational factors into the ring skeleton. The missing steric interaction between the β-substituent at the 6 position and the β-proton at the C4 position has led to a stabilization of the nonionized conformation of the molecule, resulting in the above-mentioned increased lipophilicity (PREWO et al. 1980). The sum of the effects of these variables determines the overall properties of the 6-thiatetracyclines.

6-Thiatetracyclines are the most lipophilic of all tetracyclines and yet have experienced significant improvements in their activity. This contrasts with findings for other tetracyclines which show that an increase in lipophilicity means simultaneous decrease in antibacterial activity. As already discussed earlier, the introduction of the 5a-methyl group in the tetracycline ring system for example results in a highly lipophilic 5a-methyltetracycline (273) caused by the structural effect described earlier as well as by the hydrophobic influence of the methyl group. 5a-Methyltetracycline is active against tetracycline-sensitive and tetracycline-resistant gram-positive organisms. But there is no activity against gram-negative bacteria. This finding is in agreement with other studies which have shown lipophilicity to hinder entry of molecules into gram-negative bacteria, but it stands in contrast to those of minocycline and the 6-heterotetracyclines showing that the outer membrane may not be a barrier to the entry of lipophilic tetracyclines into gram-negative bacteria and that the resistance mechanism might be less effective against more lipophilic analogues. Hence, the phenomenon exists whereby lipophilicity of the tetracyclines is of varying significance as regards their antibacterial activity.

It can be concluded that it is not lipophilicity alone which is responsible for the differences of the antibacterial activity seen for example between tetracycline, minocycline, 5a-methyltetracycline, and 6-heterotetracyclines. Indeed, besides the lipophilicity, the respective conformation of the molecule may also be an important factor in determining antibacterial activity. 6-Thiatetracyclines are active against tetracycline-resistant gram-positive and gram-negative bacteria. Since tetracycline resistance is associated with the degree of tetracycline accumulation in the cell, it can be inferred that the way the accumulation takes place for 6-thiatetracyclines is different to other tetracyclines.

It has been described (RUSSEL and AHONKHAI 1982) that plasmid-mediated resistance in gram-negative bacteria has been linked to the synthesis of novel outer and inner membrane proteins that can prevent initial tetracycline binding on the cell or tetracycline accumulation in the cell, or can promote efflux of tetracycline (CHOPRA et al. 1981).

There are indications supporting the view (BAKHTIAR and SELWYN 1983) that the presence of an R factor in the bacteria prevents the binding of tetracyclines to the bacterial cell.

Furthermore, it has been described (CHOPRA et al. 1981) that all the resistant bacteria have in common the ability to accumulate decreased amounts of tetracyclines. Where decreased accumulation is implicated there are two conceivable mechanisms: decreased uptake or increased efflux. In the case of efflux, it has been found (BALL et al. 1980; MCMARRY et al. 1980) that bacteria carrying tetracycline-resistance plasmids show increased efflux when compared with plasmidless bacteria. Both effects – uptake and efflux of tetracyclines – might operate at the same time to give an overall reduction in accumulation.

But too little is known yet about the precise role of the generally tetracycline-inducible proteins in the process of accumulation of tetracycline in the cell and therefore the picture is far from complete.

In the case of 6-thiatetracycline (327), it is postulated (RUSSEL and AHONKHAI 1982) that sufficient 6-thiatetracycline is taken up by tetracycline-resistant strains of *Escherichia coli* to "bypass" tetracycline-resistant proteins and thereby inhibit protein synthesis. Alternatively, it could be that the efflux of the accumulated 6-thiatetracycline is an inefficient process in the tetracycline-resistant strains.

Furthermore, it has been reported (NEU 1978) that the tetracyclines are not effective against resistant Enterobacteriaceae, especially *Proteus* strains, because of the cell wall structure. However, 6-thiatetracycline is evidently able to circumvent this form of resistance, to penetrate the bacterial cell wall and membrane, and to accumulate adequately inside the cell (BAKHTIAR and SELWYN 1983).

In summary, findings point to the probability that the hydrophilic/hydrophobic nature of 6-thiatetracycline permits permeation through a series of polar and nonpolar barriers as a result of structural and conformational changes within a state of equilibrium which is dependent on the nature of the solvent (HUGHES et al. 1979).

Therefore, 6-thiatetracycline should occur as an equilibrium of the zwitterionic and nonionized form and appears, in fact, to tend more toward the nonionized form than the other important tetracyclines. This stabilization of the nonionized conformation of 6-thiatetracycline leads to a more hydrophobic nature of the molecule, resulting in the increased lipophilicity which is 600 times higher than that of tetracycline and 12 times higher than that of minocycline.

According to the findings with minocycline (MACMURRY et al. 1980 and 1982) one can suggest that the high lipophilicity and certain structural and conformative features of 6-thiatetracycline may increase the rate of uptake by crossing the outer membrane more rapidly via another pathway than all the other tetracyclines and at the same time may decrease the ability of the efflux system because the active side of a possible efflux carrier or access to it may accommodate hydrophilic molecules better.

It is assumed, therefore, that the unusual structural characteristics of the 6-thiatetracyclines have led to special lipophilic characteristics and conformational peculiarities, which combine to promote penetration into the cells and to accumulate efficiently inside the cell of gram-positive and gram-negative organisms, both those which are tetracycline sensitive and those which are tetracycline resistant. This is then manifest in a broadening of the spectrum of activity and in a lessening of minimum inhibitory concentrations.

Whether these 6-thiatetracyclines, due to their changed properties, are no longer "recognized as tetracyclines" in the periplasmatic zone of the bacteria and hence no longer trigger the mechanisms which lead to changes in the permeability of the cell wall toward tetracyclines, or whether other transport routes are available to the 6-thiatetracyclines, remains an open question.

3. Pharmacodynamic and Pharmacokinetic Properties of (±)-6-Thiatetracycline (327)

A variety of reasons led to the selection of 6-thiatetracycline (327) (known in the literature as EMD 33 330) in the form of its racemate for further work leading up to clinical testing. The most important results are summarized in the following text.

a) Spectrum of Activity

The active spectrum of 6-thiatetracycline (327) was tested alongside that of tetracycline HCl, doxycycline, and minocycline against the clinically relevant gram-positive and gram-negative aerobic bacterial species. 6-Thiatetracycline was shown to cope with the bacteria normally falling within the tetracycline spectrum. Additionally, there is a broadening of the spectrum, since, unlike tetracycline, doxycycline, and minocycline, 6-thiatetracycline is also effective against *Proteus* strains (Kirchlechner et al. 1977; Rogalski 1978; Teare et al. 1981; Bakhtiar and Selwyn 1982, 1983).

b) Antibacterial Activity

Sensitivity tests were performed on 196 bacterial strains isolated from clinical material (Rogalski 1978; experimental data by H. Wahlig and E. Dingeldein). A sensitivity limit of 4 µg/ml was set for the comparative assessment of pathogen sensitivity (Table 28). In the case of gram-positive organisms, 6-thiatetracycline was effective in more than half the strains studied at concentrations of less than 4 µg/ml, in particular against *Streptococcus faecalis*, not normally within the tetracycline spectrum. Also, all 37 *Staphylococcus aureus* strains tested, even those which are regarded as being tetracycline resistant, were inhibited at concentrations of no more than 2 µg/ml. In the gram-negative range, 6-thiatetracycline was also clearly more effective against *E. coli*, *Klebsiella*, and above all *Proteus mirabilis* and indole-positive *Proteus* species than tetracycline and doxycycline. Especially to be emphasized is the clear superiority of 6-thiatetracycline against tetracycline- and doxycycline-resistant *Proteus mirabilis* strains. All of the *Haemophilus* strains tested fell within the spectrum of 6-thiatetracycline at concentrations of up to 4 µg/ml.

Table 28. Number of sensitive and resistant strains (limit value, 4 µg/ml). (Rogalski 1978; experimental data by H. Wahlig and E. Dingeldein)

Organism	Investigated strains	Thiatetracycline		Doxycycline		Tetracycline HCl	
		Sensitive	Resistant	Sensitive	Resistant	Sensitive	Resistant
Staphylococcus aureus	37 (30)	37	0	25	12	16	14
Streptococcus pyogenes/ Diplococcus pneumoniae	25 (21)	25	0	25	0	21	0
Streptococcus faecalis	12 (7)	7	5	3	9	3	4
Escherichia coli	32 (25)	32	0	25	7	16	9
Salmonella/Shigella sp.	7 (0)	7	0	7	0	–	–
Klebsiella sp.	22 (19)	17	5	9	13	11	8
Enterobacter sp.	7 (5)	3	4	2	5	3	2
Proteus mirabilis	21 (17)	20	1	1	20	0	17
Indole-positive *Proteus* sp.	18 (15)	17	1	14	4	6	9
Pseudomonas aeruginosa	15 (11)	2	13	3	12	1	10

( ) Number of strains tested against tetracycline HCl

Table 29. Bacterial efficacy of 6-thiatetracyclines (minimum bactericidal concentration) against 182 gram-positive and gram-negative clinical strains. (ROGALSKI 1978; experimental data by H. WAHLIG and E. DINGELDEIN)

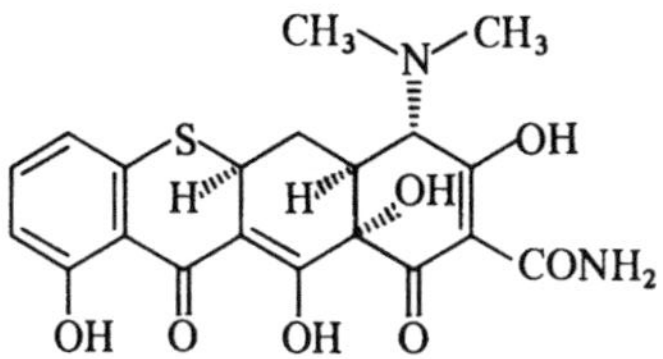

Antibiotic	Organism	Investi-gated strains	No. of killed strains, arranged acc. to MIC (μg/ml)												
			>128	128	64	32	16	8	4	2	1	0.5	0.25	0.125	≦0.063
Thiatetracycline	*Staphylococcus aureus*	32		1			13	14		4					
Doxycycline		32	7	3	12	3	5	1			1				
Tetracycline HCl		25	8		3	7	6			1					
Thiatetracycline	*Streptococcus pyogenes*	18					6	2	3	1	5	1			
Doxycycline		19	1			1	4	2	5	1	2	2	1		
Tetracycline HCl		15				3		2	2	1	2	·2	3		
Thiatetracycline	*Diplococcus pneumoniae*	6						2					2		2
Doxycycline		6							1				1		4
Tetracycline HCl		6							1	1					4
Thiatetracycline	*Streptococcus faecalis*	10					4	6							
Doxycycline		10	4	2	1	3									
Tetracycline HCl		5	3	2											

Antibiotic	Organism	Investi-gated strains	No. of killed strains, arranged acc. to MIC (μg/ml)											
			>128	128	64	32	16	8	4	2	1	0.5	0.25	0.125	≦0.063
Thiatetracycline	*Escherichia coli*	32			1			1	16	9	5				
Doxycycline		32		2	5	14	7	3		1					
Tetracycline HCl		25	7	5	9	3	1								
Thiatetracycline	*Salmonella/Shigella* sp.	7						2	2	2	1				
Doxycycline		7		1	2	1	2	1							
Tetracycline HCl		–													
Thiatetracycline	*Klebsiella* sp.	18					2	4	6	3	3				
Doxycycline		18	4	3	3	6	1				1				
Tetracycline HCl		15	5	4	2	2		1		1					
Thiatetracycline	*Enterobacter* sp.	7				1	1	5							
Doxycycline		7			3	4									
Tetracycline HCl		5	2	3											
Thiatetracycline	*Proteus mirabilis*	19			1			3	13	2					
Doxycycline		19	5	12	1	1									
Tetracycline HCl		15		10	5										
Thiatetracycline	Indole-positive *Proteus* sp.	18				1	2	3	4	3	5				
Doxycycline		18	4	1	4	7	2								
Tetracycline HCl		15	3	3	6	1	2								
Thiatetracycline	*Pseudomonas aeruginosa*	14	5	6	1	1			1						
Doxycycline		14		2	8	4									
Tetracycline HCl		10	5	5											

c) Bactericidal Effect

The bactericidal effect was tested alongside that of tetracycline and doxycycline in 182 gram-positive and gram-negative bacterial strains (Table 29; ROGALSKI 1978; experimental data by H. WAHLIG and E. DINGELDEIN). In the clinically relevant active constituent concentrations achievable in the organism, tetracyclines generally have only slight bactericidal activity, if any at all. 6-Thiatetracycline had a bactericidal effect at concentrations of up to 4 µg/ml against the majority of *E. coli, Salmonella, Klebsiella, Proteus mirabilis,* and indole-positive *Proteus* strains tested. The other substances tested came nowhere near to achieving these good results. Other comparative in vitro studies report on marked improvement of activity against gram-negative bacilli and of bactericidal effect (TEARE et al. 1981; BAKHTIAR and SELWYN 1982, 1983). Further bactericidal tests were performed to study the effect of 6-thiatetracycline on the replication rate of *Salmonella enteritidis*. 6-Thiatetracycline was shown to cause a rapid and sharp decrease in the number of replicating bacteria, with which doxycycline could not compete (Fig. 44).

d) Development of Resistance

A rapid development of resistance is frequently seen in tetracyclines used for therapeutic purposes. In in vitro investigations with a single *E. coli* strain, gradual re-

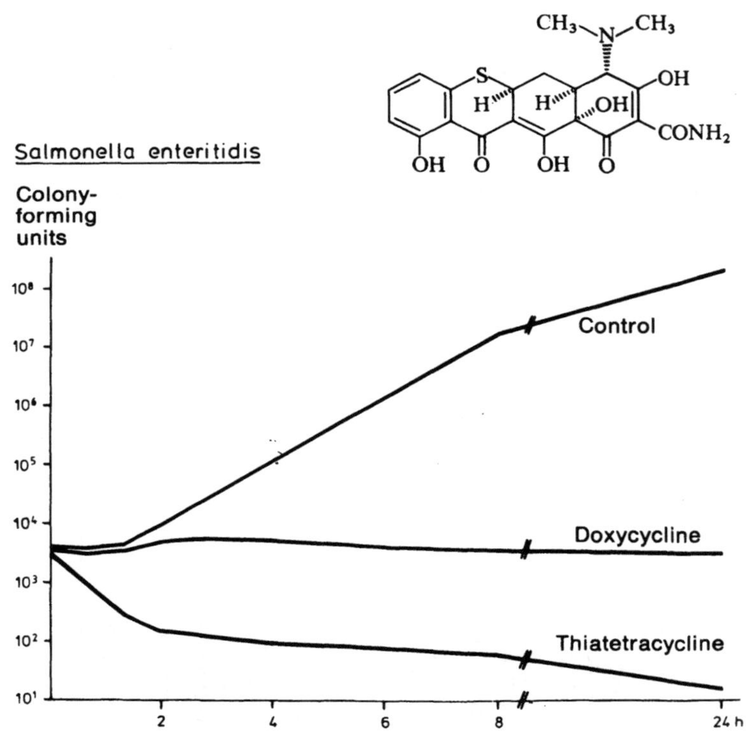

Fig. 44. Bactericidal effect of 6-thiatetracyclines. (DINGELDEIN and WAHLIG 1977)

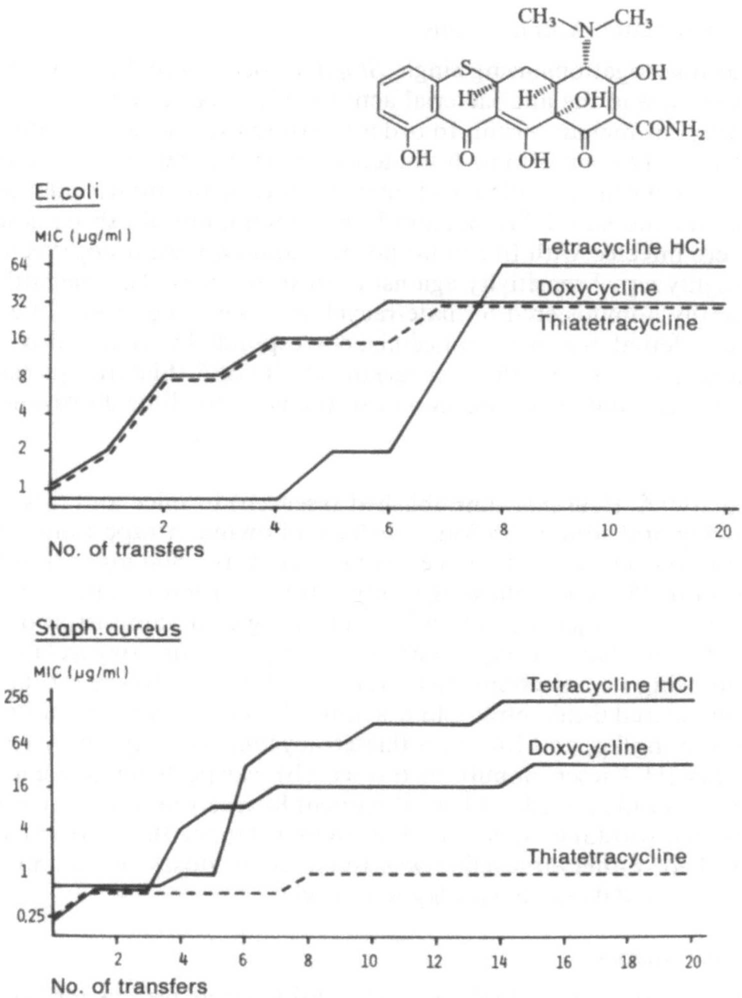

Fig. 45. Emergence of drug resistance of 6-thiatetracyclines. (DINGELDEIN and WAHLIG 1977)

sistance was developed against 6-thiatetracycline to an extent comparable with doxycycline and tetracycline. No increase in the minimum inhibitory concentrations (MICs) for three *Staphylococcus aureus* strains was observed after twenty transfers, whereas for doxycycline and tetracycline the MIC values in this trial rose to 32 and 256 µg/ml, respectively (Fig. 45; ROGALSKI 1978).

e) Protein Binding

Protein binding of 6-thiatetracycline in human and mouse serum occurs at a rate of more than 95% and in canine serum at more than 90%. Doxycycline is 90% bound and tetracycline 20%–50% bound.

f) Chemotherapeutic Animal Trials

In targeted investigations using single *Staphylococcus* and *E. coli* strains, a pronounced decrease in the antibacterial activity of 6-thiatetracycline was observed upon addition of human serum. In order to study the relevance of this phenomenon under in vivo conditions, 6-thiatetracycline was tested alongside doxycycline for its chemotherapeutic effect against an experimentally induced bacteria infection in the mouse (H. Wahlig and R. Bergmann, unpublished research). The animals were infected with five gram-positive and two gram-negative organisms having roughly equal sensitivity against both substances. The chemotherapeutic effect of orally administered 6-thiatetracycline, taking the model of experimentally induced, lethal, bacterial septicemia, corresponded to that of doxycycline. It is concluded from this that the decrease in activity of 6-thiatetracycline observed in the in vitro test following addition of serum is of no clinical relevance in vivo.

g) Toxicity

Acute toxicity (A. Heusener, unpublished research) in mice and rats was examined following oral administration as well as following intraperitoneal and intravenous injection. The LD_{50} for mice after 14 days was 1,800 mg/kg following oral administration, 95 mg/kg following intraperitoneal injection, and 73.5 mg/kg following intravenous injection. The LD_{50} following oral administration is thus of the same order as that of doxycycline (1,650 mg/kg). For doxycycline, the LD_{50} in mice following i.v. injections was given as 244 mg/kg. In the rat the LD_{50} for orally administered 6-thiatetracycline is more than 2,000 mg/kg, for i.p. 6-thiatetracycline 115 mg/kg, and for i.v. 6-thiatetracycline 44.3 mg/kg. A test for subacute toxicity (H. Kieser, unpublished research) was performed in a 4-week trial in rats (orally administered) with a subsequent 8-week observation period during which time the substance was not administered. Under the experimental conditions described, 6-thiatetracycline was tolerated in doses of 10 and 30 mg/kg, whereas doses of 100 and 300 mg/kg were toxic.

h) Pharmacokinetics

The absorption of an orally administered antibiotic as well as the intensity and duration of its serum level at above the minimum inhibitory concentrations is of tremendous importance for therapy. Table 30 shows the behavior of 6-thiatetracycline following oral administration in the mouse (DINGELDEIN and WAHLIG 1977). The results show clearly that the substance is absorbed rapidly and well; that remarkably high serum concentrations are attained after only a short time, in fact, twice as high as those for minocycline and three times as high as those for doxycycline; and that the clearly longer-persisting serum concentrations lie above the minimum inhibitory concentrations for many bacteria. Similar results were obtained in rats and dogs. The results of canine experiments are given in Table 31 (DINGELDEIN and WAHLIG 1977). In healthy subjects, the maximum serum concentration of 6-thiatetracycline following ingestion of 200 mg during a standard breakfast was 5.0 µg/ml, this being attained after about 5 h (Table 32; UNGETHÜM et al. 1980). The normal doxycycline concentration in serum was on average 3.25 µg/ml following oral administration of 200 mg and was attained roughly

Table 30. Serum concentrations (μg/ml) in mice of doxycycline, minocycline, and 6-thiatetracycline after oral application of 50 mg/kg ($N=6$). (ROGALSKI 1978; experimental data by H. WAHLIG and E. DINGELDEIN)

Antibiotic	Samples drawn after application (min)					
	Immediately before application	10	20	30	60	90
Doxycycline	0	0.31	0.83	0.86	1.38	1.41
Minocycline	0	1.04	1.48	1.93	2.25	2.10
Thiatetracycline	0	1.17	2.18	3.07	4.07	4.39

Table 31. Serum concentrations (μg/ml) in beagle dogs of doxycycline and 6-thiatetracycline after oral application of 20 mg/kg ($N=3$). (ROGALSKI 1978; experimental data by H. WAHLIG and E. DINGELDEIN)

Antibiotic	Samples drawn after application (h)								
	Immediately before application	0.25	0.5	1	1.5	2	3	4	6
Doxycycline	0	2.2	3.0	4.2	4.6	4.0	3.9	3.6	3.5
Thiatetracycline	0	1.3	3.0	5.8	7.0	8.5	7.4	7.6	7.0

Table 32. Serum concentrations (μg/ml) of doxycycline and 6-thiatetracycline following single oral administration of 200 mg given to healthy male volunteers after standardized breakfast. (UNGETHÜM et al. 1980)

Antibiotic	Times of blood sampling (h)									
	0.25	1	3	5	8	24	32	48	72	96
Doxycycline	0	0.77	2.79	2.95	2.27	1.02	0.71	0.33	0.12	0
Thiatetracycline	0	0.72	3.87	4.98	4.21	2.85	2.30	1.61	0.86	0.40

3½ h after ingestion. It is acknowledged that in the case of doxycycline the influence of food intake has a lesser effect on enteral absorption than in the case of other tetracyclines, the bioavailability of which suffers. As a sharp contrast, the relative bioavailability of 6-thiatetracycline upon administration following a meal is improved. Ingestion at breakfast, for instance, leads to a roughly 20% increase in relative bioavailability in comparison to fasting volunteers. The following elimination half-lives ($t_{50\%}$) were calculated on the basis of monitored serum concentrations: 6-thiatetracycline, 200 mg oral, about 24 h; doxycycline, 200 mg oral, about 15 h. Whereas 6-thiatetracycline still shows easily measurable serum concentrations 72 h after a single 200-mg dose (0.86 μg/ml), serum concentrations of doxycycline were, at 0.12 μg/ml, at the limit of detection 72 h after administra-

Table 33. Pharmacokinetics of EMD 33 330 in comparison to doxycycline (D) after single oral application of 100 and 200 mg EMD and 200 mg D. (Dingeldein and Ungethüm 1979)

Pharmacokinetic parameter	EMD 100 mg ($\bar{x}$)	EMD 200 mg ($\bar{x}$)	D 200 mg ($\bar{x}$)
c_{max} (μg/ml)	2.48	4.18	3.39
t_{max} (h)	2.83	3.27	2.04
$t_{1/2}$ (h)	21.889	27.314	15.313
$AUC_{0-\infty}$ ($\mu g \cdot ml^{-1} \cdot h$)	87.670	163.358	57.215
Cl_{tot} (liters/h)	1.159	1.260	3.606
Cl_{ren} (liters/h)	0.048	0.042	1.479
Renal elimination 0–96 h (% dose)	4.19	3.15	41.05

tion. Even 96 h after oral administration, 6-thiatetracycline still had measurable concentrations in serum (0.4 μg/ml).

Twenty-four after administration of 200 mg 6-thiatetracycline the serum level is still 2.85 μg/ml, so that at the time when a repeat dose is given it is still possible to reckon with pronounced antibiotic activity against the majority of potential pathogens; also, in the long term, doses can be reduced and yet effective antibiotic levels still be maintained against gram-positive and gram-negative organisms.

Measured renal elimination (0–96 h) was 3.5% of the administered dose in the case of 6-thiatetracycline, 200 mg orally; and 38.0% of the administered dose in the case of a 200-mg oral dose of doxycycline.

Furthermore a crossover study was performed on 12 healthy, fasting male volunteers to investigate serum and urine concentration during 96 h after single oral application of 100 and 200 mg 6-thiatetracycline and 200 mg doxycycline. Pharmacokinetic results are summarized in Table 33 (Dingeldein and Ungethüm 1979).

In all, three effects are observed following oral administration after a standard breakfast, as opposed to when the substance is taken by fasting persons. Firstly, the onset of 6-thiatetracycline absorption is delayed by about ¼ h; secondly, the rate of absorption is slowed down; and thirdly, the extent to which absorption occurs is improved. The overall tolerance of 6-thiatetracycline in this series of trials was found to be good.

i) Clinical Trials

As a result of the findings from the preclinical trials, 6-thiatetracycline was clinically tested in infections of the respiratory system, infections of the urogenital tract, and infections of the skin and soft tissues. Although preliminary trials in volunteers gave reason to believe that the product would be generally well tolerated, it became evident in a number of patients after only two to three doses of the product that there were considerable side effects on the CNS in some cases, so that administration of the substance was discontinued. The frequency with which these side effects occurred ultimately led the whole clinical trial to be broken off. In cases where it was not necessary to discontinue the substance, 6-thiatetracycline was seen to possess the anticipated clinical efficacy.

4. The Effect of Structural Variation on Conformational and Biological Properties

As a result of replacing the CH_2 group in the 6 position of the tetracyclic ring system by sulfur, new structural, steric, and electronic factors have been introduced into the skeleton, leading to a certain conformational change of the molecule and hence leading to new lipophilic properties.

STEZOWSKI and his research group have studied in depth the chemical-structural properties of tetracyclines by means of crystalline structure analysis and have shown that modification of the structure or changes in the stereochemistry of the BCD-ring system of tetracyclines can lead to changes in the chemical and antibacterial behavior of these compounds, these changes being again attributable to conformational properties and tautomerism of the molecule. The presence of sulfur on the C-ring of 6-thiatetracyclines endows these compounds with a structure which differs considerably from that of other tetracyclines. The effect of these structural modifications on the conformation of the free base both in the nonionized and in the zwitterionic form was investigated (PREWO and STEZOWSKI 1980; PREWO et al. 1980). The results of crystalline structure analyses have been interpreted as showing that 6-thiatetracycline is present in the nonionized form, whereby it is assumed that this is the form which is necessary for in vitro antibacterial activity to exist. Whether the zwitterionic form – necessary for the in vivo activity – is in the expected conformation is a question which has as yet not been clearly answered. Indirect substantiation for assuming the presence of the zwitterionic form is given by the ^{1}H NMR spectrum. In this, a small coupling constant is seen for the H4, H4a coupling of the 6-thiatetracycline hydrochloride. This speaks for the conformation assigned to the zwitterionic structure. Therefore, 6-thiatetracycline should occur as an equilibrium of the zwitterionic and nonionized form. 6-Thiatetracycline appears, in fact, to tend more toward the nonionized form than the other important tetracyclines. Responsibility for this is given to the lack of steric interactions between the β-substituents at the C6 atom of the natural tetracyclines and the hydrogen at C4, these normally destabilizing the conformation of the nonionized form. If the effect of the steric interactions is missing, this means that the equilibrium is shifted toward the nonionized form under physiological conditions. This again may cause 6-thiatetracycline to dwell longer in the lipophilic regions of the body and to be released more slowly to exercise its antibacterial effect than in the case of other tetracyclines. This would explain the long half-life in serum.

6-Thiatetracycline (327) and its 5a epimer (328) both have comparable in vitro activity. Both must therefore have the capability of penetrating the bacteria and of interrupting protein synthesis by reaction with the ribosomes. Both also are of comparable lipophilicity. Nevertheless, 6-thiatetracycline is active in vivo, whereas the 5a epimer is inactive. Lipophilicity is thus apparently not responsible for this descrepancy. The absence of any in vivo activity would suggest that the compound indeed does not even reach the bacterium, so that the absence of in vivo activity has something to do with the transport of the antibiotic in the blood serum. It is acknowledged that tetracyclines become bound to serum, a process which reduces their biological activity. This binding is of a hydrophobic nature.

Stezowski and co-workers have reported that in order for tetracyclines to exercise in vivo activity they must be able to assume two conformations, on the one hand that assigned to the zwitterionic and on the other that assigned to the nonionized form.

These different conformations refer to ring A, in which the hydrogens at C4 and C4a are in the one case transdiaxial, i.e., at an angle of 180° to one another, and in the other at an angle of about 60°.

In the first case the conformation is assigned to the nonionized form and in the second to the zwitterionic form. The C5a normally configured tetracycline bases and their 5a epimers have a large coupling constant in ^{1}H NMR spectroscopy in the C4,C4a transdiaxial position. The salts of the 5a-epi compounds have coupling constants of similar magnitude. This substantiates the supposition that the 5a-epi compounds in their ionized form also have the ring A conformation with transdiaxial protons. The 5a-epi compounds are hence unable in their zwitterionic form to assume the conformation assigned to this form. It is concluded that under physiological conditions either the zwitterion is not formed at all or, alternatively, it assumes a conformation not typical of the medicinally important tetracyclines.

Whatever the situation is, the implication is that the 5a epimer is bound to serum proteins in the conformation of the nonionized form. Because of its inability to assume the conformation of the zwitterionic form, the 5a epimer cannot revert from this state of affairs, so that the concentration of free, chemotherapeutic active 5a-epi-6-thiatetracycline appears to be no longer adequate to achieve bacteriostasis in the organism. It is inactive in vivo.

To summarize, investigations of the 5a-epi-6-thiatetracyclines indicated that the lack of in vivo activity was not due to its lipid absorption. It is rather the propensity of 5a-epi-6-thiatetracycline to adopt the conformation necessary for binding to serum protein which results in its reduced biological potency (PREWO et al. 1980). This explanation for the in vivo inactivity probably applies to all 5a-epi tetracyclines.

The BCD chromophore of the tetracycline structure is regarded as essential for antibacterial activity in tetracyclines. Introduction of a heteroatom in the 6 position leaves the binding geometry of the chromophore largely unaltered. The hydrogen bonds between the central carbonyl group of the chromophore and the two β-hydroxy groups is typical for those already observed in other tetracyclines (KOLLAT and STEZOWSKI 1982). It is assumed, therefore, that the introduction of the heteroatom in the 6 position primarily gives rise only to local effects in the structure of 5a-epitetracyclines.

D. Overall Structure-Activity Relationships

Studies of structure-activity relationships in the tetracyclines have shown that a number of factors are involved in determining tetracycline activity.

There are close relationships between chemical structure, configuration, conformation, and biological activity. Information available on the effects of structural modifications in the tetracyclines on biological activity points clearly to the structural features essential for tetracycline activity. The findings to date can be summed up as follows.

I. Structural Requirements for Activity

From the evidence assembled in the foregoing every tetracycline has to fulfill the following structural conditions necessary for the biological activity to exist. The linear arrangement of the rings is a fundamental prerequisite for antibacterial activity. Also, all of the medically important tetracyclines occur in the form of the di-β-hydroxyketone structure. Any interference with the keto-enol systems in ring A and rings BCD leads to a lessening of activity or to total inactivity of the tetracyclines.

The amide hydrogen can be replaced by a methyl group. Larger residues, if not rapidly cleavable in water, bring about a reduction in activity.

The C4 dimethylamino group can be replaced with a primary amino group without loss of in vitro activity. All other modifications lead to poorer activity. The presence of the 4-dimethylamino group is necessary, however, for the occurrence of the zwitterionic form, which is essential for in vivo activity in equilibrium with the nonionized form.

The configurations at the asymmetrical centers C4a, C5a, and C12a determine the conformation of the molecule. In order for optimum in vitro and in vivo activity to be unfolded, these must occur, like the center C4, in the natural α-configuration. The configurations at centers C5 and C6 are variable. For in vitro activity it is not necessary for the normal, α-configuration at center C5a to be present. The 5a β-epimers can have the same in vitro activity as their 5a α-epimers.

The hydrophobic part of the molecule from C5 to C9 is open to modification in many ways without losing antibacterial activity. Modification at C9 may be critical as steric interactions or hydrogen bonding with the oxygen atom at C10 may be detrimental to the activity. Replacement of the C6 atom through a heteroatom, in particular through sulfur, can give rise to compounds with markedly changed antibacterial and pharmacological properties. Structurally, the simplest tetracycline having a full complement of biological activity is partially synthetic 6-demethyl-6-deoxytetracycline. The simplest tetracycline with greatly improved biological activity is 6-demethyl-6-deoxy-6-thiatetracycline. Modifications at C6 and C7, in particular, have produced tetracyclines with improved antibacterial efficacy and favorable pharmacokinetics.

II. Structural Features Essential for Activity

Recent X-ray crystallographic studies (STEZOWSKI 1976, 1977; PREWO and STEZOWSKI 1977; GLATZ et al. 1979) and circular dichroism studies (MITSCHER et al. 1968, 1969, 1972) have been applied in defining the conformations and hydrogen bonding of the tetracyclines under certain conditions. The most recent papers by Stezowski and co-workers (PREWO and STEZOWSKI 1980; PREWO et al. 1980; KOLLAT and STEZOWSKI 1982), already mentioned at various points in this chapter, have considerably broadened the outlook on structure-activity relationships in tetracyclines. Although certain phenomena remain unexplained, at least much becomes more understandable and new interrelationships become clear.

Two tetracycline base structures, the zwitterionic and the nonionized forms, and the specific conformation for each of these structures are of biological significance in the medicinally important tetracyclines. Both structures are in a solvent-dependent equilibrium. The nature of this equilibrium determines the hydrophilic/hydrophobic nature of the molecule. It is assumed that for in vivo activity to exist the molecule must also have the conformation of the zwitterionic structure, while for in vitro activity a prerequisite is the nonionized structure with its associated conformation. Changes in structure and configuration can lead to conformational changes which in their turn result in changes in the equilibrium between the zwitterionic and nonionized form and thus changes in the hydrophilic/hydrophobic nature of the molecule. The degree of shift of this equilibrium is generally determined by the nature and the degree of interactions between the substituents at the C6 or 5a atoms and the hydrogen at the C4 atom.

Interactions between the β-substituents at center 6 and the proton at C4 apparently shift the equilibrium toward the zwitterionic conformation. Displacing the equilibrium toward the nonionized conformation increases the lipophilic properties of the molecule. Even in polar solvents with a high water content a not inconsiderable portion of the nonionized structure is retained in the case of the medicinally important tetracyclines (HUGHES et al. 1979). This nonionized form is readily soluble in nonaqueous organic phases, such as lipids. It can therefore be assumed that this low concentration is involved in a dynamic transport mechanism in the interface phase on the lipid membranes. Data available point to the probability that the hydrophilic/hydrophobic nature of the tetracycline molecule permits permeation through a series of polar and nonpolar barriers as a result of structural and conformational changes within a state of equilibrium.

The structural and configurative conditions at center 5a can cause far-reaching changes in the molecule. In spite of the interactions between the proton at C5a of the 5a-epi compounds and the C4 proton, there is an observed preference of the 5a epimers for the nonionized conformation, even when it is present in the structure of the ionized form (STEZOWSKI 1982). This means that the nonionized conformation is stabilized. It is thus presumed that the molecule, in departure from the equilibrium of medicinally important tetracyclines, is no longer able either to enter into the zwitterionic form under physiological conditions or to assume the conformation of the zwitterionic form. Compounds with such properties are bound to blood serum and can no longer revert from this situation owing to the lack of an equilibrium, and therefore cannot reach the actual site of action, the bacterium. These compounds are ineffectual in vivo. Larger groups, such as the methyl group, in the β-configuration at C5a cause the interactions between these and the proton at C4 to become intensified to such an extent that the molecule assumes the zwitterionic conformation. The equilibrium in such cases is probably totally in favor of the zwitterionic form. This would probably mean that the antibacterial activity is lost, since apparently the nonionized structure must also be present for in vitro antibacterial activity to exist.

If there is no β-substitution at center 6 and if, additionally, the compound has undergone a change through center 6, this can lead to a situation in which the molecule, on account of the lack of interaction between ring C and ring A, shows a great tendency to assume the conformation of the nonionized structure under physiological conditions. This then means a shift in the equilibrium of the conformations between zwitterionic and nonionized structures in favor of the nonionized one. The result would be that the compound would become increasingly lipophilic and thus become bound to a greater degree to serum. However, owing to the fact that there is an equilibrium between the zwitterionic and nonionized conformation, the tetracycline could be released slowly but steadily by unbinding from the serum proteins and thus be liberated slowly from the lipophilic regions. The product would thus have a deposition effect.

Summing up, evidence indicates (STEZOWSKI and PREWO 1980) that two chemical structures of the free base, a zwitterionic and nonionized form, are necessary to support in vivo activity and that each adopts a specific conformation. Those tetracyclines for which one or the other chemical structure or its associated conformation is not accessible are either confined to in vitro activity or are inactive.

Interactions between the tricarbonylmethane system and the dimethylamino group provide the possibility for the two chemical structures of the free base. The equilibrium between the two forms is clearly influenced by nonbonding and hydrogen-bonding interactions between the A-ring and nonchromophoric B- and C-ring moieties.

In order for the antibiotic to unfold its activity, it is absolutely essential that the site of action be reached. To do this, it must penetrate the bacterium and inhibit protein synthesis in the intracellular ribosomes.

The ability of the phenoldiketone system to donate π-electrons is important for activity (PERADEJORDI et al. 1971), since the tetracyclines apparently exercise their effect by chelating with magnesium ions, whereby the di-β-carbonyl system is regarded as being the side where chelation occurs. This complexing may be important both for the transport of the tetracycline into the cell and for its effect on the ribosomes.

The quantum mechanical approach to structure-activity relationships (PERADEJORDI et al. 1971) indicates that the variation in activity in normal tetracyclines is directly related to the electronic characteristics of the phenoldiketone and C6 molecular regions as a function of the effects of substituents. Substitutions in ring D can alter the electronic properties of the 6 center and of the phenoldiketone. Replacement of the C6 atom with a heteroatom considerably modifies the electronic properties of this center. Substitutions which raise or delocalize the charge in these two regions cause an increase to occur in in vitro antibacterial activity.

For every antibacterially active tetracycline there must apparently be certain structural and configurative requirements which are fulfilled before all the possible ring A conformations can be set up. The magnesium ion may be able to bring the tetracycline into a specific conformation through complexing, this conformation, it is assumed, being prerequisite for the activity on the ribosomes, since the conformation under physiological conditions is not necessarily the antibacterially active one.

Apart from the tetracycline-specific transport route for tetracycline into the bacterial cell via a complexing mechanism with magnesium (LAST 1969), there appear also to be unspecific possibilities for the substance to enter the bacterial cell, as already described in the case of minocycline. 6-Heterotetracyclines, in particular, appear to be able to make use of alternative transport routes. A not inconsiderable factor in these additional possible transport routes is the lipophilicity of the substance and thus certain structural and conformative features. Furthermore, a favorable combination of lipophilic and electronic properties seems to excercise some influence.

The numerous papers on the semisynthetic and totally synthetic preparation of tetracycline have shown that modifications to the structure or to the stereochemistry of the BCD chromophore cause changes in the chemical, antibacterial, and pharmacological properties, which can again be interpreted on a molecular level in terms of conformation properties and tautomerism.

III. Effect of Structural Variation on Pharmacokinetics

Prerequisite for the exercising of antibacterial activity by a substance is a sufficient concentration at the site of infection. A substance applied by the extravascular route, however, passes through the phases of absorption, dispersion, assimilation, and elimination. Thus, the drug is absorbed from the enteral or parenteral depot. It reaches the blood flow and is then partially bound to protein and other blood constituents and to the vascular walls. The bound component is antibacterially inactive. To the extent that the binding is reversible, it forms an intravascular depot. The substance is again partially bound. The nonbound portion reaches the site of action where it can unfold its activity against the organisms causing the infection. The nonbound portion also reaches the excretory organs, however, and organs in which the molecule may be converted, to be eliminated in metabolic form. This course of events in the body is just as important an aspect when one is considering structural modifications in an antibiotic as the antibacterial activity established in in vitro experiments.

Thirty years have been spent on research into tetracyclines and, despite intensive efforts, it has not proven possible to improve the spectrum and intensity of action of these drugs. It has been possible, on the other hand, to improve their pharmacokinetics. The synthesis of 6-thiatetracycline meant that for the first time structural modification led to an improvement in the spectrum and intensity of action and also in certain pharmacokinetic parameters. The pharmacokinetic parameters absorption, protein binding, half-life, elimination, and distribution in the body tissues will now be briefly examined from the point of view of structural variation. A very limited number of substances are available for comparison purposes. They comprise the natural tetracyclines which have been used in therapy, the semisynthetic tetracyclines doxycycline and minocycline, and certain data on totally synthetic 6-thiatetracycline.

The lipophilicity of tetracyclines is particularly important with regard to pharmacokinetics. Tetracyclines are known to be at their most lipophilic between pH 5 and pH 6.5. Table 28 shows the lipophilicity of tetracycline, semisynthetic methacycline, doxycycline, and minocycline, as well as that of 6-oxatetracycline and derivatives of 6-thiatetracycline in three different pH ranges.

Table 28 shows the pronounced lipophilicity of several 6-thiatetracyclines, in particular. This factor may possibly explain the properties of 6-thiatetracycline, which are reviewed below.

In acid and alkaline surroundings tetracycline and oxytetracycline have labile 6-hydroxy groups, so that in the alimentary canal already there is a breakdown of the substances into inactive and nonabsorbable tetracycline derivatives. Doxycycline and minocycline do not have these labile substituents and, furthermore, are more lipophilic. The most lipophilic compound of all, however, is 6-thiatetracycline. While the absorption rates for tetracycline and oxytetracycline are given as 58% and 77%–80%, respectively (FABRE et al. 1971), the figure for doxycycline is put at 93% (FABRE et al. 1971) and for minocycline at 100% (MACDONALD et al. 1973). Values in excess of 90% were found for 6-thiatetracycline.

The presence of ingested food especially affected the natural tetracyclines in their absorption following oral doses. Doxycycline and minocycline are reported not to be inhibited in their absorption by foodstuffs to the same extent as the natural tetracyclines (WELLING et al. 1977). By contrast, the bioavailability of 6-thiatetracycline following oral administration after breakfast rises by 20% (UNGETHÜM et al. 1980), although absorption proceeds more slowly than in the case of doxycycline, this being deduced from the time at which maximum blood levels are attained. Oral absorption of tetracyclines is dependent on the lipophilic properties of the molecule and on the stability. The far greater lipophilicity of 6-thiatetracycline has meant that the product has much improved bioavailability. This is probably attributable to the fact that 6-thiatetracycline is largely present in the duodenum, a hydrophobic zone where absorption takes place, in the nonionized conformation (STEZOWSKI 1976; PREWO and STEZOWSKI 1977; PREWO et al. 1980; COLAIZZI and KLINK 1969; BROWN and IRELAND 1978).

Numerous investigations into the serum binding of the clinically important tetracyclines have shown that the lipophilic nature of tetracyclines is the fundamental factor in deciding the extent of binding to plasma. The more lipophilic a tetracycline is, the higher is its degree of binding. Oxytetracycline is 20%–35% bound, tetracycline 25%–55%, doxycycline about 60%–90%, and minocycline 55%–75% (BROWN and IRELAND 1978), while 6-thiatetracycline with the highest lipophilicity of all tetracyclines is 95% serum bound (E. Dingeldein and H. Wahlig, unpublished research). The low degree of binding in the case of minocycline at higher lipophilicity compared with that of doxycycline is explained in terms of the steric effect of the dimethylamino group at C7.

Connected with serum binding of tetracyclines is elimination via the kidney. Seventy percent of the administered tetracycline dose, 60% of the oxytetracycline dose, 33% of the doxycycline dose, and only 11% of the minocycline dose is excreted in the urine (BROWN and IRELAND 1978). In keeping with these findings is the isolation of about 3.5% of 6-thiatetracycline, by far the most lipophilic substance, in urine (UNGETHÜM et al. 1980). This means that the greater the degree of serum binding is, the smaller is the extent of elimination via the kidney, since the protein-bound substance is not filtered into the glomeruli. Thus a considerable reduction of renal clearance takes place and, with it, reabsorption. The findings show that the lipophilicity of tetracyclines is of decisive importance in elimination of the substances.

Tetracyclines with prolonged half-lives have often been regarded as an ulterior aim, since the frequency of drug intake can be reduced, thereby affording more safety in therapy. Even 72 h after administration, 6-thiatetracycline is still present at a level of 0.8 mg/ml (UNGETHÜM et al. 1980), a level which is regarded as being just about acceptable for all tetracyclines (FABRE et al. 1971). Doxycycline is still present in a serum concentration of 0.12 μg/ml 72 h after administration under the same conditions. In the half-lives, too, it was seen that the more lipophilic the tetracycline is, the longer the half-lives are.

In summary it can be stated that the more lipophilic a tetracycline is, the better its absorption will be and the more protein-binding will increase. The consequence of this, however, is that the distribution of tetracycline into the tissue decreases and renal elimination is lessened, thereby contributing to the prolongation of the half-lives.

The factor of lipophilicity plays a decisive role in pharmacokinetics. The two lipophilic tetracyclines, minocycline and 6-thiatetracycline, exhibit CNS side effects, which are particularly noticeable in the most lipophilic of all known tetracyclines, namely 6-thiatetracycline, in fact so much so that the clinical trial had to be discontinued. It would appear that with increasing lipophilicity the concentrations in the CNS also increase, these then being responsible for the side effects.

From the point of view of pharmacokinetics, current findings would indicate that a tetracycline having a lipophilicity falling between that of tetracycline and doxycycline best satisfies all the pharmacological parameters (BROWN and IRELAND 1978).

IV. Summary

Structure-activity relationships are attributed to the interaction of three components of the tetracyclic ring system:

1. Ring A with the tricarbonylmethane chromophore and the dimethylamino group
2. The BCD chromophore
3. The nonchromophoric portions of rings B, C, and D.

Components 1 and 2, the boxed-in portion of the tetracycline molecule (350), are taboo when it comes to chemical modification, since any manipulation which produces irreversible changes in this portion of the molecule is accompanied by loss of biological activity. However, on the nonchromophoric portions of rings B, C, and D, representing the free zone in molecule (350), considerable modifications can be performed. Far-reaching substitutions as well as configurative changes and replacement of the carbon atom by heteroatoms in the 6 position are possible, with simultaneous modification of biological activity.

The precise role of the BCD chromophore, essential for the activity, is unclear, but it may be crucial to binding to the ribosome, particularly if magnesium complexation is involved (STEZOWSKI and PREWO 1980).

The A-ring of the tetracycline structure with its tricarbonylmethane chromophore and dimethylamino group which provide by their interactions the possibility for two chemical structures of the free base, a zwitterionic and a nonionized form, is of biological significance.

Also of biological significance is the specific conformation for each of these structures (STEZOWSKI and PREWO 1980).

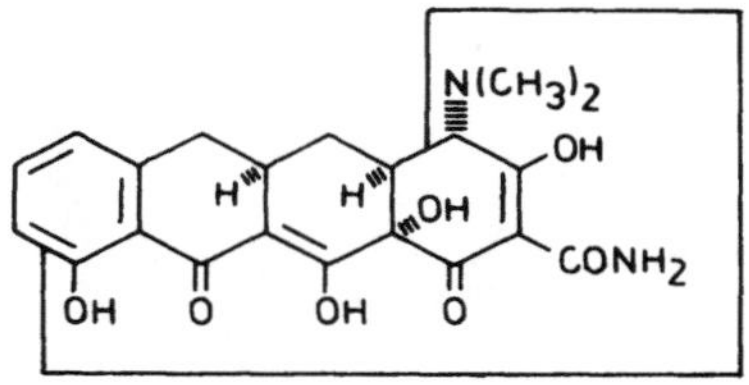

350

Evidence accumulated over the years suggests that the tetracyclines display a considerable flexibility in structure, which manifests itself in environmentally induced changes in ionization state and conformation. The finding can be interpreted in terms of a solvent-dependent equilibrium between two conformers.

$$\text{TC (nonionized enol form)} \underset{\text{lipid phase organic solvent}}{\overset{\text{aqueous or diluted acid}}{\rightleftharpoons}} \text{TC (zwitterion keto form)}$$

It is known that the extent of enolization in such a system is greatly affected by the nature of the solvent and that water tends to favor the keto form. On the other hand it could be shown that the lack of substituents at the 5, 5a, and 6 positions minimizes the influence of intramolecular repulsive forces in the determination of the conformation of the tetracyclic system. The sum of these effects determines the property of the molecule. Figure 46 shows for oxytetracycline the conformation of the zwitterionic structure (351) and the conformation of the nonionized structure (352) (PREWO and STEZOWSKI 1977).

Structure (351) presents the conformation of the zwitterionic form. The chemical structure of the zwitterion is such that both charge centers are associated with the A-ring. The positive charge is localized at the protonated dimethylamine group whereas the negative charge is distributed over the tricarbonylmethane system.

This species is highly polar and shows inter- and intramolecular hydrogen bonding.

The nonionized free base (352), shows an enolic A-ring chromophore, which is stabilized by strong hydrogen bonding between the hydroxyl group and the carbonyl moiety of the amide substituent.

The transition between the two conformers involves a twist about the bond C4a/C12a at the juncture of the A- and B-rings.

The equilibrium between these two conformers may play a significant role in their mechanism of action and is probably related to their broad antibacterial activity, membrane permeation, and pharmacokinetic properties, since there is a correlation between the conformation of the nonionized form and reported lipophilicity of tetracycline derivatives. Lipophilicity, however, is an essential factor of the biological activity.

In a presentation (STEZOWSKI 1982) about the "Intramolecular Information Transfer in Tetracycline Antibiotics" at the "Symposium on Steric Effects in Bio-

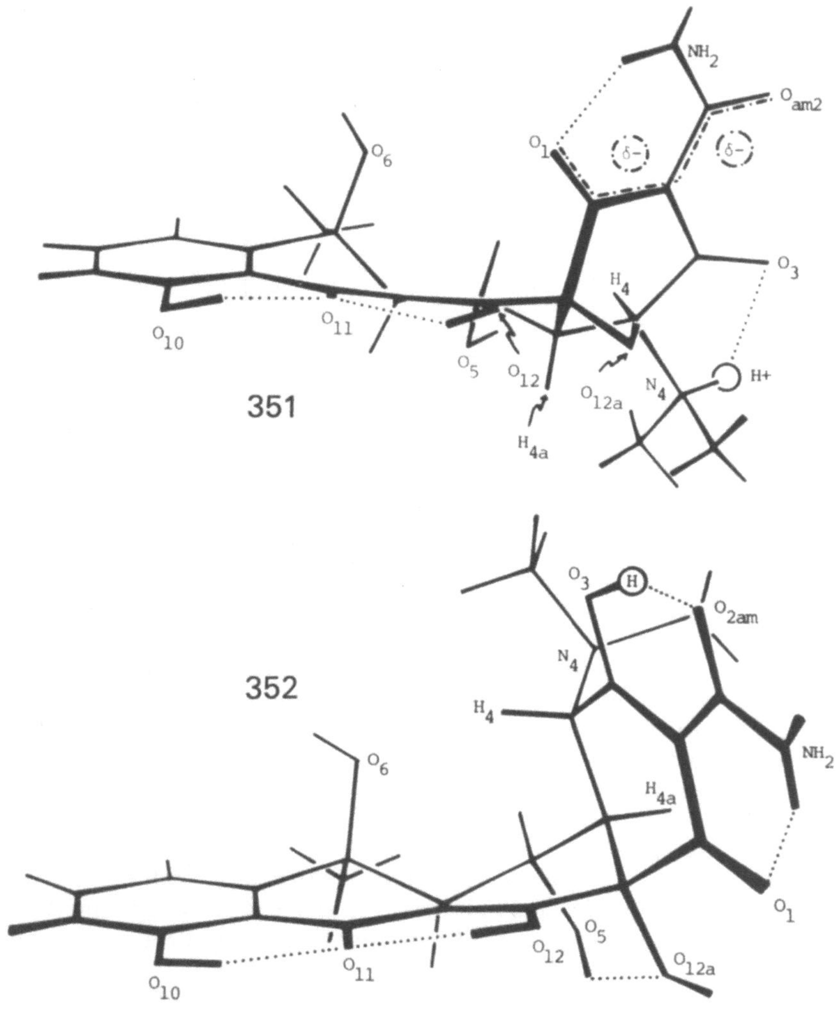

Fig. 46. The crystallographically observed conformations of oxytetracycline free bases. The drawings presented were constructed from ORTEP plots. The observed intramolecular hydrogen bonding is indicated by *dotted lines*. (PREWO and STEZOWSKI 1977)

molecules," Stezowski has summarized the results of the studies in this field as follows:

"We believe that our crystallographic work has provided insight into the effects resulting from substitution at sites 5, 6, and 7 that give rise to the differences in the relative population. Our studies reveal certain steric interactions, alluded to above, which we feel can be appropriately characterized as giving rise to an intramolecular information transfer process that directly influences the environmental dependence of the equilibrium and thereby strongly influences the antibacterial properties of a given derivative.

This theory is based upon the following concepts:

a) For tetracycline (the "parent" derivative), the low energy form for the chemical structure and conformation of an isolated molecule of the free base are those of the nonionized free base rather than those of the zwitterion,
b) That environmental effects, particularly hydration (and/or protonation), can contribute sufficient energy to give rise to the zwitterionic structure in conformation A,
c) That both species have biological importance, and
d) That steric interaction between position 6 and the hydrogen atom at position 4 strongly influences the energy difference between the tautomers."

V. Conclusions

The preceding sections have dealt with the structural features of tetracyclines necessary for biological activity. To be counted among these features are the effect of tetracyclines on the intracellular ribosomes, penetration of tetracycline through the bacterial cell wall, and transport of the substance through the body to the site of action. The structural prerequisites for antibacterial activity and for favorable pharmacokinetic properties do not always take a parallel course, so that a certain balance must be kept between these two sets of requirements. Even the best antibacterial activity is of no value if not accompanied by a maximum of clinical activity. Notari (1973), Dürckheimer (1975), and Brown and Ireland (1978) have summed up the objectives of modified tetracyclines as follows:

1. Improved antibacterial activity through a reduction of minimum inhibitory concentrations and through a broadening of the spectrum of activity
2. Good stability and solubility
3. Reduction of side effects
4. Improved pharmacokinetic properties, through an increase in the oral absorption rate and a lessening of the influence of foodstuffs on absorption, an increase in tissue distribution, a lengthening of elimination half-lives, in order to maintain a high serum level for longer, and a reduction of serum binding.

The above aims have largely been attained through the development of 6-thiatetracycline. It was the first time that molecular modification markedly improved the spectrum and intensity of the antibacterial effect and resulted in significantly improved therapeutic properties due to improved pharmacokinetics. Two of the aims have not been achieved, however; a decrease in the binding of the substance to serum and a lessening of side effects. Owing to the very high lipophilicity of 6-thiatetracycline, very high concentrations of the substance seem to enter the CNS, leading to the observed side effects. Similar side effects have also been described for minocycline, whereby this substance is reported as being the only tetracycline with satisfactory concentrations in the CNS. The increased lipophilicity of 6-thiatetracycline was without doubt one of the factors in the considerable broadening of antibacterial activity and in the favorable development of pharmacokinetic parameters such as increase of oral absorption, a lessening of the influence of foods on absorption, and a lengthening of elimination half-lives, thereby guaranteeing high serum concentrations for longer periods, leading to a reduction in dosage. The substance disregards, however, the requirement for serum binding to be reduced, since results published in the literature show that with increasing lipophilicity serum binding also increases. This is also the case in 6-thiatetracycline. Nevertheless, this effect appears not to have affected therapeutic activity.

Findings already published in the literature, namely that very lipophilic compounds also have greatly reduced antibacterial activity, were confirmed by the total synthesis of tetracycline derivatives with new structures. Minocycline, however, until then the most lipophilic compound, soon demonstrated that an increase in lipophilicity is not necessarily at the expense of antibacterial activity. 6-Thiatetracycline and other compounds from this group are by far the most lipophilic of all tetracyclines and yet have experienced a considerable broadening of the antibacterial spectrum and a lessening of minimum inhibitory concentrations in the case of gram-positive as well as and more especially in the case of gram-negative bacteria. This phenomen runs counter to the findings described in this chapter and in the literature (BLACKWOOD and ENGLISH 1970). The coincidental occurrence of favorable structural, lipophilic, and electronic factors seems to have a positive influence both on the overall antibacterial activity and on the pharmacokinetic properties of the molecule.

When the results are tabulated, one thing becomes clear. The lipophilicity is an important criterion in antibacterial activity and for pharmacokinetic properties. Since its effect can in some cases contradict notions regarding what constitutes an ideal tetracycline, it is important to define the optimum lipophilicity. The way things look today, a compromise must be found between the various ideals as to what constitutes an optimum tetracycline.

It seems barely possible to improve pharmacokinetic parameters while at the same time reducing the side effects. Also, it is quite clearly impossible to achieve lower minimum inhibitory concentrations and to broaden the spectrum of activity while maintaining the pharmacokinetics as seen in doxycycline or minocycline. In both cases lipophilicity is of crucial importance as far as we can judge today. One extremely important center for influencing this factor is position 6 and 5a in the tetracyclic ring system. The structure and configuration of these centers largely determine the conformation of the A-ring and thus also the equilibrium between the zwitterionic and the nonionized form of the molecule. The equilibrium reflects the hydrophilic and hydrophobic nature of the molecule and thus determines the antibacterial and pharmacological behavior of the substance. Position 6 in the tetracyclic ring system and its effect on the conformation of the molecule will thus remain the focus of all strategies aimed at producing new tetracyclines.

Looking back over more than 30 years of research in the tetracycline field, it is evident that it has not been possible to synthesize a tetracycline derivative which fulfills the call for an optimal tetracycline.

BROWN and IRELAND (1978) describe doxycycline and minocycline as those products on the market which best fulfill the criteria for an ideal tetracycline. It would appear as if this will remain so for some time, since apparently tetracycline research both along semisynthetic lines and along the difficult totally synthetic pathways, which culminated in the totally synthetic 6-thiatetracyclines of the research group at E. Merck, Darmstadt, has come to a halt.

References

Andre T, Ullberg S (1957) Radioactive tetracycline. J Am Chem Soc 79:494–495

Bakhtiar M, Selwyn S (1982) Comparative studies on the bactericidal activities of tetracyclines, chloramphenicol, and other "bacteriostatic" antibiotics. In: Periti P, Grassi GG (eds) Current chemotherapy and immunotherapy, proceedings of the 12th international congress of chemotherapy, vol. I. American Society for Microbiology, Washington, pp 76–77

Bakhtiar M, Selwyn S (1983) Antibacterial activity of a new thiatetracycline. J Antimicrob Chemother 11:291

Ball PR, Shales SW, Chopra I (1980) Plasmid-mediated tetracycline resistance in *Escherichia coli* involves increased efflux of the antibiotic. Biochem Biophys Res Commun 93:74–81

Barrett GC (1963) Synthesis of tetracycline analogs. J Pharm Sci 52:309–330

Beereboom JJ, Butler K (1962) Hydrolysis of 2-decarboxamido-2-cyano-6-deoxytetracycline derivatives. U.S. Patent 3,069,467

Beereboom JJ, Ursprung JJ, Rennhard HH, Stephens CR (1960) Further 6-deoxytetracycline studies: effect of aromatic substituents on biological activity. J Am Chem Soc 82:1003–1004

Berlin YA, Kolosov MN, Vasina IV, Yartseva IV (1968) The structure of chromocyclomycin. Chem Commun 762–763

Bernardelli C, Bucher G, Lauria F, Logemann W, Tosolini G, Vita G (1967) Über die Einhorn-Reaktion mit Aminosäuren. Liebigs Ann Chem 706:243–249

Bernardi L, Castiglione R De, Colonna V, Masi P, Mazzoleni R (1974) Tetracycline derivatives. I – Esters of 5-oxytetracyclines: chemistry and biological activity. Farmaco (Sci) 29:902–909

Bernardi L, Castiglione R De, Scarponi U (1975a) Simple methylation of amides. Chem Commun 320–321

Bernardi L, Castiglione R De, Colonna V, Masi P (1975b) Tetracycline derivatives. Note II. A practical synthesis of minocycline. Farmaco (Sci) 30:736–741

Bernardi L, Castiglione R De, Masi P, Mazzoleni R, Scarponi U (1975c) Tetracycline derivatives. Note III. 7- and 9-methyltetracyclines: synthesis and biological activity. Farmaco [Sci] 30:1025–1030

Bitha P, Hlavka JJ, Boothe JH (1970) 6-Fluorotetracyclines. J Med Chem 13:89–92

Blackwood RK, English AR (1970) Structure-activity relationships in the tetracycline series. Adv Appl Microbiol 13:237–266

Blackwood RK, Stephens CR (1964) Novel C-4 modified tetracycline derivatives. J Am Chem Soc 86:2736–2737

Blackwood RK, Stephens CR (1965) Some transformations of tetracycline at the 4-position. Can J Chem 43:1382–1388

Blackwood RK, Rennhard HH, Stephens CR (1960a) Some transformations at the 12a-position of the tetracyclines. J Am Chem Soc 82:745–746

Blackwood RK, Rennhard HH, Stephens CR (1960b) Some transformations at the 12a-position in the tetracycline series. J Am Chem Soc 82:5194–5197

Blackwood RK, Beereboom JJ, Rennhard HH, Schach von Wittenau M, Stephens CR (1961) 6-Methylenetetracyclines. A new class of tetracycline antibiotics. J Am Chem Soc 83:2773–2775

Blackwood RK, Beereboom JJ, Rennhard HH, Schach von Wittenau M, Stephens CR (1963) 6-Methylenetetracyclines. J Am Chem Soc 85:3943–3953

Boothe JH, Hlavka JJ (1978) Tetracyclines. Encycl Chem Tech 3:64–78

Boothe JH, Bonvicino GE, Waller CW, Petisi JP, Wilkinson RW, Broschard RB (1958) Chemistry of the tetracycline antibiotics. J Am Chem Soc 80:1654–1657

Boothe JH, Kende AS, Fields TL, Wilkinson RG (1959) Total synthesis of tetracyclines. I. (±)-Dedimethylamino-12a-deoxy-6-demethylanhydrochlorotetracycline. J Am Chem Soc 81:1006–1007

Boothe JH, Hlavka JJ, Petisi JP, Spencer JL (1960) 6-Deoxytetracyclines. I. Chemical modification by electrophilic substitution. J Am Chem Soc 82:1253–1254
Brown JR, Ireland DS (1978) Structural requirements for tetracycline activity. Pharmacol Chemother 15:161–202
Brunzell A (1962) *N*-Pyrrolidinomethyltetracycline. Stabilität in Lösungen und papierchromatographische Prüfung. Acta Chem Scand 16:245–246
Cammarata A, Yau SJ, Collett JH, Martin AN (1970) Correlation of the potencies of tetracyclines in vitro with a D-ring substituent Index. Mol Pharmacol 6:61–66
Chandra R, Dabral PK, Sharma MC, Mukerji S (1980) Water soluble tetracycline derivative: Part-II: 2-(D-glucosaminomethyl) tetracycline dihydrochloride. Indian J Pharm Sci 42:33–36
Cheney LC, Fayetteville, Risser WC, Gottstein WJ (1958) Mannich bases of tetracycline antibiotics. U.S. Patent 3,104,240
Chopra I, Howe TGB, Linton AH, Linton KB, Richmond MH, Speller DCE (1981) The tetracyclines: prospects at the beginning of the 1980s. J Antimicrob Chemother 8:5–21
Chu DTW, Huckin SN (1980) Chemistry of hexamethyldisilazane. Silylation of β-diketones and amination of β-triketones. Can J Chem 58:138–142
Chu DTW, Huckin SN, Bernstein E, Garmaise DL, Egan RS, Stanaszek RS (1981) Chemistry of chelocardin. V. Condensation with amino reagents. Can J Chem 59:763–767
Church RFR, Schaub RE, Weiss MJ (1971) Synthesis of 7-dimethylamino-6-demethyl-6-deoxytetracycline (Minocycline) via 9-nitro-6-demethyl-6-deoxytetracycline. J Org Chem 36:723–725
Cid-Dresdner H (1965) The crystal structure of terramycin hydrochloride, $C_{22}H_{24}N_2O_9 \cdot HCl$. Z Kristallogr 121:170–189
Clive DLJ (1968) Chemistry of tetracyclines. Q Rev Chem Soc 22:435–456
Colaizzi JL, Klink PR (1969) pH-partition behavior of tetracyclines. J Pharm Sci 58:1184–1189
Collett JH, Collett C, Martin AN, Cammarata A (1970) The effects of some tetracyclines on synchronously growing cultures of *Escherichia coli* B/r. J Pharm Pharmacol 22:672–678
Conover LH, Butler K, Johnston JD, Korst JJ, Woodward RB (1962) The total synthesis of 6-demethyl-6-deoxytetracycline. J Am Chem Soc 84:3222–3224
de Carneri I, Coppi G, Lauria F, Logemann W (1961) Una nouva tetraciclina solubile: la tetraciclina-L-metilenlisina. Farmaco [Prat] 16:65–79
Dingeldein E, Ungethüm W (1979) Pharmacokinetics of EMD 33330, a totally synthetic tetracycline. 11th International congress of chemotherapy and 19th interscience conference on antimicrobial agents chemotherapy, Boston, Oct 1979, Abstract 510
Dingeldein E, Wahlig H (1977) EMD 33330, a new synthetic thiatetracycline. In vitro and in vivo evaluation. XVII. Interscience conference on antimicrobial agents and chemotherapy, New York, Oct 1977; Abstract 71
Doerschuk AP, Bitler BA, McCormick JRD (1955) Reversible isomerizations in the tetracycline family. J Am Chem Soc 77:4687
Donohue J, Dunitz JD, Trueblood KN, Webster MS (1963) The crystal structure of aureomycin (chlortetracycline) hydrochloride. Configuration, bond distances and conformation. J Am Chem Soc 85:851–856
Dürckheimer W (1975) Tetracycline: Chemie, Biochemie und Struktur-Wirkungs-Beziehungen. Angew Chem 87:751–764
Esse RC, Lowery JA, Tamorria CR, Sieger GM (1964a) Tetracycloxides. I. A new class of tetracycline derivatives. J Am Chem Soc 86:3874–3875
Esse RC, Lowery JA, Tamorria CR, Sieger GM (1964b) Tetracycloxides. II. Transformations at the C-4 position. J Am Chem Soc 86:3875–3877
Fabre J, Milek E, Kalfopoulos P (1971) La cinétique des tétracyclines chez l'homme. I. Absorption digestive et concentrations sériques. Schweiz Med Wochenschr 101:593–598

Fields TL, Kende AS, Boothe JH (1960) Total synthesis of tetracyclines. II. Stereospecific synthesis of (±)-dedimethylamino-6-demethyl-6,12a-dideoxy-7-chlorotetracycline. J Am Chem Soc 82:1250–1251

Fields TL, Kende AS, Boothe JH (1961) Total synthesis of tetracyclines. V. The stereospecific elaboration of the tetracycline ring system. J Am Chem Soc 83:4612–4618

Fourtillan JB, Lefèbvre MA (1980) Corrélations structure – activité dans la famille des tetracyclines. Nouv Presse Med 9:64–70

Free SM, Wilson JW (1964) A mathematical contribution to structure-activity studies. J Med Chem 7:395–399

Glatz B, Helmchen G, Muxfeldt H, Porcher H, Prewo R, Senn J, Stezowski JJ, Stojda RJ, White DR (1979) A total synthesis and structural aspects of racemic 8-oxygenated tetracyclines. J Am Chem Soc 101:2171–2181

Gottstein WJ, Minor WF, Cheney LC (1959) Carboxamido derivatives of the tetracyclines. J Am Chem Soc 81:1198–1201

Granatek ES, Kaplan MA, Buckwalter FH (1963) *N*-(3-phthalidyl)-tetracycline, a new carboxamido derivative of tetracycline. J Med Chem 6:202

Green A, Boothe JH (1960) Chemistry of the tetracycline antibiotics. III. 12a-Deoxytetracycline. J Am Chem Soc 82:3950–3953

Green A, Wilkinson RG, Boothe JH (1960) Chemistry of the tetracycline antibiotics. II. Bromination of dedimethylaminotetracyclines. J Am Chem Soc 82:3946–3950

Gulbis J, Everett W Jr (1975) A ^{13}C Nuclear magnetic resonance analysis of the metal binding site in tetracycline. J Am Chem Soc 97:6248–6249

Gulbis J, Everett W Jr (1976) Metal binding characteristics of tetracycline derivatives in DMSO solution. Tetrahedron 32:913–917

Gurevich AI, Karapepetyan MG, Kolosov MN, Korobko VG, Onoprienko VV, Popravko SA, Shemyakin MM (1967) Synthesis of 12a-deoxy-5a,6-anhydrotetracycline. The first total synthesis of the naturally occurring tetracycline. Tetrahedron Lett 131–134

Hirokawa S, Okaya Y, Lovell FM, Pepinsky R (1959) Crystal structure of aureomycin hydrochloride. Z Krist 112:439–464

Hlavka JJ, Bitha P (1966) Photochemistry. IV. A photodeamination. Tetrahedron Lett 32:3843–3846

Hlavka JJ, Boothe JH (1973) The tetracyclines. Arzneimittelforsch 17:210–240

Hlavka JJ, Buyske DA (1960) Radioactive 7-iodo-6-deoxytetracycline in tumor tissue. Nature 186:1064–1065

Hlavka JJ, Krazinski HM (1963) The 6-deoxytetracyclines. VI. A photochemical transformation. J Org Chem 28:1422–1423

Hlavka JJ, Schneller A, Krazinski H, Boothe JH (1962a) The 6-deoxytetracyclines. III. Electrophilic and nucleophilic substitution. J Am Chem Soc 84:1426–1430

Hlavka JJ, Krazinski HM, Boothe JH (1962b) The 6-deoxytetracyclines. IV. A photochemical displacement of a diazonium group. J Org Chem 27:3674–3675

Hlavka JJ, Bitha P, Boothe JH (1968) 4-Hydroxypretetramids. J Am Chem Soc 90:1034–1037

Hochstein FA, Stephens CR, Conover LH, Regna PP, Pasternack R, Gordon PN, Pilgrim FJ, Brunings KJ, Woodward RB (1953) The structure of terramycin. J Am Chem Soc 75:5455–5475

Hochstein FA, Schach von Wittenau M, Tanner FW, Murai K (1960) 2-Acetyl-2-decarboxamidooxytetracycline. J Am Chem Soc 82:5934–5937

Holmlund CE, Andres WW, Shay AJ (1959) Chemical hydroxylation of 12a-deoxytetracycline. J Am Chem Soc 81:4748–4750

Hošťálek Z, Blumauerová M, Vaněk Z (1974) Genetic problems of the biosynthesis of tetracycline antibiotics. Adv Biochem Eng 3:13–67

Hüttenrauch R, Keiner I (1966) Epimerisierung von Mannich-Basen der Tetracyclin-Antibiotika. Naturwissenschaften 53:552

Hughes RE, Muxfeldt H, Dreele RB von (1971) Conformation of tetracycline ring systems. Structure of 5,12a-diacetyloxytetracycline. J Am Chem Soc 93:1037–1038

Hughes DW, Wilson WL, Butterfield AG, Pound NJ (1974) Stability of rolitetracycline in aqueous solution. J Pharm Pharmacol 26:79–80

Hughes LJ, Stezowski JJ, Hughes RE (1979) Chemical structural properties of tetracycline derivatives. 7. Evidence for the coexistence of the zwitterionic and nonionized forms of the free base in solution. J Am Chem Soc 101:7655–7657

Hussar DA, Niebergall PJ, Sugita ET, Doluisio JT (1968) Aspects of the epimerization of certain tetracycline derivatives. J Pharm Pharmacol 20:539–546

Jarowski CI (1963) Paper presented at the Sixth Pan American congress of pharmacy and biochemistry, Mexico City, December 1963

Jogun KH, Stezowski JJ (1976) Chemical-structural properties of tetracycline derivatives. 2. Coordination and conformation aspects of oxytetracycline metal ion complexation. J Am Chem Soc 98:6018–6026

Kelly RG (1964) Determination of anhydrotetracycline and 4-epianhydrotetracycline in a tetracycline mixture. J Pharm Sci 53:1551–1552

Kende AS, Fields TL, Boothe JH, Kushner S (1961) Total synthesis of tetracyclines. IV. Synthesis of an anhydrotetracycline derivative. J Am Chem Soc 83:439–449

Kirchlechner R (1981) Synthese von 6-Oxatetracyclin, einem weiteren Heteroanalogen Tetracyclin. Tetrahedron Lett 22/16:1497–1500

Kirchlechner R, Rogalski W (1980) Synthesis of 6-thiatetracycline, a highly active analogue of the antibiotic tetracycline. Tetrahedron Lett 21:247–250

Kirchlechner R, Seubert J (1982) Synthese von 6-Thiaminocyclin, einem Thiaanalogen des Antibiotikums Minocyclin. Arch Pharm 315:519–525

Kirchlechner R, Rogalski W, Dingeldein E, Wahlig H (1977) Thiatetracyclines, a new class of totalsynthetic tetracyclines. XVII. Interscience conference on antimicrobial agents and chemotherapy, New York, Oct 1977, Abstract 70

Kollat P, Stezowski JJ (1982) Nonionized 5a-epi-6-oxatetracycline free base. Acta Cryst B 38:2531–2533

Korst JJ (1972a) In 2-Stellung substituierte Tetracycline. Deutsche Offenlegungsschrift (Patent) 2065:149

Korst JJ (1972b) Verfahren zur Herstellung von 2-decarboxamido-2-iminotetracyclinen, bzw. ihren Säureadditionssalzen oder Metallsalzen. Deutsche Offenlegungsschrift (Patent) 2049:941

Korst JJ, Johnston JD, Butler K, Bianco EJ, Conover LH, Woodward RB (1968) The total synthesis of *d,l*-6 demethyl-6-deoxytetracycline. J Am Chem Soc 90:439–457

Koschel K. Hartmann G, Kersten W, Kersten H (1966) Die Wirkung des Chromomycins und einiger Anthracyclinantibiotica auf die DNA-abhängige Nucleinsäure-Synthese. Biochem Z 244:76–86

Last JA (1969) Studies on the binding of tetracycline to ribosomes. Biochim Biophys Acta 195:506–514

MacDonald H, Kelly RG, Allen ES, Noble JF, Kanegis LA (1973) Pharmacokinetics studies on minocycline in man. Clin Pharmacol Ther 14:852–861

Martell MJ, Boothe JH (1967) The 6-deoxytetracycline. VII. Alkylated aminotetracyclines possessing unique antibacterial activity. J Med Chem 10:44–46

Martell MJ Jr, Ross AS, Boothe JH (1967a) The 6-deoxytetracycline. IX. Imidomethylation. J Med Chem 10:359–363

Martell MJ Jr, Ross AS, Boothe JH (1967b) The 6-deoxytetracyclines. VIII. Acylaminomethylamides. J Med Chem 10:485–486

Martell MJ Jr, Ross AS, Boothe JH (1967c) The dehydrotetracyclines. I. Epimerization at C-6. J Am Chem Soc 89:6780–6781

Martin W, Hartung H, Urbach H, Dürckheimer W (1973) Synthesen in der Tetracyclinreihe. I. Totalsynthese von *d,l*-7-Chlor-6-desoxytetracyclinen und *d,l*-7-Chlor-6-desmethyl-6-desoxytetracyclinen der natürlichen, der 5a-epi- und der 6-epi-Reihe. Tetrahedron Lett 3513–3516

McCapra F, Scott AI, Delmotte P, Delmotte-Plaquée J (1964) The constitution of monorden, an antibiotic with tranquilising action. Tetrahedron Lett 869–875

McCormick JRD, Jensen ER (1968) Biosynthesis of tetracyclines. J Am Chem Soc 90:7126–7127
McCormick JRD, Fox SM, Smith LL, Bitler BA, Reichenthal J, Origoni VE, Muller WH, Winterbottom R, Doerschuk AP (1956) On the nature of the reversible isomerizations occurring in the tetracycline family. J Am Chem Soc 78:3547–3548
McCormick JRD, Fox SM, Smith LL, Bitler BA, Reichenthal J, Origoni VE, Muller WH, Winterbottom R, Doerschuk AP (1957) Studies of the reversible epimerization occurring in the tetracycline family. The preparation, properties and proof of structure of some 4-epi-tetracyclines. J Am Chem Soc 79:2849–2858
McCormick JRD, Miller PA, Growich JA, Sjolander NO, Doerschuk AP (1958) Two new tetracycline-related compounds: 7-chloro-5a(11a)-dehydrotetracycline and 5a-epi-tetracycline. A new route to tetracycline. J Am Chem Soc 80:5572–5573
McCormick JRD, Jensen ER, Miller PA, Doerschuk AP (1960) The 6-deoxytetracyclines. Further studies on the relationship between structure and antibacterial activity in the tetracycline-series. J Am Chem Soc 82:3381–3386
McCormick JRD, Winterbottom R, Bitha P (1965) Novel 7,11a-dihalotetracyclines and the process of preparing them. U.S. Patent 3,226,435
McMurry L, Petrucci RE, Levy SB (1980) Active efflux of tetracycline encoded by four genetically different tetracycline resistance determinants in *Escherichia coli*. Proceedings of the national academy of sciences 77:3974–3977
McMurry L, Cullinane JC, Levy SB (1982) Transport of the lipophilic analog minocycline differs from that of tetracycline in susceptible and resistant *Escherichia coli* strains. Antimicrob Agents Chemother 5:791–799
Miller MW, Hochstein FA (1962) Isolation and characterization of two new tetracycline antibiotics. J Org Chem 27:2525–2528
Mitscher LA (1978) The chemistry of the tetracycline antibiotics. Med Res Ser 9
Mitscher LA, Bonacci AC, Sokoloski TD (1968) Circular dichroism and solution conformation of the tetracycline antibiotics. Antimicrob Agents Chemother 78–86
Mitscher LA, Bonacci AC, Slater-Eng B, Hacker AW, Sokoloski TD (1969) Interaction of various tetracyclines with metallic cations in aqueous solutions as measured by circular dichroism. Antimicrob Agents Chemother 111–115
Mitscher LA, Rosenbrook WM Jr, Andres WW, Egan RS, Schenck J, Juvarkar JV (1970) Structure of chelocardin, a novel tetracycline antibiotic. Antimicrob Agents Chemother 38–41
Mitscher LA, Slater-Eng B, Sokoloski TD (1972) Circular dichroism measurements of the tetracyclines. IV. 5-Hydroxylated derivatives. Antimicrob Agents Chemother 2:66–72
Money T, Scott AI (1968) Recent advances in the chemistry and biochemistry of tetracyclines. Prog Org Chem 7:1–34
Muxfeldt H (1962) Synthesen der Tetracyclin-Reihe. Angew Chem 74/13:443–452
Muxfeldt H, Kreutzer A (1961) Tetracycline. II. Synthese des Desdimethylamino-anhydro-aureomycins. Chem Ber 94:881–893
Muxfeldt H, Rogalski W (1965) Tetracyclines. V. A total synthesis of (±)-6-deoxy-6-demethyltetracycline. J Am Chem Soc 87:933–934
Muxfeldt H, Hardtmann G, Kathawala F, Vedejs E, Mooberry JB (1968) Tetracyclines. VII. Total synthesis of *dl*-Terramycin. J Am Chem Soc 90:6534–6536
Muxfeldt H, Döpp H, Kaufmann JE, Schneider J, Hansen PE, Sasaki A, Geiser T (1973) Totalsynthese des Anhydro-aureomycins. Angew Chem Int Ed Engl 12:508–510
Muxfeldt H, Haas G, Hardtmann G, Kathawala F, Mooberry JB, Vedejs E (1979) Tetracyclines. 9. Total synthesis of *dl*-Terramycin. J Am Chem Soc 101:689–701
Neu HC (1978) Symposium on the tetracyclines: a major appraisal. Bulletin NY Acad Med 54:141–145
Nikaido H, Nakae T (1979) The outer membrane of gram-negative bacteria. Adv Microb Physiol 20:163–250
Notari RE (1973) Pharmacokinetics and molecular modification: implications in drug design and evaluation. J Pharm Sci 62:865–880

Oliver TJ, Prokop JF, Bower RR, Otto RH (1962) Chelocardin, a new broad-spectrum antibiotic. I. Discovery and biological properties. Antimicrob Agents Chemother 583–591

Pelcak E, Dornbush A (1948) Aureomycin – a new antibiotic. Ann NY Acad Sci 51:218

Peradejordi F, Martin AN, Cammarata A (1971) Quantum chemical approach to structure-activity relationships of tetracycline antibiotics. J Pharm Sci 60:576–582

Petisi J, Spencer JL, Hlavka JJ, Boothe JH (1962) 6-Deoxytetracyclines. III. Nitrations and subsequent reactions. J Med Pharm Chem 5:538–546

Prewo R, Stezowski JJ (1977) Chemical structural properties of tetracycline derivatives. 3. The integrity of the conformation of the nonionized free base. J Am Chem Soc 99:1117–1121

Prewo R, Stezowski JJ (1980) Chemical-structural properties of tetracycline derivatives. 9. 7-Chlorotetracycline derivatives with modified stereochemistry. J Am Chem Soc 102:7015–7020

Prewo R, Stezowski JJ, Kirchlechner R (1980) Chemical-structural properties of tetracycline derivatives. 10. The 6-thiatetracyclines. J Am Chem Soc 102:7021–7026

Purcell WP, Bass GE, Clayton JM (1973) Strategy of drug design, a molecular guide to biological activity. Wiley, New York

Purich SD, Colaizzi JL, Poust RI (1973) pH-partition behaviour of amino acid-like β-lactum antibiotics. J Pharm Sci 62:545–549

Redin GS (1966) Antibacterial activity in mice of minocycline, a new tetracycline. Antimicrob Agents Chemother 371–376

Remmers EG, Sieger GM, Doerschuk AP (1963) Some observations on the kinetics of the C-4 epimerization of tetracycline. J Pharm Sci 52:752–756

Rennhard HH, Blackwood RK, Stephens CR (1961) Fluortetracyclines. I. Perchloryl fluoride studies in the tetracycline series. J Am Chem Soc 83:2775–2777

Rigler NE, Bag SP, Leyden DE, Sudmeier JL, Reilley CN (1965) Determination of a protonation scheme of tetracycline using nuclear magnetic resonance. Anal Chem 37:872–875

Rogalski W (1978) Structure-activity relationships of thiatetracyclines. XVIII. Interscience conference on antimicrobial agents and chemotherapy, Atlanta, Oct 1978

Russell AD, Ahonkhai I (1982) Antibacterial activity of a new thiatetracycline antibiotic, thiacycline, in comparison with tetracycline, doxycycline and minocycline. J Antimicrob Chemother 9:445–449

Schach von Wittenau M, Beereboom JJ, Blackwood RK, Stephens CR (1962) 6-Deoxytetracyclines. III. Stereochemistry at C-6. J Am Chem Soc 84:2645–2647

Schach von Wittenau M, Hochstein FA, Stephens CR (1963) Tautomerism of 5a-11a-dehydro-7-chlorotetracycline. Preparation of 5-alkoxy-7-chloranhydrotetracyclines. J Org Chem 28:2454–2456

Schach von Wittenau M, Blackwood RK, Conover LH, Glavert RH, Woodward RB (1965) The stereochemistry at C-5 in oxytetracycline. J Am Chem Soc 87:134–135

Schach von Wittenau M, Blackwood RK (1966) Proton magnetic resonance; spectra of tetracyclines. J Org Chem 31:613–615

Schwarz JSP, Applegate HE (1967) Chemistry of tetracyclines. II. Allotetracycline and allooxytetracycline. J Org Chem 32:1241–1243

Schwarz JSP, Applegate HE, Bouchard JL, Weisenborn FL (1967) Chemistry of tetracyclines. I. Mercuric acetate oxidation of tetracycline. J Org Chem 32:1238–1241

Scott AI, Bedford CT (1962) Simulation of the biosynthesis of tetracyclines. A partial synthesis of tetracycline from anhydroaureomycin. J Am Chem Soc 84:2271–2274

Shu P (1966) Oxidative preparation of 9-hydroxytetracyclines. J Am Chem Soc 88:4529–4530

Siedel W, Söder A, Lindner F (1958) Die Aminomethylierung der Tetracycline. Zur Chemie des Reverin. Münch Med Wochenschr 17:661–663

Sinclair AC, Schenck JR, Post GG, Cardinal EV, Burokas S, Fricke HH (1962) Chelocardin, a new broad-spectrum antibiotic. II. Isolation and characterization. Antimicrob Agents Chemother 592–595
Spencer JL, Hlavka JJ, Petisi J, Krazinski HM, Boothe JH (1963) 6-Deoxytetracyclines. V. 7,9-Disubstituted products. J Med Chem 6:405–407
Steigbigel NH, Reed CW, Finland M (1968) Susceptibility of common pathogenic bacteria to seven tetracycline antibiotics in vitro. Am J Med Sci 255:179–195
Stephens CR (1962) U.S. Patent 3028409 (assigned to Chas. Pfizer and Co., Inc.)
Stephens CR, Conover LH, Pasternack R, Hochstein FA, Moreland WT, Regna PP, Pilgrim FJ, Brunings KJ, Woodward RB (1954) The structure of aureomycin. J Am Chem Soc 76:3568–3575
Stephens CR, Bianco EJ, Pilgrim FJ (1955) A new reagent for dehydrating primary amides under mild conditions. J Am Chem Soc 77:1701–1702
Stephens CR, Conover LH, Gordon PN, Pennington FC, Wagner RL, Brunings KJ, Pilgrim FJ (1956) Epitetracycline – the chemical relationship between tetracycline and "Quatrimycin". J Am Chem Soc 78:1515–1516
Stephens CR, Beereboom JJ, Rennhard HH, Gordon PN, Murai K, Blackwood RK, Schach von Wittenau M (1963) 6-Deoxytetracyclines. IV. Preparation, C-6 stereochemistry, and reactions. J Am Chem Soc 85:2643–2652
Stezowski JJ (1976) Chemical-structural properties of tetracycline derivatives. 1. Molecular structure and conformation of the free base derivatives. J Am Chem Soc 98:6012–6018
Stezowski JJ (1977) Chemical-structural properties of tetracycline antibiotics. 5. Ring A tautomerism involving the protonated amide substituent as observed in the crystal structure of α-6-deoxytetracycline hydrohaldes. J Am Chem Soc 99:1122–1129
Stezowski JJ (1982) Steric effects – Intramolecular information transfer in tetracycline antibiotics. In: Náray-Szabó (ed) Proceedings of the symposium on steric effects in biomolecules. Academia IAI Kiadó, Budapest, 1982, pp 3–13
Stezowski JJ, Prewo R (1980) Chemical-structural properties of tetracycline derivatives. Abstr Pap Am Chem Soc Meet Phys 179:87
Takeuchi Y, Buerger MJ (1960) The crystal structure of Terramycin hydrochloride. Proc Natl Acad Sci USA 46:1366–1370
Tamorria CR, Esse RC (1965) Alkoxyalkyltetracyclines. J Med Chem 8:870–872
Teare EL, Bakhtiar M, Selwyn S (1981) Comparative in vitro studies of a new thiatetracycline and three existing tetracyclines. Drugs Exp Clin Res VII (3):307–311
Terada H, Inagi T (1975) Proposed partition mechanism of tetracycline. Chem Pharm Bull 23:1960–1968
Toon S, Rowland M (1979) Quantitative structure pharmacokinetic activity relationships with some tetracyclines. J Pharm Pharmacol [Suppl] 31:43P
Tritton TR (1977) Ribosome-tetracycline interactions. Biochemistry 16:4133–4138
Tubaro E, Banci F (1964) The pharmacology of chlormethylenecycline, a new chlortetracycline. Arzneimittelforsch 5:95–100
Tute MS (1975) Lipophilicity. Chem Ind (Lond) 100–105
Ungethüm W, Dingeldein E, Pabst J, Leopold G, Diekmann H (1980) Clinical pharmacokinetics of EMD 33330, a new totally synthetic tetracycline. World conference on clinical pharmacology and therapuetics, London, 3rd–9th August 1980. Abstract No. 0438
Urbach H, Hartung H, Martin W, Dürckheimer W (1973) Synthesen in der Tetracyclinreihe. II. Totalsynthese von *d,l*-4-Amino-7-chlor-2-*N*-methylcarbamyl-2-descarbamyl-4-desdimethylamino-6-desmethyl-6-desoxytetracyclin. Tetrahedron Lett 1973:4907–4910
Valcavi U, Campanella G, Pacini N (1963) Pirazolderivati della tetracyclina e clorotetracyclina. Gazz Chim Ital 93:916–928
Valcavi U, Brandt A, Corsi GB, Minoja F, Pascucci G (1981) Chemical modifications in the tetracycline series. J Antibiotics 34:34–39
Vaněk Z, Cudlin J, Blumauerova M, Hošt'álek Z (1974) How many genes are required for the synthesis of chlortetracycline? Folia Microbiol (Prague) 16:225–240

van den Hende JH (1965) The crystal and molecular structures of 7-chloro- and 7-bromo-4-hydroxytetracycloxide. J Am Chem Soc 87:929–931
von Dreele RB, Hughes RE (1971) Crystal and molecular structure of 5,12a-diacetyloxytetracycline. J Am Chem Soc 93:7290–7296
Welling PG, Koch PA, Lau CC, Craig WA (1977) Bioavailability of tetracycline and doxycycline in fasted and nonfasted subjects. Antimicrob Agents Chemother 11:462–469
Wilkinson RG, Boothe JH (1961) Deutsches Patentamt (GP) Auslegeschrift 1, 1088, 481: Verfahren zur Herstellung neuer Verbindungen der Tetracylinreihe
Williamson DE, Everett W Jr (1975) A proton nuclear magnetic resonance study of the site of metal binding in tetracycline. J Am Chem Soc 97:2397–2405
Woodward RB (1963) The total synthesis of a tetracycline. Pure Appl Chem 6:561–573

CHAPTER 6

Mode of Action of the Tetracyclines and the Nature of Bacterial Resistance to Them

I. CHOPRA

A. Introduction

In an introductory chapter to a symposium on biochemical studies of antimicrobial drugs, GALE (1966) suggests that advances in the development or use of a particular antibiotic will depend upon answers to at least five questions:

1. What is the precise mechanism of the (selectively) toxic action?
2. What is the site of the toxic action within the sensitive cell?
3. Why is the action selective?
4. What is the relationship between the chemical structure of the drug and the chemistry of the sensitive site?
5. By what mechanisms do normally sensitive (microbial) cells become resistant to the toxic action?

In this chapter an attempt is made to address each of these points in the context of the tetracyclines. Previous reviews have dealt with most of these aspects, but generally have not been sufficiently comprehensive to cover all five points. Thus the mode of action of the tetracyclines was reviewed by FRANKLIN (1966), LASKIN (1967), GALE et al. (1972), MITSCHER (1978), and KAJI and RYOJI (1979), and the nature of resistance by LEVY et al. (1977), CHOPRA and HOWE (1978), and CHOPRA et al. (1981 a). This chapter permits an extensive review on both the

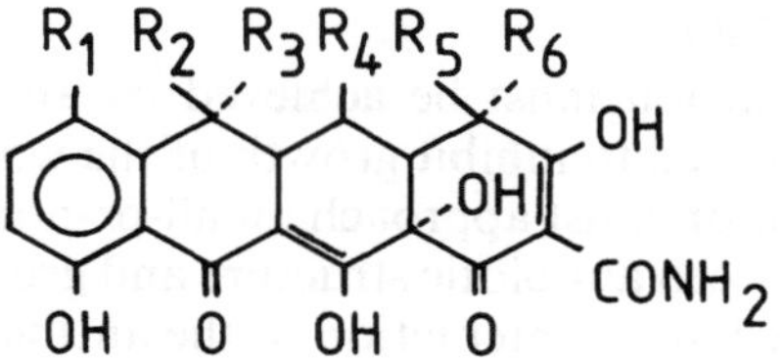

	R_1	R_2	R_3	R_4	R_5	R_6
Tetracycline	H	OH	CH_3	H	H	$N(CH_3)_2$
Oxytetracycline	H	OH	CH_3	OH	H	$N(CH_3)_2$
Chlorotetracycline	Cl	OH	CH_3	H	H	$N(CH_3)_2$
Demethylchlorotetracycline	Cl	OH	H	H	H	$N(CH_3)_2$
Doxycycline	H	H	CH_3	OH	H	$N(CH_3)_2$
β-Chelocardin	H	H	CH_3	H	NH_2	H
Minocycline	$N(CH_3)_2$	H	H	H	H	$N(CH_3)_2$

Fig. 1. Tetracyclines widely employed in studies of drug action and bacterial resistance

mode of action of the tetracyclines and the nature of bacterial resistance to them. Figure 1 lists those tetracyclines which have been extensively used for these studies.

B. Mode of Action of the Tetracyclines: Studies Before 1964

I. Introduction

The antibiotic era, ushered in by the clinical application of penicillins and sulphonamides, was soon followed by the introduction of the tetracyclines. Chlorotetracycline (Fig. 1) was the first member of the tetracycline series to be used clinically (DUGGAR 1948); this was followed by the introduction of tetracycline, oxytetracycline, demethylchlorotetracycline and more recently minocycline (Fig. 1). Following the discovery that these compounds exhibited selective toxicity towards infecting microorganisms, numerous experiments have been conducted to elucidate the basis by which the tetracyclines inhibit microbial growth. These experiments are summarized in the following sections.

II. Early Studies (1948–1953) on the Mode of Action of Tetracyclines

Investigators concerned with mechanisms of antibiotic action have always been aware of the difficulties in defining the primary site of action of a drug. Indeed, in order to avoid confusion regarding unimportant or secondary effects, HAHN (1959) produced a set of criteria to judge whether an inhibited reaction constituted the primary target:

1. The inhibited reaction must be vital to the survival or growth of the microorganism.
2. Inhibition of the reaction must occur in all those organisms known to be susceptible to the antibiotic.
3. Inhibition of the reaction must be achieved by an antibiotic concentration equivalent to that needed to inhibit growth of the whole microorganism.
4. The degree of inhibition must approach an all-or-none effect.
5. The relationship between antibiotic structure and growth inhibitory properties must also be reflected in the interaction of the antibiotic with its target site.

A survey of early work on the mode of action of tetracyclines and application of criteria 1–4 leads to an almost bewildering array of potential target sites for the tetracyclines (Table 1).

III. Studies (1953–1964) Identifying Protein Synthesis as the Primary Target for the Action of Tetracyclines

Studies in the 1950s and early 1960s identified protein synthesis as the primary target of tetracycline action. GALE and FOLKES (1953) made the important discovery that protein synthesis in washed cells of *Staphylococcus aureus* was far more

Table 1. Effects of tetracyclines on microbial systems[a]

Process inhibited	Organism studied	Tetracycline analogue used	Amount of antibiotic (μg/ml) required to achieve inhibitory effect
Oxidative and energy-producing reactions	Various	TC, CTC, OTC	0.12–1,000
Enzyme synthesis	Various	TC, CTC, OTC	0.02– 250
Enzyme activity	Various	TC, CTC, OTC	0.1 –1,000
Cell wall biosynthesis	*Escherichia coli* *Staphylococcus aureus*	CTC, OTC	2.5 – 100
Solute transport	*Escherichia coli* *Shigella flexneri*	CTC, OTC	0.3 – 100

TC, tetracycline; CTC, chlorotetracycline; OTC, oxytetracycline
[a] References to this early work can be found in the reviews by FRANKLIN (1966) and LASKIN (1967)

Table 2. Effect of chlorotetracycline and oxytetracycline on the growth and metabolism of *Staphylococcus aureus*[a]. [Based on the data of GALE and FOLKES (1953)]

Antibiotic	Antibiotic concentration (μg/ml) that inhibits growth	Antibiotic concentration (μg/ml) causing a 50% inhibition of			
		Protein synthesis	Nucleic acid synthesis	Glutamic acid transport	Catabolism of glucose
Chlorotetracycline	0.5–1.0	0.2	50	50	200
Oxytetracycline	0.5–1.0	0.4	300	500	600

[a] Metabolic studies performed on washed cell suspensions

susceptible to inhibition by tetracycline or oxytetracycline than other metabolic processes (Table 2). HASH et al. (1964) confirmed and extended the results of GALE and FOLKES (1953) by showing that the speed and extent to which tetracyclines inhibited protein synthesis in *S. aureus* was far in excess of effects on the synthesis of other macromolecules. The concentrations of tetracycline that caused cessation of protein synthesis are bacteriostatic to whole bacteria (HEMAN-ACKAH 1976).

C. Current Views on the Nature of Bacterial Protein Synthesis

I. Introduction

Current views (1964-present) on the manner by which tetracyclines inhibit bacterial protein synthesis will be considered in Sects. D–F. However, before discussing this work it seems appropriate to present a brief description of the structure of bacterial ribosomes and the nature of bacterial protein synthesis. Comprehensive treatment of these subjects is clearly beyond the scope of this chapter, but several reviews on these topics have recently appeared (BRIMACOMBE 1978; BRIMACOMBE et al. 1976, 1978; CHAMBLISS et al. 1979; GRUNBERG-MANAGO and GROS 1977; GRUNBERG-MANAGO et al. 1978; WEISSBACH and PESTKA 1977), to which the reader is referred for further information.

II. Structure of Ribosomes

Bacterial ribosomes have a sedimentation coefficient of 70S and are composed of two subunits with sedimentation coefficients of 30S and 50S. The composition of bacterial ribosomes, especially those of *Escherichia coli,* has been the subject of extensive investigations [in particular see contributions in WEISSBACH and PESTKA (1977) and CHAMBLISS et al. (1979)]. *E. coli* 30S subunits contain one molecule of 16S RNA (molecular weight, 5.5×10^5) and 21 proteins (designated S1, S2, etc.) whereas 50S subunits contain one molecule each of 5S RNA (molecular weight, 4×10^4) and 23S RNA (molecular weight, 1.1×10^6) together with 32 proteins (designated L1, L2, etc.).

In conjunction with a number of other components, including mRNA, aminoacyl tRNA and soluble factors (see Sect. C.III), ribosomes conduct the synthesis of proteins. Figures 2–4 show models of the *E. coli* ribosomal subunits and the 70S ribosome which have been constructed from electron microscopic studies.

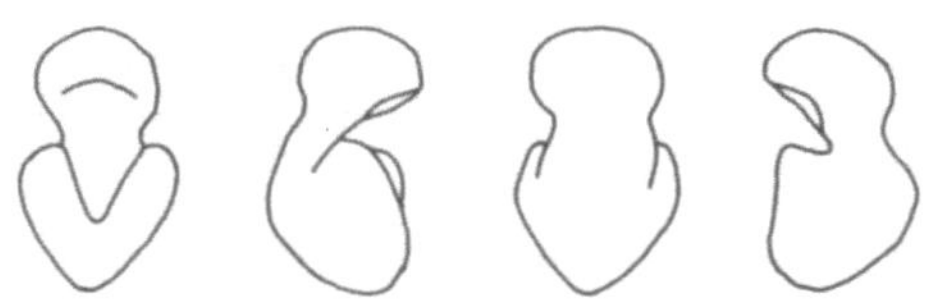

Fig. 2. Model of the *Escherichia coli* 30S ribosomal subunit. The four views are derived by successive rotation through an angle of 90°. [Based on STOFFLER and WITTMANN (1977)]

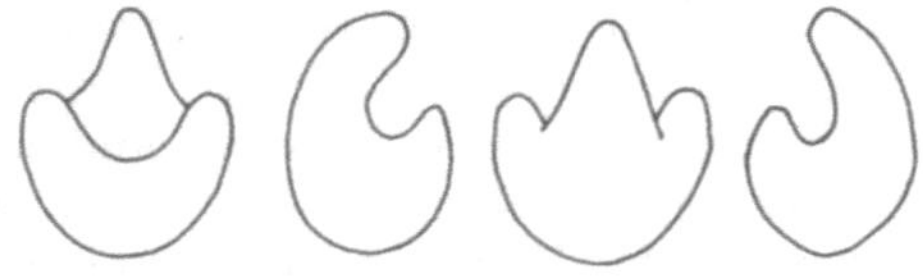

Fig. 3. Model of the *Escherichia coli* 50S ribosomal subunit. The four views are derived by successive rotation through an angle of 90°. [Based on STOFFLER and WITTMANN (1977)]

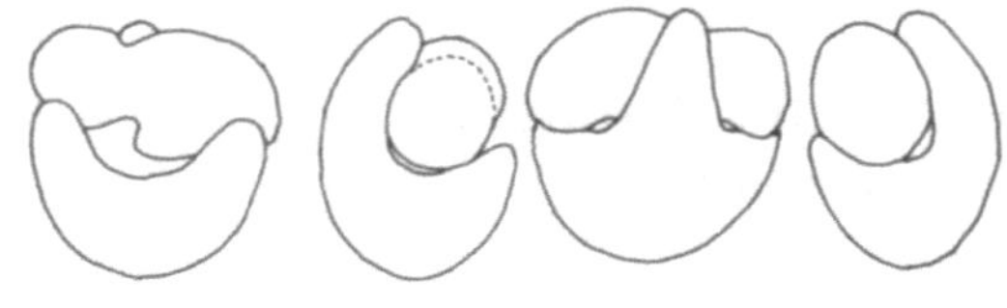

Fig. 4. Model of the *Escherichia coli* 70S ribosome with the 30S subunit lying on the 50S subunit. The four views are derived by successive rotation through an angle of 90°. [Based on STOFFLER and WITTMANN (1977)]

The groove formed between the two subunits in the 70S ribosome (Fig. 4) probably accommodates the mRNA (SZEKELY 1980). Ribosomes have two adjacent sites for the binding of tRNA during protein synthesis: the A-site (or aminoacyl) tRNA binding site) and the P-site (or peptidyl tRNA binding site). As discussed in subsequent sections the tetracyclines primarily inhibit the binding of aminoacyl tRNA to the A-site.

III. Initiation of Protein Synthesis (Fig. 5A, Steps I–IV)

Initiation of protein synthesis involves a series of reactions during which:

1. The 30S ribosomal subunit binds to the region of the mRNA containing the initiation codon AUG.

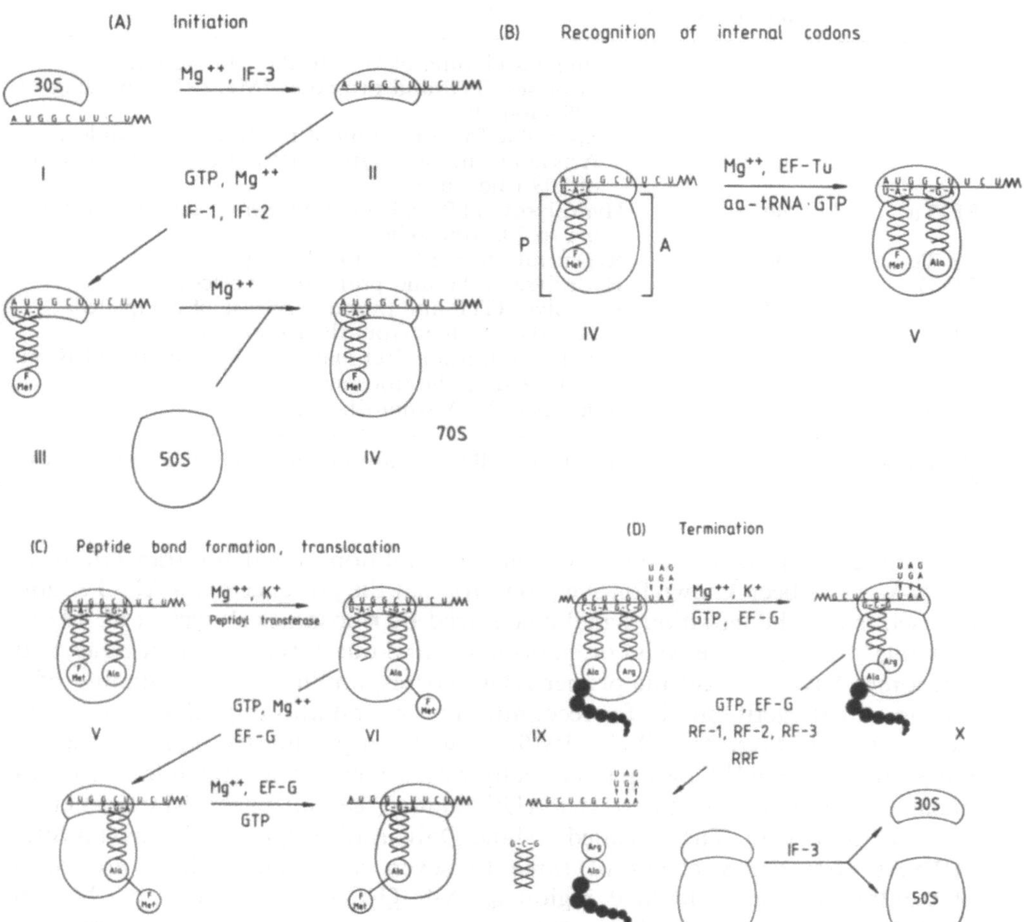

Fig. 5 A–D. Schematic summary of protein synthesis in *Escherichia coli*. Details of the individual steps are described in the text and the nature of the soluble protein factors (IF-1, IF-2 etc.) in Table 3. *P*, peptidyl site; *A*, acceptor site

2. Formylmethionyl tRNA (f-Met-tRNA$_f^{Met}$) is attached to the 30S-mRNA complex in response to the codon AUG. The resultant complex is called "the 30S initiation complex."
3. The 50S ribosomal subunit is added to form "the 70S initiation complex."

Several initiation factors (i.e. proteins playing an important role in initiation, but only transiently bound to the ribosomes) are involved in the above steps. Their properties and modes of action are summarized in Table 3 and Fig. 5A.

Table 3. Soluble protein factors involved in the synthesis of polypeptides in *Escherichia coli*. [Based on WEISSBACH (1980) and HIRASHIMA and KAJI (1972)]

Name of factor	Molecular weight (daltons × 10^3)	Function
IF-1	9	Stimulates binding of IF-2 to the 30S subunit
IF-2	118	Hydrolyses GTP and promotes fMet-tRNA binding to 30S subunits
IF-3	22	Responsible for formation of mRNA. 30S complex. Acts as an anti-association factor preventing formation of 70S ribosomes
EF-Tu	44	Hydrolyses GTP and promotes aminoacyl-tRNA binding to 70S ribosomes
EF-Ts	30	Regeneration of Ef-Tu. GTP complex
EF-G	80	Hydrolyses GTP and promotes translocation
RF-1	44	Hydrolyse GTP and promote release of completed peptidyl residues from the ribosome
RF-2	47	
RF-3	?	Function uncertain, but may stimulate binding of RF-1 and RF-2 to the ribosome
RRF	18	Releases mRNA from ribosomes

IF, initiation factor; EF, elongation factor; RF, release factor; RRF, ribosome-release factor

Although the codon AUG acts as the initiation signal for translation of mRNA, it has been known for over 10 years that the presence of an AUG codon by itself is not the initiation signal recognized by ribosomes (REVEL et al. 1970). Obviously the sequence AUG often occurs in and out of phase in a message, and ribosomes have to select the proper AUG corresponding to the beginning of a cistron. An attractive model for recognition of the initiation signal was proposed by SHINE and DALGARNO (1974, 1975), in which a pyrimidine-rich sequence at the 3′ end of 16S RNA base pairs directly with a polypurine stretch found 10–14 nucleotides upstream of the starter AUG codon (see GRUNBERG-MANAGO et al. 1978 for a review). The so-called "Shine-Dalgarno" sequences in prokaryotic mRNAs comprise stretches of three to seven nucleotides which are complementary to the underlined region $_{HO}$ A-U-U-C-C-U-C-C-A $_{(5')}$ of the 16S RNA. In addition to the "Shine-Dalgarno" region, nucleotides upstream from this area are probably important for the binding of mRNA to ribosomes (SCHERER et al. 1980). These nucleotides, some of which comprise translated codons, probably stabilize the 30S-mRNA complex by interaction with ribosomal proteins. In *E. coli* the proteins S1, S4, S12, S18, and S21 are particularly important in this context (GRUNBERG-MANAGO et al. 1978).

In conclusion, mRNA selection by ribosomes depends on a large number of variables involving both ribosomes and mRNA structure. This topic will be reconsidered in Sect. XV when the possible origin of plasmid-located tetracycline resistance genes is discussed.

IV. Recognition of Internal Codons (Fig. 5 B, Steps IV, V)

Upon addition of the 50S ribosomal subunit the 70S initiation complex is prepared for recognition of internal codons. The P-site is occupied by fMet-$tRNA_f^{Met}$ and the A-site is vacant. The codon present in the A-site (Fig. 5 B) determines the binding of cognate aminoacyl-tRNA to the ribosome. The affinity of aminoacyl-tRNA itself for the A-site is low and the aminoacyl-tRNA binding reaction involves a protein elongation factor (EF-Tu in *E. coli*) (Table 3). Aminoacyl-tRNA becomes bound to the A-site in the form of the ternary complex EF-Tu · aminoacyl-tRNA · GTP. Formylmethionyl transfer RNA (fMet-$tRNA_f^{Met}$) does not react with EF-Tu · GTP so that individual formylmethionine residues never enter the ribosomal A-site (see GRUNBERG-MANAGO et al. 1978).

Codon-anticodon interaction in the A-site is accompanied by hydrolysis of one molecule of GTP for every molecule of aminoacyl-tRNA bound. This reaction results in release of EF-Tu · GDP from the ribosome. The binary complex itself cannot bind aminoacyl-tRNA, but regeneration of EF-Tu · GDP to EF-Tu · GTP is mediated by the elongation factor EF-Ts (Table 3), which, incidentally, never binds to the ribosome. Thus GTP and GDP are allosteric effectors of EF-Tu: the EF-Tu · GDP complex cannot bind aminoacyl-tRNA and cannot be retained in the ribosome, whereas the EF-Tu · GTP complex binds aminoacyl-tRNA to form a ternary complex which interacts with the ribosomal A-site.

V. Peptide Bond Formation and Translocation (Fig. 5 C, Steps V–VIII)

Following release of the EF-Tu · GDP complex from the ribosome, the formylmethionine residue (or peptidyl residue in subsequent chain elongation cycles) is cleaved from its tRNA in the P-site and transferred to the aminoacyl-tRNA in the A-site. The reaction is catalysed by peptidyltransferase which is located in the 50S subunit. The P-site is now occupied by a deacylated tRNA and the A-site contains peptidyl-tRNA that has been elongated by one aminoacyl residue. Several coordinated processes now occur known collectively as "translocation":

1. Deacylated tRNA is released from the P-site.
2. The peptidyl-tRNA moves from the A- to the P-site, where it remains linked to the mRNA via codon-anticodon interaction.
3. Movement of mRNA and ribosome with respect to each other causes a new codon to enter the A-site.

The starting point for recognition of a further internal codon is therefore reached and the sequence of events (V–VIII, Fig. 5 C) repeated.

Maximum rates of translocation depend upon elongation factor EF–G (Table 3) and GTP. Although GTP is converted to GDP during translocation, the purpose of the hydrolysis is not fully understood (BROT 1977). Factor EF–G and GTP interact with ribosomes to form unstable ternary complexes that contain GDP. This indicates that hydrolysis of GTP occurs during, or shortly after, complex formation. Possibly translocation occurs as a result of binding of EF–G to the ribosome and hydrolysis of GTP is required to release EF–G for its recycling. Thus GTP may also be an allosteric effector of elongation factor EF–G.

VI. Termination of Protein Synthesis (Fig. 5 D, Steps IX–XII)

Termination involves the appearance of termination codons (UAG, UGA or UAA) in the A-site and the release factors RF-1, RF-2, and RF-3 (Table 3). RF-1 (in the presence of UAG or UAA) and RF-2 (in the presence of UGA or UAA) promote cleavage of the completed peptidyl residue from tRNA by activating peptidyl transferase. The peptide leaves the ribosome and adopts the conformation of an active protein. Release of the deacylated tRNA and mRNA from the 70S ribosome also occur at this stage. These steps probably require EF–G, hydrolysis of GTP and the additional factor RRF (ribosome-release factor) (Table 3). Initiation factor IF3 (Table 3) prevents reassociation of subunits to form 70S ribosomes, thus permitting the start of another initiation cycle.

D. Effects of Tetracyclines on Protein Synthesis in Prokaryotes

I. Effects of Tetracyclines on the Synthesis of Protein In Vivo

Elucidation of the mode of action of tetracyclines has been derived primarily from in vitro studies. However, before discussing this work it is important to consider experiments which examined the effects of tetracycline upon protein synthesis in vivo. This is a useful approach because the in vivo effects can then be related to the observations made in vitro.

CUNDLIFFE (1967) developed a system using *Bacillus* protoplasts which permitted investigation of the effects of antibiotics on polysome metabolism. This approach is particularly useful for indicating those antibiotics which selectively inhibit peptide chain elongation. Such drugs, at some concentration, will cause release of ribosomes from polysomes, but the extent of this release should not exceed 50%. The reasoning behind this statement (see CUNDLIFFE 1967; GALE et al. 1972) is as follows. Polysomes are formed by the successive attachment of ribosomes to the 5′ end of mRNA to produce complexes consisting on average of 15–20 ribosomes [based on the calculations of LEIJ et al. (1979) and assuming (MCQUILLEN 1966) that the molecular weight of an average protein is 50,000]. Inhibition of chain elongation will prevent movement of ribosomes along the mRNA, but any unaffected ribosomes on the 3′ side of inhibited ribosomes should be able to complete their nascent proteins and become released from the mRNA. Assuming that the binding of drug to the ribosome is random, concentrations of the drug resulting in one interaction per polysome would release about 50% of the component ribosomes. In contrast, drugs having selective effects upon initiation should cause release of more than 50% of the ribosomes, and drugs which preferentially inhibit termination should prevent polysome breakdown.

Low concentrations of chlorotetracycline (1–5 μg/ml) caused polysome breakdown in metabolically active *Bacillus* protoplasts and released about 50% of the ribosomes from mRNA (CUNDLIFFE 1967). These findings are consistent with inhibition of chain elongation by chlorotetracycline. At higher drug concentrations (150 μg/ml) polysome breakdown was reduced (CUNDLIFFE 1967). This result is predictable as higher drug concentrations lead to inactivation of more than one ribosome per polysome. GURGO et al. (1969) performed experiments analogous to those of CUNDLIFFE (1967), but found that high concentrations of tetracycline (100 μg/ml) caused polysome breakdown. The data on polysome metabolism (CUNDLIFFE 1967; GURGO et al. 1969) could therefore be interpreted to indicate that tetracyclines inhibit both polypeptide chain elongation and initiation.

Further in vivo studies (CUNDLIFFE and MCQUILLEN 1967) showed that inhibition of chain elongation did not result from inhibition of peptidyl transferase. Puromycin, by acting as an analogue of aminoacyl-adenosine, causes release of nascent peptides (as peptidyl-puromycin) from tRNA bound to ribosomes. The so-called "puromycin reaction" requires participation of peptidyl transferase (GALE et al. 1972). In *Bacillus* protoplasts chlorotetracycline failed to inhibit the "puromycin reaction," thereby implying that the drug does not directly prevent peptide bond formation (CUNDLIFFE and MCQUILLEN 1967).

II. Effects of Tetracyclines on the Synthesis of Protein In Vitro

1. Tetracyclines Do Not Inhibit Aminoacyl-tRNA Formation

Formation of aminoacyl-tRNA proceeds in two stages. In the first stage the amino acid is activated, i.e. linked, to adenosylmonophosphate by an acid anhydride bond. In the second stage the aminoacyl residue is transferred to a tRNA molecule. These processes are not inhibited by the tetracyclines (FRANKLIN 1963; LASKIN and CHAN 1964).

2. Tetracyclines Do Not Inhibit Attachment of mRNA to 30S Ribosomal Subunits

Although SUAREZ and NATHANS (1965) and HIEROWSKI (1965) demonstrated that tetracyclines do not inhibit association of poly U with *E. coli* ribosomes, other experiments (summarized by FRANKLIN 1966) suggested that attachment of mRNA to ribosomes might indeed be prevented. This possibility was re-examined by FRANKLIN (1966). *E. coli* ribosomes depleted of endogenous mRNA were incubated with exogenous messenger RNA in the presence of soluble factors capable of promoting protein synthesis. Chlorotetracycline added before, together with, or after the addition of exogenous mRNA had an equivalent inhibitory effect on protein synthesis. FRANKLIN (1966) therefore concluded that chlorotetracycline does not inhibit protein synthesis by preventing attachment of mRNA to the ribosome.

3. Tetracyclines Do Not Inhibit Translocation or Peptidyl Transferase Activity

It is generally agreed that tetracyclines do not inhibit translocation or peptidyl transferase reactions in vitro (Gale et al. 1972; Kaji and Ryoji 1979). In those cases where peptidyl transferase is inhibited by tetracycline in vitro, high drug concentrations ($>10^{-3}$ *M*) are usually required (Traut and Monro 1964). The results of Cerna et al. (1969) indicating inhibition of peptidyl transferase in vitro at tetracycline concentrations of only 10^{-4} *M* are thought to be atypical (see Gale et al. 1972).

4. Tetracyclines Inhibit Binding of Aminoacyl-tRNA to the Ribosomal A-Site: The Major Mode of Action

As noted in Sect. C.IV binding of aminoacyl-tRNA to the ribosomal A-site in vivo involves formation of the complex EF-Tu · aminoacyl-tRNA · GTP. Although the non-enzymatic binding is slower than the process catalysed by EF-Tu (Gavrilova et al. 1976) amino acids which bind to ribosomes in the absence of the elongation factor can participate in peptide bond formation (Igarashi and Kaji 1967). Before the involvement of EF-Tu in protein synthesis was recognized, two groups demonstrated that tetracycline inhibits the non-enzymatic binding of aminoacyl-tRNA to ribosomes (Suarez and Nathans 1965; Hierowski 1965). The existence of two ribosomal binding sites for tRNA (corresponding to the A- and P-sites) was recognized by 1965 and indeed Suarez and Nathans (1965) correctly deduced that tetracycline preferentially inhibits the binding of aminoacyl-tRNA to one of them (now recognized as the A-site).

Gottesman (1967) considerably clarified the mode of action of tetracyclines. Polylysyl-tRNA and lysyl-tRNA were isolated from *E. coli*. Their binding to 70S ribosome-poly A complexes and ability to form additional peptide bonds were examined. Neither binding of polylysyl-tRNA to ribosomes, nor the ability of polylysine to participate in the "puromycin reaction," were affected by chlorotetracycline. Unlike polylysyl-tRNA, lysyl-tRNA added subsequently did not react with puromycin. Furthermore the subsequent binding of lysyl-tRNA to the ribosome was inhibited by chlorotetracycline. Gottesman (1967) interpreted the results as follows:

1. Binding of polylysyl-tRNA occurs at the P-site in a manner unaffected by chlorotetracycline.
2. In ribosomes containing polylysyl-tRNA in the P-site, lysyl-tRNA binds to the A-site. Binding of lysyl-tRNA to the A-site is inhibited by chlorotetracycline.
3. Peptide bond formation is not directly inhibited by chlorotetracycline.

After the role of EF-Tu in the binding of aminoacyl-tRNA to the A-site was recognized (Ravel 1967), several groups convincingly demonstrated that enzymic (EF-Tu mediated) in vitro binding of aminoacyl-tRNA is strongly inhibited by tetracyclines (Lucas-Lenard and Haenni 1968; Gordon 1969; Ravel et al. 1969; Skoultchi et al. 1970). Furthermore, reduced binding of aminoacyl-tRNA to the ribosome was not caused simply by lack of formation of the EF-Tu · aminoacyl-tRNA · GTP complex (Jerez et al. 1969).

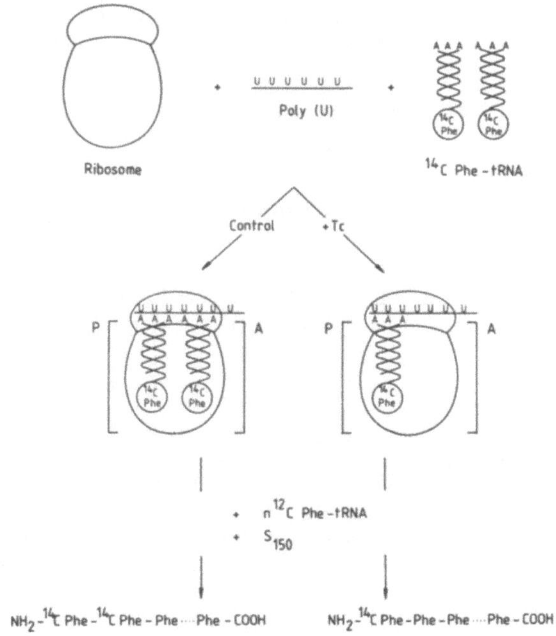

Fig. 6. Summary of experiments performed by IGARASHI and KAJI (1970) to demonstrate preferential inhibition by tetracycline of aminoacyl-tRNA binding to the ribosomal A-site. *P*, peptidyl site; *A*, acceptor site; *S150*, soluble protein fraction obtained after centrifugation of *Escherichia coli* extracts at 150,000 g. [Based on Fig. 2 in KAJI and RYOJI (1979)]

Although the involvement of EF-Tu in protein synthesis was recognized in 1967, valuable experiments concerning the action of tetracyclines have nevertheless been conducted in its absence. An example is provided by the elegant studies of IGARASHI and KAJI (1970) (Fig. 6). Non-enzymic binding of aminoacyl-tRNA to mRNA-70S ribosome complexes is affected by the concentration of Mg^{2+} (IGARASHI et al. 1969; IGARASHI and KAJI 1970). At Mg^{2+} concentrations greater than 12 m*M*, aminoacyl-tRNA enters both the P- and the A-site, but below 10 m*M* Mg^{2+} only the P-site is utilized. IGARASHI and KAJI (1970) produced 70S-poly U-^{14}C-phenylalanine-tRNA complexes in the presence of 13 m*M* Mg^{2+}. Under these conditions the ^{14}C-labelled aminoacyl-tRNA was located in both the P- and the A-sites. The complex containing ^{14}C-labelled phenylalanine was then mixed with non-radioactive phenylalanine-tRNA and the formation of peptide bonds permitted by addition of the soluble protein fraction (S-150). N-terminal analysis of the resultant polyphenylalanine revealed, as expected, that the N-terminal residue and its adjoining neighbour were radioactive, whereas all the other phenylalanine residues were unlabelled. When tetracycline was present during formation of the 70S-poly U-^{14}C-phenylalanine-tRNA complexes a different result was obtained (Fig. 6). In this case the radioactivity was located predominantly in the N-terminal phenylalanine residue. These results show that tetracycline preferentially inhibits the binding of aminoacyl-tRNA to the ribosomal A-site.

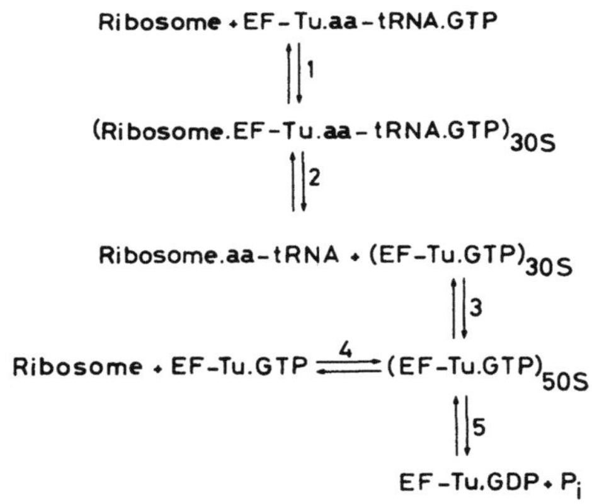

Fig. 7. Possible interactions of binary and ternary complexes containing EF-Tu with 70S ribosomes. The scheme shown is speculative. In step *1* (inhibited by tetracyclines) the ternary complex binds to that part of the A-site located in the 30S subunit. In step *2* the aminoacyl-tRNA becomes stabilized and the EF-Tu · GTP complex becomes transferred (step *3*) to the 50S subunit. Step *4* shows direct binding of the binary complex to the 50S subunit. Step *5* shows hydrolysis of GTP and release of EF-Tu · GDP from the ribosome

As noted in Sect. C.IV the GTPase activity associated with EF-Tu is normally dependent upon both charged tRNA and ribosomes. Despite the ability of tetracyclines to prevent binding of the EF-Tu-aminoacyl-tRNA · GTP complex, they do not inhibit the GTPase activity of EF-Tu (GORDON 1969; LUCAS-LENARD et al. 1969). This led to the suggestion (SKOULTCHI et al. 1969) that tetracyclines might permit a loose binding of the ternary complex to the ribosome, sufficient to promote GTP cleavage, but not stable enough to permit detection of the binding by methods normally used. In fact, the results of GORDON (1969) and LUCAS-LENARD et al. (1969) are probably explained by the finding that the binary complex EF-Tu · GTP can interact with ribosomes and cause GTP hydrolysis (see GRUNBERG-MANAGO et al. 1978). One must assume therefore that tetracyclines do not inhibit the binding of EF-Tu · GTP nor the subsequent ability of the ribosome to activate the GTPase site on the soluble factor. Because the ribosomal site which activates GTPase is located on the 50S subunit (GORDON 1969) and the binding site for tetracycline is probably located in the 30S subunit (see Sect. E.II), the interactions of the binary and ternary complexes with 70S ribosomes may proceed as shown in Fig. 7.

5. Tetracyclines Inhibit Reactions at the P-Site and Affect Polypeptide Initiation: Minor Modes of Action

In growing bacteria the majority of ribosomes are engaged in protein synthesis and the peptidyl sites are occupied either by peptidyl-tRNA or deacylated tRNA. Hence incoming aminoacyl-tRNA binds only to the A-sites. Therefore the statement that tetracyclines prevent the binding of aminoacyl-tRNA during chain elongation means that the inhibitory action is primarily upon the A-site.

Tetracyclines can, however, under certain circumstances, affect the ribosomal P-site. TANAKA et al. (1972) indirectly monitored the effect of tetracycline upon the binding of phenylalanyl-tRNA to the A- and P-sites of 70S-poly U ribosomal complexes. Tetracycline inhibited significantly the binding of phenylalanyl-tRNA at the P-site as well as the A-site in the presence of high concentrations (13 m*M*) of Mg^{2+}. Although the region on the 30S subunit into which fMet-$tRNA_f^{Met}$ binds during polypeptide chain initiation (see Fig. 5 A) is not considered to comprise the P-site as such, it does form part of the P-site following completion of the 70S-initiation complex. In view of the results of TANAKA et al. (1972) it is therefore not surprising to find that tetracyclines inhibit the non-enzymic binding of phenylalanyl-tRNA to 30S · poly U ribosomal complexes (PESTKA and NIRENBERG 1966; SUZUKA et al. 1966). Action on the 30S subunit also probably explains why tetracycline prevents the AUG-dependent binding of fMet-$tRNA_f^{Met}$ to ribosomes (SARKER and THACH 1968). The ability of tetracyclines to affect initiation of protein synthesis could explain the polysome degradation observed in vivo by GURGO et al. (1969) (see Sect. D.I).

6. Tetracyclines Inhibit Chain Termination: A Minor Mode of Action

As noted in Sect. C.VI chain termination involves release of completed polypeptides from tRNA and ribosomes, and dissociation of 70S ribosomes into 50S and 30S subunits. Inhibitory effects of tetracycline on termination have been shown by SCOLNICK et al. (1968) and UEHARA et al. (1976) and probably result from the inability of release factors to interact with the termination codons in the A-site (KAJI and RYOJI 1979). The interaction between release factors RF-1 and RF-2 and the ribosome is codon specific and in *E. coli* involves proteins L7 and L12 (WEISSBACH 1980), so that binding of tetracyclines to the acceptor site may alter ribosomal configuration and (a) directly prevent the binding of release factors (KAJI and RYOJI 1979) or (b) cause interference with the positioning of the termination codon in the A-site which indirectly leads to poor binding of release factors (KAJI and RYOJI 1979). In essence both these inhibitory effects represent A-site interactions and are probably analogous to the action of tetracyclines on the binding of aminoacyl-tRNA to ribosomes. Reactions involving ribosome release factor are also sensitive to tetracyclines, but these steps are not thought to be major targets for tetracycline action (see KAJI and RYOJI 1979).

E. Binding of Tetracyclines to Macromolecules

I. Introduction

Tetracyclines bind to proteins, DNA, synthetic polynucleotides, ribosomes, and tRNA (GALE et al. 1972; KAJI and RYOJI 1979). Therefore the inhibitory effects of tetracyclines upon aminoacyl-tRNA binding could be exerted by attachment of drug to ribosomes, to mRNA within ribosomes, to aminoacyl-tRNA, or to elongation factor EF-Tu. However, only the interaction with ribosomes is considered to result in inhibition of protein synthesis (see KAJI and RYOJI 1979). Consequently, there has been much interest in the number and nature of tetracycline-binding sites within bacterial ribosomes.

II. Binding of Tetracyclines to Ribosomes

Many studies on the binding of tetracyclines to bacterial ribosomes have been performed (Connamacher and Mandel 1965, 1968; Day 1966a, b; Maxwell 1968; White and Cantor 1971; Kersten and Fey 1971; Fey et al. 1973; Strel'tsov et al. 1975; Tritton 1977; Goldman et al. 1980, 1983). A consensus has emerged on the existence of a single strong binding site for tetracycline per 70S ribosome with a dissociation constant (K_d) for binding between 1 and 30×10^{-6} M (Strel'tsov et al. 1975; Tritton 1977). These values fall within the range observed for the functional binding of other antibiotics to intact ribosomes or ribosomal subunits (Cundliffe 1980). For tetracycline there are also a large number (several hundred) of weaker binding sites, with an approximate K_d of 6×10^{-2} M (Strel'tsov et al. 1975).

The weak binding sites occur on both ribosomal subunits (Fey et al. 1973), but it is not known whether the strong binding site is also shared by both subunits. Some studies show that when 70S ribosome-tetracycline complexes are dissociated into subunits by suspension in buffers containing low levels of Mg^{2+}, most, but not all, of the tightly bound tetracycline is associated with the 30S subunit (Connamacher and Mandel 1965, 1968; Maxwell 1968). Aryl ketones have been used as photolabile groups in the photoaffinity labelling of *E. coli* ribosomes (e.g. see Cooperman 1979). The presence of such a group in the tetracycline molecule, together with the known photolability of tetracycline (Leeson and Weidenheimer 1969; Hlavka and Bitha 1966), led to experiments using radioactively labelled [^3H]tetracycline as a photoaffinity label for ribosomes (Cooperman 1980a; Goldman et al. 1980, 1983). Photoincorporation of tetracycline into 70S ribosomes resulted in preferential labelling of the 30S subunit. Analysis of proteins from the 30S subunit showed considerable labelling of proteins S18 and S4 with minor labelling of S7, S13, and S14 (Goldman et al. 1980).

In a subsequent study (Goldman et al. 1983) a more detailed examination of the photoincorporation process was presented. These recent studies revealed that tetracycline photodecomposes appreciably during a typical photoincorporation experiment. The covalent incorporation observed on irradiation of tetracycline and ribosomes results not only from light-dependent incorporation of tetracycline, but also from light-dependent and -independent incorporation of tetracycline photoproducts. This re-evaluation of the photoincorporation experiments now demonstrates that protein S7 is the major protein labelled by native tetracycline. The previously reported high labelling of proteins S18 and S4 (Goldman et al. 1980) is now believed to result from the incorporation of tetracycline photoproducts (Goldman et al. 1983).

In contrast to the above findings, which suggest that the strong binding site is located in the 30S subunit, other studies show that isolated 30S and 50S subunits are both capable of strong tetracycline binding (Day 1966a, b; Fey et al. 1973). The situation could be rationalized by proposing that both ribosomal subunits contribute to the single strong binding site for tetracyclines on 70S ribosomes. Evidence consistent with this proposal was obtained by WERNER et al. (1975), who showed that 70S ribosomes were more effective than 30S or 50S subunits in alleviating inhibition of cell-free protein synthesis by oxytetracycline.

F. Molecular Basis of Tetracycline Action

The results obtained from both in vivo and in vitro work argue that tetracyclines act predominantly by inhibiting the binding of aminoacyl-tRNA to the ribosomal A-site. How is this achieved in molecular terms and what is the relationship between the ribosomal binding sites for tetracycline and the action of the drug?

Despite confusing and conflicting reports a consensus has emerged that the single tight binding of tetracycline per 70S ribosome is sufficient to inhibit the A-site function of aminoacyl-tRNA binding, whereas at high concentrations association of tetracycline with the weaker non-specific binding sites can cause inhibition of other ribosomal functions (KAJI and RYOJI 1979; NIERHAUS and WITTMANN 1980).

HOGENAUER and TURNOWSKY (1972) suggest that a tetracycline molecule binds to a ribosome in such a way that the codon-anticodon interaction between the tRNA and the mRNA in the A-site is disrupted. A less attractive hypothesis, in view of the model presented earlier (Fig. 7), would be that tetracycline directly interrupts the interaction of EF-Tu at the A-site. Assuming that HOGENAUER and TURNOWSKY (1972) are correct, then we might expect protein S7 to be located at the site of codon-anticodon interaction. Although not directly located at this site, protein S7 by interacting with the 3′ (aminoacyl) end of tRNA probably plays an important role in the positioning of the aminoacyl-tRNA at the time of codon-anticodon recognition (GRUNBERG-MANAGO et al. 1978; OFENGAND 1980; COOPERMAN 1980b). The correlation between the labelling of S7 by native tetracycline and its probable involvement in codon-anticodon interaction or tRNA alignment implies a direct causal relationship between the sets of observations. In support of this reasoning GOLDMAN et al. (1983) demonstrated that photolabelling of ribosomes by native tetracycline was accompanied by loss of binding activity for phenylalanyl-tRNA. Although the photoincorporation experiments (GOLDMAN et al. 1983) demonstrate a role for protein S7 in the binding of tetracycline to bacterial ribosomes, mutational studies show that at least one other ribosomal protein may comprise part of the antibiotic binding site. Thus WILLIAMS and SMITH (1979) isolated a tetracycline-resistant mutant of *Bacillus subtilis* that possessed an altered 30S subunit protein, S10. In *E. coli* this protein is located on the external surface of the 30S subunit and like S7 has been implicated in the process of tRNA binding/alignment (KAHAN et al. 1981).

The preceding discussion in this section has not considered the manner by which tetracyclines interact with ribosomal components. SMYTHIES et al. (1972) presented a theoretical model (Fig. 8) to explain binding of tetracyclines to ribosomes which involve only drug-RNA interactions. Clearly this model (Fig. 8) could be reconciled with the results of photolabelling if the initial binding of tetracyclines to ribosomal RNA produces conformational changes which then allow protein S7 (possibly also S10) to bind the drug. Although this suggestion is

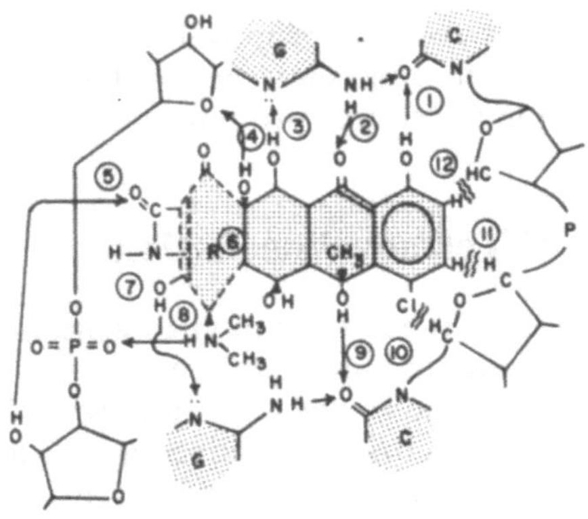

Fig. 8. A model for the binding of tetracyclines to ribosomal RNA. A composite tetracycline molecule is shown based on the structures for tetracycline, chlorotetracycline, oxytetracycline, and rolitetracycline. The composite molecule is inverted relative to the normal presentation for tetracyclines (see Fig. 1). The 5OH is found only in oxytetracycline and the 7Cl only in chlorotetracycline. The substituent R at position 2 is H, apart from rolitetracycline where it is $NH \cdot CH_2 \cdot N$. Binding is as follows (hydrogen bonds except where stated): *1*, 10OH group to cytosine O; *2*, 11=O to guanine NH; *3*, 12OH to guanine 3N; *4*, the OH between C_{12} and C_1 to ribose ring O; *5*, the C=O at position 2 to a ribose OH (weak interaction); *6*, the NH_2 group (or $NH \cdot CH_2 \cdot N$ of rolitetracycline) intercalates between the purine clouds; *7*, the 3OH to the guanine (or adenine) 3N; *8*, the basic NH^+ to phosphate O^- (ionic); *9*, the 6OH to =O on cytosine (or uracil); *10, 11, 12*, the 7, 8, 9 hydrogens (or 7Cl of chlorotetracycline) make hydrophobic interactions with ribose methyl groups. *G*, guanine; *C*, cytosine. (SMYTHIES et al. 1972)

highly speculative, it is at least consistent with the observation that protein S7 interacts with ribosomal RNA (GRUNBERG-MANAGO et al. 1978; OFENGAND 1980; COOPERMAN 1980b). Nevertheless, as noted by MITSCHER (1978), the model of SMYTHIES et al. (1972) (Fig. 8) does not account for the role of cations in the binding of tetracyclines to ribosomes (COIBION and LASZLO 1979), nor does it explain why seemingly trivial changes to tetracycline structure (e.g. isomerization of C4 to produce 4-epitetracycline) should render the drug inactive. Further consideration of the structural features of the tetracycline molecule required for activity are considered in the next section.

G. Relation Between Structure and Activity in the Tetracyclines

Since the appearance of chlorotetracycline in the late 1940s (DUGGAR 1948), a large number of derivatives and degradation products have been produced (BLACKWOOD and ENGLISH 1977; MITSCHER 1978). Examination of the antibiotic activities of these compounds permits some generalizations regarding those parts of the molecule that are necessary for biological activity. Only a brief discussion is presented here and the reader is referred to the extensive reviews of BLACKWOOD and ENGLISH (1977), MITSCHER (1978) and VALCAVI (1981) for further details.

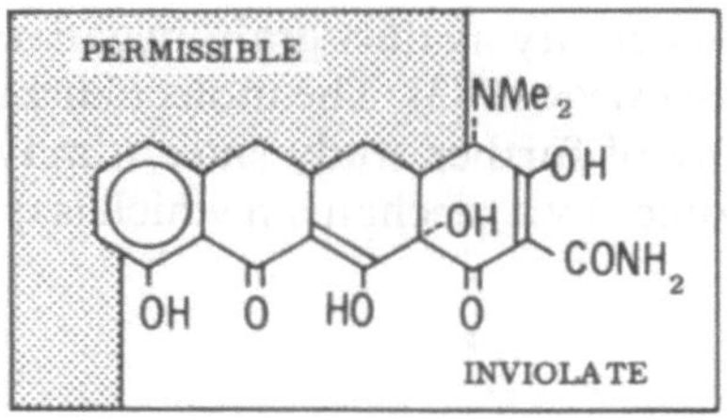

Fig. 9. Minimum structural requirement for tetracycline activity and those portions of the molecule which are inviolate or where changes are permissible. Based on BLACKWOOD and ENGLISH (1977) and MITSCHER (1978). The figure is reproduced from MITSCHER (1978)

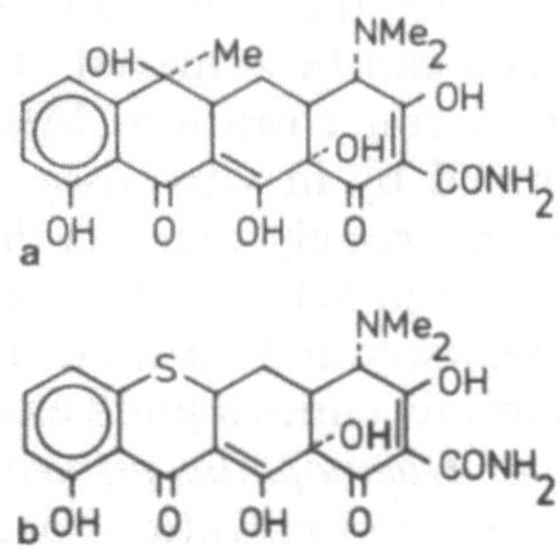

Fig. 10. Structural formulae of tetracycline **a** and 6-thia-tetracycline **b**

Most of the experiments on structure-activity relationships have relied upon determination of the ability of tetracyclines to inhibit growth of whole bacteria, rather than the efficacy upon protein synthesis in vitro. Thus poor inhibition of bacterial growth by a derivative could relate to failure of drug transport rather than inability to inhibit protein synthesis. Clearly those compounds that show antibacterial activity are transported into the cell and inhibit protein synthesis, so that those regions of the molecule required in common for both functions can be defined. Consideration of all known tetracycline derivatives allows definition of the minimum structural requirement for activity, together with those regions of the molecule where changes are permissible (Fig. 9). Permissible changes relate primarily to pendant groups, but even substitution of C6 with sulphur to produce 6-thiatetracycline (Fig. 10) does not result in loss of activity (PREWO et al. 1980). Although Fig. 9 indicates the general regions of the molecule where changes either do or do not abolish antimicrobial activity, it should be noted that modifications at positions 4a, 8 (permissible region) and 3, 10 (inviolate region) have not been achieved (VALCAVI 1981).

One study (TRITTON 1977) permits direct evaluation of tetracycline structure in relation to inhibitory activity at the ribosome. Differences in the ability of tetracyclines to inhibit protein synthesis in vitro were noted, with tetracycline the least potent and minocycline the most potent of six tetracyclines tested. Although these results might imply that some tetracyclines bind covalently to ribosomes and exert bactericidal effects, there is in fact little evidence for this as most tetracyclines act in a bacteriostatic manner (FEDORKO et al. 1968; BAKHTIAR and SELWYN 1983). Nevertheless, the thiatetracyclines (e.g. 6-thiatetracycline, Fig. 10) apparently have bactericidal activity against gram-negative, but not gram-positive, bacteria (Bakhtiar and Selwyn 1983). The molecular basis of the cidal response is unknown, but is worthy of further study since it may imply that thiatetracyclines interact with ribosomes by a mechanism which is qualitatively distinct from other tetracyclines.

H. Effects of Growth in the Presence of Low Tetracycline Concentrations on Microbial Metabolism

For many years it has been assumed that antibiotics eradicate infections because the concentration of drug which can be achieved at the site of infection in vivo exceeds the minimum inhibitory concentration (MIC) or minimum bactericidal concentration (MBC) determined by in vitro assays. However, there is now a growing body of evidence which strongly suggests that antibiotic concentrations below the conventionally determined MIC or MBC levels can be effective in treatment (see Ahlstedt 1981; Atkinson and Amaral 1982; O'Grady 1982, for recent reviews). With regard to tetracyclines a good example of the situation is provided by considering therapy of *Haemophilus influenzae* infections. When the tetracyclines are used their sputum concentrations are frequently below the MIC for *Haemophilus influenzae*, yet these antibiotics are nevertheless successfully used for the treatment of infections caused by this organism (O'Grady 1982). Other clinical studies illustrate that many patients receive higher levels of antibiotics than are actually required to arrest an infection and that shorter dosing periods or smaller antibiotic concentrations could well achieve similar results (O'Grady 1982). A similar situation also exists in veterinary medicine where antibiotics are deliberately administered at low levels for purposes of growth promotion, which presumably results principally from suppression of microbial growth.

The therapeutic effects of low antibiotic levels have been variously ascribed to inhibition of toxin synthesis, interference with bacterial adhesion and enhanced sensitivity to host defence mechanisms (Ahlstedt 1981; Atkinson and Amaral 1982). Interference with bacterial adhesion appears to be a particularly important inhibitory target for tetracyclines administered at low levels (Eisenstein et al. 1982; Vosbeck et al. 1982). Although the underlying molecular events responsible for the inhibition of adhesion are unknown (Atkinson and Amaral 1982), the inhibitory effects may be related to the preferential activity of tetracyclines against the synthesis of envelope proteins that has been reported by some authors (Hirashima et al. 1973; Piovant et al. 1978).

I. Selective Toxicity of the Tetracyclines

I. Introduction

The concept of antimicrobial chemotherapy, i.e. "the problem of internal disinfection, of destroying living parasites within the infected body" was first formulated by Ehrlich (see Himmelweit 1960). Following their discovery in the 1950s it was soon clear that the tetracyclines constituted an example of Ehrlich's "magic bullets." The selective action of tetracyclines against prokaryotic cells might result from:

1. Inability of the drugs to enter eukaryotic cells.
2. Inability of tetracyclines to inhibit protein synthesis in eukaryotic cells.

These aspects are considered below.

II. Entry of Tetracyclines into Eukaryotic Cells

Some intact eukaryotic microorganisms are impermeable to tetracycline (SCHWARTZ et al. 1972), but this is not a general feature of eukaryotic cells. Thus tetracyclines penetrate into most organs of the body (see MITSCHER 1978) and inhibit the growth of cultured cells in vitro at concentrations comparable to those required for inhibition of bacterial growth (KAJI and RYOJI 1979). Although the nature of tetracycline transport across eukaryotic membranes has not been investigated in detail, it may resemble the process in bacteria (see Sect. J) because at lest some mammalian cells actively accumulate tetracycline (BANERJEE and CHAKRABARTI 1976). Furthermore, the sensitivity of chlamydial infections to tetracycline implies the drug can cross the eukaryotic host cell membrane to inhibit the intracellular microorganisms.

III. Effect of Tetracyclines on Eukaryotic Protein Synthesis

Initially tetracyclines were thought to be inactive towards eukaryotic protein synthesis (RENDI and OCHOA 1961). Subsequent work (see BEARD et al. 1969 for a review) proved that this was untrue and indeed recent studies show that isolated rat liver ribosomes are readily photolabelled by tetracycline (REBOUD et al. 1982). The eukaryotic ribosomes studied by REBOUD et al. (1982) comprised cytoplasmic ribosomes but mitochondrial ribosomes also contain binding sites for tetracyclines (BOYNTON et al. 1980).

IV. Selective Toxicity of the Tetracyclines – The Apparent Paradox Explained

The tetracyclines are apparently able both to enter eukaryotic cells and inhibit protein synthesis within them. At first sight it therefore seems difficult to explain their selective action against microorganisms. Recent studies by VAN DEN BOGERT and KROON (1981) have considerably clarified this apparent paradox. Tetracyclines in the doses normally used in antibiotic therapy have no effect on the synthesis of cytoplasmic proteins, but do to some extent inhibit mitochondrial protein synthesis. The observation that tetracyclines have no serious side effects notwithstanding this inhibitory action has, of course, to be explained. It seems that even a 50% decrease in the activity of the terminal enzyme of the respiratory chain does not lead to the situation that oxidative phosphorylation becomes rate limiting for adequate functioning of most tissues and organs. Provided synthesis of this key enzyme is not substantially inhibited then no serious side effects of tetracycline therapy occur in the host.

J. Transport of Tetracyclines into Bacteria

I. Introduction

Clearly, in order to inhibit protein synthesis tetracyclines must enter the bacterial cell. To reach their target in gram-negative bacteria the tetracyclines cross two membranes (the outer and cytoplasmic membranes), whereas in gram-positive bacteria transport across only one membrane (the cytoplasmic membrane) is re-

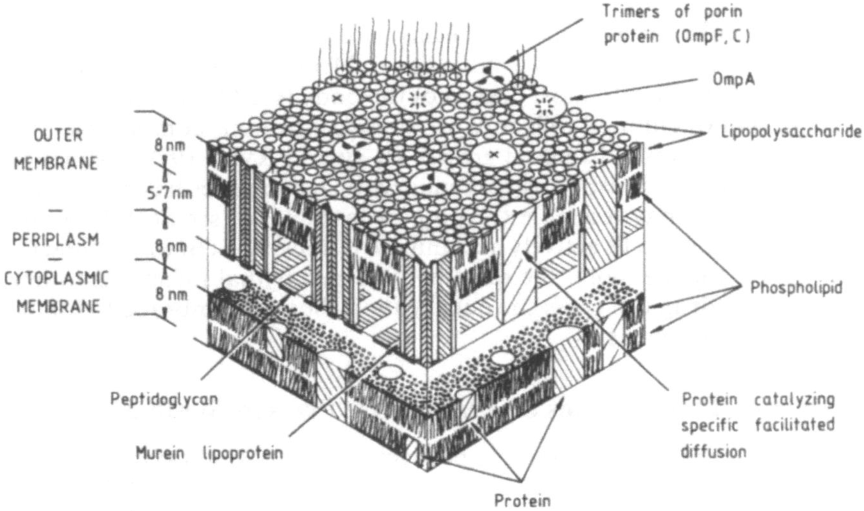

Fig. 11. Model of envelope structure in gram-negative bacteria. Based on NIKAIDO and NAKAE (1979). See NIKAIDO and NAKAE (1979), NIKAIDO et al. (1980), and OSBORN and WU (1980) for information on the structure and function of the outer membrane, and SALTON and OWEN (1976) for similar information on the cytoplasmic membrane

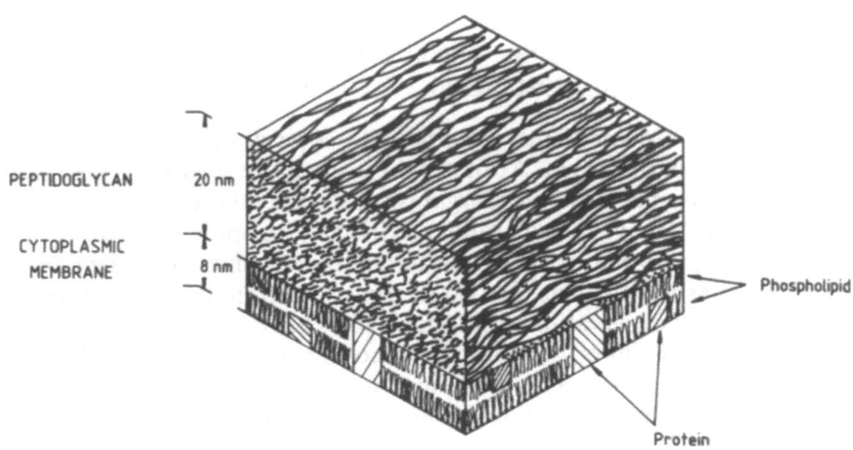

Fig. 12. Model of envelope structure in gram-positive bacteria. [Based on COSTERTON and CHENG (1975)]

quired (Figs. 11 and 12). Transport of tetracyclines (and other antibiotics) has been the subject of a recent review (CHOPRA and BALL 1982), so that only a summary of the topic is presented here, together with some recent advances.

II. Transport of Tetracyclines Across the Gram-Negative Outer Membrane

Information on this topic has been derived almost exclusively from studies with *E. coli*. Passage of tetracyclines across the outer membrane appears to occur predominantly by passive diffusion with no evidence for involvement of facilitated diffusion systems (CHOPRA and HOWE 1978). There are two routes for the non-specific diffusion of tetracyclines across the outer membrane (BALL et al. 1977):

1. Through hydrophilic transmembrane protein pores with a preference for those formed by the *ompF* porin (Fig. 11) (CHOPRA and ECCLES 1978)
2. Through apolar membrane regions.

By analogy with other substrates (NIKAIDO 1976) we would expect hydrophilic tetracyclines (e.g. tetracycline) (Table 4) to diffuse through porins and hydrophobic tetracyclines (e.g. minocycline) (Table 4) to cross by the second route. These assertions are supported by some experimental data (BALL et al. 1977; CHOPRA

Table 4. Partition coefficients of some of the tetracyclines. (CHOPRA and HOWE 1978)

Antibiotic	Partition coefficient	
	Chloroform/water	Octanol/water
Minocycline	30	1.1
Doxycycline	0.48	0.60
Tetracycline	0.09	0.036
Oxytetracycline	0.007	0.025

Molecules with octanol/water partition coefficient > about 0.07 are regarded as hydrophobic (NIKAIDO 1976; NIKAIDO and NAKAE 1979)

Table 5. Susceptibility of *Escherichia coli* and *Bacillus subtilis* to tetracyclines

Organism	Concentrations of antibiotic (μg/ml ± 1 standard deviation) required to cause a 50% reduction in growth rate	
	Tetracycline	Minocycline
Escherichia coli K-12 JC3272	0.29 ± 0.02[a]	0.42 ± 0.08[a]
Bacillus subtilis NCIB10106	0.35 ± 0.01[b]	0.025 ± 0.005[c]

[a] SHALES et al. (1980)
[b] ECCLES et al. (1981)
[c] I. CHOPRA (unpublished data)

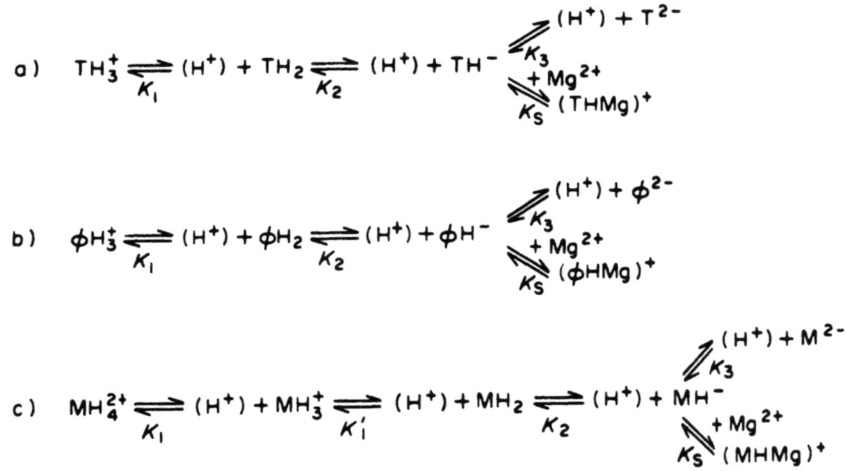

Fig. 13. Dissociation schemes for **a** tetracycline hydrochloride, **b** oxytetracycline hydrochloride, and **c** minocycline hydrochloride. [Based on CHOPRA and HOWE (1978) and data of BARRINGER et al. (1974)]

and ECCLES 1978; CHOPRA and SHALES 1981; LEIVE et al. 1984), but the studies to date suffer from the inability to obtain direct estimates for the diffusion rates of tetracyclines across the outer membrane. Although minocycline can cross the outer membrane, comparison of its activity against *B. subtilis* and *E. coli* (Table 5) implies that the outer membrane does constitute a considerable permeability barrier to its entry (CHOPRA and SHALES 1981). Its behaviour therefore conforms to the pattern observed for other hydrophobic drugs (NIKAIDO 1976). Indeed this conclusion has recently been confirmed by LEIVE et al. (1984).

PIOVANT et al. (1978) proposed that when hydrophobic antibiotics enter *E. coli* they do so by diffusion through regions that connect the cytoplasmic and outer membranes. The preferential activity of hydrophobic inhibitors of protein synthesis against membrane-bound ribosomes (HIRASHIMA et al. 1973; PIOVANT et al. 1978) is assumed by PIOVANT et al. (1978) to reflect the proximity of junction points to the sites of synthesis of envelope polypeptides. Diffusion of minocycline through apolar outer membrane regions could therefore locate the antibiotic at sites favourable for entry across the cytoplasmic membrane via junction points. Recently, CHOPRA and SHALES (1981) tested this model for minocycline uptake by determining its activity against the synthesis of cytoplasmic and envelope proteins, but found no evidence for preferential entry through junction regions.

The tetracyclines are acids which can ionize in aqueous solution (Fig. 13, Table 6). At neutral pH the forms TH_2, TH^- and OH_2, OH^- predominate for tetracycline and oxytetracycline (see CHOPRA and HOWE 1978), whereas for minocycline MH_2 is the major species (BARRINGER et al. 1974). Although a Donnan equilibrium exists across the outer membrane (negative charge inside) (STOCK et al. 1977) it will not hinder diffusion of the uncharged species, and indeed the forms TH_2, OH_2 and MH_2 probably enter gram-negative bacteria (see CHOPRA and HOWE 1978). However, diffusion of the anionic species across the outer mem-

Table 6. Ionization constants (K_1, K_1', K_2, K_3) of tetracycline, oxytetracycline and minocycline hydrochlorides and stability constants K_s of complexes with magnesium (BARRINGER et al. 1974; CHOPRA and HOWE 1978)

Antibiotic	pK_1	pK_1'	pK_2	pK_3	pK_s
Tetracycline	3.3	–	7.7	9.7	4.16–4.29
Oxytetracycline	3.3	–	7.3	9.1	3.80–3.96
Minocycline	2.8	5.0	7.8	9.5	ND[a]

[a] Not determined, but minocycline does form magnesium chelates (BARRINGER et al. 1974)

brane is likely to be severely hindered. Binding of divalent cations by the TH^- and OH^- anions will lead to the formation of cationic chelates (Fig. 13) that should be able to cross the outer membrane in response to the Donnan equilibrium. Nevertheless, the sensitivity of a number of bacteria to tetracycline is reduced in the presence of increasing concentrations of Mg^{2+} (see CHOPRA and HOWE 1978). This may be due to the reduced solubility of tetracycline-metal chelates compared with the free antibiotics (BARRINGER et al. 1974).

Although many questions remain concerning the molecular basis by which tetracyclines cross the outer membrane, their passage across this structure has recently been used as a probe for detecting certain outer membrane changes in *E. coli* (LEIVE et al. 1984). Since the rate of uptake of tetracyclines is limited by the outer membrane (MCMURRY et al. 1982; LEIVE et al. 1984) changes in the interaction of these antibiotics with *E. coli* can be used to detect overall changes in outer membrane composition (LEIVE et al. 1984). The method depends upon sensitivity testing with a series of tetracycline analogues of varying hydrophobicities and measurement of alterations in fluorescent properties of tetracyclines (see Sect. J.IV) upon interaction with bacteria. Although this new method has not yet been widely applied, its originators (LEIVE et al. 1984) claim that it may prove as useful as an analogous method used to measure access of β-lactam antibiotics across the gram-negative outer membrane (see CHOPRA and BALL 1982).

III. Transport of Tetracyclines Across the Cytoplasmic Membrane of Gram-Positive and -Negative Bacteria

Although a variety of tetracycline analogues exist, detailed studies on transport of these antibiotics across the bacterial cytoplasmic membrane have been confined mostly to tetracycline itself.

In susceptible *E. coli* (and probably also other organisms), passage of tetracycline across the cytoplasmic membrane occurs both by energy-independent and energy-dependent uptake systems and each uptake system contributes towards inhibition of protein synthesis (MCMURRAY and LEVY 1978). Energy-independent uptake most likely represents passive diffusion of drug through the membrane (MCMURRY and LEVY 1978). This view is further supported by the recent findings of ARGAST and BECK (1984), showing that tetracycline diffuses through phospholipid bilayers in liposomes. Clearly these findings support the contention that passive diffusion of tetracycline occurs during accumulation of the antibiotic by whole bacteria. Much effort has been devoted towards understanding the molecular basis of energy-dependent uptake both in *E. coli* (CHOPRA and BALL 1982; FRANKLIN and HIGGINSON 1970; LEVY 1981; MCMURRY and LEVY 1978; MCMURRY et al. 1981a, b; SMITH and CHOPRA 1984) and other organisms (FAYOLLE et al. 1980).

Since tetracycline is a hydrophilic molecule (Table 4 and MCMURRY et al. 1982), the simplest explanation for energy-dependent passage across the membrane and subsequent concentration in the cell (MCMURRY and LEVY 1978; MCMURRY et al. 1982) would lie in the use of an active, carrier-mediated transport system. Active transport systems in *E. coli* can generally be classified into two types: (a) osmotic-shock-resistant systems which are coupled to the proton-motive force and (b) osmotic-shock-sensitive systems which are coupled to phosphate-bond hydrolysis (for reviews see BOOTH and HAMILTON 1980; ROSEN and KASHKET 1978; WEST 1980). In their recent studies on active tetracycline transport in *E. coli*, MCMURRY et al. (1981b) concluded that tetracycline transport was coupled primarily to the proton-motive force. Nevertheless, earlier studies (MCMURRY and LEVY 1978) imply that tetracycline transport may also be coupled to phosphate-bond hydrolysis. In general the studies conducted so far on the nature of energy coupling to tetracycline transport are difficult to interpret because tetracycline uptake has not usually been directly compared with transport of solutes with known modes of energy coupling. Such comparisons are necessary to show that the experimental conditions used lead to the expected changes in energy available to drive proton-motive-force- and phosphate-bond-dependent transport. Recently SMITH and CHOPRA (1984) re-evaluated aspects of tetracycline transport by comparing antibiotic transport directly with that of proline (proton-motive force dependent) and glutamine (phospate-bond dependent). We obtained evidence that tetracycline transport is coupled to phosphate-bond hydrolysis, but nevertheless is not completely sensitive to osmotic shock (SMITH and CHOPRA 1984). These results could be explained by supposing that tetracycline utilizes two transport systems, one coupled to phosphate-bond hydrolysis and sensitive to osmotic shock, and the other coupled to the proton-motive force and shock resistant. This conclusion is at least consistent with the reported energy requirements of tetracycline transport (MCMURRY and LEVY 1978; LEVY 1981; MCMURRY et al. 1981a, b; SMITH and CHOPRA 1984).

The observations on energy coupling to transport in *E. coli* imply that two distinct carrier systems may operate for tetracycline accumulation. These carriers have very low affinities for tetracycline because saturation kinetics have not been reported in *E. coli* (MCMURRY and LEVY 1978; SMITH and CHOPRA 1983; Fig. 14). Saturation kinetics have been reported in other bacteria but even in these cases the K_m values are high (540–2,5000 μM) (WECKESSER and MAGNUSON 1976; HEDSTROM et al. 1982), again implying poor affinity of carrier proteins for the antibiotic. The membrane-located tetracycline transport systems have not been identified. Nevertheless, MITSCHER (1978) has drawn attention to a weak structural analogy between part of the tetracycline molecule and L-amino acids, particularly glutamate (Fig. 15). Glutamate transport is itself a proton-motive-force-dependent system (ROSEN and KASHKETT 1978) and the suggestion that tetracyclines

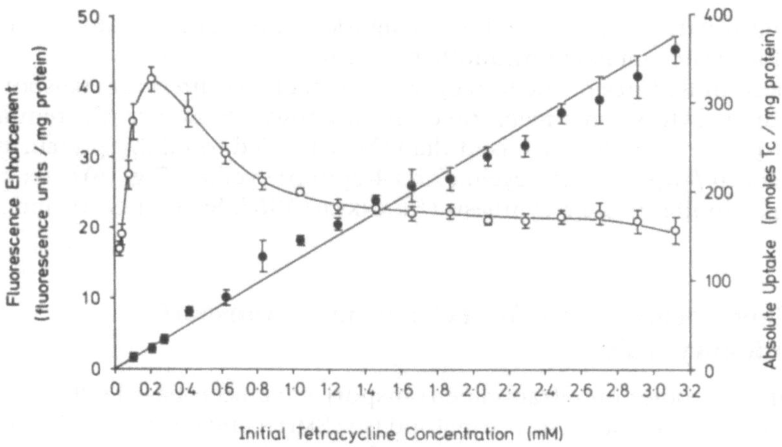

Fig. 14. Absolute uptake of tetracycline (●) and fluorescence enhancement (○) after exposure of *Escherichia coli* K12 to various concentrations of tetracycline for 1 min. The method employed for absolute drug uptake is considered equivalent to a radioactive transport assay (see SMITH and CHOPRA 1983). Values are the means of at least six independent determinations ±1 standard error of the mean. (SMITH and CHOPRA 1983)

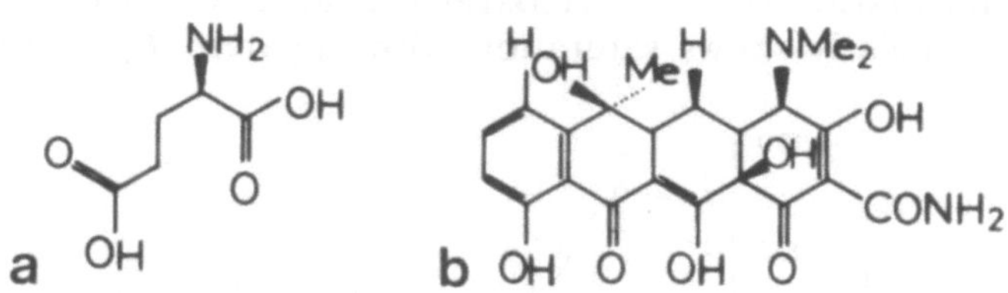

Fig. 15. Structural analogy between L-glutamate **a** and tetracycline **b**. The dimethylamino group in the tetracycline molecule corresponds to the amino group in L-glutamate. [Modified from MITSCHER (1978)]

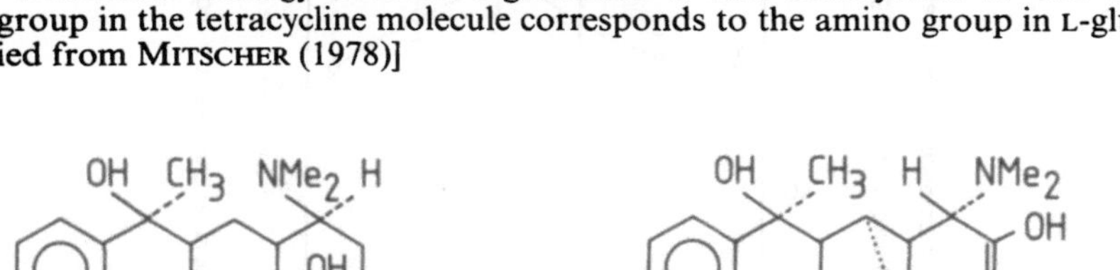

Fig. 16. Structure of 4-epitetracycline **a** and β-apo-oxytetracycline **b**. [Based on structures in MITSCHER (1978)]

utilize this amino acid transport system is therefore consistent with the partial involvement of the proton-motive force in tetracycline accumulation. The apparent use of more than one transport system by tetracycline may explain why it has not proved possible to isolate chromosomal mutants resistant to high levels of tetracycline (CHOPRA and HOWE 1978; MCMURRY and LEVY 1978). Thus a mutation in one of the carriers would not lead to high-level resistance because the antibiotic would still be accumulated by another system.

Structural features of the tetracycline molecule required for transport across the bacterial cytoplasmic membrane are unknown. However, the requirements for transport may be less stringent than those needed to inhibit protein synthesis because both β-apo-oxytetracycline and 4-epitetracycline (Fig. 16) enter bacteria, but do not inhibit protein synthesis (FRANKLIN 1967; SOMPOLINSKY and KRAUSZ 1973).

IV. Fluorescence Assay for Tetracycline Transport – A Cautionary Tale

Most of the studies on tetracycline transport have been based either upon a radioactive assay or a fluorescence method (see SMITH and CHOPRA 1983). The latter depends on fluorescence enhancement of the antibiotic as it enters the cell. The fluorescence method has potential advantages over the radioactive method because it permits studies on the accumulation of tetracycline analogues that are not readily available in a radioactive form. However, the two types of assay cannot necessarily be assumed to give comparable results. For example there are only two reports using radioactive antibiotic where saturation kinetics are observed (WECKESSER and MAGNUSON 1976; HEDSTROM et al. 1982), whereas the fluorescence method regularly shows saturation with apparent K_ms between 38 and

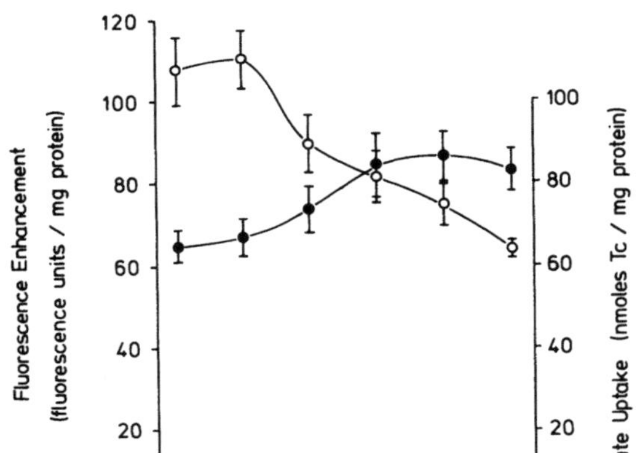

Fig. 17. pH dependence of tetracycline uptake by *Escherichia coli* K-12. Bacteria were grown in a minimal medium and then resuspended in phosphate buffer containing glycerol at the pH values indicated. Bacteria were equilibrated with tetracycline (200 $\mu M/5 \times 10^9$ cells) and samples removed to measure both fluorescence (○) and absolute amounts of accumulated drug (●). The method employed for absolute drug uptake is considered equivalent to a radioactive transport assay (see SMITH and CHOPRA 1983). Values are the means of at least seven independent determinations ±1 standard error of the mean. (SMITH and CHOPRA 1983)

400 μ*M* (see CHOPRA and BALL 1982). The apparent saturation of transport using the fluorescence method was also considered in the recent studies of SMITH and CHOPRA (1983). In these experiments the two types of transport assay were compared directly and found to give dissimilar results for uptake into *E. coli* (Fig. 14). No evidence for saturation was obtained using an absolute transport method, but fluorescence enhancement decreased between 0.4 and 1.0 m*M* tetracycline and was approximately constant thereafter up to 3.2 m*M* tetracycline (Fig. 14). Fluorescence enhancement and uptake of tetracycline are therefore correlated only when external levels up to about 0.4 m*M* (approximately 100 μg/ml) are used (Fig. 14). Differences were also noted with respect to the apparent pH optimum for transport into *E. coli* (Fig. 17).

A number of problems are therefore associated with the fluorescence assay, which does not necessarily estimate true intracellular drug concentrations (SMITH and CHOPRA 1983). This may explain other apparent anomalies reported in the literature. For example, the conflicting data concerning competitive inhibition by minocycline on tetracycline uptake may be resolved as follows. DEL BENE and ROGERS (1975) reported no competitive inhibition by minocycline on tetracycline uptake using [^{3}H]tetracycline. Nevertheless, SAMRA et al. (1978) reported competitive inhibition by minocycline using the fluorescence assay. Possibly SAMRA et al. (1978) were observing apparent competitive inhibition by increasing concentrations of minocycline owing to increased quenching of tetracycline fluorescence by minocycline.

Because of difficulties associated with the fluorescence method, interpretation of data using this method can be uncertain. For this reason the description of tetracycline transport given in the previous sections has not been based on results derived from fluorescence assays. The fluorescence assay has also been used in studies on tetracycline resistance and its reliability in this context will be considered in Sect. K.XI.

V. Transport of Tetracycline Across the Bacterial Cytoplasmic Membrane: Conclusion

Despite problems associated with the use of fluorescence assays to investigate transport of tetracyclines into bacteria (see Sect. J.IV) studies using this method continue to be reported (LINDLEY et al. 1984; MUNSKE et al. 1984). Unfortunately the conclusions reached by these authors, particularly in relation to the apparent saturation kinetics of tetracycline transport into bacteria, must be treated with caution for the reasons already outlined in the previous section.

In 1978 this author mentioned that many questions remained concerning the nature of tetracycline transport across the bacterial cytoplasmic membrane (CHOPRA and HOWE 1978). Although many advances have been made since 1978 one puzzling fact remains unanswered: although tetracycline transport is energy dependent no proteins which function as membrane carriers have so far been identified. In this respect tetracyclines may resemble other lipid-soluble ions (e.g., dibenzyl-dimethylammonium), which can be accumulated in a thermodynamically passive way, but are nevertheless dependent upon cellular energy for uptake (ALTENDORF et al. 1975; GRININVIENE et al. 1974; HAROLD and PAPINEAU 1972a, b).

K. Plasmid-Determined Resistance to the Tetracyclines

I. Occurrence of Plasmids in Natural Bacterial Isolates

Tetracycline resistance genes in many bacterial species are located on plasmids. Bukhari et al. (1977) provide a comprehensive list of those species from which tetracycline-resistance plasmids had been isolated up to the mid-1970s. Since then tetracycline-resistance plasmids have also been found in a number of other species and the current situation is summarized in Table 7.

Table 7. Natural bacterial isolates that contain tetracycline-resistance plasmids

Achromobacter liquefaciens	Providencia sp.
Aerobacter cloacae	*Salmonella panama*
Bacillus cereus[a]	*Salmonella paratyphi* B
Bacillus stearothermophilus[b]	*Salmonella typhi*
Bacteroides fragilis[c]	*Salmonella typhimurium*
Campylobacter fetus sub sp. *jejuni*[d]	*Shigella dysenteriae*
Corynebacterium xerosis[e]	*Shigella flexneri*
Escherichia coli	*Shigella sonnei*
Haemophilus influenzae[f]	*Staphylococcus aureus*
Klebsiella pneumoniae	*Streptococcus agalactiae*
Pseudomonas aeruginosa	*Streptococcus faecalis*
Proteus mirabilis	*Streptococcus faecalis* sub sp. *var zymogenes*
Proteus morganii	*Vibrio cholerae*
Proteus rettgeri	

[a] Bernhard et al. (1978)
[b] Bingham et al. (1979)
[c] Privitera et al. (1979), Fayolle et al. (1980)
[d] Taylor et al. (1980), Tenover et al. (1983)
[e] Kono et al. (1983)
[f] Kaulfers et al. (1978), Jahn et al. (1979)

See Bukhari et al. (1977) for details of plasmids isolated from other organisms.

II. Tetracycline-Resistance Determinants: Transposable and Amplifiable Sequences

The tetracycline-resistance genes in several plasmids are contained within transposons and amplifiable DNA sequences (Table 8). The amplifiable DNA sequences may themselves occur within transposons, or within other regions not capable of transposition (e.g. in pAMα1) (Table 8). The molecular basis of amplification has been studied in Tn*1721* and pAMα1. In both cases the tetracycline-resistance determinants are flanked by direct repeats (Figs. 18 and 19) which permit amplification by recombination. Various models have been proposed for amplification of resistance genes in pAMα1 (Fig. 19), but there is no evidence yet favouring one model over another. Higher degrees of amplification than those depicted may arise from repetition of the basic processes. The phenotypic effects of *tet* gene amplification are considered in a separate section (Sect. K.VIII).

A transposable genetic element conferring tetracycline resistance has been detected in the chromosome of *Streptococcus faecalis* (Franke and Clewell 1981) and there is also tentative evidence for a chromosomally integrated tetracycline-

Table 8. Tetracycline-resistance determinants: transposable and amplifiable sequences. (CHOPRA et al. 1981a)

Plasmid	Organism within which plasmid characterized	Transposon[a]	Amplifiable sequence	References
R100	*E. coli*	Tn*10*; 6·2 Mdal		FOSTER et al. (1975); KLECKNER et al. (1975)
pIP69	*E. coli*	Tn*805*; 6·2 Mdal		COHEN (1976); MENDEZ et al. (1980). Eccles, Howe, Bennett and Chopra (unpublished results)
pUB889	*E. coli*	'Tn*tet*'; c. 6 Mdal		BENNETT et al. (1980)
pRSD1	*E. coli*	Tn*1721*; 7·2 Mdal	3·55 Mdal sequence within Tn*1721*	SCHMITT et al. (1979)
pFS402	*E. coli*	Tn*1771*; 7·1 Mdal	3·5 Mdal sequence within Tn*1771*	SCHOFFL and PÜHLER (1979a, b)
pR1234	*Haemophilus influenzae*	Tn*Tc*+Tn*Cm*?; total 7·5 Mdal	Tn*Tc*+Tn*Cm*?	JAHN et al. (1979)
pFR16017	*H. influenzae*	Tn*Tc*; 6·3 Mdal	4 Mdal sequence within TN*Tc*	JAHN et al. (1979)
pAM α1	*Streptococcus faecalis*		2·65 Mdal sequence	CLEWELL et al. (1975); YAGI and CLEWELL (1976); CLEWELL and YAGI (1977); YAGI and CLEWELL (1977)

[a] Tn*Tc*, transposon conferring tetracycline resistance; Tn*Cm*, transposon conferring chloramphenicol resistance. Tn*1721* and Tn*1771* are now believed to be identical (SCHOFFL et al. 1981)

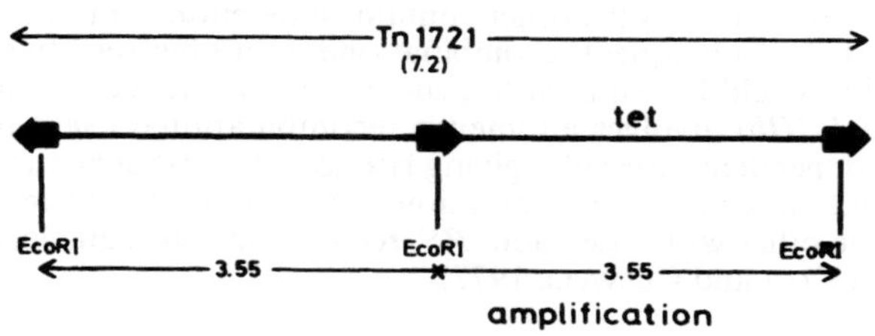

Fig. 18. Model of Tn*1721* comprising three symmetrically arranged repeats characterized by *Eco*RI sites. The tetracycline-resistance region (*tet*) is flanked by two direct repeats which provide sequence homology for amplification. The third repeat is inverted and provides the basis for transposition. Dimensions are marked in Mdals. (SCHMITT et al. 1979)

resistance transposon in *Staphylococcus aureus*. Resistance controlled by the chromosomal genes in *S. aureus* is qualitatively different from that mediated by staphylococcal plasmids: plasmid determinants confer inducible resistance to tetracycline but not to minocycline, whereas the chromosomal genes confer either constitutive or inducible resistance to both drugs or constitutive resistance to minocycline alone (CHOPRA et al. 1974; ASHESHOV 1975; SCHAEFLER et al. 1976). The precise relationship between the chromosomal and plasmid-linked determi-

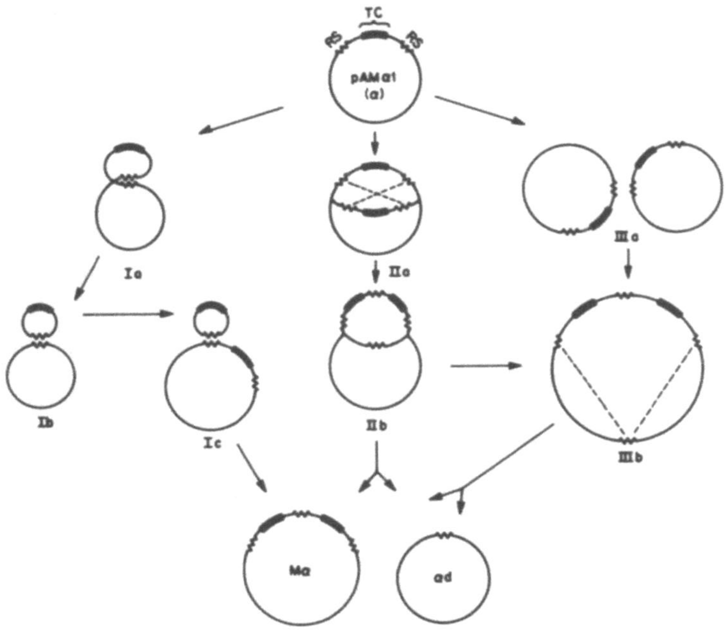

Fig. 19. Models for the generation of plasmid DNA molecules with a deletion or repeats of the tetracycline-resistance region of pAMα1. In *Ia through Ic* an intramolecular recombinational event results in the looping out of a small 2.65-megadalton circle, which then recombines with an intact molecule of pAMα1, resulting in a duplication. *IIa through IIb* represent an uneven recombinational event between RS sequences on the daughter strands of a partially replicated plasmid. Depending on the nature of events that follow, this structure could give rise to a dimeric structure (*IIIb*) or two independent molecules, one of which contains a duplication, whereas the other contains a deletion. In the case where a dimeric structure is generated, a subsequent recombinational event between two RS sequences (see *dashed lines in IIIb*) would be required to generate two independent molecules. The third model (*IIIa through IIIb*) involves an uneven recombinational event between the RS sequences of two independent molecules giving rise to a dimeric structure. A subsequent recombination would be required for generation of two independent molecules, one with a duplication and the other with a deletion. *RS*, recombination sequences; *TC*, tetracycline-resistance region. (YAGI and CLEWELL 1977)

nants is unknown, but they appear to code for related products which are membrane located (SOMPOLINSKY et al. 1979). The different phenotypes in *S. aureus* might be explained by assuming that the resistance genes are contained in a transposon, the expression of which is altered by integration into the chromosome. Genes for resistance to some other antibiotics are parts of transposons in *S. aureus* (PHILLIPS and NOVICK 1979).

Transposition of tetracycline-resistance genes between plasmids is an important means for their dissemination within bacterial populations because transposons can transfer from one replicon to another independently of the *rec*A$^+$-mediated recombination system of bacteria. This subject will be considered briefly in Sect. K.XIV.

III. Genetic Comparison of Regions Coding for Tetracycline Resistance

Although plasmids which confer resistance to tetracyclines have been found in virtually all bacterial species (Table 7) detailed studies on the nature of resistance have been confined to determinants from the *Enterobacteriaceae* and *Bacilli*. The nature of the regions coding for tetracycline resistance can be studied by analysis both of the resistance genes themselves and the nature of the products coded by the genes. The latter is considered in Sect. K.IV. This section considers information obtained from tests for location of sites sensitive to restriction endonucleases (restriction mapping) and for homology between DNA base sequences.

Restriction maps of several tetracycline-resistance determinants are available (e.g. MATTES et al. 1979; BENNETT et al. 1980; JORGENSEN et al. 1979; TAIT and BOYER 1978b; BINGHAM et al. 1980) but the maps are usually only of limited value for comparison of common nucleotide regions because each group of workers has used a different set of restriction endonucleases. Valid comparisons are possible, however, between the tetracycline-resistance regions of RP1, R222 (containing TN*10*) and pSC101, where the data indicate dissimilarity of nucleotides between the determinants (Table 9).

Table 9. Sites for certain restriction endonucleases within the tetracycline-resistance determinants of R222 (containing Tn*10*), RP1 and pSC101

Enzyme	Recognition sequence[a]	Cleavage site in tetracycline-resistance-determinant of[b]		
		R222	RP1	pSC101
*Bam*HI	G↓GATCC	+	–	+
*Hpa*I	GTT↓AAC	+	–	–
*Sal*I	G↓TCGAC	–	+	+
*Sma*I	CCC↓GGG	–	+	–

[a] Recognition sequences are abbreviated so that only one strand (5' → 3') is indicated. The point of cleavage is indicated by an arrow (↓) (ROBERTS 1980)
[b] Based on MENDEZ et al. (1980). +, –, presence or absence of cleavage site

A superior method for establishing relationships between tetracycline-resistance determinants involves DNA-DNA hybridization. The technique permitted MENDEZ et al. (1980) to classify the tetracycline-resistance determinants found in gram-negative bacteria into four groups (A–D, Table 10) between which it can be assumed that there is less than 85% base matching (HOWLEY et al. 1979). Some *TetA* and *TetB* determinants reside in transposons, e.g. Tn*1771* and Tn*1721* (*TetA*), Tn*10*, and Tn*805* (*TetB*), but determinants of class C and D have not yet been reported in transposons (MENDEZ et al. 1980). The incidence of determinants A–C amongst naturally occurring tetracycline-resistant strains of *E. coli* has been determined (LEVY 1981; MARSHALL et al. 1983). Bacteria containing *TetA* or *TetB* determinants comprised about 85% of the resistant isolates, a finding consistent with the location of these determinants in transposons.

Table 10. Classification of tetracycline-resistance determinants found in gram-negative bacteria

Class		Prototype plasmid	Resistance levels (μg/ml)[a]		
CHABBERT and SCAVIZZI (1976)	MENDEZ et al. (1980)		Tetra-cycline	Mino-cycline[b]	β-Chelocardin[b] (cetocycline)
TetA	A	RP1	75–150	5–10	<5
TetB	B	R100	150–200	≧10	≧5
?	C	pSC101[c]	≦ 25	< 5	<5
?	D	RA1	100	< 5	<5

[a] MENDEZ et al. (1980)
[b] Plasmidless host has a resistance level <5 μg/ml
[c] Origin of the tetracycline-resistance determinant in pSC101 is unknown; see COHEN and CHANG (1977)

Studies comparable to those of MENDEZ et al. (1980) have also been conducted with tetracycline-resistance determinants found in streptococci (BURDETT et al. 1982). At least two plasmid-located determinants have been identified (*TetL* and *TetN*) which are genetically distinct and also confer different levels of resistance to minocycline. Neither of the determinants found in streptococci, nor indeed any plasmid determinants from gram-positive species, hybridize with the class A–C determinants of gram-negative bacteria (LEVY 1981; SMITH et al. 1981; BURDETT et al. 1982; ECCLES and CHOPRA 1984). In contrast to the heterogeneity of tetracycline-resistance determinants in gram-negative bacteria and streptococci, those found in spore-forming soil bacilli comprise a related group (POLACK and NOVICK 1982; ECCLES and CHOPRA 1984). These results suggest that a single *tet* determinant may have become dispersed in a family of plasmids which collectively are responsible for much of the naturally occurring tetracycline-resistance in *Bacillus* species. Nevertheless there is no homology between the tetracycline-resistance determinants found in *Bacillus* and those found in staphylococci, streptococci or, as mentioned above, gram-negative bacteria (POLACK and NOVICK 1982; ECCLES and CHOPRA 1984).

IV. Proteins Synthesized by Tetracycline-Resistance Determinants: General Nature of the Proteins and Organization of the Genes Which Encode Them

1. Introduction

The first attempts to identify plasmid-determined proteins concerned with tetracycline-resistance were made by VAN EMBDEN and COHEN (1973) and FRANKLIN and ROWND (1973). Both groups demonstrated enrichment of proteins following induction of cells or minicells harbouring resistance plasmids, but the data obtained from these early studies are very limited; for instance, not even the molecular weights of the enriched polypeptides are quoted.

A group of workers from Israel were the first authors to claim isolation of proteins specified by plasmid-located tetracycline-resistance determinants (WOJDANI et al. 1976). In *E. coli* they detected an envelope protein of molecular weight 50,000 (encoded by an uncharacterized plasmid originally isolated in *Salmonella typhi*) and in *Staphylococcus aureus* a membrane protein of molecular weight 32,000 in two separate tetracycline-resistant strains. The staphylococcal studies employed the strains V738 and 111, both of which were assumed to contain plasmids. Tentative evidence for plasmid-borne resistance to tetracycline in strain 111 has been obtained (MAY et al. 1964), but the nature of the genes encoding resistance in strain V738 is unknown. In a previous review (CHOPRA and HOWE 1978) we stated that it was difficult to assign either of these proteins as products of tetracycline-resistance genes. However, a more recent publication from the group in Israel (SOMPOLINSKY et al. 1979) which has answered some of our earlier criticisms presents data which are somewhat more convincing. However, in view of the advances made in the genetic characterization of plasmid-located tetracycline-resistance genes it is unfortunate that the group in Israel has concentrated on studies with relatively obscure plasmids whose genetic relationship with other determinants is unknown.

Other studies have convincingly established the nature of proteins encoded by the *TetA–C* determinants found in gram-negative bacteria and the *Bacillus* plasmid pAB124 (Table 11). The organization of these determinants and the proteins they encode are discussed more fully in the following sections.

2. *TetA* Determinants

The tetracycline-resistance determinants of plasmid RP1 and transposon Tn*1721* have been studied in considerable detail. Although these determinants are closely related, and classified as *TetA*, they do in fact differ from each other to a small extent (WATERS et al. 1983).

BENNETT and SHALES (1981) mapped the tetracycline-resistance determinant of RP1. The resistance determinant is located approximately 14 kb from the *Eco*RI site of the plasmid. The structural genes comprise a nucleotide sequence of about 1.3 kb and adjacent to this is a region of about 500 bp which encodes a repressor. More extensive studies have been conducted with the *TetA* determinant found in Tn*1721* (ALTENBUCHNER et al. 1983; Fig. 20). The genes encoding resistance are located in a 2.1 kb portion of the transposon and by the use of various mutants two genes were characterized and mapped (Fig. 20). The gene responsible for resistance encompasses 1,250 bp and codes for a membrane-located protein of apparent molecular weight 34K. The second gene, about 650 bp long, codes for a soluble 26K protein which was identified as a repressor. The genes are adjacent to each other and have opposite transcriptional polarity which suggests that the operators controlling their expression are located in a small intercistronic region between the genes (Fig. 20).

Recently the DNA sequences of the *tet* determinants in RP1 and Tn*1721* have been obtained (WATERS et al. 1983). An open reading frame potentially encoding a 42K protein (molecular weight calculated from the nucleotide sequence data) is located in the right half of each determinant.

Table 11. Membrane proteins encoded by different tetracycline-resistance determinants that are involved in active efflux of tetracyclines

Determinant[a]	Prototype plasmid	Properties of the proteins			Tetracyclines extruded							References
		Mol. wt. (K) from		Amino acid residues	Tc	OTc	CTc	DCTc	DDHMTc	Doxy	Min	
		Gel electrophoresis	DNA sequences									
TetA	RP1	34	42	399	+	+	+					ALTENBUCHNER et al. (1983); BALL et al. (1980); MCMURRY et al. (1980, 1982); CHOPRA et al. (1982)
TetB	R100	36	43	401	+	+	+	+	+	+	+	WATERS et al. (1983); HILLEN and SCHOLLMEIER (1983)
TetC	pBR322	34	42	396	+	+	+	+	+			TAIT and BOYER (1978a); CHOPRA et al. (1982); PEDEN (1983)
	pAB124	32			+	+						ECCLES and CHOPRA (1984)

Tc, tetracycline; OTc, oxytetracycline; CTc, chlortetracycline; DCTc, demethylchlortetracycline; DDHMTc, 6-demethyl-6-deoxy-5-hydroxy-6-methylenetetracycline; Doxy, doxycycline; Min, minocycline

[a] Classification according to the scheme of MENDEZ et al. (1980)

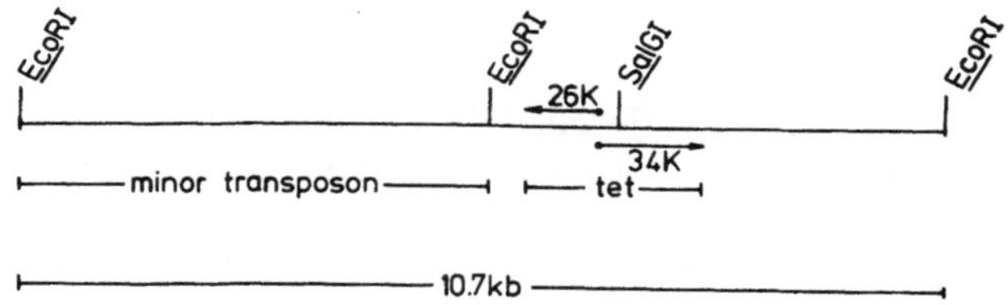

Fig. 20. Transcriptional and restriction site map of the *tet* region in Tn*1721*. *Arrows above and below the map* indicate genes encoding proteins involved in tetracycline resistance (34K) or its control (26K) (see text). *kb*, kilobases; ←, promoter. [Based on the data of ALTENBUCHNER et al. (1983)]

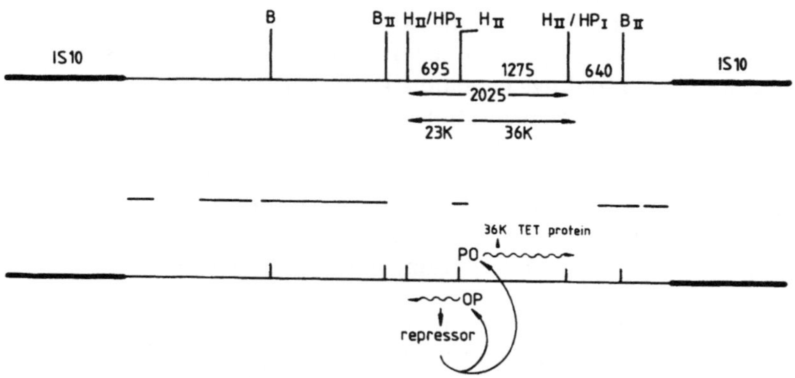

Fig. 21. Transcriptional and restriction site maps of the resistance region of Tn*10* (*TetB*). *The vertical lines above the upper map* show some of the restriction endonuclease cleavage sites located in Tn*10*. *Numbers (not followed by the letter K)* refer to the length of DNA regions in base pairs. *Below the upper map* the regions which code for the tetracycline-inducible 36K resistance protein and the autogenously controlled 23K repressor protein are indicated, together with their directions of transcription. *Horizontal lines* designate the general location of RNA polymerase binding sites. *The lower map* shows the probable organization of the regulatory elements controlling expression of the 23K repressor and 36K resistance protein (synonym TET protein). *B*, *Bam*HI; B_{II}, *Bgl*II; H_{II}, *Hinc*II; HP_I, *Hpa*I. The models are based on the data of JORGENSEN et al. (1978, 1979), JORGENSEN and REZNIKOFF (1979), WRAY et al. (1981), BERTRAND et al. (1981), and HILLEN et al. (1982).

3. *TetB* Determinants

The *TetB* determinant located in transposon Tn*10* has been extensively studied. Deletion analysis shows that the structural gene for a 36K membrane-located resistance protein resides mainly within *Hinc*II fragment 1,275 and the structural gene for a 23K repressor within *Hinc*II fragment 695 (Fig. 21) (JORGENSEN and REZNIKOFF 1979; WRAY et al. 1981). The *Hinc*II site at the junction between fragments 695 and 1,275 (Fig. 21) lies within the promotor controlling transcription of the 36K proton (JORGENSEN and REZNIKOFF 1979; WRAY et al. 1981). Evidence supporting this view is as follows.

1. Prior incubation of Tn*10* DNA with RNA polymerase in vitro inhibits *Hinc*II cleavage at the site between fragments 695 and 1,275 (JORGENSEN and REZNIKOFF 1979).

2. Several promoters are known to contain *Hinc*II cleavage sites (see WRAY et al. 1981 for a discussion).
3. Tn*10* recombinants having different DNA sequences on the upstream side of the RNA polymerase protected *Hinc*II site have altered levels of the 36K resistance protein (WRAY et al. 1981).

In vitro studies (BERTRAND et al. 1981) indicate that the transcription initiation site for the repressor is located only 15–20 base pairs away from the initiation site for the 36K protein. Since the promoter controlling repressor synthesis does not lie within fragment 695 (WRAY et al. 1981) this implies that the promoters overlap (Fig. 21). Furthermore, separate operators exist in this region because uninduced minicells containing Tn*10* produce repressor, but not the 36K protein (WRAY et al. 1981). The arrangement of promoters dictates that transcription of the repressor and the 36K protein occurs in opposite directions (Fig. 21). Most of WRAY et al. (1981) findings have now been confirmed by BECK et al. (1982).

Recently, genetic complementation data (CURIALE and LEVY 1982; COLEMAN et al. 1983) have suggested that two resistance proteins are produced by the *TetB* determinant in Tn*10*. Nevertheless these results appear to result from intragenic complementation between missense mutations in different domains of the single (36K) polypeptide (CURIALE et al. 1984). Furthermore, nucleic acid sequencing has revealed only one open reading frame in the *TetB* determinant, potentially encoding a 44K polypeptide.

From studies on ribosome binding sites in Tn*10*, CALAME et al. (1978) concluded that products of the Tn*10* resistance region are transcribed from one DNA strand. These results conflict with the more recent data on transcription in the resistance region (Fig. 21), which imply that the repressor and 36K protein are transcribed from separate DNA strands.

4. *TetC* Determinants

The *TetC* determinant in the plasmid pSC101 and its derivative pBR322 has been extensively studied. *E. coli* strains carrying pSC101 synthesize four membrane-located proteins apparently concerned with tetracycline resistance – 34K, 26K, 18K, and 14K (Table 12). Apart from the 18K protein, synthesis of these polypeptides is inducible. Both the 26K and 18K proteins may require the presence of the 34K protein before they can function. The plasmid pBR322 contains part of the tetracycline-resistance region from pSC101, but in this case only the 34K and 18K proteins are synthesized and their expression is constitutive (BOYER et al. 1977).

The tetracycline-resistance region of pBR322 was first sequenced by SUTCLIFFE (1978) and from the data he predicted the amino acid sequences of seven hypothetical proteins (A-179, B-112, B-125, C-338, D-82, E-152, F-99) that could be produced and concerned with expression of resistance. Which of these proteins are synthesized and what is their relation to the products observed in minicells harbouring pSC101 or pBR322? On the basis of size the hypothetical proteins A-179, B-112, B-125, D-82, E-152, and F-99 are all too small to account for the 34K protein resolved by polyacrylamide gel electrophoresis. SUTCLIFFE (1978) therefore reasoned that the 34K protein corresponded to the hypothetical protein C-

Table 12. Properties of tetracycline-resistance proteins specified by pSC101

Protein molecular weight (kilodaltons) From gel electrophoresis	Regulation of synthesis	Location	Possible function	Comments	References
34	Inducible	Cytoplasmic membrane	Prevents Tc accumulation		Tait and Boyer (1978a)
26	Inducible	Cytoplasmic membrane	Unknown	May require 34K protein to function	Gayda and Markovitz (1978)
18	Constitutive	Envelope	Prevents Tc accumulation	May require 34K protein to function	Gayda et al. (1979)
14	Inducible	Envelope	Prevents initial binding of Tc to cell		

338. There is good correlation between the predicted molecular weight of hypothetical protein A-179 and the 18K protein observed in bacteria. The sequence predicts a molecular weight of 22K including a hydrophobic leader sequence of 3.5K. Cleavage of the leader sequence would therefore yield a product whose molecular weight is very close to that of the 18K protein (presumed to be fully processed) found in minicells. Despite this evidence favouring a connection between the 18K protein and A-179 other data (see below) show that protein A-179 may only be a hypothetical pBR322 product.

Information concerning the possible arrangement of the structural genes for tetracycline resistance in pSC101 comes from a variety of sources. Restriction endonuclease analysis of pSC101 (and the derivative plasmid pMB9) permitted coding regions to be assigned to the four proteins involved in pSC101-mediated resistance (Tait and Boyer 1978b) (Fig. 22). Because synthesis of the 18K protein is constitutive (Table 12), the model implies that transcriptional control of the genes coding for the 34K, 26K, and 14K proteins is not achieved by regulating the synthesis of a single polycistronic mRNA molecule. Nothing is known about the direction of transcription of the genes coding for the 14K and 26K proteins, but models for the 34K and 18K proteins have been proposed.

By employing RNA polymerase binding and restriction endonuclease digestion several authors demonstrated that the region in and around the *Hin*dIII site of pBR322 constitutes a promotor (position 0, Fig. 23) (Rodriguez et al. 1979; West and Rodriguez 1980). This location for a promotor is also consistent with electron microscopic analysis of in vitro transcriptional complexes of pBR322 (Stuber and Bujard 1981). The structural gene for the 34K protein produced in minicells lies to the "right" of the promoter region at the *Hin*dIII site because insertions at the *Bam*HI site (position 347, Fig. 23) reduce the size of the 34K protein (Rambach and Hogness 1977). Since the nucleotide sequence of the region in Fig. 23 is known (Sutcliffe 1978), it should be possible to predict the exact lo-

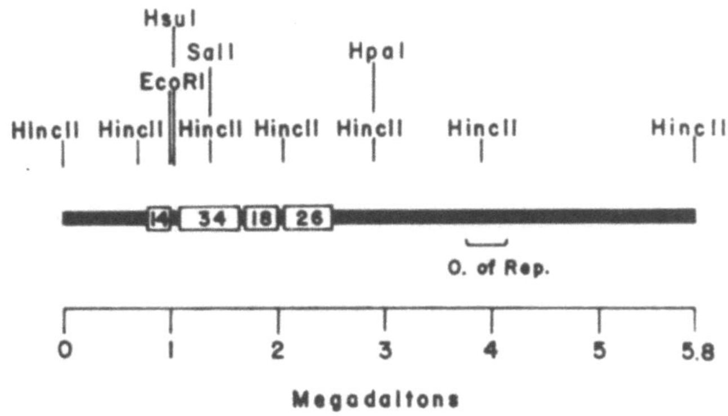

Fig. 22. Map of the tetracycline-resistance region of pSC101. The genes for the four polypeptides involved in tetracycline resistance have been positioned on the restriction map of pSC101. The approximate origin of replication of pSC101 is indicated by *O. of Rep.* (TAIT and BOYER 1978b)

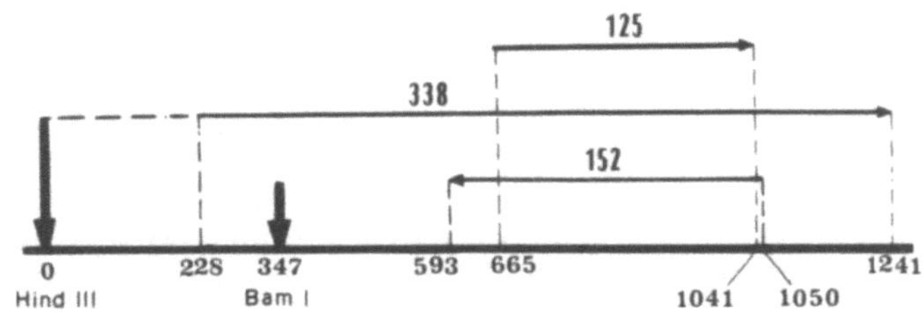

Fig. 23. Model for the possible organization of tetracycline-resistance genes in pBR322. *The numbers along the map (0 to 1241)* indicate the distance in base pairs from the *Hind*III site at position 0 which itself corresponds to position 30 in the numbering system of SUTCLIFFE (1978). *347, Bam*HI restriction endonuclease site. *593, 1041, 1241,* sites of putative termination codons respectively for hypothetical resistance proteins E-152, B-125, and C-338. *228, 665, 1050,* sites of putative initiation codons respectively for hypothetical resistance proteins C-338, B-125, and E-152. (KOPYLOVA-SVIRIDOVA et al. 1979)

cation of the structural gene for the 34K protein. Initiation signals for translation (ATG or GTG) occur only at two sites close to the "right" of the *Hind*III site, one at a distance of 51 base pairs from the *Hind*III site and the other at a distance of 228 base pairs. Initiation at the second site (position 228, Fig. 23) seems more probable as the calculated size of the protein (43.3K; 338 amino acid residues) is closer to the observed molecular weight of 34K than the hypothetical protein initiated at position 51, which would have 397 amino acid residues. Synthesis of the 338 amino acid residue protein (C-338) in the manner described predicts a long region (approximately 228 base pairs) between promoter and starting triplets. However, this is not uncommon in prokaryotes [see KOPYLOVA-SVIRIDOVA et al. (1979) for a discussion]. Surprisingly, in vitro transcriptional analysis indicates a terminator at or near position 680 (Fig. 23), which is within the proposed structural gene for the 34K protein (STUBER and BUJARD 1981). Termination of hypothetical gene C-338 at this point would produce a polypeptide of molecular weight 19K. The function of the termination site is unclear, but the sequence around it (positions 648–696, Fig. 23) may contain an attenuator (STUBER and

BUJARD 1981). Therefore in pSC101 (which contains a repressor structural gene) synthesis of the 34K protein may be subject to more than one form of transcriptional control.

TAIT and BOYER (1978b) suggest that the structural gene for the 18K protein is adjacent and to the "right" of the gene encoding the 34K protein (Fig. 22). This would agree with the hypothetical location and direction of transcription of pBR322 gene E-152 (Fig. 23) (SUTCLIFFE 1978), giving rise to a protein of 152 amino acid residues and with a molecular weight close to the observed value of 18K. However, no promoter has been located in or around position 1,050 (Fig. 23) (STUBER and BUJARD 1981). The product of hypothetical gene B-125 might correspond to the 18K product seen in vivo, but again there is no promoter at position 665 (Fig. 23) (STUBER and BUJARD 1981). Some evidence favouring the 18K protein as a product of pBR322 hypothetical gene A-179 has already been considered. According to SUTCLIFFE (1978) this protein would be initiated from position 117–119 (initiator codon ATG) and its structural gene would therefore contain the *Bam*HI site at position 347 (Fig. 23). However, DNA insertions at the *Bam*HI site do not eliminate the synthesis of the 18K protein in minicells containing the recombinant plasmids (KOPYLOVA-SVIRIDOVA et al. 1979). Furthermore, Sutcliffe's hypothesis for the location of gene A-179 implies that translation of the 179 amino acid residue protein might obstruct binding of ribosomes to the mRNA of the 338-residue protein (C-338). This is not consistent with data showing that minicells containing pBR322 produce the larger protein (34K) in much greater amounts than the smaller (18K) protein (KOPYLOVA-SVIRIDOVA et al. 1979; SANCAR et al. 1979).

From the foregoing discussion it can be observed that the structural gene for the 18K pBR322 protein cannot easily be located in the tetracycline-resistance region. In fact recent sequencing data are not consistent with the observation that the 18K protein is a product of the tetracycline-resistance region. Recently, a correction has been made to the pBR322 DNA sequence previously reported by Sutcliffe. An additional CG base pair has now been inserted at position 526, which lies within the tetracycline-resistance region (LIVNEH 1983; PEDEN 1983). This change adjusts the published sequence to allow an open reading frame from nucleotides 86–1,273 (new number) coding for a hypothetical protein of 396 amino acids and molecular weight 41.5K (PEDEN 1983; NGUYEN et al. 1983; WATERS et al. 1983). The addition of the single nucleotide pair to the sequence causes a change in the reading frames so that Sutcliffe's predicted protein A-179 now becomes part of the predicted protein C-338 (PEDEN 1983). The recent corrections to the pBR322 nucleotide sequence which predict that a single polypeptide encodes pBR322-mediated resistance to tetracycline have recently been confirmed by BACKMAN and BOYER (1983). These authors demonstrated that small deletions in pBR322 which abolished tetracycline resistance also resulted in the absence or alteration of the 34K pBR322-encoded protein.

5. The Tetracycline-Resistance Determinant of Bacillus Plasmid pAB124

Plasmid pAB124 was originally isolated in *Bacillus stearothermophilus* (see ECCLES et al. 1981). The tetracycline-resistance determinant from this plasmid has

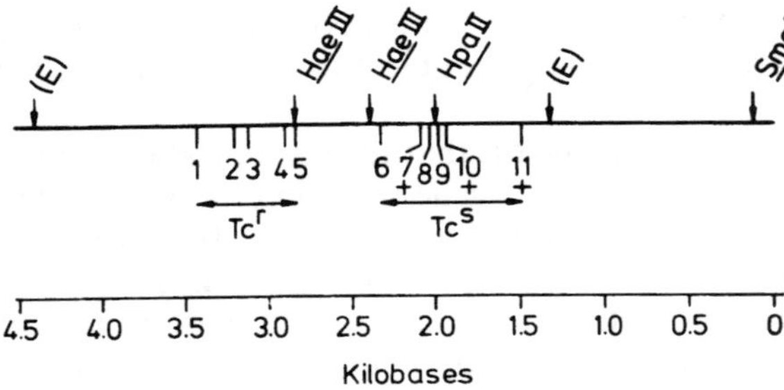

Fig. 24. Restriction map of the tetracycline-resistance determinant from *Bacillus* plasmid pAB124. A fragment of pAB124 carrying the genes encoding tetracycline resistance was cloned into the *Escherichia coli* plasmid pSF2124 (ECCLES et al. 1981) thereby producing pUB1721. Plasmid pUB1721 confers only a low level of tetracycline resistance in *E. coli*, but a mutant was obtained (pUB1730) which expresses high-level resistance in this host (ECCLES and CHOPRA 1984). The above map shows the tetracycline-resistance region of pUB1731 which is a derivative of pUB1730 from which *Eco*RI sites (*E*) have been removed. The *horizontal line* represents a region of pUB1731 DNA. *Arrows* above this line indicate restriction sites. *Vertical lines* below the horizontal line represent the location of various insertion mutations. The regions in which insertions cause tetracycline resistance or sensitivity are indicated. The mutants followed by the symbol + are unable to cause tetracycline efflux. The other mutants have not been tested for their ability to cause tetracycline efflux. (ECCLES and CHOPRA 1984)

been cloned both in *B. subtilis* and *E. coli* and extensively characterized in the latter host (ECCLES et al. 1981; ECCLES and CHOPRA 1984). A restriction map of the determinant is presented in Fig. 24. Although the resistance determinant does not hybridize with any of the *TetA-TetD* determinants found in gram-negative bacteria it encodes a membrane-located resistance protein which has a similar molecular weight to those encoded by *TetA* and *TetB* (Table 11).

V. Mode of Action of Membrane-Located Resistance Proteins

The mechanism by which the plasmid-encoded membrane proteins confer tetracycline resistance has emerged gradually during the past decade. Initially, decreased accumulation was explained solely by reduced antibiotic influx, with no apparent evidence for efflux (YOUNG and HUBBALL 1976). This led to a theory suggesting that membrane-located resistance proteins chelate cations involved in tetracycline transport (BOCHNER et al. 1980; HERRIN et al. 1982). Thus the resistance proteins are assumed to lower the free metal ion concentration in the membrane and prevent entry of tetracycline. However, such theories are no longer tenable and there is now little doubt that the membrane-located resistance proteins promote enery-dependent tetracycline efflux (BALL et al. 1980; MCMURRY et al. 1980; MCMURRY et al. 1982; HEDSTROM et al. 1982). Strong evidence that these proteins are involved in efflux is provided by tetracycline accumulation studies with derivatives in which the respective structural genes have been deleted or mutated (TAIT and BOYER 1978a; COLEMAN et al. 1983; ECCLES and CHOPRA 1984) (Figs. 24 and 25) and by the observation that the content of wild-type *TetB* pro-

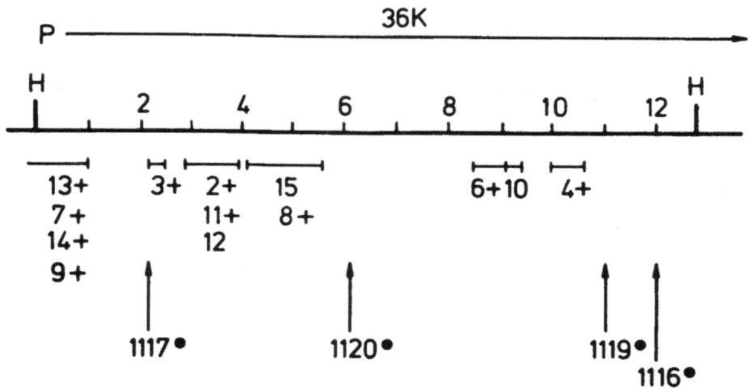

Fig. 25. Map of mutations in the tetracycline-resistance region of Tn*10* (TetB). The *horizontal line in the centre* depicts the 1275-bp *Hin*cII fragment that carries the structural gene for the 36K membrane-located protein involved in tetracycline efflux. The *numbers above this line* are physical coordinates in hundreds of base pairs. The *lower horizontal lines* indicate regions in which *tet* point mutants have been isolated. Those mutants followed by *the symbol* + (e.g. *13*) have decreased capacity to cause tetracycline efflux. The *vertical lines* show the positions of various insertions of transposon Tn*5* into the *tet* region. These insertions result in the production of truncated derivatives of the 36K protein (symbolized ●). The numbers *1116–1120* refer to the insertion mutants (see COLEMAN et al. 1983). *P*, promoter for 36K resistance protein; *H*, *Hin*cII site). [Based on COLEMAN et al. 1983)]

tein in the membrane correlates with the ability of cells to prevent tetracycline accumulation (CHOPRA et al. 1983) (Fig. 26).

Since tetracycline uptake into sensitive bacteria involves active transport (Sect. J.III) do the resistance proteins interact directly with the transport sites to reverse the influx system of the host cell? This possibility has been eliminated by use of membrane vesicles which show that the active efflux systems in resistant bacteria differ from the active influx system in sensitive cells. Thus, the systems differ with respect to kinetic constants, pH and magnesium requirements (Table 13). We can conclude from these data that the plasmid-encoded membrane resistance proteins represent saturable carriers promoting efflux of tetracyclines. The nature of energy coupling to efflux has not been explored in detail, but it appears to be driven by the proton-motive force (MCMURRY et al. 1980).

Table 13. Properties of tetracycline influx and efflux systems in membrane vesicles from *Pseudomonas putida* (HEDSTROM et al. 1982) and *Escherichia coli*. (MCMURRY et al. 1980, 1981b)

System	Kinetic constants		Optima for influx/efflux	
	K_m (μM)	V_{max} (nmol/min/mg protein)	pH	[Mg^{2+}] (mM)
Pseudomonas putida influx	2,500	50	NE	NE
Escherichia coli influx	ND	ND	6.9	1
P. putida, TetA-mediated efflux	2.0–3.5	0.15	NE	NE
E. coli. TetB-mediated efflux	6	0.1–1	7.7	3–10

ND, not determinable; NE, not estimated

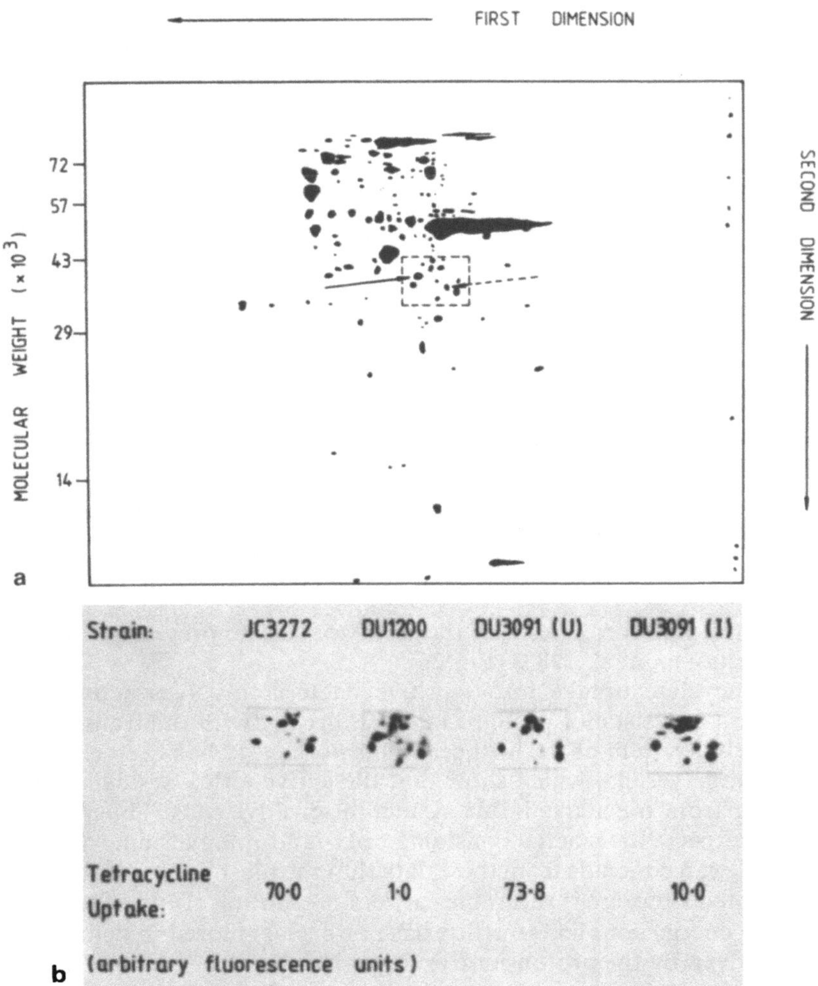

Fig. 26 a, b. Detection of the Tn*10*-determined 36-kilodalton resistance protein (pI, 6.4) in the cytoplasmic membrane of *Escherichia coli* and correlation of its content with reduced tetracycline accumulation (CHOPRA et al. 1983). Cytoplasmic membranes were fractionated using Sarkosyl and polypeptides resolved by two-dimensional electrophoresis as described by CHOPRA and SHALES (1980). **a** Diagrammatic representation of proteins from the inner membrane of DU1200 (chromosomally integrated Tn*10*; constitutive expression of resistance) separated by two-dimensional electrophoresis. Basic proteins are located to the right, acidic proteins to the left. *The solid line within the boxed area* shows the 36K *"Tet"* protein and *the broken line* a normal host product that is enriched in cells expressing high-level resistance (See **b**). The significance of the latter change is unknown. **b** Inner membrane proteins (molecular weights, 32–43K; pIs, 6.0–6.6) from several *E. coli* strains. Proteins shown are equivalent to those found in the *boxed area* of **a** above. *JC3272*, tetracycline-sensitive parental strain; *DU1200*, chromosomally integrated Tn*10*: constitutive expression of resistance; *DU3091*, chromosomally integrated Tn*10*: inducible expression of resistance. *U*, uninduced; *I*, induced. Tetracycline uptake was determined by fluorescence spectroscopy (BALL et al. 1980; SHALES et al. 1980)

VI. Membrane Architecture in Relation to the Binding and Function of Plasmid-Determined Tetracycline-Resistance Proteins

The membrane proteins involved in resistance presumably integrate with and assume specific configurations within bacterial cell envelopes in order to function. Several studies suggested that phospholipid and fatty acid metabolism might be altered in bacteria containing tetracycline-resistance plasmids (DUNNICK and O'LEARY 1970; KUZINA et al. 1977; RINGROSE and HIGGINS 1974; SULING and O'LEARY 1977). Although the changes could reflect formation of new membrane domains to accommodate the resistance proteins, we have been unable to find evidence to support this hypothesis. Thus, tetracycline-resistance can be induced in the absence of lipid synthesis (CHOPRA 1975, 1978) and no differences in phospholipid or fatty acid content were noted in *E. coli* strains isogenic apart from possession of a Tn*10* mutant in which expression of tetracycline-resistance is constitutive (CHOPRA and ECCLES 1977; CHOPRA 1978). The reported changes in the lipid content of strains harbouring tetracycline-resistance plasmids may therefore be non-specific. Acquisition of plasmids invariably leads to an alteration in the growth rate of the bacterial cell (ZUND and LEBEK 1980) which could indirectly lead to altered lipid metabolism.

However, one situation does illustrate that certain membrane properties must exist in order that resistance proteins can function. In minicells expression of plasmid-determined tetracycline resistance is defective (FRANKLIN and FOSTER 1974; LEVY 1975), which implies that certain membrane components required for resistance protein activity are not distributed into minicells at the time of their formation.

VII. Membrane-Located Resistance Proteins: Specific Properties and Comparisons Between Proteins Encoded by Different Determinants

Data on the amino acid compositions of the resistance proteins obtained either by direct analysis (Table 14) or by deduction from nucleotide sequencing data (Fig. 27) permit characterization of protein polarities (Table 15) and relatedness. The polarities of the resistance proteins are consistent with their reported location in membranes since soluble proteins show values above 47 (CAPALDI and VANDERKOOI 1972). A general method is available for estimation of the degree of homology between proteins (MARCHALONIS and WELTMAN 1971). On this basis neither the *Staphylococcus aureus* 32K protein nor the *E. coli* 50K protein are related to each other. Furthermore these proteins show no homology with the *TetA* 34K protein, the *TetB* 36K protein or the pBR322 34K protein. On the other hand the *TetA, TetB,* and pBR322 resistance proteins are related to each other since they have many amino acid residues in common (Fig. 27; see also WATERS et al. 1983; NGUYEN et al. 1983).

The molecular weights of the *TetA, TetB,* and pBR322 proteins predicted from the DNA sequences are greater than the apparent molecular weights observed by separation on polyacrylamide gels (Table 11). This discrepancy might be explained in two ways: either the resistance proteins are synthesized as molecules which are reduced in length on insertion into the membrane, or the electro-

Table 14. Amino acid composition (residues/100 residues) of proteins probably involved in expression of tetracycline resistance in *Staphylococcus aureus* and *Escherichia coli.* (Wojdani et al. 1976)

Amino acid	Protein	
	Staphylococcus aureus 32K	*Escherichia coli* 50K
Lys	1.56	5.28
His	2.58	2.02
Arg	6.90	4.24
Asp	10.28	9.69
AspN	–	–
Thr	4.56	5.43
Ser	7.10	5.28
Glu	12.41	11.41
GluN	–	–
Pro	5.39	2.91
Gly	17.05	10.39
Ala	9.49	13.15
Cys	1.06	0.45
Val	3.72	7.03
Met	1.21	3.51
Isoleu	2.81	5.11
Leu	4.63	8.42
Tyr	12.15	2.42
Phe	1.63	3.26
Trp	ND	ND

ND, not determined

phoretic mobility of the proteins is anomalous. The second explanation is more likely because several membrane proteins have been reported to migrate in gels with a higher mobility than would be expected from their known molecular weights (e.g., see Noel et al. 1979). The variable migration of the *TetB* membrane protein in different electrophoresis systems (see Chopra et al. 1981) also lends support to the idea that the electrophoretic mobility of the resistance proteins is anomalous.

Some cytoplasmic membrane proteins are synthesized as pre-proteins, i.e., with hydrophobic N-terminal leader sequences of about 20 amino acids (Pratt et al. 1981). Leader sequences are required for insertion and translocation of these proteins within the envelope but the pre-proteins are subsequently processed to remove the leader sequences and generate the mature product. The nucleotide sequences at the beginning of the *TetA, B,* and pBR322 structural genes do not predict involvement of leader sequences for membrane insertion of the resistance proteins (Nguyen et al. 1983). Furthermore, the *TetB* protein has the same electrophoretic mobility whether isolated from minicells or synthesized in vitro (Yang et al. 1976), again suggesting that this protein is not processed in vivo. Similar experiments conducted with the pAB124-encoded efflux protein also provide no evidence for leader sequences in this system (Eccles and Chopra 1984).

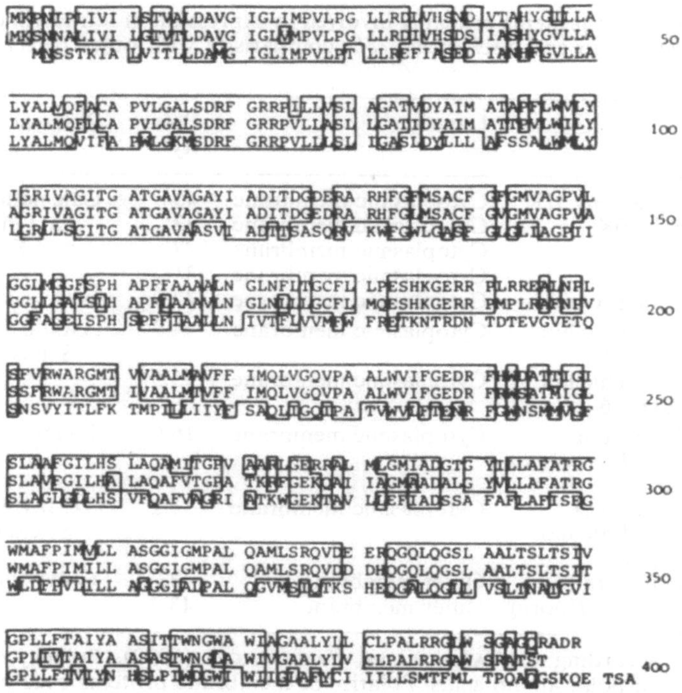

Fig. 27. Predicted amino acid sequences of membrane proteins coded by the *Escherichia coli TetA*, pBR322, and *TetB* determinants. The amino acid sequences of membrane-located resistance proteins coded by *TetA* (*upper*), pBR322 (*middle*), and *TetB* (*lower*) are shown, aligned for maximum homology. The proteins are believed to correspond to those in Table 11 and the protein sequences are given by the one-letter amino acid code (IUPAC-IUB Commission 1969). Amino acid sequences are those reported by WATERS et al. (1983) (*TetA*), PEDEN (1983) (pBR322), and HILLEN and SCHOLLMEIER (1983) (*TetB*). Homologous residues are indicated by *boxes*

Since hybridization experiments revealed that the *TetA, TetB,* and pBR322 determinants are distinct due to lack of DNA homology (MENDEZ et al. 1980), one would also predict that the amino acid sequences of the resistance proteins will differ. Nevertheless, since these proteins are able in common to promote tetracycline efflux, conserved amino acid sequences may exist. Alignment of the *TetA, TetB,* and pBR322 membrane protein sequences to produce maximum homology (Fig. 27) indicates that the proteins, as anticipated, are dissimilar. Despite differences between the proteins, several amino acid sequences are common to each, particularly in some localized regions of each protein (Fig. 27). Some, or all, of these conserved regions are therefore likely to be involved in promoting tetracycline efflux. The ability of *Tet* determinants to confer resistance to different tetracycline analogues has been known for some time (MENDEZ et al. 1980; CHOPRA et al. 1982) and this is apparently reflected by differences in the capacity of the membrane-resistance proteins to promote efflux of the analogues (Table 11). Differences in the ability to extrude tetracycline analogues is presumably related

Table 15. Polarity of proteins probably involved in expression of tetracycline resistance in *Staphylococcus aureus* and *Escherichia coli:* comparison with other bacterial membrane proteins

Protein	Location	Polarity[a]	References
Staphylococcus aureus 32K	Cytoplasmic membrane	45	Calculations based on data in Table 14 and Fig. 27
Escherichia coli 50K	Cytoplasmic membrane	43	
34K *TetA*	Cytoplasmic membrane	27	
36 K *TetB*	Cytoplasmic membrane	31	
34K pBR322 *tet* protein	Cytoplasmic membrane	27	
Escherichia coli penicillin binding protein 5	Cytoplasmic membrane	44.9	AMANUMA and STROMINGER (1980)
Escherichia coli penicillin binding protein 6	Cytoplasmic membrane	45.5	
Carbodiimide-reactive component of *Escherichia coli* ATPase	Cytoplasmic membrane	16.0	FILLINGAME (1976)
Staphylococcus aureus C55-isoprenoid alcohol phosphokinase	Cytoplasmic membrane	31.2	SANDERMANN and STROMINGER (1971)
Escherichia coli OmpA	Outer membrane	43.3	GARTEN et al. (1975)
Escherichia coli OmpF porin	Outer membrane	43.4	

[a] Calculated according to CAPALDI and VANDERKOOI (1972). Polarity, sum of mole percentages of polar amino acids. Polarity of membrane proteins usually <47

to differences in amino acid sequence within the proteins, but at present it is difficult to predict which polypeptide regions are involved in recognition of different tetracyclines.

VIII. Gene Copy Number and Decreased Tetracycline Accumulation

Gene amplification (i.e. an increase in number) of plasmid-located antibiotic resistance determinants frequently leads to increased levels of antibiotic resistance, e.g. to ampicillin, chloramphenicol and streptomycin (UHLIN and NORDSTROM 1977). In most cases increased resistance results from elevated levels of soluble enzymes, but in the case of tetracycline-resistance the anticipated increase in efflux upon increasing the gene copy number is not realized. As discussed below this implies that the number of functional binding sites within the membrane that can accommodate the plasmid-specified proteins is limited.

WEIBAUER et al. (1981) studied tetracycline gene amplification in *E. coli* using the *TetA* determinant in transposon Tn*1721*. The transposable element consists of a "minor transposon" encoding functions required for transposition and a separate tetracycline-resistance determinant (Figs. 18 and 20). As already noted the latter is flanked by two direct repeats which provide sequence homology for amplification of tetracycline-resistance genes. Multiple tandem repeats of the resistance determinant were generated to study the relationship between gene dosage and reduced tetracycline accumulation, but increased efflux of the antibiotic was not observed with increasing number of resistance genes in the range of 1–36 copies per chromosome (Weibauer et al. 1981). Although these data imply a limited number of membrane sites at which the resistance proteins can integrate, increased osmotic lability of cells was observed upon increasing the gene copy number. This probably indicates that an excess of resistance protein is accumulating in the cell envelope, leading to instability. Therefore, although the ability of the cytoplasmic membrane to accommodate the *TetA*-determined resistance protein may not be limited per se, the number of functional sites from which tetracycline efflux can be promoted is probably saturable at the level of one determinant per chromosome.

Studies on gene dosage effects with the *TetB* determinant have also been conducted, but this has involved cloning the determinant into plasmid vectors having different numbers of copies per chromosome (Chopra et al. 1981 b; Coleman and Foster 1981). The effect of increasing the number of *TetB* determinants per cell is more complex than the situation which occurs with *TetA*. In the case of *TetB*, increased copy numbers lead to decreased expression of resistance associated with reduced expression of the efflux system (Chopra et al. 1981 b). The molecular basis of this response is poorly understood, but may represent a regulatory mechanism to prevent overproduction of the membrane-located resistance protein (Coleman and Foster 1981).

Although reduced *tet* gene expression can, in principle, provide an explanation for the reduced tetracycline-resistance of multicopy *TetB* strains, several recent observations are not consistent with a regulatory model (Moyed and Bertrand 1983; Moyed et al. 1983). Indeed, it is now proposed that the relative sensitivity of multicopy *TetB* strains to tetracycline is caused by the synthesis of multiple copies of the 36K protein (Moyed and Bertrand 1983; Moyed et al. 1983). Overproduction of the resistance protein may lead to membrane destabilization, thereby lowering the efficiency of the tetracycline efflux system.

The reason that *TetA* and *TetB* determinants show different responses with respect to gene dosage is not clear, but could be related to the ability of *TetB* determinants to encode minocycline resistance (Chopra et al. 1981 b).

IX. Are the Membrane-Located Resistance Proteins That Mediate Efflux the Only Products Responsible for Resistance?

Several investigators have commented that the observed decrease in tetracycline accumulation seems insufficient to explain the levels of tetracycline-resistance encoded by plasmids (Levy 1981; Eccles et al. 1981; McMurry et al. 1980; Shales et al. 1980). Although the determinant in pSC101 (*TetC*) apparently specifies four proteins involved in resistance (Table 12), the other determinants appear to encode only a single product (other than repressor proteins), i.e. the membrane-located resistance proteins described above. As already noted genetic complementation data (Curiale and Levy 1982; Coleman et al. 1983) have suggested that two resistance proteins are produced by the *TetB* determinant, but these results could nevertheless be explained by intragenic complementation between missense mutations in different domains of a single polypeptide. Furthermore, nucleic acid sequencing has revealed only one open reading frame in the *TetB* determinant, potentially encoding the 44K polypeptide (HILLEN and SCHOLLMEIER 1983; NGUYEN et al. 1983). The apparent discrepancy between resistance levels mediated by plasmids and the decreased tetracycline accumulation they cause may be explained by the involvement of *tet* gene repressors in resistance, i.e. by binding tetracycline the repressors may actually contribute to resistance themselves (BECK et al. 1982).

In previous publications we reported that tetracycline-resistance determinants express up to three phenotypic mechanisms of resistance (SHALES et al. 1980; CHOPRA et al. 1983). In the light of new findings described in this article we can now suggest that mechanism 1 is mediated by repressors (BECK et al. 1982) and mechanism 2 entails antibiotic efflux promoted by the membrane-located proteins (Table 11). Mechanism 3 (coded by the *TetB* determinant) was previously thought to involve ribosomal alterations (YANG et al. 1976; LEVY et al. 1977; SHALES et al. 1980). This, however, is not the case (S. W. Shales, I. Chopra, unpublished work) and the phenotype, like that conferred by mechanism 2, results from minocycline efflux promoted by the membrane-located resistance protein (MCMURRY et al. 1982). The inability of *TetA* and *TetC* determinants to express minocycline resistance probably results from failure of the respective resistance proteins to promote efflux of the antibiotic (Table 11).

Apart from regulatory proteins it is clear that for each of the tetracycline-resistance determinants examined in detail (i.e. *TetA, TetB,* pBR322, and *Bacillus* plamid pAB124) only one polypeptide is specified. In each case these polypeptides alone are sufficient to express resistance. Furthermore the polypeptides have similar molecular weights, are membrane-located and function to promote energy-dependent efflux of tetracyclines. Although the *TetC* determinant in pBR322 encodes a single polypeptide concerned with resistance, the *TetC* determinant in pSC101 from which pBR322 was derived was initially reported to encode four proteins concerned with resistance, i.e. with molecular weights of 34K, 26K, 18K, and 14K (Table 12). Although the role of the 18K protein as a product concerned with resistance has now been discounted (see Sect. K.IV.4), the possibility remains that pSC101-mediated tetracycline-resistance involves the participation of the 26K and 14K proteins in addition to the 34K polypeptide (BACKMAN and BOYER 1983). On the other hand it is unclear why expression of pSC101-mediated tetracycline-resistance should require several products whereas other well-characterized determinants appear to encode only a single product which is sufficient for expression of resistance. Clearly further work is required on the nature of pSC101-encoded products to resolve the problems raised, but in this author's opinion the other pSC101 products apparently involved in resistance may either prove to be artifacts or not concerned with expression of resistance. At the time of writing it therefore seems more probable that resistance specified by tetracycline determinants results in each case from the synthesis of a single membrane polypeptide that causes tetracycline efflux from the cell. The further possibility that repressor molecules contribute to resistance needs to be examined in more detail.

X. Therapeutic Consequences of Tetracycline-Resistance Gene Amplification

The high prevalence of plasmid-determined tetracycline-resistance has undoubtedly reduced the value of tetracyclines for human and veterinary medicine (CHOPRA et al. 1981 a). Selection pressure with tetracycline in vitro may cause multiplication of resistance gene copies in those plasmids containing amplifiable DNA sequences (Table 8). Although such amplification may raise resistance levels due to elevated repressor levels (WIEBAUER et al. 1981), increased quantities of resistance proteins in the membrane may cause physiological problems for the cell, e.g. membrane destabilization (WIEBAUER et al. 1981; MOYED and BERTRAND 1983; MOYED et al. 1983). Thus even though bacteria harbouring amplifiable tetracycline determinants may possess the capacity to undergo an increase in resistance, in some clinical conditions it may be disadvantageous for them to do so.

XI. Use of the Fluorescence Assay for Tetracycline for Studies on Plasmid-Determined Resistance

In addition to its use for studies on the nature of tetracycline transport into sensitive bacteria, the tetracycline fluorescence assay has been used extensively for studies on plasmid-determined tetracycline resistance. As noted in a previous section (J.IV) this assay has certain limitations for studies on tetracycline transport. Nevertheless, the technique has been successfully used to study resistance. In this context the following can be noted:

1. In cells harbouring Tn*10* or the plasmids pIP7 and RP1, there is a precise correlation between decreased uptake measured by the fluorescence assay and increased antibiotic resistance (SHALES et al. 1980).
2. Studies utilizing either the fluorescence or labelled drug technique both show the involvement of accelerated drug efflux in resistance (BALL et al. 1980; MCMURRY et al. 1980).
3. Use of the fluorescence assay with tetracycline analogues has permitted phenotypic differentiation of various gram-negative tetracycline-resistance determinants known to differ genetically (CHOPRA et al. 1982, see also Table 11).

XII. Inducibility of Plasmid-Determined Resistance to Tetracycline

1. Introduction

As already mentioned several tetracycline-resistance determinants are now known to encode repressor proteins that regulate transcription of tetracycline-resistance genes. Earlier studies on the nature of plasmid-determined tetracycline-resistance in *E. coli* and *Staphylococcus aureus* had already indicated the likely involvement of repressors because the character was generally found to be inducible, i.e. the level of resistance increases in response to the presence of subinhibitory concentrations of the drug (see CHOPRA and HOWE 1978). However, this does not necessarily mean that all the components contributing to resistance are also inducible, e.g. one of the "resistance" proteins encoded by pSC101 is expressed constitutively (TAIT and BOYER 1978a). The only naturally occurring plasmid-linked determinant where the products are all expressed constitutively is that of plasmid pAMα1 found in *Streptococcus faecalis* (CLEWELL et al. 1975).

2. The Basis of Regulatory Control

Expression of inducible resistance is under negative regulatory control, i.e. there is a regulatory gene the product of which controls one or more structural genes that are coordinately expressed. The evidence for negative regulatory control can be summarized as follows.

1. Constitutive mutants can be isolated, both of the repressor-negative type and operator-constitutive type (REEVE and ROBERTSON 1975; FOSTER 1977).
2. Fusion of the tetracycline-resistance region of Tn*10* to an external gene, *lacZ*, demonstrates that the structural region is under the control of a tetracycline repressor (BECK 1979).
3. Proteins with repressor-like properties have been isolated from extracts of *E. coli* harbouring Tn*10* (YANG et al. 1976; HILLEN et al. 1982) and pSC101 (TAIT and BOYER 1978a).

Recent studies (ZUPANCIC et al. 1980; BERTRAND et al. 1981; WRAY et al. 1981; BECK et al. 1982; HILLEN and UNGER 1982; HILLEN et al. 1982, 1983) on the regulatory control of resistance in Tn*10* have led to the following conclusions:

1. The structural gene for the repressor is adjacent to that encoding the membrane-located 36K efflux protein (Fig. 21).
2. The structural genes for the repressor and the adjacent resistance protein are transcribed in opposite directions form functionally overlapping promoters (Fig. 21).
3. The repressor negatively regulates transcription of its own structural gene as well as the structural gene for the resistance protein (Fig. 21).
4. The stoichiometry for the TET repressor-TET operator interaction is one repressor molecule per operator, the functional repressor being a dimer.
5. The repressor may be envelope associated.

Presumable negative autogenous control of repressor synthesis ensures that the concentration of repressor is limited. This probably permits rapid de-repression and hence expression of resistance when bacteria encounter tetracycline. The ability of the Tn*10*-encoded TET system to respond to minimal amounts of the drug is also achieved by a comparatively high association constant for the TET repressor-tetracycline complex (HILLEN et al. 1982, 1983). The association constant for the TET repressor-tetracycline complex is greater than the association constant for the TET repressor-TET operator complex (HILLEN et al. 1982, 1983). These properties differ from those of other regulatory systems, e.g. the *lac* operon, where the repressor-operator interaction is more stable than the repressor-lactose interaction (see HILLEN et al. 1982). These differences are presumably related to the functions of the regulatory systems. The *lac* genes code for metabolizing enzymes and should not therefore become derepressed before adequate amounts of substrate accumulate. This situation is achieved by a relatively low association constant for the repressor-lactose complex. In contrast, the tetracycline-resistance determinant should respond to minimal amounts of the drug in order to protect the cell from inhibition. This is achieved by a high association constant for the TET repressor-tetracycline complex.

Our understanding of the regulatory properties of the Tn*10* repressor is complicated by its location in the cell envelope (BECK et al. 1982). Although such a location is unusual it is not unique because the *traJ* protein, which is located in the *E. coli* outer membrane, is required for transcription of the *tra* genes (ACHTMAN et al. 1979). One reason that the Tn*10* tetracycline gene repressor is envelope located may possibly relate to an active role in resistance where the repressor protein cooperates with the membrane-located efflux protein (36K) (see BECK et al. 1982 and Sect. K.IX).

Experiments on the regulation of Tn*1721*-mediated tetracycline-resistance have identified a repressor with a molecular weight similar to that observed for Tn*10* (ALTENBUCHNER et al. 1983). Furthermore, transcriptional control of the tetracycline-resistance determinant appears to be identical with that of Tn*10*, i.e. involving overlapping promoters.

3. Are Repressor Molecules Heterogeneous?

The classification of tetracycline-resistance determinants by MENDEZ et al. (1980) (Table 10) did not consider whether repressor molecules were also heterogeneous. Repressors controlling expression of determinants A–C are not inactivated by chelocardin (Table 16), but extensive studies on repressor-drug interaction have not been conducted so that heterogeneity of repressors cannot yet be inferred from this type of data. Nevertheless, data derived from examination of plasmid diploids, and more recently direct assays for repressor binding to *tet* gene operators, support some degree of repressor heterogeneity amongst tetracycline-resistance determinants found in gram-negative bacteria (REEVE and ROBERTSON 1975; REEVE 1978; WRAY and REZNIKOFF 1983).

Table 16. Induction of resistance to tetracycline (Tc) or minocycline (Min) in *Escherichia coli* containing determinants of groups A–C

Inducer	*TetA*		*TetB*		*TetC*	References
	Tc	Min[a]	Tc	Min	Tc	
Tetracycline	+	+	+	+	+	FOSTER and WALSH (1974)
Oxytetracycline	ND	+	ND	+	ND	CHABBERT and SCAVIZZI (1976)
Minocycline	ND	+	ND	+	ND	SHALES et al. (1980)
Chelocardin	–	–	–	–	–	MENDEZ et al. (1980)

ND, not determined
[a] *TetA* determinants only confer low-level resistance to minocycline (see Table 10)

Table 17. Activity of tetracycline analogues as growth inhibitors and inducers of plasmid-determined tetracycline resistance in *Staphylococcus aureus*. [Based on SOMPOLINSKY and KRAUSZ (1973) and INOUE et al. (1977)]

Analogue	Activity as	
	Antibacterial agent[a]	Inducer
Tetracycline	+	+
Oxytetracycline	+	+
Minocycline	+	+
Chelocardin	+	−
Chlorotetracycline	+	+
Doxycycline	+	+
6-Methyleneoxytetracycline	+	+
6-Demethyl-7-chlorotetracycline	+	+
6-Demethyltetracycline	+	+
6-Deoxy-6-methylenetetracycline	+	+
6-Demethyl-6-deoxytetracycline	+	+
5a,6-anhydrotetracycline	+	+
5a,11a-Dehydro-7-chlorotetracycline	−	Poor
2-Acetyl-2-decarboxyamidetetracycline	Poor	+
2-Acetyl-2-decarboxyamide-5-hydroxytetracycline	Poor	Poor
7-Nitro-6-methyl-6-deoxytetracycline	+	+
12a-Deoxy-5a,6-anhydrotetracycline	+	−
4-Epitetracycline	Poor	+
4a, 12a-Anhydro-6-demethyl-6-deoxytetracycline	−	−
12a-Deoxytetracycline	−	−
4a,12a-Anhydro-4-desdimethylaminotetracycline	−	−

+, active; −, not active
[a] Determined using a plasmid-free strain

4. Tetracyclines That Inactivate Repressors

As noted above, extensive studies on repressor-tetracycline interactions have not been conducted with plasmids found in gram-negative bacteria. However, comprehensive studies were performed by SOMPOLINSKY and KRAUSZ (1973) and INOUE et al. (1977) using staphylococci. Apart from chelocardin and 12a-deoxy-5a,6 anhydrotetracycline, all tetracyclines with inhibitory activity also acted as inducers (Table 17). The situation with chelocardin in *Staphylococcus aureus* therefore resembles that found with resistance determinants from gram-negative bacteria. Tetracycline analogues which are themselves poor inhibitors of growth can nevertheless induce resistance to tetracycline, as shown by 4-epitetracycline (Fig. 16) and 2-acetyl-2-decarboxyamide tetracycline in *Staphylococcus aureus* (Table 17) (SOMPOLINSKY and KRAUSZ 1973). In *E. coli* plasmid-determined tetracycline resistance is induced by β-apo-oxytetracycline (Fig. 16) (FRANKLIN 1967), an analogue without effect on protein synthesis. This further confirms that derivatives lacking inhibitory activity can nevertheless induce resistance and therefore the receptors for induction must differ from those required to inhibit protein synthesis.

Table 18. Sensitivity of tetracycline-resistant (Tn*10* determined) and -sensitive *Escherichia coli* to chelating agents and picolinic acid analogues. (BOCHNER et al. 1980)

Compound (generic name)	Sensitivity or resistance[a]
1. Tetracycline	R
2. 8-Hydroxyquinoline	S
3. 1,10-Phenanthroline	S
4. 2,2′-Bipyridine	S
5. Thenoyltrifluoroacetone	S
6. Ethylenediamine tetraacetic acid (EDTA)	S
7. Ethyleneglycol-bis (*β*-aminoethyl ether) *N,N′*tetraacetic acid (EGTA)	–
8. Ethylenediamine di (o-hydroxyphenyl acetic acid) (EDDA)	S
9. Pyridine-2-carboxylic acid (picolinic acid)	S
10. 2-Methyl pyridine (2-picoline)	–
11. Pyridine-2-acetic acid (2-pyridylacetic acid)	–
12. Pyridine-3-carboxylic acid (nicotinic acid)	R
13. Pyridine-2,3-dicarboxylic acid (quinolinic acid)	R
14. Pyrazine-2-carboxylic acid (2-pyrazine carboxylic acid)	R
15. Pyrrole-2-carboxylic acid	S
16. Quinoline-2-carboxylic acid (quinaldic acid)	S
17. 5-Butyl picolinic acid (fusaric acid)	S
18. Picolinic acid *N*-oxide	S
19. 2-Mercaptopyridine *N*-oxide	S
20. O-Amino benzoic acid (anthranilic acid)	–

[a] S indicates that the tet^r strain is more sensitive than the tet^s strain; R indicates that the tet^r is more resistant than the tet^s strain; – indicates identical sensitivity of the tet^r and tet^s strain

XIII. Expression of Tetracycline Resistance in Escherichia coli Renders Cells Hypersensitive to Lipophilic Chelating Agents

During studies designed to develop a method for the direct selection of tetracycline-sensitive *E. coli* from a predominantly resistant population, BOCHNER et al. (1980) found tetracycline-resistant cells (carrying Tn*10* or pBR322) to be preferentially inhibited by a variety of lipophilic compounds (Table 18). The findings of BOCHNER et al. (1980) were confirmed by MALOY and NUNN (1981). The molecular basis of hypersensitivity to the lipophilic compounds is unclear, but BOCHNER et al. (1980) suggest that the response is due to chelation of essential membrane cations the level of which has already been reduced following insertion of resistance proteins into the envelope. However, as already noted, there is little experimental evidence to support the hypothesis of BOCHNER et al. (1980).

XIV. Epidemiology of Tetracycline Resistance

This subject has recently been reviewed elsewhere (CHOPRA et al. 1981 a) and so will not be considered in detail here.

There is abundant evidence that use of tetracyclines rapidly selects for resistant bacterial populations. This occurs in humans receiving tetracyclines for therapeutic purposes and also in animals receiving the antibiotics either prophylactically or therapeutically. The emergence of resistant populations under these conditions is due to elimination of sensitive competitors by the antibiotic and their replacement by resistant bacteria. Transfer of resistance genes to a species in which they have not previously occurred results either from conjugation or, particularly for the staphylococci, by transduction.

The plasmids which specify tetracycline resistance in *Staphylococcus aureus* have a similar size (2.7–2.9 Mdal) and confer similar levels of resistance to the antibiotic (LACEY 1975; BUKHARI et al. 1977; WILSON and BALDWIN 1978; POLACK and NOVICK 1982). This suggests that one plasmid containing the same tetracycline-resistance determinant has spread throughout the staphylococci (LACEY 1975). In support of this hypothesis several tetracycline-resistance plasmids produce identical cleavage patterns when treated with the same group of restriction endonucleases (WILSON and BALDWIN 1978; POLACK and NOVICK 1982). In contrast to this situation the four major classes of resistance determinant in gram-negative bacteria (Table 10) are widely distributed among the various plasmid incompatibility groups. The wide dissemination of some of these determinants results from the presence of the resistance genes within transposons (Table 8). Transposons can transfer from one plasmid to another independently of the *rec*A$^+$-mediated recombination systems of bacteria and their primary function is therefore to recombine non-homologous DNAs. Transposons are bounded by the so-called "inverted repeats," polynucleotide sequences which are rotationally symmetrical (though not necessarily identical) at the extremes of the piece of DNA that is transposed. Although transposable resistance genes have a substantial role in the evolution of plasmids coding for multiple antibiotic resistance (e.g. see RUBENS et al. 1979), a detailed description of transposition is beyond the scope of this review. For further information the reader is referred to the review articles by COHEN (1976), KLECKNER (1977), STARLINGER (1980), and CALOS and MILLER (1980).

A new, and potentially disturbing, aspect of tetracycline resistance transfer has recently emerged. In 1978 PETIT et al. speculated that there may be resistance factors whose conjugative abilities are inducible by the antibiotic to which they mediate resistance. Such a mechanism would result in efficient spread of the plasmid and thus a rapid adaptation of a bacterial population to changes in environmental conditions. Subsequently PRIVITERA et al. (1979, 1981) found such a system in *Bacteroides fragilis,* where transfer of tetracycline-resistance plasmids depends on induction by subinhibitory concentrations of tetracycline. Increased conjugal activity in the presence of tetracycline is not, however, due directly to expression of resistance as there is independent control of both resistance and its transferability (PRIVITERA et al. 1981). A distinct, but related, phenomenon may apply to transposition of the tetracycline-resistance genes contained in transposon Tn*10*. SCHMIDT et al. (1981) detected a tetracycline-inducible RNA species encoded by the inverted repeat of Tn*10*, which they suggest may be involved in the transposition process itself. Thus low concentrations of tetracycline may increase the transposition frequency of Tn*10*.

XV. Origin of Plasmid-Located Tetracycline-Resistance Genes

1. Introduction

The presence of antibiotic resistance plasmids in clinical and veterinary isolates poses the question of where the plasmids originated from. When considering this question it is useful to remember:

1. That the current emergence of resistant bacteria invariably results from transfer of resistance genes from one organism to another, followed by selection of resistant cells under conditions of antibiotic challenge (see Sect. K.XIV).
2. That transfer of genes is particularly favourable when they are plasmid located.
3. That a plasmid location for resistance genes can be beneficial to the host because it frequently permits higher levels of resistance than could be attained by a single copy of a chromosomal gene. This relates to the finding that many plasmids have copy numbers greater than one per chromosome (BUKHARI et al. 1977) and that a positive gene dosage response occurs for many plasmid-mediated antibiotic resistance mechanisms (see Sect. K.VIII).

A popular theory for the evolution of plasmid-determined antibiotic resistance relates the origin of the resistance genes to those soil organisms that produce antibiotics, or share the same ecological niche as the antibiotic producers (BENVENISTE and DAVIES 1973; DAVIES and SMITH 1978). By virtue of points 1–3 above we could anticipate that resistance plasmids evolved in soil microorganisms either to protect the antibiotic producers from self-destruction or to permit survival of the coinhabitants. [For alternative views on this contentious topic see GOTTLIEB (1976) and HOPWOOD (1981).] Although it will be difficult to find firm evidence that plasmid resistance genes in clinical isolates derived originally from soil species, the hypothesis can be assessed by consideration of the following questions:

1. Were resistance plasmids present in microorganisms before the advent of antimicrobial chemotherapy?
2. Have resistance plasmids been isolated from soil microorganisms?
3. Could resistance plasmids, or resistance genes, have been transferred from soil species to an animal commensal or pathogen and then disseminated to a wide range of bacterial species?
4. What are the prospects for expression of a "foreign" gene in a new host?

These questions are addressed in the following sections, with special emphasis, where possible, on the origins of plasmid-determined tetracycline resistance.

2. Were Resistance Plasmids Present in Microorganisms Before the Widespread Use of Tetracyclines by Man?

A strain of *E. coli* isolated in 1937 (before the antibiotic era) and kept as a stock culture until lyophilized in 1946 was found (in 1967) to contain a plasmid encoding tetracycline resistance (SMITH 1967). Tetracyclines were introduced into developed communities during the 1950s, but there are still parts of the world where there is little or no use of these antibiotics. Nevertheless, tetracycline-resistant organisms have been isolated from humans and animals in these remote areas, and the genes for resistance are frequently plasmid located (MARE 1968; GARDNER et al. 1969; DAVIS and ANANDAN 1970; MARCOS and WOODS 1973; BURT and WOODS 1976). These findings suggest that even where drugs are not used for therapeutic or veterinary purposes, resistance plasmids do exist.

3. Are Tetracycline-Resistance Plasmids Present in Soil Microorganisms?

Tetracyclines are produced by two soil microorganisms: *Streptomyces aureofaciens* and *S. rimosus* (HOPWOOD and MERRICK 1977), both of which are assumed to protect themselves from their own product (DEMAIN 1974). Efflux of tetracycline may play a role in *S. aureofaciens* because a strain producing 2 mg tetracycline/ml possesses ribosomes that are 50% inhibited in vitro by only 50 μg antibiotic/ml (MIKULIK et al. 1971).

In *S. rimosus* the resistance genes could be plasmid located because non-reverting oxytetracycline-sensitive mutants arose both spontaneously and with increased frequency after acridine dye treatment (BORONIN and SADOVNIKOVA 1972). The putative plasmid encoding tetracycline resistance in *S. rimosus* appears unrelated to the plasmid SRP1 which is also found in this species, because SRP1 has only fertility properties (FRIEND et al. 1978). A plasmid (molecular weight 5.2×10^6) which may determine resistance to tetracycline was recently isolated from a non-antibiotic-producing, but otherwise uncharacterized strain of *Streptomyces* (BRANDSCH et al. 1980) (Table 19). Members of the genus *Bacillus* are another group of soil organisms which have been examined for the presence of tetracycline-resistance plasmids. In contrast to the situation with *Streptomyces* there are sound data to favour the presence of tetracycline-resistance plasmids in a variety of soil bacilli (Table 19). Furthermore, plasmid-determined tetracycline resistance in bacilli is known to involve antibiotic efflux (see Sect. K.V).

4. Is There Gene Transfer from Soil Microorganisms to Bacteria That Inhabit Man or Animals?

The term gene transfer encompasses two processes:

1. The actual transfer of DNA from one cell to another
2. The establisment of some (or all) of the genetic information in the recipient cell.

A variety of transfer mechanisms exist for gene transfer between microorganisms that include transformation, transduction, and conjugation (LOW and PORTER 1978). Although there are no documented cases of natural gene transfer between soil prokaryotes and other microorganisms, transformation has been suggested as a possibility (BENVENISTE and DAVIES 1973). The maintenance of resistance genes in a "foreign" species is most likely to result from recombination with an existing replicon, i.e. the bacterial chromosome, or an existing plasmid. In some cases recombination requires extensive homology between the parental DNA molecules (general recombination), but in other cases, particularly involving transposons, there is little or no requirement for homology between the participating DNA sequences (LOW and PORTER 1978). Transposition might there-

Table 19. Plasmids found in natural soil isolates that have been correlated with expression of tetracycline resistance

Micro-organism	Plasmid	Plasmid molecular weight (daltons × 10^6)	Evidence for involvement of plasmid in expression of tetracycline resistance	References
Streptomyces	Nomenclature not assigned	5.2	Equivocal	BRANDSCH et al. (1980)
Bacillus cereus	pBC16	2.8	Unequivocal	BERNHARD et al. (1978)
Bacillus stearothermophilus	pAB124	2.9	Unequivocal	BINGHAM et al. (1979)

fore have been an important means for the evolutionary dissemination of tetracycline-resistance genes. This hypothesis is consistent with the location of several tetracycline-resistance determinants in transposons (Table 8).

5. Expression of "Foreign" Prokaryotic Genes in New Bacterial Hosts

Assuming that a gene from a "foreign" species is stably maintained in a new host, then phenotypic expression of its product will depend upon:

1. Transcription of the gene into mRNA
2. Translation of mRNA into protein
3. The provision by the host of any necessary products required for post-transcriptional processing of the "foreign" product
4. The provision by the new host of any necessary receptor site for the protein, e.g. a specific domain within the cytoplasmic membrane.

These points are discussed separately below.

a) Transcription of the Gene into mRNA

Transcription produces an exact copy of a continuous stretch of DNA and depends upon:

1. A specific start point of transcription, i.e. association of RNA polymerase with a promoter region on the DNA
2. Precise copying of the DNA sequence on the basis of complementarity of nucleotides
3. A specific termination site of transcription.

All known cellular RNA polymerases carry out the same reaction (i.e. step 2), but steps 1 and 2 can be host specific (SZEKELY 1980; OLD and PRIMROSE 1980). Indeed failure to initiate transcription is responsible for the lack of expression of ampicillin- and chloramphenicol-resistance genes from Enterobacteriaceae in *Bacillus subtilis* (KREFT et al. 1983). Poor transcription might also be responsible for failure to express staphylococcal genes for erythromycin and sulphonamide resistance in *E. coli* (COURVALIN and FIANDT 1980). Lack of transcription of *Bacillus* tetracycline-resistance genes in *E. coli* has been reported (ECCLES et al. 1981), but application of selection pressure to *E. coli* leads to a mutation where transcription of the "foreign" tetracycline-resistance genes is achieved by use of *E. coli* promoters surrounding the cloned resistance genes (ECCLES and CHOPRA 1984).

b) Translation of mRNA into Protein

Translation in heterologous systems can depend upon the nature of initiation factors, with IF-3 being particularly important for mRNA selection by ribosomes (SZEKELY 1980). Furthermore the structure of mRNA may itself control the efficiency of initiation and therefore translation of a gene into protein (SCHERER et al. 1980). In recent years the question of whether ribosomes posses an inherent specificity for translation of certain mRNA species has been addressed. Although the composition of ribosomes from microorganisms can differ considerably (BRIMACOMBE et al. 1978; OSAWA and HORI 1980), *Bacillus stearothermophilus* provides the only well-documented case in which binding of mRNA depends upon ribosome structure. *B. stearothermophilus* ribosomes only interact weakly with *E. coli* mRNA (STEITZ 1973; GOLDBERG and STEITZ 1974; HELD et al. 1974; ISONO and ISONO 1976) and this was attributed to lack of the protein S1 in the 30S ribosomal subunit of *B. stearothermophilus*. In view of the findings made by ECCLES and CHOPRA (1984) on expression of *Bacillus* tetracycline-resistance genes in *E. coli* this is unlikely to be a regular barrier to expression of foreign tetracycline-resistance genes.

c) Post-transcriptional Processing of Proteins

The best-documented example of post-transcriptional processing of proteins in bacteria involves cleavage of N-terminal signal sequences from certain secreted and membrane-located polypeptides. The signal sequences are implicated in the transport of these proteins into or across membranes. Removal of the signal sequence from the nascent polypeptide by endopeptidase activity is probably crucial to the accurate placement of protein in the membrane, or to the final liberation of a secreted protein (INOUYE and HALEGOUA 1980). Since the membrane-located resistance proteins involved in tetracycline efflux probably do not contain leader sequences (see Sect. K.VII) failure to process membrane-resistance proteins seems an unlikely barrier to the ancestral spread of tetracycline resistance.

d) Provision of Receptor Sites

Host-specific membrane domains for expression of tetracycline resistance seem unlikely in view of the findings made by ECCLES and CHOPRA (1984), which demonstrate functional expression of a *Bacillus* tetracycline efflux protein in *E. coli*.

6. Conclusions

Despite potential barriers to phenotypic expression in a "foreign" microorganism there are several examples where successful interspecies expression of antibiotic resistance has been achieved (Table 20). The data concerning expression of tetracycline resistance are tenable with the hypothesis that resistance in clinical isolates

Table 20. Examples of gene expression in heterologous species involving resistance to antibiotics

DNA investigated	Original DNA source	Gene expression in	References
β-Lactamase genes	pI258 from *Straphylococcus aureus*	Original host and *Escherichia coli*	CHANG and COHEN (1974)
	Chromosome of *Bacillus licheniformis*	Original host and *Escherichia coli, Bacillus subtilis*	BRAMMAR et al. (1980) GRAY and CHANG (1981)
Chloramphenicol-resistance genes	pUB112, pSA2100, pCM194, pCW6, pCW8, pC221, pSC194, pC223, all from *Staphylococcus aureus*	Original host and *Bacillus* species	EHRLICH (1977) GRYCZAN et al. (1978) GOEBEL et al. (1979) BROWN and CARLTON (1980) DANCER (1980)
Fusidic-acid-resistance genes	pUB101 from *Staphylococcus* aureus	Original host and *Bacillus subtilis*	GRYCZAN et al. (1978)
Aminoglycoside-resistance genes	pUB110, pK545, pSH2, pSA2100, RN1956, pWA1, all from *Staphylococcus aureus*	Original host, *Escherichia coli* and *Bacillus* species	GRYCZAN et al. (1978) COURVALIN and FIANDT (1980) BROWN and CARLTON (1980)
Tetracycline-resistance genes	pT127 from *Staphylococcus aureus*	Original host and *Bacillus subtilis*	EHRLICH (1977)
	pBC16 from *Bacillus cereus*	Original host and *Bacillus* species. Partial expression in *Escherichia coli*	KREFT et al. (1978) BROWN and CARLTON (1980)
	pAB124 from *Bacillus stearothermophilus*	Original host and *Bacillus subtilis*. Expression in *Escherichia coli* after plasmid mutation	ECCLES et al. (1981) ECCLES and CHOPRA (1984)
	pBR322[a]	Enterobacteriaceae and *Bacillus subtilis*	GOEBEL et al. (1979) KREFT et al. (1983)

[a] The tetracycline-resistance genes in pBR322 are derived from pSC101 (SUTCLIFFE 1978), but the origin of the resistance determinant in pSC101 is unknown (COHEN and CHANG 1977). However, the tetracycline-resistance determinant in pSC101 is homologous with determinants found in plasmids isolated from *Salmonella* species (MENDEZ et al 1980)

originated from soil microorganisms, e.g. bacilli or streptomyces. In both cases resistance mechanisms have been invoked which are analogous to these specified by plasmids in clinical isolates. Furthermore, BASSETT et al. (1980) indicate conditions that existed in A.D. 350 that may have favoured transfer of tetracycline-resistance plasmids from soil microorganisms to human pathogens or commensals. Our observations on expression of a *Bacillus* tetracycline-resistance determinant in *E. coli* (ECCLES et al. 1981; ECCLES and CHOPRA 1984) indicate that there may be initial barriers to expression of tetracycline resistance in a "foreign" host due to lack of transcription of resistance genes. However, this deficiency can be readily overcome (at least in laboratory studies) by a mutation which places the "foreign" tetracycline-resistance genes under the control of a host promoter.

Although tetracycline-resistance genes may well have originated in soil microorganisms, there is no homology between plasmid-located tetracycline-resistance determinants found in soil bacilli and clinical isolates of staphylococci, streptococci, or several gram-negative bacteria. This implies that the products mediating tetracycline resistance in bacilli differ from those in other bacterial species. This pattern is also exhibited by other products mediating antibiotic resistance. For instance, aminoglycoside-modifying enzymes in *Streptomyces* do not cross-react immunologically with those enzymes having a similar function in clinical isolates (DAVIES and SMITH 1978). Nevertheless, plasmid pBC16 from *Bacillus cereus* and pUB110 from *Staphylococcus aureus* are homologous except for the regions conferring antibiotic resistance, a finding which suggests the occurrence of natural plasmid transfer between soil bacilli and staphylococci (POLACK and NOVICK 1982).

Although plasmids may well have been involved in the evolutionary dissemination of tetracycline-resistance genes it seems likely that the ultimate origin of these genes was chromosomal DNA. Recent evidence to support this hypothesis has been obtained by studies on chromosomal mutation to tetracycline resistance (GEORGE and LEVY 1983a, b). These findings are considered in the Sect. L. It is clear, however, that if there was a single ancestral tetracycline-resistance determinant, e.g. in soil bacilli, then it has diverged to the extent that even among closely related species such as the coliforms and streptococci a variety of different tetracycline-resistance determinants exist.

L. Chromosomal Mutation to Tetracycline Resistance

Although high-level resistance to tetracyclines usually results from acquisition of plasmids or transposition of genes to the chromosome, several examples of chromosomal mutation to resistance have been reported. Some of these mutations can confer a considerable increase in resistance so that if they occur naturally they could significantly affect the therapeutic outcome of treatment with tetracyclines.

Mutation at the *cml*B locus in *E. coli* leads to a low level (two- to threefold) increase in resistance to both tetracycline and chloramphenicol (REEVE 1966, 1968; FOSTER 1975). The mutation results in loss of the outer membrane porin *omp*F, through which both drugs normally diffuse across the outer membrane (CHOPRA and ECCLES 1978) (see also Sect. J.II). More recently other types of chromosomal mutation conferring tetracycline resistance in *E. coli* have been identified. GEORGE and LEVY (1983a, b) demonstrated that several separate mutations contributed to expression of tetracycline resistance presumably in an additive or synergistic cooperation between different loci. Resistance appears to involve a tetracycline efflux system and is therefore likely to be mediated at the level of the cytoplasmic membrane. In view of the phenotypic similarity between this newly discovered chromosomally mediated system and that encoded by resistance plasmids, it is plausible to postulate an evolutionary link in the context of the origin of plasmid-resistance genes (GEORGE and LEVY 1983a).

Apart from chromosomal mutations which render resistance to tetracycline by virtue of membrane changes, ribosomal mutation to resistance also occurs. WILLIAMS and SMITH (1979) isolated two types of chromosomal mutant in *Bacillus subtilis* that survived in the presence of high concentrations of drug (>50 μg/ml). *TetA* mutants mapped in a region adjacent to known ribosomal genes and resulted from alteration in the 30S ribosomal protein S10 (also see Sect. F), whereas *TetB* mutants probably resulted from loss of ability to transport tetracycline into the cell. Note that the designations *TetA* and *TetB* used by WILLIAMS and SMITH are not synonymous with those used by MENDEZ et al. (1980) in the classification of plasmid-located tetracycline-resistance determinants. Chromosomal mutation to resistance involving altered ribosomes had previously been reported in *E. coli* by CRAVEN et al. (1969), but the nature of the alteration was not determined and the mutants are now no longer available for study (G. R. Craven, personal communication).

M. Conclusions

Although the mode of action of tetracyclines was established more than 10 years ago a precise understanding of how they inhibit protein synthesis is still lacking. Nevertheless, the prospects for defining the molecular basis of tetracycline action are promising, partly because of increasing knowledge of ribosome structure and also because of photolabelling techniques using tetracyclines.

The evolution of plasmid-determined tetracycline resistance in bacteria is intriguing because it is clear that the majority of tetracycline-resistance determinants differ from each other, and that a series of distinct membrane-located resistance proteins with similar functions has therefore evolved. Nevertheless the overall similarity in the organization of several different tetracycline-resistance determinants suggests that they arose from a common ancestor. This hypothesis is strengthened by other data. The nucleotide sequences for the genes encoding the *E. coli TetA*, *TetB*, and pBR322 tetracycline efflux proteins have been compared (Table 21). The observed homologies are sufficient to account for divergent evo-

Table 21. Nucleotide sequence homologies between the genes coding for *Escherichia coli* tetracycline efflux proteins. [Based on data of WATERS et al. (1983) and NGUYEN et al. (1983)]

Tet sequences compared	Nucleotide homology (%)
TetA/pBR322	74
TetA/*TetB*	48
TetB/pBR322	49

lution from a common ancestral gene (WATERS et al. 1983; NGUYEN et al. 1983). Greater sequence homology exists between the *TetA* and pBR322 genes than between these genes and that in *TetB* (Table 21). These comparisons suggest an early divergence of *TetB* from the ancestral gene with a much later divergence of *TetA* and the pBR322 resistance genes (WATERS et al. 1983). At least three of the existing resistance proteins therefore seem to have arisen as a consequence of divergent evolution. The reasons for this are unknown and thus there is a major gap in our understanding of how plasmid-determined resistance has evolved in response to the use of tetracyclines.

Acknowledgements. I am indebted to the following: Dr. E. Cundliffe and Dr. T.G.B. Howe for comments on the manuscript, Stuart Shales for help with artwork, Betty Fry for photographic assistance and Sheila Travers for secretarial assistance. I also thank several colleagues for the provision of data before publication. Much of the author's original research work has been supported by grants from the United Kingdom Medical Research Council (programme grant G970/107/B to Professor M.H. Richmond and project grants G975/100/C, G978/67/SB, G978/834/S, and G979/642/SB to the author).

References

Achtman M, Manning PA, Edelbluth C, Herrlich P (1979) Export without proteolytic processing of inner and outer membrane proteins encoded by the F sex factor *tra* cistrons in *Escherichia coli* minicells. Proc Natl Acad Sci USA 76:4837–4841

Ahlstedt S (1981) The antibacterial effects of low concentrations of antibiotics and host defence factors: a review. J Antimicrob Chemother 8:59–70

Altenbuchner J, Schmid K, Schmitt R (1983) Tn1721-encoded tetracycline resistance: mapping of structural and regulatory genes mediating resistance. J Bacteriol 153:116–123

Altendorf K, Hirata H, Harold FM (1975) Accumulation of lipid-soluble ions and of rubidium as indicators of the electrical potential in membrane vesicles of *E. coli*. J Biol Chem 250:1405–1412

Amanuma H, Strominger JL (1980) Purification and properties of penicillin-binding proteins 5 and 6 from *Escherichia coli* membranes. J Biol Chem 255:11173–11180

Argast M, Beck CF (1984) Tetracycline diffuses through phospholipid bilayers and binds to phospholipids. Antimicrob Agents Chemother: 26:263–265

Asheshov EH (1975) The genetics of tetracycline resistance in *Staphylococcus aureus*. J Gen Microbiol 88:132–140

Atkinson BA, Amaral L (1982) Sublethal concentrations of antibiotics, effects on bacteria and the immune system. CRC Crit Rev Microbiol 9:101–138

Backman K, Boyer HW (1983) Tetracycline resistance determined by pBR322 is mediated by one polypeptide. Gene 26:197–203

Bakhtiar M, Selwyn S (1983) Antibacterial activity of a new thiatetracycline. J Antimicrob Chemother 11:291

Ball PR, Chopra I, Eccles SJ (1977) Accumulation of tetracyclines by *Escherichia coli* K-12. Biochem Biophys Res Commun 77:1500–1507

Ball PR, Shales SW, Chopra I (1980) Plasmid-mediated tetracycline resistance in *Escherichia coli* involves increased efflux of the antibiotic. Biochem Biophys Res Commun 93:74–81

Banerjee S, Chakrabarti K (1976) The transport of tetracyclines across the mouse ileum in vitro: the effects of cations and other agents. J Pharm Pharmacol 28:133–138

Barringer WC, Shultz W, Sieger GM, Nash RA (1974) Minocycline hydrochloride and its relationship to other tetracycline antibiotics. Am J Pharm 146:179–191

Bassett EJ, Keith MS, Armelagos GJ, Martin DL, Villanueva AR (1980) Tetracycline-labeled human bone from ancient Sudanese Nubia. Science 209:1532–1534

Beard NS, Armentrout SA, Weisberger AS (1969) Inhibition of mammalian protein synthesis by antibiotics. Pharmacol Rev 21:213–245

Beck CF (1979) A genetic approach to analysis of transposons. Proc Natl Acad Sci USA 76:2376–2380

Beck CF, Mutzel R, Barbe J, Muller W (1982) A multifunctional gene (*tetR*) controls Tn10 encoded tetracycline resistance. J Bacteriol 150:633–642

Bennett PM, Shales SW (1981) Characterization of the tetracycline resistance region of the IncP plasmid RP1. In: Levy SB (ed) Molecular biology, pathogenicity and ecology of bacterial plasmids. Plenum, New York, p 581

Bennett PM, Richmond MH, Petrocheilou V (1980) The inactivation of *tet* genes on a plasmid by the duplication of one inverted repeat of a transposon-like structure which itself mediates tetracycline resistance. Plasmid 3:135–149

Benveniste R, Davies J (1973) Aminoglycoside antibiotic-inactivating enzymes in actinomycetes similar to those present in clinical isolates of antibiotic-resistant bacteria. Proc Natl Acad Sci USA 70:2276–2280

Bernard K, Schrempf H, Goebel W (1978) Bacteriocin and antibiotic resistance plasmids in *Bacillus cereus* and *Bacillus subtilis*. J Bacteriol 133:879–903

Bertrand K, Postle K, Wray L, Reznikoff W (1981) Regulation of transposon Tn10 tetracycline resistance. In: Levy SB (ed) Molecular biology, pathogenicity and ecology of bacterial plasmids. Plenum, New York, p 582

Bingham AHA, Bruton CJ, Atkinson T (1979) Isolation and partial characterisation of four plasmids from antibiotic resistant thermophilic bacilli. J Gen Microbiol 114:401–408

Bingham AHA, Bruton CJ, Atkinson T (1980) Characterisation of *Bacillus stearothermophilus* plasmid pAB124 and construction of deletion variants. J Gen Microbiol 119:109–115

Blackwood RK, English AR (1977) Structure-activity relationships in the tetracycline series. In: Perlman D (ed) Structure-activity relationships in the semisynthetic antibiotics. Academic, London, p 397

Bochner BR, Huang H-C, Schieven GL, Ames BN (1980) Positive selection for loss of tetracycline resistance. J Bacteriol 143:926–933

Booth IR, Hamilton WA (1980) Energetics of bacterial amino acid transport. In: Payne JW (ed) Microorganisms and nitrogen sources. Wiley, Chichester, p 171

Boronin AM, Sadovnikova LG (1972) Elimination by acridine dyes of oxytetracycline resistance in Actinomyces rimosus. Genetika 8:174–176

Boyer HW, Betlach M, Bolivar F, Rodriguez RL, Heyneker HL, Shine J, Goodman HM (1977) The construction of molecular cloning vehicles. In: Beers RF, Bassett EG (eds) Recombinant molecules: impact on science and society. Raven, New York, p 9

Boynton JE, Gillham NW, Lambowitz AM (1980) Biogenesis of chloroplast and mitochondrial ribosomes. In: Chambliss G, Craven GR, Davies J, Davis K, Kahan L, Nomura M (eds) Ribosomes: structure, function and genetics. University Park Press, Baltimore, p 903

Brammar WJ, Muir S, McMorris A (1980) Molecular cloning of the gene for the beta-lactamase of *Bacillus licheniformis* and its expression in *Escherichia coli*. Mol Gen Genet 178:217–224

Brandsch R, Hefco E, Brandsch C, Rotinberg P, Keleman S (1980) Possible plasmid control of sporulation, soluble pigment production and tetracycline resistance in a wild *Streptomyces* sp. strain. J Antibiot 33:1204–1205

Brimacombe R (1978) The structure of the bacterial ribosome. In: Stanier RY, Rogers HJ, Ward JB (eds) Relations between structure and function in the prokaryotic cell. Twenty-eighth symposium of the Society for General Microbiology. Cambridge University Press, Cambridge, p 1

Brimacombe R, Nierhaus KH, Garrett RA, Wittman HG (1976) The ribosome of *Escherichia coli*. Progr Nucleic Acid Res 18:1–44

Brimacombe R, Stoffler G, Wittmann HG (1978) Ribosome structure. Annu Rev Biochem 47:217–249

Brot N (1977) Translocation. In: Weissbach H, Pestka S (eds) Molecular mechanisms of protein biosynthesis. Academic, New York, p 375

Brown BJ, Carlton BC (1980) Plasmid-mediated transformation in *Bacillus megaterium*. J Bacteriol 142:508–512

Bukhari AI, Shapiro JL, Adhya SL (1977) DNA insertion elements, plasmids and episomes. Cold Spring Harbor Laboratory, Cold Spring Harbor

Burdett V, Inamine J, Rajagopalan S (1982) Heterogeneity of tetracycline resistance determinants in *Streptococcus*. J Bacteriol 149:995–1004

Burt SJ, Woods DR (1976) Evolution of transferable antibiotic resistance in coliform bacteria from remote environments. Antimicrob Agents Chemother 10:567–568

Calame K, Nakada D, Ihler G (1978) Location of ribosome-binding sites on the tetracycline resistance transposon Tn10. J Bacteriol 135:668–674

Calos MP, Miller JH (1980) Transposable elements. Cell 20:579–595

Capaldi RA, Vanderkooi G (1972) The low polarity of many membrane proteins. Proc Natl Acad Sci USA 69:930–932

Cerna J, Rychlik I, Pulkrabek P (1969) The effect of antibiotics on the coded binding of peptidyl-tRNA to the ribosome and on the transfer of the peptidyl residue to puromycin. Eur J Biochem 9:27–35

Chabbert YA, Scavizzi MR (1976) Chelocardin-inducible resistance in *Escherichia coli* bearing R plasmids. Antimicrob Agents Chemother 9:36–41

Chambliss G, Craven GR, Davies J, Davis D, Kahan L, Nomura M (1979) Ribosomes, structure, function and genetics. University Park Press, Baltimore

Chang ACY, Cohen SH (1974) Genome construction between bacterial species in vitro: replication and expression of *Staphylococcus plasmid* genes in *Escherichia coli*. Proc Natl Acad Sci USA 71:1030–1034

Chopra I (1975) Induction of tetracycline resistance in *Staphylococcus aureus* in the absence of lipid synthesis. J Gen Microbiol 91:433–436

Chopra I (1978) Plasmid determined tetracycline resistance in *Escherichia coli* K12: lack of evidence that resistance is related to changes in lipid metabolism. Biochem Soc Trans 6:431–433

Chopra I, Ball PR (1982) Transport of antibiotics into bacteria. Adv Microb Physiol 23:183–240

Chopra I, Eccles SJ (1977) Tetracycline resistance in *Escherichia coli* K12 is not associated with a decrease in cyclopropane fatty acid content. J Gen Microbiol 103:393–396

Chopra I, Eccles SJ (1978) Diffusion of tetracycline across the outer membrane of *Escherichia coli* K-12: involvement of protein Ia. Biochem Biophys Res Commun 83:550–557

Chopra I, Howe TGB (1978) Bacterial resistance to the tetracyclines. Microbiol Rev 42:707–724

Chopra I, Shales SW (1980) Comparison of the polypeptide composition of *Escherichia coli* outer membranes prepared by two methods. J Bacteriol 144:425–427

Chopra I, Shales SW (1981) Susceptibility of protein synthesis in *Escherichia coli* to tetracycline and minocycline. J Gen Microbiol 124:187–189

Chopra I, Lacey RW, Connolly J (1974) Biochemical and genetic basis of tetracycline resistance in *Staphylococcus aureus*. Antimicrob Agents Chemother 6:397–404

Chopra I, Howe TGB, Linton AH, Linton KB, Richmond MH, Speller DCE (1981 a) The tetracyclines: prospects at the beginning of the 1980s. J Antimicrob Chemother 8:5–21

Chopra I, Shales SW, Ward JM, Wallace LJ (1981 b) Reduced expression of Tn10 mediated tetracycline resistance in *Escherichia coli* containing more than one copy of the transposon. J Gen Microbiol 126:45–54

Chopra I, Shales SW, Ball PR (1982). Tetracycline resistance determinants from groups A to D vary in their ability to confer decreased accumulation of tetracycline derivatives by *Escherichia coli*. J Gen Microbiol 128:689–692

Chopra I, Shales SW, Ball PR (1983) Methods for studying bacterial resistance to the tetracyclines. In: Skinner FA, Russell AD, Quesnel LB (eds) Technical series of the Society for Applied Bacteriology, vol 18. Academic, London, p 223

Clewell DB, Yagi Y (1977) Amplification of the tetracycline resistance determinant on plasmid pAMα1 in *Streptococcus faecalis*. In: Bukhari AI, Shapiro JA, Adhya L (eds) DNA insertion elements, plasmids and episomes. Cold Spring Harbor Laboratory, Cold Spring Harbor, p 235

Clewell DB, Yagi Y, Bauer B (1975) Plasmid-determined tetracycline resistance in *Streptococcus faecalis:* evidence for gene amplification during growth in the presence of tetracycline. Proc Natl Acad Sci USA 72:1720–1724

Cohen SN (1976) Transposable genetic elements and plasmid evolution. Nature 263:731–738

Cohen SN, Chang ACY (1977) Revised interpretation of the origin of the pSC101 plasmid. J Bacteriol 132:734–737

Coibion C, Laszlo P (1979) Binding of the alkali metal cations to tetracycline. Biochem Pharmacol 28:1367–1372

Coleman DC, Foster TJ (1981) Analysis of the reduction in expression of tetracycline resistance determined by transposon Tn10 in the multicopy state. Molec Gen Genet 182:171–177

Coleman DC, Chopra I, Shales SW, Howe TGB, Foster TJ (1983) Analysis of tetracycline resistance encoded by transposon Tn10: deletion mapping of tetracycline-sensitive point mutations and identification of two structural genes. J Bacteriol 153:921–929

Connamacher RH, Mandel HG (1965) Binding of tetracycline to the 30S ribosomes and polyuridilic acid. Biochem Biophys Res Commun 20:98–103

Connamacher RH, Mandel HG (1968) Studies on the intra-cellular localization of tetracycline in bacteria. Biochem Biophys Acta 166:475–486

Cooperman BS (1979) Photoaffinity labelling of ribosomes. In: Grossman L, Moldave K (eds) Methods in enzymology, vol 59. Academic, New York, p 796

Cooperman BS (1980a) Photolabile antibiotics as probes of ribosomal structure and function. Ann NY Acad Sci 346:302–323

Cooperman BS (1980b) Functional sites on the *Escherichia coli* ribosome as defined by affinity labeling. In: Chambliss G, Craven GR, Davies J, Davis K, Kahan L, Nomura M (eds) Ribosomes: structure, function and genetics. University Park Press, Baltimore, p 531

Costerton JW, Cheng K-J (1975) The role of the bacterial cell envelope in antibiotic resistance. J Antimicrob Chemother 1:363–377

Courvalin P, Fiandt M (1980) Aminoglycoside-modifying enzymes of *Staphylococcus aureus:* expression in *Escherichia coli*. Gene 9:247–269

Craven GR, Gavin R, Fanning T (1969) The transfer RNA binding site of the 30S ribosome and the site of tetracycline inhibition. Cold Spring Harbor Symp Quant Biol 34:129–137

Cundliffe E (1967) Antibiotics and polyribosomes, chlorotetracycline and polyribosomes of *Bacillus megaterium*. Mol Pharmacol 3:401–411

Cundliffe E (1980) Antibiotics and prokaryotic ribosomes: action, interaction, and resistance. In: Chambliss G, Craven GR, Davies J, Davis K, Kahan L, Nomura M (eds) Ribosomes: structure, function and genetics. University Park Press, Balitore, p 555

Cundliffe E, McQuillen K (1967) Bacterial protein synthesis: the effects of antibiotics. J Mol Biol 30:137–146

Curiale MS, Levy SB (1982) Two complementation groups mediate tetracycline resistance determined by Tn10. J Bacteriol 151:209–215

Curiale MS, McMurry LM, Levy SB (1984) Intracistronic complementation of the tetracycline resistance membrane protein of Tn*10*. J Bacteriol 157:211–217

Dancer BN (1980) Transfer of plasmids among bacilli. J Gen Microbiol 121:263–266

Davies J, Smith DI (1978) Plasmid-determined resistance to antimicrobial agents. Annu Rev Microbiol 32:469–518

Davis CE, Anandan J (1970) The evolution of an R factor: a study of a preantibiotic community in Borneo. N Engl J Med 282:117–122

Day LE (1966a) Tetracycline inhibition of cell-free protein synthesis. I. Binding of tetracycline to components of the system. J Bacteriol 91:1917–1923

Day LE (1966b) Tetracycline inhibition of cell-free protein synthesis. II. Effects of the binding of tetracycline to the components of the system. J Bacteriol 92:197–203

DelBene VE, Rogers M (1975) Comparison of tetracycline and minocycline transport in *Escherichia coli*. Antimicrob Agents Chemother 7:801–806

Demain AL (1974) How do antibiotic producing micro-organisms avoid suicide? Ann NY Acad Sci 235:601–612

Duggar BM (1948) Aureomycin: a product of the continuing search for new antibiotics. Ann NY Acad Sci 51:177–181

Dunnick JK, O'Leary WM (1970) Correlation of bacterial lipid composition with antibiotic resistance. J Bacteriol 101:892–900

Eccles SJ, Chopra I (1984) Biochemical and genetic characterization of the *tet* determinant of *Bacillus* plasmid pAB124. J Bacteriol 158:134–140

Eccles S, Docherty A, Chopra I, Shales S, Ball P (1981) Tetracycline resistance genes from *Bacillus* plasmid pAB124 confer decreased accumulation of the antibiotic in *Bacillus subtilis* but not in *Escherichia coli*. J Bacteriol 145:1417–1420

Ehrlich SD (1977) Replication and expression of plasmids from *Staphylococcus aureus* in *Bacillus subtilis*. Proc Natl Acad Sci USA 74:1680–1682

Eisenstein BI, Beachey EH, Ofek I (1982) Differential effects of antibiotics on adhesins of antibiotic resistant strains of *Escherichia coli*. Scand J Infect Dis [Suppl] 33:108–114

Fayolle F, Privitera G, Sebald M (1980) Tetracycline transport in *Bacteroides fragilis*. Antimicrob Agents Chemother 18:502–505

Fedorko J, Katz S, Allnoch H (1968) In vitro activity of minocycline, a new tetracycline. Am J Med Sci 255:252–258

Fey G, Reiss M, Kersten H (1973) Interaction of tetracyclines with ribosomal subunits from *Escherichia coli*. A fluorometric investigation. Biochemistry 12:1160–1164

Fillingame RH (1976) Purification of the carbodiimide-reactive protein component of the ATP energy-transducing system of *Escherichia coli*. J Biol Chem 251:6630–6637

Foster TJ (1975) R-factor tetracycline and chloramphenicol resistance in *Escherichia coli* K12 *cmlB* mutants. J Gen Microbiol 90:303–310

Foster TJ (1977) Isolation and characterisation of mutants of R100-1 which express tetracycline resistance constitutively. FEMS Micro Lett 2:271–274

Foster TJ, Walsh A (1974) Phenotypic characterization of R-factor tetracycline resistance determinants. Genet Res 24:333–343

Foster TJ, Howe TGB, Richmond KMV (1975) Translocation of the tetracycline resistance determinant from R100-1 to the *Escherichia coli* K-12 chromosome. J Bacteriol 124:1153–1158

Franke AE, Clewell DB (1981) Evidence for a chromosome-borne resistance transposon (Tn916) in *Streptococcus faecalis* that is capable of "conjugal" transfer in the absence of a conjugative plasmid. J Bacteriol 145:494–502

Franklin TJ (1963) The inhibition of incorporation of leucine into protein of cell-free systems from rat liver and *Escherichia coli* by chlorotetracycline. Biochem J 87:449–453

Franklin TJ (1966) Mode of action of the tetracyclines. In: Newton BA, Reynolds PE (eds) Biochemical studies of antimicrobial drugs. Sixteenth symposium of the Society for General Microbiology. Cambridge University Press, Cambridge, p 192

Franklin TJ (1967) Resistance of *Escherichia coli* to tetracyclines. Changes in permeability to tetracyclines in *Escherichia coli* bearing transferable resistance factors. Biochem J 105:371–378

Franklin TJ, Foster SJ (1974) Expression of R-factor-mediated resistance to tetracycline in *Escherichia coli* minicells. Antimicrob Agents Chemother 5:194–195

Franklin TJ, Higginson B (1970) Active accumulation of tetracycline by *Escherichia coli*. Biochem J 116:287–297

Franklin TJ, Rownd R (1973) R-factor-mediated resistance to tetracycline in *Proteus mirabilis*. J Bacteriol 115:235–242

Friend EJ, Warren M, Hopwood DA (1978) Genetic evidence for a plasmid controlling fertility in an industrial strain of *Streptomyces rimosus*. J Gen Microbiol 106:201–206

Gale EF (1966) The object of the exercise. In: Newton BA, Reynolds PE (eds) Biochemical studies of antimicrobial drugs. Sixteenth symposium of the Society for General Microbiology. Cambridge University Press, Cambridge, p 1

Gale EF, Folkes JP (1953) The assimilation of amino acids by bacteria. 15. Actions of antibiotics on nucleic acid and protein synthesis in *Staphylococcus aureus*. Biochem J 53:493–498

Gale EF, Cundliffe E, Reynolds PE, Richmond MH, Waring MJ (1972) The molecular basis of antibiotic action. Wiley, London

Gardner P, Smith DH, Beer H, Moellering RC (1969) Recovery of resistance (R) factors from a drug-free community. Lancet 2:774–776

Garten W, Hindennach I, Henning U (1975) The major proteins of the *Escherichia coli* outer cell envelope membrane. Characterization of proteins II* and III, comparison of all proteins. Eur J Biochem 59:215–221

Gavrilova LP, Kostiashkina OE, Koreliansky VE, Rutkevitch NM, Spirin AS (1976) Factor-free (non enzymic) and factor dependent systems of translation of polyuridylic acid by *Escherichia coli* ribosomes. J Mol Biol 101:537–552

Gayda RC, Markovitz A (1978) A cloned DNA Fragment specifying major outer membrane protein a in *Escherichia coli* K-12. J Bacteriol 136:369–380

Gayda RC, Tanabe JH, Knigge KM, Markovitz A (1979) Identification by deletion analysis of an inducible protein required for pSC101-mediated tetracycline resistance. Plasmid 2:417–425

George AM, Levy SB (1983 a) Amplifiable resistance to tetracycline, chloramphenicol, and other antibiotics in *E. coli:* involvement of a non-plasmid-determined efflux of tetracycline. J Bacteriol 155:531–540

George AM, Levy SB (1983 b) Genes in the major cotransduction gap of the *E. coli* K12 linkage map required for the expression of chromosomal resistance to tetracycline and other antibiotics. J Bacteriol 155:541–548

Goebel W, Kreft J, Burger KJ (1979) Molecular cloning in *Bacillus subtilis*. In: Timmis KN, Puhler A (eds) Plasmids of medical, environmental and commercial importance. Elsevier, Amsterdam, p 471

Goldberg ML, Steitz JA (1974) Cistron specificity of 30S ribosomes heterologously reconstituted with components from *Escherichia coli* and *Bacillus stearothermophilus*. Biochemistry 13:2123–2129

Goldman RA, Cooperman BS, Strycharz WA, Williams BA, Tritton TR (1980) Photoincorporation of tetracycline into *Escherichia coli* ribosomes. Identification of labeled proteins and functional consequences. FEBS Lett 118:113–118

Goldman RA, Hasan T, Hall CC, Strycharz WA, Cooperman BS (1983) Photoincorporation of tetracycline into *Escherichia coli* ribosomes. Identification of the major proteins photolabeled by native tetracycline and tetracycline photoproducts and implications for the inhibitory action of tetracycline on protein synthesis. Biochemistry 22:359–368

Gordon J (1969) Hydrolysis of guanosine 5′-triphosphate associated with binding of aminoacyl transfer ribonucleic acid to ribosomes. J Biol Chem 244:5680–5686

Gottesman ME (1967) Reaction of ribosome-bound peptidyl transfer ribonucleic acid with aminoacyl transfer ribonucleic acid or puromycin. J Biol Chem 242:5564–5571

Gottlieb D (1976) The production and role of antibiotics in soil. J Antibiot 29:987–1000

Gray O, Chang S (1981) Molecular cloning and expression of *Bacillus licheniformis* β-lactamase gene in *Escherichia coli* and *Bacillus subtilis*. J Bacteriol 145:422–428

Grininviene B, Chmieliauskaite V, Grinius L (1974) Energy-linked transport of permeant ions in *E. coli* cells: evidence for membrane potential generation by proton pump. Biochem Biophys Res Commun 56:206–213

Grunberg-Manago M, Gros G (1977) Initiation mechanisms of protein synthesis. In: Cohn W (ed) Progress in nucleic acid research and molecular biology, vol 20. Academic, New York, p 209

Grunberg-Manago M, Buckingham RH, Cooperman BS, Hershey JWB (1978) Structure and function of the translation machinery. In: Stanier RY, Rogers HJ, Ward JB (eds) Relations between structure and function in the prokaryotic cell. Twenty-eight symposium of the Society for General Microbiology. Cambridge University Press, Cambridge, p 27

Gryczan TJ, Contente S, Dubnau D (1978) Characterization of *Staphylococcus aureus* plasmids introduced by transformation into *Bacillus subtilis*. J Bacteriol 134:318–329

Gurgo C, Apirion D, Schlessinger D (1969) Polyribosome metabolism in *Escherichia coli* treated with chloramphenicol, neomycin, spectinomycin or tetracycline. J Mol Biol 45:205–220

Hahn FE (1959) Mode of action of antibiotics. Proc Fourth Intern Congr Biochem 5:104

Harold FM, Papineau D (1972a) Cation transport and electrogenesis by *Streptococcus faecalis*. I. The membrane potential. J Membrane Biol 8:27–44

Harold FM, Papineau D (1972b) Cation transport and electrogenesis by *Streptococcus faecalis*. II. Proton and sodium extrusion. J Membrane Biol 8:45–62

Hash JH, Wishnick M, Miller PA (1964) On the mode of action of the tetracycline antibiotics in *Staphylococcus aureus*. J Biol Chem 239:2070–2078

Hedstrom RC, Crider BP, Eagon RG (1982) Comparison of kinetics of active tetracycline uptake and active tetracycline efflux in sensitive and plasmid RP4-containing *Pseudomonas putida*. J Bacteriol 152:255–259

Held WA, Gette WR, Nomura M (1974) Role of 16S ribosomal ribonucleic acid and the 30S ribosomal protein S12 in the initiation of natural messenger ribonucleic acid translation. Biochemistry 13:2115–2122

Heman-Ackah SM (1976) Comparison of tetracycline action on *Staphylococcus aureus* and *Escherichia coli* by microbial kinetics. Antimicrob Agents Chemother 10:223–228

Herrin GL, Russell DR, Bennett GN (1982) A stable derivative of pBR322 conferring increased tetracycline resistance and increased sensitivity to fusaric acid. Plasmid 7:290–293

Hierowski M (1965) Inhibition of protein synthesis by chlorotetracycline in the *Escherichia coli* in vitro system. Proc Natl Acad Sci USA 53:594–599

Hillen W, Schollmeier K (1983) Nucleotide sequence of the Tn10 encoded tetracycline resistance gene. Nucleic Acid Res 11:525–539

Hillen W, Unger B (1982) Binding of four repressors to double stranded *tet* operator region stabilizes it against thermal denaturation. Nature 297:700–702

Hillen W, Klock G, Kaffenberger I, Wray LV, Reznikoff WS (1982) Purification of the TET repressor and TET operator from the transposon Tn10 and characterization of their interaction. J Biol Chem 257:6605–6613

Hillen W, Gatz C, Altschmied L, Schollmeier K, Meier I (1983) Control of expression of the Tn*10*-encoded tetracycline resistance genes. Equilibrium and kinetic investigation of the regulatory reactions. J Mol Biol 169:707–721

Himmelweit F (1960) The collected papers of Paul Ehrlich, vol 3, Pergamon, London

Hirashima A, Kaji A (1972) Purification and properties of ribosome-releasing factor. Biochemistry 11:4037–4044

Hirashima A, Childs G, Inouye M (1973) Differential inhibitory effects of antibiotics on the biosynthesis of envelope proteins of *Escherichia coli*. J Mol Biol 79:373–389

Hlavka JJ, Bitha P (1966) Photochemistry IV. A photodeamination. Tetrahedron Lett 32:3843–3846

Hogenauer G, Turnowsky F (1972) The effects of streptomycin and tetracycline on codon-anticodon interactions. FEBS Lett 26:185–188

Hopwood DA (1981) Genetic studies of antibiotics and other secondary metabolites. In: Glover SW, Hopwood DA (eds) Genetics as a tool in microbiology, 31st symposium of the Society for General Microbiology. Cambridge University Press, Cambridge, p 187

Hopwood DA, Merrick MJ (1977) Genetics of antibiotic production. Bacteriol Rev 41:595–635

Howley PM, Israel MA, Low M-F, Martin MA (1979) A rapid method for detecting and mapping homology between heterologous DNAs. Evaluation of polyomavirus genomes. J Biol Chem 254:4876–4883

Igarashi K, Kaji A (1967) On the nature of two ribosomal sites for specific sRNA binding. Proc Natl Acad Sci USA 58:1971–1976

Igarashi K, Kaji A (1970) Relationship between sites 1, 2 and acceptor, donor sites for the binding of aminoacyl tRNA to ribosomes. Eur J Biochem 14:41–46

Igarashi K, Ishitsuka H, Kaji A (1969) Comparative studies on the mechanism of action of lincomycin, streptomycin and erythromycin. Biochem Biophys Res Commun 37:499–504

Inoue M, Kazawa T, Mitsuhashi S (1977) Antibacterial and inducer activities for tetracycline resistance by its derivatives and analogues. Microbiol Immunol 21:59–67

Inouye M, Halegoua S (1980) Secretion and membrane localization of proteins in *Escherichia coli.* CRC Crit Rev Biochem 7:339–371

Isono K, Isono S (1976) Lack of ribosomal protein S1 in *Bacillis stearothermophilus.* Proc Natl Acad Sci USA 73:767–770

IUPAC-IUB Commission on Biochemical Nomenclature (1969) A one letter notation for amino acid sequences, tentative rules. Biochem J 113:1–4

Jahn G, Laufs R, Kaulfers P-M, Kolenda H (1979) Molecular nature of two *Haemophilus influenzae* R factors containing resistances and the multiple integration of drug resistance transposons. J Bacteriol 138:584–597

Jerez C, Sandoval A, Allende J, Henes C, Ofengand J (1969) Specificity of the interaction of aminoacyl ribonucleic acid with a protein-guanosine triphosphate complex from wheat embryo. Biochemistry 8:3006–3014

Jorgensen RA, Reznikoff WS (1979) Organization of structural and regulatory genes that mediate tetracycline resistance in transposon 10. J Bacteriol 138:705–714

Jorgensen RA, Berg D, Reznikoff W (1978) Genetic organization in the transposable tetracycline resistance determinant Tn10. In: Schlessinger D (ed) Microbiology 1978. American Society for Microbiology, Washington, p 181

Jorgensen RA, Berg DE, Allet B, Reznikoff WS (1979) Restriction enzyme cleavage map of Tn10, a transposon which encodes tetracycline resistance. J Bacteriol 137:681–685

Kahan L, Winkelmann DA, Lake JA (1981) Ribosomal proteins S3, S6, S8 and S10 of *Escherichia coli* localized on the external surface of the small subunit by immune electron microscopy. J Mol Biol 145:193–214

Kaji A, Ryoji M (1979) Tetracycline. In: Hahn FE (ed) Antibiotics, vol 5, Springer, Berlin Heidelberg New York, p 304

Kaulfers KM, Laufs R, Jahn G (1978) Molecular properties of transmissible R factors of *Haemophilus influenzae* determining tetracycline resistance. J Gen Microbiol 105:243–252

Kersten H, Fey G (1971) On the mechanism of tetracycline action and resistance: association of tetracyclines with ribosomes and ribosomal subunits studied by a fluorometric method. In: Krčméry V, Rosival L, Watanabe T (eds) Bacterial plasmids and antibiotic resistance. First international symposium on infectious antibiotic resistance. Springer, Berlin Heidelberg New York, p 399

Kleckner N (1977) Translocatable elements in procaryotes. Cell 11:11–23

Kleckner N, Chan RK, Tye B-K, Botstein D (1975) Mutagenesis by insertion of a drug-resistance element carrying an inverted repetition. J Mol Biol 97:561–575

Kono M, Sasatsu M, Aoki T (1983) R plasmids in *Corynebacterium xerosis* strains. Antimicrob Agents Chemother 23:506–508

Kopylova-Sviridova TN, Soukovatitsin VV, Fodor I (1979) Synthesis of proteins coded by plasmid vectors of pcv series (Ap^R, Tc^R) and their recombinant derivatives (pDm) in *Escherichia coli* minicells. Gene 7:121–139

Kreft J, Bernhard K, Goebel W (1978) Recombinant plasmids capable of replication in *Bacillus subtilis* and *Escherichia coli.* Molec Gen Genet 162:59–67

Kreft J, Burger KJ, Goebel W (1983) Expression of antibiotic resistance genes from *Escherichia coli* in *Bacillus subtilis.* Molec Gen Genet 190:384–389

Kuzina ZA, Belousova II, Tereshin IM (1977) Lipid composition of tetracycline-sensitive and -resistant *Escherichia coli* cells. Microbiology 46:210–214

Lacey RW (1975) Antibiotic resistance plasmids of *Staphylococcus aureus* and their clinical importance. Bacteriol Rev 39:1–32

Laskin AI (1967) Tetracyclines. In: Gottlieb D, Shaw PD (eds) Antibiotics, vol 1. Springer, Berlin Heidelberg New York, p 331

Laskin AI, Chan WM (1964) Inhibition by tetracyclines of polyuridylic acid directed phenylalanine incorporation in *Escherichia coli* by cell-free extracts. Biochem Biophys Res Commun 14:137–142

Leeson LJ, Weidenheimer JF (1969) Stability of tetracycline and riboflavin. J Pharm Sci 58:355–357

Leij LD, Kingma J, Witholt B (1979) Nature of the regions involved in the insertion of newly synthesized protein into the outer membrane of *Escherichia coli*. Biochim Biophys Acta 553:224–234

Leive L, Telesetsky S, Coleman WG, Carr D (1984) Tetracyclines of various hydrophobicities as a probe for permeability of *E. coli* outer membranes. Antimicrob Agents Chemother 25:539–544

Levy SB (1975) The relation of a tetracycline-induced R factor membrane protein to tetracycline resistance. In: Mitsuhashi S, Rosival L, Kremery V (eds) Drug-inactivating enzymes and antibiotic resistance. Springer, Berlin Heidelberg New York, p 215

Levy SB (1981) The tetracyclines: microbial sensitivity and resistance. In: Grassi GG, Sabath LD (eds) New trends in antibiotics: research and therapy. Elsevier, Amsterdam, p 27

Levy SB, McMurry L, Onigman P, Saunders RM (1977) Plasmid-mediated tetracycline resistance in *Escherichia coli*. In: Drews J, Hogenauer G (eds) Topics in infectious diseases, vol II. Springer, Berlin Heidelberg New York, p 177

Lindley EV, Munske GR, Magnuson JA (1984) Kinetic analysis of tetracycline accumulation by *Streptococcus faecalis*. J Bacteriol 158:334–336

Livneh Z (1983) Directed mutagenesis method for analysis of mutagen specificity: application to ultra-violet induced mutagenesis. Proc Natl Acad Sci USA 80:237–241

Low KB, Porter DD (1978) Modes of gene transfer and recombination in bacteria. Annu Rev Genet 12:249–287

Lucas-Lenard J, Haenni AL (1968) Requirement of guanosine 5′-triphosphate for ribosomal binding of aminoacyl-sRNA. Proc Natl Acad Sci USA 59:554–559

Lucas-Lenard J, Tao P, Haenni AL (1969) Further studies on bacterial polypeptide elongation. Cold Spring Harbour Symp Quant Biol 34:455–462

Maloy SR, Nunn WD (1981) Selection for loss of tetracycline resistance by *Escherichia coli*. J Bacteriol 145:1110–1112

Marchalonis JJ, Weltman JK (1971) Relatedness among proteins: a new method of estimation and its application to immunoglobulins. Comp Biochem Physiol 38B:609–625

Marcos D, Woods DR (1973) Ecology of R factors: a study of urban and remote communities and their environments. S Afr Med J 47:340–341

Mare IJ (1968) Incidence of R factors among Gram-negative bacteria in drug-free human and animal communities. Nature 220:1046–1047

Marshall B, Tachibana C, Levy SB (1983) Frequency of tetracycline resistance determinants among lactose-fermenting coliforms. Antimicrob Agents Chemother 24:835–840

Mattes R, Burkardt HJ, Schmitt R (1979) Repetition of tetracycline resistance determinant genes on R plasmid pRSD1 in *Escherichia coli*. Molec Gen Genet 168:173–184

Maxwell IH (1968) Studies of the binding of tetracyclines to ribosomes in vitro. Mol Pharmacol 4:25–37

May JW, Houghton RH, Perret CJ (1964) The effect of growth at elevated temperatures on some heritable properties of *Staphylococcus aureus*. J Gen Microbiol 37:157–169

McMurry LM, Levy SB (1978) Two transport systems for tetracycline in sensitive *Escherichia coli:* critical role for an initial rapid uptake system insensitive to energy inhibitors. Antimicrob Agents Chemother 14:201–209

McMurry L, Petrucci RE, Levy SB (1980) Active efflux of tetracycline encoded by four genetically different tetracycline resistance determinants in *Escherichia coli*. Proc Natl Acad Sci USA 77:3974–3977

McMurry L, Cullinane J, Petrucci R, Levy SB (1981 a) Active uptake of tetracycline in membrane vesicles of sensitive *Escherichia coli*. In: Levy SB (ed) Molecular biology, pathogenicity and ecology of bacterial plasmids. Plenum, New York, p 633

McMurry LM, Cullinane JC, Petrucci RE, Levy SB (1981 b) Active uptake of tetracycline by membrane vesicles from susceptible *Escherichia coli*. Antimicrob Agents Chemother 20:307–313

McMurry LM, Cullinane JC, Levy SB (1982) Transport of the lipophilic analog minocycline differs from that of tetracycline in susceptible and resistant *Escherichia coli* strains. Antimicrob Agents Chemother 22:791–799

McQuillen K (1966) The physical organization of nucleic acid and protein synthesis. In: Pollock MR, Richmond MH (eds) Function and structure in micro-organisms. Fifteenth symposium of the Society for General Microbiology. Cambridge University Press, Cambridge, p 134

Mendez B, Tachibana C, Levy SB (1980) Heterogeneity of tetracycline resistance determinants. Plasmid 3:99–108

Mikulik K, Karnetova J, Quyen N, Blaumerova M, Komersova I, Varek Z (1971) Interaction of tetracycline with protein synthesizing system of *Streptomyces aureofaciens*. J Antibiot 24:801–809

Mitscher LA (1978) The chemistry of the tetracycline antibiotics. Dekker, New York

Moyed HS, Bertrand KP (1983) Mutations in multicopy Tn*10 tet* plasmids that confer resistance to inhibitory effects of inducers of *tet* gene expression. J Bacteriol 155:557–564

Moyed HS, Nguyen TT, Bertrand KP (1983) Multicopy Tn*10 tet* plasmids confer sensitivity to induction of *tet* gene expression. J Bacteriol 155:549–556

Munske GR, Lindley EV, Magnuson JA (1984) *Streptococcus faecalis* proton gradients and tetracycline transport. J Bacteriol 158:49–54

Nguyen TT, Postle K, Bertrand KP (1983) Sequence homology between the tetracycline-resistance determinants of Tn*10* and pBR322. Gene 25:83–92

Nierhaus KH, Wittmann HG (1980) Ribosomal function and its inhibition by antibiotics in prokaryotes. Naturwissenschaften 67:234–250

Nikaido H (1976) Outer membrane of *Salmonella typhimurium*. Transmembrane diffusion of some hydrophobic substances. Biochim Biophys Acta 433:118–132

Nikaido H, Nakae T (1979) The outer membrane of Gram-negative bacteria. Adv Microb Physiol 20:163–250

Nikaido H, Luckey M, Rosenberg EY (1980) Non-specific and specific diffusion channels in the outer membrane of *Escherichia coli*. J Supramol Struct 13:305–313

Noel D, Nikaido K, Ames F-L (1979) A single amino acid substitution in a histidine-transport protein drastically alters its mobility in sodium dodecyl sulfate polyacrylamide gel electrophoresis. Biochemistry 18:4159–4165

Ofengand J (1980) The topography of tRNA binding sites on the ribosome. In: Chambliss G, Craven GR, Davies J, Davis K, Kahan L, Nomura M (eds) Ribosomes: structure, function and genetics. University Park Press, Baltimore, p 497

O'Grady F (1982) Antibiotics in the 1980s. Adv Med 18:55–71

Old RW, Primrose SB (1980) Principles of gene manipulation: an introduction to genetic engineering. Blackwell, Oxford

Osawa S, Hori H (1980) Molecular evolution of ribosomal components. In: Chambliss G, Craven GR, Davies J, Davis K, Kahan L, Nomura M (eds) Ribosomes: structure, function and genetics. University Park Press, Baltimore, p 333

Osborn MJ, Wu HCP (1980) Proteins of the outer membrane of Gram-negative bacteria. Annu Rev Microbiol 34:369–422

Peden KWC (1983) Revised sequence of the tetracycline-resistance gene of pBR322. Gene 22:277–280

Pestka S, Nirenberg M (1966) Codeword recognition on 30S ribosomes. Cold Spring Harbour Symp Quant Biol 31:641–656

Petit A, Tempe J, Kerr A, Holsters M, Montagu M van, Schell J (1978) Substrate induction of conjugative activity of *Agrobacterium tumefaciens* Ti plasmids. Nature 271:570–571

Phillips S, Novick RP (1979) Tn 554 – a site-specific repressor-controlled transposon in *Staphylococcus aureus*. Nature 278:476–478

Piovant M, Varenne S, Pages JM, Lazdunski C (1978) Preferential sensitivity of syntheses of exported proteins to translation inhibitors of low polarity in *Escherichia coli*. Mol Gen Genet 164:265–274

Polak J, Novick RP (1982) Closely related plasmids from *Staphylococcus aureus* and soil bacilli. Plasmid 7:152–162

Pratt JM, Holland IB, Spratt BG (1981) Precursor forms of penicillin binding proteins 5 and 6 of the *Escherichia coli* cytoplasmic membrane. Nature 293:307–309

Prewo R, Stezowski JJ, Kirchlechner R (1980) Chemical-structural properties of tetracycline derivatives. 10. The 6-thiatetracyclines. J Am Chem Soc 102:7021–7026

Privitera G, Sebald M, Fayolle F (1979) Common regulatory mechanism of expression and conjugative ability of a tetracycline resistance plasmid in *Bacteroides fragilis*. Nature 278:657–659

Privitera G, Fayolle F, Sebald M (1981) Resistance to tetracycline, erythromycin and clindamycin in the *Bacteroides fragilis* group: inducible versus constitutive tetracycline resistance. Antimicrob Agents Chemother 20:314–320

Rambach A, Hogness DS (1977) Translation of *Drosophila melanogaster* sequences in *Escherichia coli*. Proc Natl Acad Sci USA 74:5041–5045

Ravel JM (1967) Demonstration of a guanosine triphosphate-dependent enzymatic binding of aminoacyl-ribonucleic acid to *Escherichia coli* ribosomes. Proc Natl Acad Sci USA 57:1811–1816

Ravel JM, Shorey RL, Garner CW, Dawkins RC, Shive W (1969) The role of an aminoacyl-tRNA-GTP-protein complex in polypeptide synthesis. Cold Spring Harbour Symp Quant Biol 34:321–330

Reboud A-M, Dubost S, Reboud J-P (1982) Photoincorporation of tetracycline into rat-liver ribosomes and subunits. Eur J Biochem 124:389–396

Reeve ECR (1966) Characteristics of some single step mutants to chloramphenicol resistance in *Escherichia coli* K12 and their interactions with R-factor genes. Genet Res 7:281–286

Reeve ECR (1968) Genetic analysis of some mutations causing resistance to tetracycline in *Escherichia coli* K12. Genet Res 11:303–309

Reeve ECR (1978) Evidence that there are two types of determinant for tetracycline resistance among R-factors. Genet Res 31:75–84

Reeve ECR, Robertson JM (1975) The characteristics of eleven mutants of R-factor R57 constitutive for tetracycline resistance, selected and tested in *Escherichia coli* K12. Genet Res 25:297–312

Rendi R, Ochoa S (1961) Enzyme specificity in activation and transfer of amino acids to ribonucleoprotein particles. Science 133:1367

Revel M, Greenshpan H, Herzberg M (1970) Specificity in the binding of *Escherichia coli* ribosomes to natural messenger RNA. Eur J Biochem 16:117–122

Ringrose PS, Higgins JE (1974) The interrelationship of tetracycline resistance, decynoyl-*N*-acetyl cysteamine and membrane fatty acid composition in *Escherichia coli*. J Antibiot 27:833–837

Roberts RJ (1980) Directory of restriction endonucleases. In: Grossman L, Moldave K (eds) Methods in enzymology, vol 65. Academic, New York, p 1

Rodriguez RL, West RW, Heyneker HL, Bolivar F, Boyer HW (1979) Characterizing wild-type and mutant promoters of the tetracycline resistance gene in pBR313. Nucleic Acids Res 6:3267–3287

Rosen BP, Kashkett ER (1978) Energetics of active transport. In: Rosen BP (ed) Bacterial transport. Dekker, New York, p 559

Rubens CE, McNeill WF, Farrar WE (1979) Evolution of multiple-antibiotic-resistance plasmids mediated by transposable plasmid deoxyribonucleic acid sequences. J Bacteriol 140:713–719

Salton MRJ, Owen P (1976) Bacterial membrane structure. Annu Rev Microbiol 30:451–482

Samra Z, Krausz-Steinmetz J, Sompolinsky D (1978) Transport of tetracyclines through the bacterial cell membrane assayed by fluorescence: a study with susceptible and resistant strains of *Staphylococcus aureus* and *Escherichia coli*. Microbios 21:7–22

Sancar A, Hack AM, Rupp WD (1979) Simple method for identification of plasmid-coded proteins. J Bacteriol 137:692–693

Sandermann H, Strominger JL (1971) C_{55}-isoprenoid alcohol phosphokinase: an extremely hydrophobic protein from the bacterial membrane. Proc Natl Acad Sci USA 68:2441–2443

Sarker S, Thach RE (1968) Inhibition of formylmethionyl-transfer RNA binding to ribosomes by tetracycline. Proc Natl Acad Sci USA 60:1479–1486

Schaefler S, Francois W, Ruby CL (1976) Minocycline resistance in *Staphylococcus aureus:* effect on phage susceptibility. Antimicrob Agents Chemother 9:600–613

Scherer GFE, Walkinshaw MD, Arnott S, Marre DJ (1980) The ribosome binding site recognized by *Escherichia coli* ribosomes have regions with signal character in both the leader and protein coding segments. Nucleic Acids Res 8:3895–3907

Schmidt FJ, Jorgensen RA, Wilde M De, Davies JE (1981) A specific tetracycline-induced, low-molecular weight RNA encoded by the inverted repeat of Tn10 (IS10). Plasmid 6:148–150

Schmitt R, Bernard E, Mattes R (1979) Characterization of Tn1721, a new transposon containing tetracycline resistance capable of amplification. Mol Gen Genet 172:53–65

Schoffl F, Pühler A (1979 a) Intramolecular amplification of tetracycline resistance determinant of transposon Tn1771 in *Escherichia coli*. Genet Res 33:253–260

Schoffl F, Pühler A (1979 b) The plasmid system of *Escherichia coli* strain UR12644. Genet Res 34:287–301

Schoffl F, Arnold W, Pühler A, Altenbuchner J, Schmitt R (1981) The tetracycline resistance transposons Tn1721 and Tn1771 have 3 38-base-pair repeats and generate 5-base-pair direct repeats. Mol Gen Genet 181:87–94

Schwartz SN, Medoff G, Kobayashi GS, Kwan CN, Schlessinger D (1972) Antifungal properties of polymyxin B and its potentiation of tetracycline as an antifungal agent. Antimicrob Agents Chemother 2:36–40

Scolnick E, Tompkins R, Caskey T (1968) Release factors differing in specificity for termination codon. Proc Natl Acad Sci USA 61:768–774

Shales SW, Chopra I, Ball PR (1980) Evidence for more than one mechanism of plasmid-determined tetracycline resistance in *Escherichia coli*. J Gen Microbiol 121:221–229

Shine J, Dalgarno L (1974) The 3′-terminal sequence of *Escherichia coli* 16S ribosomal RNA: complementarity to nonsense triplets and ribosome binding sites. Proc Natl Acad Sci USA 71:1342–1346

Shine J, Dalgarno L (1975) Determinant of cistron specificity in bacterial ribosomes. Nature 254:34–36

Skoultchi A, Ono Y, Waterson J, Lengyel P (1969) Peptide chain elongation. Cold Spring Harbour Symp Quant Biol 34:437–454

Skoultchi A, Ono Y, Waterson J, Lengyel P (1970) Peptide chain elongation: indications for the binding of an amino acid polymerization factor, guanosine 5′-triphosphate-aminoacyl transfer ribonucleic acid complex to the messenger-ribosome complex. Biochemistry 9:508–514

Smith DH (1967) R factor infection of *Escherichia coli* lyophilized in 1946. J Bacteriol 94:2071–2072

Smith MCM, Chopra I (1983) Limitations of a fluorescence assay for studies on tetracycline transport into *Escherichia coli*. Antimicrob Agents Chemother 23:175–178

Smith MCM, Chopra I (1984) Energetics of tetracycline transport into *Escherichia coli*. Antimicrob Agents Chemother 25:446–449

Smith MD, Hazum S, Guild WR (1981) Homology among "tet" determinants in conjugative elements of streptococci. J Bacteriol 148:232–240

Smythies JR, Benington F, Morin RD (1972) On the molecular mechanism of action of the tetracyclines. Experientia 28:1253–1254

Sompolinsky D, Krausz J (1973) Action of 12 tetracyclines on susceptible and resistant strains of *Staphylococcus aureus*. Antimicrob Agents Chemother 4:237–247
Sompolinsky D, Samra Z, Steinmetz-Krausz J, Assaf O, Passal T (1979) Studies on plasmid-borne resistance to tetracycline. In: Shafferman A, Cohen A, Smith SR (eds) Extrachromosomal inheritance in bacteria. Karger, Basel, p 198
Starlinger P (1980) 1S elements and transposons. Plasmid 3:241–259
Steitz JA (1973) Specific recognition of non-initiator regions in RNA bacteriophage messengers by ribosomes of *Bacillus stearothermophilus*. J Mol Biol 73:1–16
Stock JB, Rauch B, Roseman S (1977) Periplasmic space in *Salmonella typhimurium* and *Escherichia coli*. J Biol Chem 252:7850–7861
Stoffler G, Wittman HG (1977) Primary structure and three dimensional arrangement of proteins within the *Escherichia coli* ribosome. In: Weissbach H, Pestka S (eds) Molecular mechanisms of protein biosynthesis. Academic, New York, p 117
Strel'tsov SA, Kukhanova MK, Gurskii GV, Kraerskii AA, Belyavskaya IV, Viktorova LS, Treboganov AD, Gottikh BD (1975) Binding of hydroxytetracycline to *E. coli* ribosomes. Mol Biol 9:729–738 (English edition)
Stuber D, Bujard H (1981) Organization of transcriptional signals in plasmids pBR322 and pACYC184. Proc Natl Acad Sci USA 78:167–171
Suarez G, Nathans D (1965) Inhibition of aminoacyl tRNA binding to ribosomes by tetracycline. Biochem Biophys Res Commun 18:743–750
Suling WJ, O'Leary WM (1977) Lipids of antibiotic-resistant and -susceptible members of the Enterobacteriaceae. Can J Microbiol 23:1045–1051
Sutcliffe JG (1978) Complete nucleotide sequence of the *Escherichia coli* plasmid pBR322. Cold Spring Harbor Symp Quant Biol 43:77–90
Suzuka I, Kaji H, Kaji A (1966) Binding of specific sRNA to 30S ribosomal subunits: effects of 50S ribosomal subunits. Proc Natl Acad Sci USA 55:1483–1490
Szekely M (1980) From DNA to protein, the transfer of genetic information. Macmillan, London
Tait RC, Boyer HW (1978a) On the nature of tetracycline resistance controlled by the plasmid pSC101. Cell 13:73–81
Tait RC, Boyer HW (1978b) Restriction endonuclease mapping of pSC101 and pMB9. Mol Gen Genet 164:285–288
Tanaka S, Igarashi K, Kaji A (1972) Studies on the action of tetracycline and puromycin. J Biol Chem 247:45–50
Taylor DE, DeGrandis SA, Karmali MA, Fleming PC (1980) Transmissible tetracycline resistance in *Campylobacter jejuni*. Lancet II:797
Tenover FC, Bronsdon MA, Gordon KP, Plorde JL (1983) Isolation of plasmids encoding tetracycline resistance from *Campylobacter jenuni* strains isolated from simians. Antimicrob Agents Chemother 23:320–322
Traut RR, Monro RE (1964) The puromycin reaction and its relation to protein synthesis. J Mol Biol 10:63–72
Tritton TR (1977) Ribosome-tetracycline interaction. Biochemistry 16:4133–4138
Uehara Y, Hori M, Umezawa H (1976) Specific inhibition of the termination process of protein synthesis by negamycin. Biochim Biophys Acta 442:251–262
Uhlin BE, Nordstrom K (1977) R plasmid gene dosage effects in *Escherichia coli* K12: copy mutants of the R plasmid R1 *drd*-19. Plasmid 1:1–7
Valcavi U (1981) Tetracyclines: chemical aspects and some structure-activity relationships. In: Grassi GG, Sabath LD (eds) New trends in antibiotics: research and therapy. Elsevier, Amsterdam, p 3
van den Bogert C, Kroon AM (1981) Tissue distribution and effects on mitochondrial protein synthesis of tetracyclines after prolonged continuous intravenous administration to rats. Biochem Pharmacol 30:1706–1709
van Embden J, Cohen SN (1973) Molecular and genetic studies of an R factor system consisting of independent transfer and drug resistance plasmids. J Bacteriol 116:699–709
Vosbeck K, Mett H, Huber U, Bohn J, Petignat M (1982) Effects of low concentrations of antibiotics on *Escherichia coli* adhesion. Antimicrob Agents Chemother 21:864–869

Waters SH, Rogowsky P, Grinsted J, Altenbuchner J, Schmitt R (1983) The tetracycline resistance determinants of RP1 and Tn*1721:* nucleotide sequence analysis. Nucleic Acid Res 11:6089–6105

Weckesser J, Magnuson JA (1976) Light-induced tetracycline accumulation by *Rhodopseudomonas sphaeroides.* J Supramol Struct 4:515–520

Weissbach H (1980) Soluble factors in protein synthesis. In: Chambliss G, Craven GR, Davies J, Davis K, Kahan L, Nomura M (eds) Ribosomes: structure, function and genetics. University Park Press, Baltimore, p 377–411

Weissbach H, Pestka S (1977) Molecular mechanisms of protein biosynthesis. Academic, New York

Werner R, Kollack A, Nierhaus D, Schreiner G, Nierhaus KH (1975) Experiments on the binding sites and the action of some antibiotics which inhibit ribosomal functions. In: Drews J, Hahn FE (eds) Topics in infectious diseases, vol 1. Springer, Vienna New York, p 217

West IC (1980) Energy coupling in secondary active transport. Biochim Biophys Acta 604:91–126

West RW, Rodriguez RL (1980) Construction and characterization of *Escherichia coli* promoter-probe plasmid vectors. II. RNA polymerase binding studies on antibiotic-resistance promoters. Gene 9:175–193

White JP, Cantor CR (1971) Role of magnesium in the binding of tetracycline to *Escherichia coli* ribosomes. J Mol Biol 58:397–400

Wiebauer K, Schraml S, Shales SW, Schmitt R (1981) The tetracycline resistance transposon Tn1721; RecA-dependent gene amplification and expression of tetracycline resistance. J Bacteriol 147:851–859

Williams G, Smith I (1979) Chromosomal mutations causing resistance to tetracycline in *Bacillus subtilis.* Mol Gen Genet 177:23–29

Wilson CR, Baldwin JN (1978) Characterization and construction of molecular cloning vehicles within *Staphylococcus aureus.* J Bacteriol 136:402–413

Wojdani A, Avtalion RR, Sompolinsky D (1976) Isolation and characterization of tetracycline resistance proteins from *Staphylococcus aureus* and *Escherichia coli.* Antimicrob Agents Chemother 9:526–534

Wray LV, Reznikoff WS (1983) Identification of repressor binding sites controlling expression of tetracycline resistance encoded by Tn*10.* J Bacteriol 156:1188–1191

Wray LV, Jorgensen RA, Reznikoff WS (1981) Identification of the tetracycline resistance promoter and repressor in transposon Tn10. J Bacteriol 147:297–304

Yagi Y, Clewell DB (1976) Plasmid determined tetracycline resistance in *Streptococcus faecalis:* randomly repeated resistance determinants in amplified forms of pAMα1 DNA. J Mol Biol 102:583–600

Yagi Y, Clewell DB (1977) Identification and characterization of a small sequence located at two sites on the amplifiable tetracycline resistance plasmid pAMα1 in *Streptococcus faecalis.* J Bacteriol 129:400–406

Yang HL, Zubay G, Levy SB (1976) Synthesis of an R plasmid protein associated with tetracycline resistance is negatively regulated. Proc Natl Acad Sci USA 73:1509–1512

Young TW, Hubball SJ (1976) R-factor mediated resistance to tetracycline in *Escherichia coli* K-12. An R factor with a mutation to temperature sensitive tetracycline resistance. Biochem Biophys Res Commun 70:117–124

Zupancic TJ, King SR, Pogue-Geile KL, Jaskunas SR (1980) Identification of a second tetracycline-inducible polypeptide encoded by Tn10. J Bacteriol 144:346–355

Zund P, Lebek G (1980) Generation time-prolonging R plasmids: correlation between increases in the generation time of *Escherichia coli* caused by R plasmids and their molecular size. Plasmid 3:65–69

Note Added in Proof

Following completion of this chapter two important articles concerning the genetic and biochemical basis of *TetB* mediated tetracycline resistance have been published. Both papers (BRAUS et al. 1984; SCHOLLMEIER and HILLEN 1984) provide evidence for two further structural genes in addition to that encoding the well-characterized 36K efflux protein (see Sect. K.IV). The newly identified genes, termed *tetC* and *tetD*, encode proteins of apparent subunit molecular weights of 23,000 and 18,000 respectively, the lower molecular weight protein being membrane associated (BRAUS et al. 1984). Seemingly the *tetC* and *tetD* encoded proteins do not contribute to expression of *TetB* mediated resistance in *E. coli* K-12, but may nevertheless be important for expression of resistance in other gram-negative bacteria (BRAUS et al. 1984). Possibly the 26K and 14K proteins encoded by the *TetC* determinant in plasmid pSC101 (see Sects. K.IV and K.IX) fall into the same category, i.e. these proteins contribute little to expression of tetracycline resistance in *E. coli* K-12, but may be important for expression of resistance in other bacterial hosts.

References

Braus G, Argast M, Beck CF (1984) Identification of additional genes on transposon Tn*10*: *tetC* and *tetD*. J Bacteriol 160:504–509

Schollmeier K, Hillen W (1984) Transposon Tn*10* contains two structural genes with opposite polarity between *tetA* and IS10_R. J Bacteriol 160:499–503

CHAPTER 7

Clinical Uses of the Tetracyclines

B. A. CUNHA

A. Antimicrobial Activity

The first tetracycline to be discovered, chlortetracycline, was isolated from *Streptomyces aurefaciens* in 1944. Since 1944, several tetracycline analogues have been developed including oxytetracycline, which was introduced in 1950, tetracycline hydrochloride in 1953, and demethylchlortetracycline (demeclocycline). In the late 1950s it was discovered that the 6-hydroxyl group could be removed from the basic tetracycline group, which resulted in the 6-deoxytetracyclines, with significantly different microbiological and pharmacokinetic properties. In the 1960s the so-called "second generation" or long-acting tetracyclines were introduced. Doxycycline was isolated in 1962 (SCHACH VON WITTENAU et al. 1962) and minocycline was introduced in 1967 (REDIN 1967). Although all tetracyclines inhibit bacterial protein synthesis, there are significant differences in inherent antibacterial activity between the short-acting and long-acting tetracyclines.

Most members of the *Klebsiella-Enterobacter* group are susceptible to doxycycline. The activity of doxycycline against *Enterobacter* is species specific, i.e., *Enterobacter aerogenes* is in general more sensitive [minimal inhibitory concentration (MIC) range, 12.5–25 μg/ml] when compared with *E. cloacae*, which requires a higher concentration. Susceptibilities also vary with the serotype of the organism. Eight percent of *Klebsiella pneumoniae* strains are inhibited by concentrations of approximately 50 μg/ml, which is not clinically achievable. However, doxycycline is more active against *Klebsiella* species than other tetracycline analogues (STEIGBIGEL et al. 1968; GRABER et al. 1969). With respect to *Escherichia coli* susceptibility to doxycycline is also highly strain dependent. Sensitive strains of *E. coli* are usually inhibited by concentrations of 1.6–12.5 μg/ml. Strains of *E. coli* resistant to conventional tetracycline may be inhibited by doxycycline at clinically achievable concentrations. Doxycycline is more active than conventional tetracycline against *Hemophilus influenzae*. Most strains of *H. influenzae* are inhibited by 1–6 μg doxycycline (STEIGBIGEL et al. 1968; NEU 1978).

Neisseria species are highly susceptible to all strains of tetracycline, and doxycycline is active against some sulfur-resistant strains. Doxycycline is also highly active against *Neisseria gonorrhoeae*; the MIC is approximately 0.4 μg/ml (NEU 1978). The susceptibility of other gram-negative organisms to doxycycline is variable. Usually *Shigella, Vibro,* and *Acinetobacter* species are sensitive (STEIGBIGEL et al. 1968). Doxycycline shares with the other tetracyclines essentially no activity against *Proteus mirabilis* and *Pseudomonas aeruginosa* (ISENBERG 1967).

Doxycycline is highly active against *Bacteriodes fragilis* in vitro. Thirty percent of *B. fragilis* isolates are inhibited by $\geqq 0.4$ µg/ml doxycycline. Sixty percent of strains of *B. fragilis* are susceptible to 2.5 µg/ml, and 90% of strains are inhibited by 4–8 µg/ml doxycycline, which is readily achievable when the drug is given intravenously or orally (Thadepalli et al. 1978). Anaerobic gram-positive bacilli are also as susceptible to doxycycline. The majority of clostridial species and lactobacilli are inhibited by concentrations of doxycycline $\geqq 2.5$ µg/ml (Chow et al. 1974).

The gram-positive organisms are more susceptible to doxycycline when compared with conventional tetracycline. Group D streptococci, e.g., *Enterococcus*, are in general resistant to the tetracyclines. However, doxycycline is the most active tetracycline with respect to Group D streptococci (Steigbigel et al. 1968). Doxycycline is more active against *Streptococcus aureus* and *S. epidermidis* than are the conventional tetracyclines (Lewis et al. 1976). Eighty-five percent of strains are inhibited by $\geqq 8$ µg/ml doxycycline. Thirty-two percent of strains are inhibited by >1 µg/ml doxycycline.

Against hemolytic streptococci tetracyclines were highly active compounds. Unfortunately, because of widespread resistance the tetracyclines are now inactive against approximately 25% of these organisms. Against susceptible strains of beta-hemolytic streptococci the mean MIC of doxycycline is usually approximately 0.5 µg/ml (Finland et al. 1976). In addition, doxycycline is highly active against the pneumococcus and *Corynebacterium diphtheriae*. MIC ranges of doxycycline against *S. pneumoniae* are between 0.2 and 12 µg/ml. It should be noted that doxycycline is twice as active against the pneumococcus as is conventional tetracycline (Cunha 1979).

Minocycline shares in common with doxycycline much of the same spectrum of enhanced antimicrobiological activity with certain important exceptions. Against strains of *N. gonorrhea* minocycline is the most active tetracycline, 80% of strains being inhibited by >0.4 µg/ml. No tetracycline analogue has activity against penicillinase-producing strains of *N. gonorrhea* because of cross-resistance to the penicillin compounds (Steigbigel et al. 1968). Against anaerobic bacteria minocycline is the most highly active tetracycline with respect to *Bacteroides fragilis*. Seventy percent of strains are sensitive to >3 µg/ml; therefore, minocycline is 4 times more active than doxycycline and 13 times more active against this organism than conventional tetracycline (Chow et al. 1975).

Minocycline is highly susceptible to nonaeruginosa strains of *Pseudomonas*. Nearly all strains are inhibited by >2 µg/ml minocycline. Minocycline is also considerably more active than doxycycline in this respect (Tilton and Ryon 1978).

With respect to gram-positive organisms minocycline is the most active tetracycline against *S. aureus*. This may be explained in part by the ability of minocycline to penetrate the cell wall of the organism. Against the pneumococcus the activity of minocycline is comparable to that of doxycycline but it is considerably less active than doxycycline against enterococci (Steigbigel et al. 1968).

Compared with the other tetracyclines minocycline has comparable activity against *Rickettsia, Chlamydia, Microplasma,* and *Legionella* species (Steigbigel et al. 1968).

The activity of the tetracycline analogues, their safety and their pharmacokinetic profiles determine their clinical usefulness. Tetracyclines have proved to be immensely useful antibiotics since their introduction because of their unusually wide spectrum of activity. Tetracycline should be avoided if possible in pregnant women and in children less than 8 years of age. Depending on the tetracycline analogue, these agents must be used with caution in patients with hepatic or liver disease.

B. Clinical Uses

Tetracyclines are the antibiotics of choice against a variety of organisms. They are also effective alternative agents against a variety of other microorganisms and finally are effective in treating a variety of infectious disease syndromes. Each of these general areas will be considered sequentially and areas where tetracyclines are suboptimal therapy will also be included.

C. Treatment of First Choice

The tetracyclines have traditionally been the preferred therapeutic agents against *Pasteurella* infections. *Pasteurella pestis* may be treated with tetracycline alone, but most authorities prefer to combine streptomycin with tetracycline in the treatment of bubonic plague (BUTLER et al. 1974). Streptomycin is also effective for the treatment of tularemia due to *P. tularensis*, but treatment with a tetracycline is preferred by most infectious disease experts. Tetracyclines have also been used successfully over the years against *P. multocida*; there is no advantage in using any particular tetracycline analogue against these organisms, although minocycline is the most active compound in vitro against *P. multocida*.

Tetracyclines have been used successfully to treat brucellosis. Once again, some authorities prefer to add streptomycin to the tetracycline regimen in seriously ill patients. Ordinarily brucellosis is treated for 2- to 4-week period because of the high incidence of relapse with this interesting cellular organism (WHO 1977).

The organism responsible for relapsing fever, *Borrelia recurrentis*, is also highly sensitive to tetracycline therapy. Interestingly, relapsing fever has ben cured with a single-dose tetracycline or erythromycin. However, it is suggested that treatment ordinarily be given for 2 weeks because of the propensity of this organism to recur; hence the name relapsing fever. Therapy may be given parenterally or orally depending upon the severity of the disease.

Melioidosis, the etiological agent of which is *Pseudomonas pseudomallei*, is another unusual infectious disease well handled by the tetracyclines. Considerable experience in treating melioidosis was gained as the result of the conflict in Vietnam during the 1960s. High doses of tetracyclines for 3–4 weeks have been proven effective. A few strains of *P. pseudomallei* are resistant to the tetracyclines, but no drug has uniform activity against this organism. Some authorities prefer to use tetracycline in combination with chloramphenicol or trimethoprimsulfamethoxazole (SPONITZ et al. 1967).

Against *Vibrio cholerae,* the organism responsible for cholera, tetracyclines have been useful early in the course of the disease, which is primarily a toxin-mediated process, and for this reason antibiotic therapy is only useful during the early stages. Replacement of fluid and electrolyte losses are of critical importance. Conventional tetracycline has been successful in the first 48 h of the disease. Doxycycline may have an advantage since single-dose cures of cholera have been reported using doxycycline (300-mg dose for adults) (De et al. 1976). Minocycline is as clinically effective as tetracycline in the treatment of cholera but does not result in elimination of the organism from the feces as rapidly as conventional tetracycline (Mazumder et al. 1974).

Mycoplasma pneumoniae infections are best treated with tetracyclines. Therapy should be continued for at least 2 weeks to prevent relapse. The ability of the antibiotic to eliminate the organism for oropharyngeal secretions is variable. Minocycline and doxycycline are more likely to eliminate the carrier state of the organisms than is conventional tetracycline because of their superior penetration into oropharyngeal secretions (Smith et al. 1967).

For many years tetracyclines were used extensively to treat pertussis. However, because this is primarily a disorder of young children tetracyclines are relatively contraindicated in this clinical setting. Erythromycin is now considered by many to be the drug of choice in treating pertussis. Neither the tetracyclines nor erythromycin alter the natural course of the illness, but eliminate the carriage of the organism and oropharyngeal secretions (Bass et al. 1969).

One of the most important uses for the tetracyclines has been in the treatment of rickettsial infections. Some clinicians prefer to use chloramphenicol in the treatment of Rocky Mountain spotted fever, but the majority of physicians prefer a tetracycline derivative. Rocky Mountain spotted fever may be treated orally or parenterally depending upon the severity of the illness of the patient. Ordinarily treatment should be continued for 2–4 weeks because the organisms are obligate intracellular parasites, and shorter therapeutic courses have been associated with clinical relapse (Woodward 1980; Beltran and Cunha 1983).

Tetracyclines are also the preferred antibiotics for the treatment of murine, scrub, and epidemic typhus. Tetracyclines have also been useful in the treatment of rickettsial pox (Mull 1966; Berman and Kundin 1973). In the treatment of typhus, therapy is usually continued until 48 h after the patient has become afebrile. Q fever is a benign self-limiting infectious disease and therapy is best reserved for chronic Q fever. In the event of cardiac involvement, i.e., Q fever endocarditis, prolonged high-dose therapy with minocycline or doxycycline has the best chance of effecting cure. Valve replacement may become necessary if antibiotic control of the infection is unsuccessful or if hemodynamic deterioration occurs.

In treating *Shigella* dysentery single-dose therapy is effective. There is no therapeutic difference among the various forms of the tetracyclines, but since high intralumenal concentrations of antibiotic are desirable a shorter-acting tetracycline would have a theoretical advantage in eliminating the organism from the stool. Unfortunately, resistance has become an increasing problem so that at the present time approximately 60% of the strains of *Shigella* are resistant to all of the tetracyclines (Pickering et al. 1978).

Currently tetracyclines enjoy widespread usage in the treatment of chlamydial infections. It has recently been realized that psittacosis occasionally presents as an atypical pneumonia. The tetracyclines are the most effective drugs against *Chlyamidia psittaci*. Psittacosis therapy should be ordinarily continued for 3–4 weeks since the relapse rate is high when a shorter course of treatment is given (WHO 1977; JAWETZ 1969). It is important to appreciate that erythromycin is relatively inactive, given in the usual fashion, in patients with psittacosis (JONAS and CUNHA 1981).

Inclusion conjunctivitis and trachoma have traditionally been successfully treated with tetracyclines. Prolonged therapy as in other chlamydial infections for at least 3 weeks and occasionally 6 weeks has been recommended. Trachoma has also been treated topically using tetracycline eye ointment given daily over a 6-week period. Efficacy is not as great as with the usual treatment but it is useful in selected situations. Ophthalmia neonatorum due to the trachoma agent is preventable if treatment is begun during the first 2 weeks of life. Prolonged therapy for as long as 6 weeks may be required (DAWSON et al. 1971; DUNLOP 1977).

The L-serotypes of *Chlamydia* are responsible for lymphogranuloma venereum. All of the serotypes are highly sensitive to the tetracyclines. Therapy is usually continued for at least 2 weeks. Minocycline and doxycycline have the advantage of less frequent dosing and improving patient compliance (VALASCO et al. 1972).

The largest single area of use for the tetracyclines has recently been in the treatment of nonspecific ureteritis due to *Chlamydia* or *Ureaplasmas*. The most effective drugs for the treatment of nonspecific urethritis have been the tetracyclines. Treatment with tetracyclines usually yields a 70% cure rate after a 2-week therapeutic course. As with other chlamydial or mycoplasmal infections prolonged therapy with a long-acting tetracycline provides the best chance of clinical cure. If prolonged therapy is required single-dose minocycline or doxycycline regimens may be safely given for several weeks (EDWARDS and ROOT 1979; SCHACHTER 1978).

Although the tetracyclines are consistently active against the *Chlamydia* when they are responsible for a nonspecific urethritis the mycoplasma may occasionally be resistant (BOWIE et al. 1976). Such strains are usually sensitive to erythromycin. In pregnant females with gonococcal urethritis erythromycin may be substituted for the tetracyclines.

Although penicillin G is the preferred drug for established syphilis, tetracyclines given prophylactically will kill incubating spirochetes and have been used as alternative therapy in treating penicillin-sensitive patients with the disease. Early syphilis less than 1 year in duration may be treated for 2 weeks. Long-standing syphilis treatment should be continued for at least 30 days. Because of their pharmacokinetic properties, minocycline and doxycycline are the most likely of the tetracycline compounds to effect cure on a theoretical basis (KNOX and MONTGOMERY 1959; CDC 1978). Doxycycline "single-session therapy" has been used to treat gonorrhea. Minocycline has also been similarly used for the same purpose. Both antibiotics employed in this fashion are less effective than when given daily for a period of 1 week. Tetracyclines should not be used to treat penicillinase-producing strains of *Neisseria gonorrhea* because of cross-resistance. Although penicillin remains the drug of choice in the treatment of gonorrhea, comparable results in penicillin-allergic patients have been achieved with the tetracyclines and derivatives (WIESNER et al. 1973; BAYTCH 1974; CDC 1983). Tetracyclines have been suggested by some authorities as the preferred treatment for gonococcal urethritis because of the coexistence of *Chlamydia* or *Ureaplasma* organisms in such patients. The tetracyclines are active against all of these organisms while penicillin derivatives are only active against the gonococcus.

In terms of prophylaxis doxycycline has been used extensively in the prevention of traveler's diarrhea due to toxicogenic strains of *E. coli.* Doxycycline has the advantage of being active against *Vibrio cholerae, Shigella* dysentery, *Campylobacter, Yersinia, Salmonella,* and to a lesser extent *Entomoeba histolytica.* For this reason it is an ideal drug for travelers to take in areas where these enteric pathogens are prevalent (SACK et al. 1978).

Minocycline has been especially useful in the prevention of meningococcal infections by elimination of the organism in the carrier. Minocycline is approximately as good as rifampin in eradicating sufanilamide-sensitive and -resistant meningococci from the oropharynx. Minocycline is the only tetracycline that should be employed for this purpose because of its superior penetration into the oropharyngeal secretions (DEVINE et al. 1971; JONAS and CUNHA 1981).

D. Effective Alternative Treatment

Tetracyclines have been used in a variety of circumstances when the patient is unable to take the drug of choice or for pharmacokinetic reasons (CUNHA et al. 1982a, b).

The tetracyclines are highly active against the pneumococcus; due to resistance short-acting tetracyclines should not be used in penicillin-allergic patients to treat serious pneumococcal sepsis. There is essentially no resistance to the longer-acting tetracyclines when used against *S. pneumoniae* (DEVINE et al. 1971).

Tetracyclines have been used as alternative therapy against *Listeria.* However, the drug of choice remains ampicillin if the patient is not penicillin allergic.

The tetracyclines have proved quite useful against *Hemophilus influenzae,* especially the longer-acting tetracyclines. *H. Influenzae* is usually found in upper respiratory tract secretions, i.e., sinus fluid, bronchial secretions, or middle ear fluid. The longer-acting tetracyclines producing higher blood and tissue levels offer the therapeutic advantage in treating these infections due to *H. influenzae.* While the second-generation tetracyclines are no more active than the shorter-acting tetracyclines against *Hemophilus,* the superior tissue penetration ability of doxycycline and minocycline confer an advantage at the tissue level compared with ampicillin or the oral cephalosporin (STEIGBIGEL et al. 1968; CUNHA et al. 1982b).

Hemophilus ducreyi, the organism responsible for chancroid, is also very sensitive to tetracycline derivatives. Once again, the longer-acting tetracyclines are preferred because their pharmacokinetic properties of once or twice daily dosing are important in increasing patient compliance.

Doxycycline and minocycline are reasonably active agents against *Bacteroides fragilis*. At clinically achievable concentrations the shorter-acting tetracyclines inhibit only 30% of *B. fragilis*. In contradistinction, doxycycline and minocycline inhibit over 80% of *B. fragilis* strains at clinically achievable concentrations. Since the longer-acting tetracyclines have a limited but important gram-negative spectrum they are ideal drugs when oral monotherapy of mild to moderately severe pelvic or abdominal infections is indicated. For life-threatening *B. fragilis* sepsis, other antibiotics such as metronidizole, chloramphenicol, or clindamycin in combination with TMP-SMX or an aminoglycoside would be preferred (CUNHA et al. 1982b).

The tetracyclines have been useful as alternative therapy in *Yersina enterocolitica* infections (ERIKSSON and OLCEN 1975). Ordinarily, *Y. enterocolitica* bacteremia is treated with an aminoglycoside. Alternatively, in addition to the use of a tetracycline, chloramphenicol is favored by the majority of clinicians to treat this infection when an aminoglycoside cannot be used.

Tetracyclines have been used adjunctively in the treatment of amebic dysentery. Tetracyclines are used to treat the intestinal phase of amebic dysentery but are ineffective in systemic or hepatic amebiasis. Metronidazole is the preferred drug at the present time for intestinal, systemic, and hepatic amebiasis. Tetracyclines are active against other parasitic organisms, primarily malaria organisms of the *Plasmodium falciparum* variety. Tetracyclines have been used in combination with quinine in the treatment of chloroquine-resistant *P. falciparum* malaria. Tetracycline used alone is ineffective. Treatment is ordinarily continued for 2 weeks.

Staphylococcal infections of the skin have been successfully treated by longer-acting tetracyclines. There are many tetracycline-resistant strains of staphylococci but these are usually sensitive to minocycline. Minocycline has more inherent antistaphylococcal activity than does doxycycline or erythromycin. Therefore, in penicillin-allergic patients it is frequently used to treat soft tissue infections due to staphylococci in the absence of bacteremia. If a patient has staphylococcal bacteremia, then an antistaphylococcal penicillin is usually used. Alternatively cephaloporin or vancomycin therapy has been successful in this clinical situation (PHAIR et al. 1974; ALLEN 1976).

Tetracyclines in general and doxycycline in particular have been useful in alternative therapy in the treatment of legionnaire's disease. Although erythromycin is ordinarily the preferred drug in the treatment of known *Legionella pneumophila* infections, tetracycline derivatives are effective in vitro and in vivo. Doxycycline may be employed in patients having moderately severe diarrhea secondary to the disease process where therapy with erythromycin may exacerbate the problem. Alternatively, if the patient presents with atypical pneumonitis and legionnaire's disease in one of several diagnostic possibilities then doxycycline would be the preferred empirical therapy since it is active against all the organisms causing atypical pneumonitis (*Myoplasma* pneumonia, Q fever, tularemia pneumonia, psitticosis, *Legionella* pneumophilia). As with erythromycin, therapy should be prolonged because of the intracellular preference of the organism. Doxycycline therapy is usually continued for a total of 4–6 weeks (CUNHA and QUINTILIANI 1979; JONAS et al. 1981).

Against unusual organisms such as *Flavobacterium meningosepticum,* which has occasionally been associated with nosocomial meningitis, minocycline has proved to be effective therapy. Minocycline possesses a high degree of microbiological activity against the organisms and in addition penetrates into the CSF in adequate concentration (MADERAZO et al. 1975). Tetracyclines have been used in a variety of infections due to other unusual organisms such as *Bacillus anthracis, Erysipelothrix,* etc., but experience with these agents in such infections is limited and standard sources should be consulted to determine the optimal therapy against unusual organisms.

E. Treatment of Clinical Syndromes

One of the most common uses of the tetracyclines is in treating the syndrome of chronic bronchitis. An exacerbation of chronic bronchitis is usually initially due to a viral organism but in the majority of cases there is a secondary bacterial invader responsible for the inflammatory response and bronchial edema. The organisms usually incriminated in exacerbation of chronic bronchitis are the pneumococcus, group A streptococci, or *Hemophilus influenza.* The tetracyclines, especially minocycline or doxycycline, are useful in treating exacerbations of chronic bronchitis due to these organisms because of their microbiological activity and penetration into the secretions of the respiratory tract. Alternative treatment with TMP-SMX, amoxicillin, or becampilcillin have also been used in this clinical setting. Shorter-acting tetracyclines should not be used because of the likelihood of tetracycline-resistant strains of streptococci, pneumococci, or *Hemophilus influenzae* (CUNHA 1982a, b).

Long-acting tetracyclines have been used in the treatment of abdominal and pelvic peritonitis. Doxycycline and minocycline have been used alone successfully for prophylaxis in pelvic and abdominal procedures. The longer-acting tetracyclines have also been used in combination with an aminoglycoside in the therapy of intraabdominal or pelvic infections. In life-threatening infections of the pelvis or abdomen, tetracyclines should not be included in the regimen. Short-acting tetracyclines because of their relative inactivity against *Bacteroides fragilis* should not even be used prophylactically (KLEIN et al. 1977; KLASTERSKY et al. 1977).

Tetracyclines have a limited use in treating urinary tract infections. Tetracyclines are more active in an acid urine. First-generation tetracyclines especially tetracycline hydrochloride are excreted in high concentration in the urine. Therefore in the treatment of lower urinary tract infections involving the bladder, doxycycline and minocycline may be used but provide lower albeit adequate urinary concentrations. Because the short-acting tetracyclines concentrate to such a higher degree in the urine they may be used in unusual circumstances to treat organisms such as *Pseudomonas* one can find in the urinary tract. Conventional sensitivity testing suggests that these organisms are resistant to tetracycline, but such testing does not take into account the very high levels achieved in the urine when short-acting tetracyclines are given by mouth. In patients with renal insufficiency where short-acting tetracyclines are contraindicated minocycline or doxycycline may be used to advantage in selected situations (CUNHA et al. 1982b; MUSHER et al. 1975).

Long-term low-dosage tetracycline therapy has been used successfully for years to treat patients with mild to moderately severe acne. Tetracyclines penetrate into the lipid-rich layers of the dermis and inhibit the primary organism responsible for acne, *Corynebacterium acnes*. Tetracycline is excreted in the sebum by binding to epithelial cells. The antibiotic is eliminated through the sebum or via desquamation and exerts its effect by reducing the inflammatory effect of oleosa-produced acid in the sebum. Long-term therapy may be continued for months or years without major side effects. Because the antibiotic concentrates in the dermis, 250 mg orally once daily is adequate. In the few cases that do not respond to conventional tetracycline therapy, minocycline should be tried because of its superior penetration into the lipid layers of the skin. Minocycline is clearly superior to doxycycline in this respect and may also have to be used for a prolonged period at a low dose of 100 mg/day (POCHI 1976; BAER et al. 1976).

Tetracyclines have also been used to treat acute and chronic prostatitis. Parenchymal cells of the prostate represent a penetration barrier to most antibiotics because of their high lipid content. Doxycycline has been used successfully, especially in the treatment of chronic prostatitis, because of its penetration into the parenchyma of the subacutely inflammed prostate. The organisms usually responsible for prostatitis are the aerobic gram-negative coliforms and, to a lesser extent, chlamydia. Since treatment is ordinarily continued for at least 3 months a drug such as doxycycline is ideal because it may be given once daily with few or no side effects. Theoretically minocycline, because of its lipid solubility characteristics, would be comparable to or better than doxycycline, but little clinical experience of the use of this antibiotic exists (RISTUCCIA and CUNHA 1982).

A new clinical entity has recently been described which has been termed acute urethal syndrome. Acute urethal syndrome has been associated with three organisms, i.e., *E. coli, Staphylococcus saprophyicus*, and *Chlamydia*. Doxycycline is the preferred drug in treating this urethal syndrome because of its activity against all of the organisms and its penetration into the secretions of the distal urethra. Therapy should be continued for 2 weeks since shorter courses of therapy are associated with a relatively high relapse rate.

Tropical sprue and Whipple's disease have been successfully treated with tetracycline derivatives. No studies have shown any difference between the long- and shorter-acting tetracyclines in this regard but the longer tetracyclines would offer a theoretical advantage based upon their tissue penetration ability. Although no etiological agent has been associated with either of these situations, clinical response is usually noted after 4 weeks of therapy. Therapy may have to be continued indefinitely (CLANCY et al. 1975; RICKELS et al. 1972).

F. Ineffective Treatment

Except during unusual circumstances tetracyclines should not be used to treat serious staphylococcal infections, endocarditis, gram-negative bacteremias, meningitis, septic arthritis or osteromyelitis, leptospirosis, or tuberculosis. Although tetracyclines have occasionally been used to treat these infections other agents are preferable and standard texts should be consulted in the individual case.

G. Dosage and Duration of Therapy

To avoid redundancy in the text specific dosing information with each infection has been purposely omitted unless it varies from the usual daily dose or mode of administration. The great majority of infectious disease processes are treated for 1–2 weeks with tetracyclines or any other antibiotic. Exceptions to this rule occur and are specifically mentioned in association with each organism or syndrome. Table 1 indicates the usual dosing information on the short-acting and long-acting tetracyclines which the reader should use unless the text specifically states an exception. It should also be noted that the dosages given are for patients with normal hepatic and renal function with normal host defense mechanisms. Changes may need to be made in patients with a variety of abnormal disease states. Obese patients, patients with ascites, burn patients, etc. may need to have special modifications of the usual dosing regimens. Patients that are compromised hosts may need to be treated for longer than usual with tetracyclines or any other antibiotic given. As mentioned previously, tetracyclines should not be used if the organism is known to be resistant to the antibiotic, if the patient is less than 8 years of age, or if the patient is pregnant. Taking into account all of these special situations, the tetracyclines have proven to be immensely useful drugs in a wide variety of infectious diseases. If administered selectively and appropriately these drugs will continue to be an important part of the clinician's armamentarium.

Table 1. Mean minimum inhibitory concentrations

	Tetracycline (μg/ml)	Doxycline (μg/ml)	Minocycline (μg/ml)
Gram-positive bacteria			
Staphylococcus pyogenes	3.1	1.6	0.78
Streptococcus pyogenes (group A)	0.78	0.39	0.39
Streptococcus pneumoniae	0.8	0.2	0.2
Streptococcus viridans spp.	3.1	0.39	0.39
Streptococcus faecalis (Enterococcus, group D)	>100	50	100
Gram-negative bacteria			
Escherichia coli	12.5	12.5	6.3
Enterobacter	25	25	12.5
Klebsiella	50	50	25
Serratia	200	50	25
Proteus mirabilis	>100	>100	>100
Neisseria gonorrhoeae	0.78	0.39	0.39
N. meningitidis	0.8	1.6	1.6
Hemophilus influenzae	1.6	1.6	1.6
Mycoplasma and *Chlamydia*			
M. pneumoniae	1.6	1.6	1.6
Ureaplasma urealyticum	0.4	0.1	0.13
Chlamydia	0.6	0.06	0.02
Legionella			
L. pneumophila	5.2	1.0	0.43

References

Allen JC (1976) Drugs five years later: minocycline. Ann Intern Med 85:482
Baer RL, Leshaw SM, Shalita AR (1976) High-dose tetracycline therapy in severe acne. Arch Dermatol 112:479
Bass JW, Klenk EL, Kotheimer JB, Linnemann CC, Smith MHD (1969) Antimicrobial treatment of pertussis. J Pediatr 75:786
Baytch H (1974) Minocycline in single dose therapy in the treatment of gonococcal urethritis in male patients. Med J Aust 1:831
Beltran MD, Cunha BA (1983) Rocky mountain spotted fever: varied presentations. Medical Journal of Nassau Hospital 5:10
Berman SJ, Kundin WD (1973) Scrub typhus in South Vietnam. A study of 87 cases. Ann Intern Med 79:26
Bowie WR, Alexander ER, Floyd JF, Holmes J, Miller Y, Holmes KK (1976) Differential response of chlamydial and ureaplasma-associated urethritis to sulphafurazole (sulfisoxazole) and aminocyclitols. Lancet 2:1276
Butler T, Bell WR, Linh NN, Tiep ND, Arnold K (1974) *Yersinia pestis* infection in Vietnam. I. Clinical and hematological aspects. J Infect Dis [Suppl] 129:78
Center for Disease Control (1978) Penicillinase-(beta-lactamase) producing *Neisseria gonorrhoeae* – worldwide. Morbidity and Mortality Weekly Report 27:10
Chow AW, Pattern V, Guze L (1974) In vitro activity of doxycycline against anaerobic bacteria. In: Doxycycline (Vibramycin): recent investigations and clinical experience. Pfizer, New York, p 9
Chow AW, Pattern V, Guze LB (1975) Comparative susceptibility of anaerobic bacteria to minocycline, doxycycline, and tetracycline. Antimicrob Agents Chemother 7:46
Clancy RL, Tomkins WAF, Muckle TJ, Richardson H, Rawls WE (1975) Isolation and characterization of an aetiological agent in Whipple's disease. Br Med J 3:568
Cunha BA (1979) Pharmacokinetics of doxycycline. Postgrad Med Commun Sept:63
Cunha BA, Quintiliani R (1979) The atypical pneumonias: a diagnostic and therapeutic approach. Postgrad Med 66:95
Cunha BA, Sibley C, Ristuccia AM (1982 a) Doxycycline. Ther Drug Monit 4:115
Cunha BA, Comer J, Jonas M (1982 b) The tetracyclines. Med Clin North Am 66:293–302
Dawson CR, Ostler HB, Hanna L, Hoshiwara I, Jawetz E (1971) Tetracyclines in the treatment of chronic trachoma in American Indians. J Infect Dis 124:255
De S, Chaudhuri A, Dutta P, Dutta D, De SP, Pal SC (1976) Doxycycline in the treatment of cholera. Bull WHO 54:177
Devine LF, Johnson DP, Hagerman CR, Pierce WE, Rhode SL, Peckinpaugh RO (1971) The effect of minocycline on meningococcal nasopharyngeal carrier state in naval personnel. Am J Epidemiol 93:337
Dunlop EMC (1977) Treatment of patients suffering from chlamydial infections. J Antimicrob Chemother 3:377
Edwards L, Root T (1979) Comparison of two recent studies in nongonococcal urethritis. In: Proceedings of symposium on sexually transmitted disease. Reappraisal of the role of Vibramycin (doxycycline). Science and Medicine, New York, p 35
Eriksson M, Olcen P (1975) Septicemia due to *Yersinia enterococlitica* in a noncompromised host. Scand J Infect Dis 7:78
Finland M, Garnes C, Wilcox C et al. (1976) Susceptibility of beta-hemolytic streptococci to 65 antibacterial agents. Antimicrob Agents Chemother 9:11
Graber CD, Jervery LP, Martin F et al. (1969) In vitro and in vivo sensitivity of staphylococci and selected bycteria to minocycline, tetracycline, and doxycycline. J SC Med Assoc 65:187
Isenberg HD (1967) In vitro activity of doxycycline against bacteria from clinical material. Appl Microbiol 15:1074
Jawetz E (1969) Chemotherapy of chlamydial infections. Adv Pharmacol Chemother 7:253
Jonas M, Cunha BA (1981) Legionnaire's disease treated with doxycycline. Lancet 1:1107

Klastersky J, Husson M, Weerts-Ruhl D, Daneau D (1977) Anaerobic wound infections in cancer patients: comparative trail of clindamycin, trindazole and doxycycline. Antimicrob Agents Chemother 12:523

Klein RA, Busch DF, Wilson SE, Flora DJ, Finegold SM (1977) Doxycycline in abdominal surgery. JAMA 238:1933

Knox JM, Montgomery CH (1959) Antibiotics other than penicillin in the treatment of syphilis. N Engl J Med 261:277

Lewis SA, Altemeier WA (1976) Correlation of in vitro resistance of *Staphylococcus aureus* to tetracycline, doxycycline, and minocycline with in vivo use. Chemotherapy (Basel) 22:319

Maderazo EG, Quintiliani R, Tilton RC, Bartlett R, Joyce NC, Andriole, VT (1975) Activity of minocycline against *Acinetobacter calcoacetics* var *anitratus* (syn *Herellea vaginicola*) and *Serratia marcescens*. Antimicrob Agents Chemother 8:54

Mazumder DNG, Sirkar BK, De SP (1974) Minocycline in the treatment of cholera. A comparison with tetracycline. Indian J Med Res 6:712

Mull MM (1966) The tetracyclines, a critical reappraisal. Am J Dis Child 112:483

Musher DM, Minuth JN, Thorsteinsson SB, Holmes T (1975) Effectiveness of achievable urinary concentrations of tetracyclines against tetracycline-resistant pathogenic bacteria. J Infect Dis [Suppl] 131:40

Neu HC (1978) A symposium on the tetracyclines: a major appraisal. Bull NY Acad Med 54:141 (second series)

Phair JP, Hartman RE, Carleton J (1974) Evaluation of the efficacy of minocycline therapy for staphylococcal soft-tissue infection. Antimicrob Agents Chemother 6:551

Pickering LK, DuPont HL, Olarte J (1978) Single-dose tetracycline therapy for shigellosis in adults. JAMA 239:853

Pochi PE (1976) Editorial. Antibiotics in acne. N Engl J Med 294:43

Redin GS (1967) Antibacterial activity in mice of minocycline, a new tetracycline. Antimicrob Agents Chemother, p 371

Rickels FR, Klipstein FA, Tomasini J, Corcino JJ, Maldonado N (1972) Long-term follow-up of antibiotic-treated tropical sprue. Ann Intern Med 76:203

Ristuccia AM, Cunha BA (1982) Current concepts in the treatment of prostatitis. J Urol 20:338

Sack DA, Kaminsky DC, Sack RB, Itotia JN, Arthur RR, Kapikian A, Orskov F, Orskov I (1978). Prophylactic doxycycline for travelers' diarrhea. Results of a prospective double-blind study of Peace Corps Volunteers in Kenya. N Engl J Med 298:758

Schach von Wittenau, Beereboom JJ, Blackwood RK et al. (1962) 6 Deoxytetracyclines. III. Stereochemistry at C.6. J Am Chem Soc 84:2645

Schachter J (1978) Chlamydial infections (second of three parts). N Engl J Med 298:490

Smith CB, Friedewald WT, Chanock RM (1967) Shedding of *Mycoplasma pneumoniae* after tetracycline and erythromycin therapy. N Engl J Med 276:1172

Sponitz M, Rudnitzky J, Rambaud JJ (1967) Melioidosis pneumonitis. JAMA 202:950

Steigbigel NH, Reed CW, Finland M (1968) Susceptibility of common pathogenic bacteria to seven tetracycline antibiotics in vitro. Am J Med Sci 255:179

Thadepalli H, Webb D, Guang JT (1978) Anaerobic lung infections treated with doxycycline. Bull NY Acad Med 54:165

Tilton RC, Ryon RW (1978) Susceptibilities of *Pseudomonas* species to tetracycline/gentamicin and tobra. Am J Clin Pathol 69:410

Velasco JE, Miller AE, Zaias N (1972) Minocycline in the treatment of venereal disease. JAMA 220:1232

WHO (1977) *Chlamydia* surveillance. Wkly Epidem Reports 52:230

Wiesner PJ, Holmes KK, Sparling PF, Maness MJ, Bear DM, Gutman LT, Karney WW (1973) Single doses of methacycline and doxycycline for gonorrhea: a cooperative study of the frequency and cause of treatment failure. J Infect Dis 127:461

Woodward TE (1980) Rocky Mountain spotted fever. In: Isselbacher KJ, Adams RD, Braunwald E, Petersdorf R (eds) Harrision's principles of internal medicine. McGraw Hill, New York, p 750

CHAPTER 8

Nonmedical Uses of the Tetracyclines

R. H. GUSTAFSON and J. S. KISER

A. Historical

It was first reported in 1946 that an antibiotic, streptomycin, in a chick's diet could improve the rate of growth. MOORE et al. (1946) suggested that antimicrobials could inhibit certain bacterial groups which might decrease the growth of the animal. The purpose of their work with chicks was to inactivate completely all bacteria in the intestinal tract so that vitamin requirements could be studied experimentally, uncomplicated by the animals' native microflora. The implications of this observation and the potential uses of antibiotics in livestock production were largely overlooked.

In 1949, it was demonstrated that chlortetracycline at rather low levels in livestock rations beneficially affected rate of growth and feed utilization. Jukes and his group (STOKSTAD et al. 1949) were searching for low-cost sources of vitamin B_{12} for use in poultry diets. Since Lederle Laboratories were developing Aureomycin chlortetracycline for human use at that time the mash from fermentations of this antibiotic was considered as a possible source of B_{12} (JUKES 1977). The first laboratory experiments showed a remarkable and consistent improvement in growth of chicks produced by this fermentation by-product. It was quickly determined that the antibiotic residue in the mash was largely responsible for this effect.

The initial observations in chickens were confirmed and extended to swine and cattle by BARTLEY et al. (1950), CUNHA et al. (1950a), LOOSLI and WALLACE (1950), MCGINNIS et al. (1950), RUSOFF (1950), and STOKSTAD and JUKES (1950). The potential utility of these observations was immediately recognized.

Exhaustive laboratory and field experiments led to the development of Aureomycin chlortetracycline as an important tool in the rapidly changing field of animal agriculture. This was followed by similar studies for oxytetracycline, penicillin, streptomycin, and bacitracin, and these antibiotics soon became available as animal feed additives.

Within a short time it was apparent that the use of several of the growth-promoting antibiotics reduced the incidence and severity of endemic bacterial disease in livestock. This coincided with the increasing use of confinement rearing of meat animals, a trend which diminished the need for space and labor but increased the risk of debilitating infections in livestock and poultry. During the 1950s the initial high costs of feed antibiotics were sharply reduced as a consequence of improved production efficiency and the rapidly expanding market worldwide. Whereas the initial growth-promoting levels of tetracyclines ranged from 11 to 55 mg/kg feed, the declining costs made it economically practicable to use disease prevention levels as high as 220 mg/kg. Combinations of feed antimicrobials were developed and registered worldwide in order to provide broader protection against disease and to achieve maximum growth promotion and feed efficiency. In the American swine industry a current widely used combination product contains chlortetracycline at 110 mg/kg, sulfamethazine or sulfathiazole at 110 mg/kg, and penicillin at 55 mg/kg. Tylosin with sulfamethazine and penicillin with streptomycin are also antibacterials long in use as combinations in animal feeds.

B. Growth Promotion and Improved Feed Efficiency in Livestock

I. Poultry

The discovery of the property of chlortetracycline which improves the rate of weight gain and increases the amount of animal produced per kilogram of feed consumed was made by Jukes and his group when they tested the dried mash from the fermentation by *Streptomyces aureofaciens* which produced chlortetracycline (then known as Aureomycin). They discovered that this produced even better growth than that caused by liver extract, crystalline animal protein factor (APF), or vitamin B_{12} (Stokstad et al. 1949). When they tested crystalline chlortetracycline they found that it promoted growth to a greater degree than streptomycin or 3-nitro-4-hydroxyphenylarsonic acid, even in the presence of adequate vitamin B_{12} (Stokstad and Jukes 1950). The growth-promoting effect of chlortetracycline was quickly confirmed by Whitehill et al. (1950), but their results with penicillin and streptomycin were equal to those with chlortetracycline. Chloramphenicol was less effective.

The question of the mode of action of chlortetracycline has never been conclusively answered but it is probable that improvement in performance is a consequence of suppression of deleterious organisms in the animal's intestine. Bird et al. (1952) found that chicks raised in an environment where poultry had not previously been raised grew faster than similar chicks produced in an environment previously used for chick-rearing.

The addition of chlortetracycline to the ration of birds in both the "new" and "old" environments resulted in an increased rate of growth. A more direct substantiation of the theory was supplied by Sieburth et al. (1952), who fed fresh feces to turkey poults. This resulted in growth slower than that of birds not so treated. However, the addition of oxytetracycline, penicillin, or a combination of the two reversed this effect and resulted in greater growth than that of untreated controls.

It was postulated early in the use of antibiotics in animal feeds that if the growth effect was due to the suppression of deleterious organisms in the intestines of the animals that those organisms would become resistant to the antibiotic and the growth effect would be lost. Indeed, Waibel et al. (1954) noted a disappearance of the growth effect of penicillin and chlortetracycline in an "old" environment after several years of use of these antibiotics. They attributed this to possible elimination of the harmful bacteria from the environment of the chicks. LIBBY and SCHAIBLE (1955) observed that between 1950 and 1954 there was a progressive decrease in the magnitude of the growth response of birds given antibiotics compared with controls given no antibiotics but they also noted the apparent reduction in antibiotic action was a result of improved performance in the controls during these years. This suggested that in this environment the prevalence of organisms which inhibited growth may have been reduced. This was further substantiated by a decrease in mortality among these battery-raised chicks from 8.5% in 1950 to 2.8% in 1954.

HETH and BIRD (1962) compared the growth responses of chicks given chlortetracycline or oxytetracycline at 10–35 mg/kg feed in two periods, 1950–1954 and 1955–1960. The average response was 112.3% during the first period and 110.2% for the second, not a significant difference.

WAIBEL et al. (1960) compared the effectiveness of several levels of erythromycin with that of arsanilic acid, procaine penicillin, oleandomycin, a mixture of streptomycin sulfate, procaine penicillin and sulfaquinoxaline at several levels, or chlortetracycline on the growth and feed efficiency of turkey poults. Erythromycin gave a dose response, over the range of 4.4–55 mg/kg, of 5.8%–15.2%. The response to the combination of streptomycin, penicillin, and sulfaquinoxaline was flat over the range of 11–55 mg/kg but increased from 7.0% to 13.4% from 55 to 110 mg/kg. Oleandomycin and chlortetracycline both gave more than an 8% improvement in growth response while arsanilic acid and procaine penicillin each gave less than a 5% improvement. Feed efficiency was not improved by any of the treatments.

BIRD (1968) reviewed the literature on the effect of bacitracin, penicillin, oxytetracycline, and chlortetracycline on the growth and feed efficiency of chickens and concluded that there was no evidence of a trend toward decreased effectiveness of any of these four antibiotics. He particularly emphasized work which showed that the effect lasted over the entire life of the broiler rather than being confined to the first 3 or 4 weeks. The maximum effect is usually seen during the first 3 weeks with the degree of improvement somewhat reduced by the 6th–8th week of the broiler's life.

Chlortetracycline was shown to increase growth rate and efficiency of feed and energy utilization in experiments reported by BEGIN (1971). There was no effect on metabolizable energy derived from the diet or on the total intake of feed or energy. The responses were equivalent at all doses from 50 to 200 mg/kg feed. These experiments were done in facilities in which chlortetracycline had been used for many years.

Fifty-five antimicrobial substances were tested for their ability to promote growth of chickens in a series of experiments by BUNYAN et al. (1977). The substances included cephalosporins, semisynthetic penicillins, aminoglycosides, macrolides, chlor- and oxytetracyclines, as well as bacitracin, virginiamycin, flavomycin, chloramphenicol, lincomycin, novobiocin, and spectinomycin. All of the antibiotics approved for chick growth promotion in the United States were active in these tests. Chloramphenicol and novobiocin were inactive as were neomycin and kanamycin. The latter two antibiotics are aminoglycosides related to streptomycin, which was highly active.

Chlortetracycline is well known as an active chelator of calcium. Since chicken feeds contain fairly large amounts of calcium it was hypothesized that reducing the amount of calcium in the feed would increase the activity of the drug (KISER 1961). Experiments were done in which the regular feed, which contained 1.33% calcium, was replaced by a similar feed which contained only 0.21%. Chlortetracycline was added at levels of 220, 440, or 880 mg/kg and weight gains, feed consumption, and plasma concentrations were measured. Feed consumption of regular- and low-calcium feed was the same; and there was no significant difference in the gains of birds on any of the three levels of antibiotic in either feed. There was a significant increase in plasma concentration of chlortetracycline in birds on the low-calcium feed at all levels and at 24, 48, and 72 h. This increased plasma concentration was reflected in an increased survival time of birds experimentally infected with *Salmonella gallinarum*.

Recently, BIRD (1980) reviewed the literature on the use of chlortetracycline, oxytetracycline, and penicillin as growth promoters for chickens and concluded that after 30 years of use they were still effective.

II. Cattle

The ability of chlortetracycline to improve the rate of growth and reduce scouring in dairy calves was first reported in 1950. BARTLEY et al. (1950) found that chlortetracycline given at the rate of 15 mg/head per day for 42 days, by capsule, improved the weight gain of calves from birth to 42 days by 70%. They attributed this effect to prevention of scours. This work was expanded (BARTLEY et al. 1953) and the effect of withdrawing the chlortetracycline when the calves were 7 weeks of age versus continuing its use to 12 weeks of age was observed. The rate of gain of the calves decreased following withdrawal of the antibiotic.

LOOSLI and WALLACE (1950) added chlortetracycline, either as APF or as crystalline chlortetracycline, to the feed at the rate of 10 mg/kg of total dry matter. In all cases the calves on chlortetracycline gained more rapidly and had less scours than the control calves.

LASSITER (1955) reviewed the available publications and concluded that chlortetracycline was effective in improving weight gains and reducing scours in calves.

A mixture of bacitracin and penicillin proved less effective than chlortetracycline or streptomycin in improving weight gains or feed efficiency of dairy calves but it was equally effective in controlling the incidence of diarrhea (HOGUE et al. 1957).

LASSITER et al. (1957) compared the effects of chlortetracycline, erythromycin, and hygromycin on the growth rate and well-being of young dairy calves. They found that chlortetracycline and erythromycin increased the growth rate and feed consumption of the calves and reduced the incidence of scours. Hygromycin did not improve the growth rate but it decreased feed consumption. It also reduced the incidence of scours. It should be noted that the hygromycin used in this work was probably not the same as hygromycin B, which is an anthelmintic with little or no antibacterial activity.

BOLSEN et al. (1968) studied the effect of various levels of chlortetracycline on the performance of feedlot cattle being fed all concentrate rations, i.e., rations containing very high levels of energy, usually from corn or milo. The levels of chlortetracycline used were 11, 22, or 44 mg/kg ration. No liver abscesses were found in any of the animals on chlortetracycline but 5 of 30 controls had liver abscesses. The animals on chlortetracycline made better average daily weight gains than those that received no antibiotic but there was no significant difference between the gains of the animals on the higher versus the lower levels of drug.

Another experiment with heifers in a feedlot was done by UTLEY et al. (1972). They fed oxytetracycline at 75 mg/head per day or melangesterol acetate (MGA) at 0.4 mg/head per day, or a combination of the two, to heifers for 110 days. The oxytetracycline did not improve the growth rate, feed efficiency, or carcass characteristics of the cattle in this trial. The group on both oxytetracycline and MGA had a slightly better feed to gain ratio than either treatment alone.

The effect of chlortetracycline alone and in combination with various levels of copper sulfate in the feed was studied by FELSMAN et al. (1973). They found that chlortetracycline at 22 mg/kg feed of calves fed from less than a week of age to 98 days produced a better rate of gain than in those not given chlortetracycline. Calves getting both copper and chlortetracycline grew at the same rate or more slowly than those getting chlortetracycline alone.

In 1977, MORRILL et al. (1977) investigated the effect of oxytetracycline on the growth rate of calves with or without milk fermented by two *Lactobacillus* species ("probiotics"). Low levels of antibiotics had been used in the feed of calves at this location for many years. In these trials the calves fed the antibiotic gained faster, consumed more calf starter, and had firmer feces than those without antibiotic. This was not true of calves that were given the "probiotics."

III. Horses

TAYLOR et al. (1954) showed that chlortetracycline, given at the rate of 100 mg/foal per day from birth to 3 months of age and 200 mg/foal per day from 3 to 9 months of age resulted in an increase of more than 10% in absolute rate of growth. The improvement in rate of growth was even more impressive when expressed as the relative growth rate, which takes into account the weight at birth. In this case the improvement was more than 30% for the first 21 weeks and 27% for 39 weeks.

IV. Swine

1. Effect on Growth and Feed Efficiency

JUKES et al. (1950) were the first to show that chlortetracycline in the feed of young pigs would significantly improve the rate of growth. They also noted that scours, of undetermined etiology, occurred in control but not in medicated pigs and that the rate of weight gain was highest in the pigs receiving the largest amount of chlortetracycline. CARPENTER (1950a) made much the same observations and he also observed that the feed efficiency of the pigs on chlortetracycline was improved. CATRON (1950a) and CUFF et al. (1950) emphasized the decrease in scouring and improvement in growth rate of runt pigs. CUNHA et al. (1949, 1950a, 1950b) reported results similar to those of JUKES. They also stated that penicillin did not stimulate growth of the pigs and that streptomycin was less effective than chlortetracycline. WHITEHAIR et al. (1951) fed groups of pigs with persistent diarrhea of undetermined etiology with feed containing chlortetracycline, streptomycin, penicillin, or APF (containing chlortetracycline). The performance of all the medicated pigs was improved and mortality was reduced. SPEER et al. (1950) reported that healthy pigs under good management conditions showed less response to chlortetracycline in the feed than did less healthy pigs under less optimal management. CATRON et al. (1951) was able to demonstrate that increasing levels of chlortetracycline resulted in increasing rates of gain and feed efficiency. TERRILL et al. (1952) compared chlortetracycline with bacitracin for effect on rate of gain and feed efficiency. Chlortetracycline at 1 mg/kg feed gave significantly better rates of gain and feed efficiency than bacitracin at the same level. A review of the value of antibiotics by BRAUDE et al. (1953) summarized the work to that time and clearly demonstrated the value of chlortetracycline in improving the performance of swine.

ELLIOTT et al. (1964) showed that the addition of sulfamethazine, 100 g, and penicillin G (as procaine penicillin), 50 g, to chlortetracycline, 110 mg/kg feed, further improved the performance of young pigs. In one experiment the pigs were inoculated with a culture of *Salmonella choleraesuis* var. *kunzendorf* and two groups were given feed medicated with the combination either 7 days before or at the time of inoculation. Both groups of medicated pigs grew faster than nonmedicated, noninoculated controls and the group given medicated feed before inoculation demonstrated better feed efficiency than the nonmedicated, noninoculated group.

In 1966, TEAGUE et al. (1966) summarized the results of 25 experiments done at one location during the period from the fall of 1950 to the summer of 1963. In only four experiments did chlortetracycline fail to increase the rate of gain of the pigs by 2%–12% and in four experiments it failed to increase feed efficiency by 1%–8%; but in only one experiment did it fail to increase one or the other of these parameters. It was hypothesized, early in the use of antibiotics, that improvement in the performance of pigs was due to the suppression of certain elements of the microbial flora and that in time this effect would disappear because of development of antibiotic resistance. The work of TEAGUE et al. (1966) suggests that antibiotic efficacy had been maintained.

A more recent study (CLAWSEN and ALSMEYER 1973) showed that oxytetracycline at 330 g/ton feed, alone or in combination with neomycin at the same level, and the combination of chlortetracycline 110 g, sulfathiazole 110 g, and penicillin 55 mg/kg feed were effective in improving the rate of weight gain and feed efficiency of young pigs. This advantage was usually maintained to market weight when the drugs were withdrawn from the feed after being fed for 4 or 5 weeks. In another experiment WAHLSTROM and LIBAL (1975) fed pigs furazolidone 165 mg, oxytetracycline 110 mg, and arsanilic acid 99 mg/kg feed or chlortetracycline 110 mg, sulfamethazine 110 mg, and penicillin 55 mg/kg feed for 37 days. Both combinations significantly improved rates of weight gain and feed efficiency during the medication period. In general, pigs given medicated feed during the earlier part of the trial continued to gain faster than controls after the drugs were withdrawn.

2. Effect on Reproduction

CARPENTER (1950 b) studied the effect of chlortetracycline in the feed of gestating and lactating sows. He found that pigs from sows given chlortetracycline during the 56-day lactation period averaged 44% heavier at weaning than control pigs.

MESSERSMITH et al. (1966) did two series of experiments to determine the effect of feeding chlortetracycline at high levels during the prebreeding and breeding period. In the first series of experiments sows were fed 440 mg chlortetracycline/kg feed, equivalent to about 1 g/head per day for periods ranging from 32 to 64 days. Sixty-two percent of the control sows farrowed versus 99% of the treated group. In the second series of experiments, in which sows were given feed with 220 mg chlortetracycline/kg, equivalent to 0.5 g/sow per day, 74% of control sows farrowed versus 86% of the treated group. There were no significant differences in average litter size between control and treated sows in either series of experiments nor were the number of stillborn pigs or those dying within the first 3 weeks significantly different between control and treated animals.

RUIZ et al. (1968) studied the effect of a combination of chlortetracycline 0.5 g, sulfamethazine 0.5 g, and penicillin 0.25 g/sow per day for a 4-week period starting 1 week before and continuing for 3 weeks during the breeding period. They found that the antibiotic-treated sows farrowed more pigs than the nontreated group and that both the conception rate and farrowing rate were significantly improved. They also attempted to learn whether the antibiotic treatment would change the vaginal microflora of the sows. The bacteria studied were hemolytic and nonhemolytic micrococci, nonhemolytic streptococci and *Corynebacterium* spp., alpha- and beta-hemolytic streptococci and *Corynebacterium* spp., *Bacillus* spp., and *Escherichia coli*. The methods used failed to reveal any changes in the vaginal population of these organisms.

A comprehensive study was conducted under the direction of Dr. Virgil Hays at the University of Kentucky to learn the influence of chlortetracycline in the feed on the reproductive performance of swine and on the incidence and persistence of antibiotic-resistant enteric bacteria (LANGLOIS et al. 1978). This study involved two sow herds in different locations. One herd received no antibiotic for any purpose for a period of more than 3½ years. The other was given 110 mg chlortetracycline/kg feed continuously. The breeding record of the herd not given antibiotics was available for a previous 9-year period during which antibiotics had been used. Compared with the average performance over this 9-year period, after antibiotic withdrawal the conception rate, litter size at birth and weaning, pig survival, and average pig weight at weaning declined linearly with time. Postweaning gains of pigs were also significantly less when antibiotics were not fed. Litter size at birth and at weaning was greater in the herd given antibiotics than in that not given antibiotics. These authors used a disk method for measuring sensitivity to chlortetracycline and it was found that more than 90% of the enteric bacteria isolated from the pigs on chlortetracycline were resistant to the drug, but approximately 50% of isolates continued to be resistant to chlortetracycline after the pigs had received no antibiotic for 42 months.

C. Disease Prevention Effects of Chlortetracycline and Oxytetracycline

I. Poultry

1. Mycoplasma

Mycoplasma gallisepticum is one component of a combination of infectious agents which causes chronic respiratory disease (CRD, air sac disease) of chickens and infectious sinusitis of turkeys. The other components are *E. coli* and infectious bronchitis virus. CRD is characterized by a very high morbidity within a flock. Mortality is usually low but may be very high in young broilers where all three organisms are present. Symptoms within a flock may be mild or severe but the disease may cause substantial economic loss due to retarded growth, poor feed conversion, and downgrading or condemnation of carcasses.

The tetracyclines are effective in control of mycoplasmal infections. A substantial degree of control has been achieved by serological testing of flocks used to produce eggs for hatching of broilers. Serologically positive birds are eliminated until a serologically negative flock is obtained. This technique has been successful in eliminating the disease in both chicken and turkey flocks (YODER 1978).

Mycoplasma meleagridis causes an air sac infection in young poults. The disease is very widespread but less serious than that caused by *M. gallisepticum*. The most effective control measure is to inject the small end of the embryonated egg with a solution containing a combination of gentamicin and tylosin (YAMAMOTO 1978).

WONG and JAMES (1953) showed that chlortetracycline and oxytetracycline were active against *M. gallisepticum*, the agent of infectious sinusitis of turkeys, which had just been isolated and identified at that time. Similar results were obtained by GROSS and JOHNSON (1953) with organisms from both chickens and turkeys. These results of in ovo tests were confirmed and extended in vivo by WHITE-STEVENS and ZEIBEL (1954). In field trials involving several thousand birds, chlortetracycline in the feed resulted in higher final weights and better feed efficiency than in untreated birds, both in experimentally and naturally infected flocks.

Spiramycin, leucomycin, and erythromycin were compared with chlortetracycline for their ability to control an experimental *M. gallisepticum* infection in chicks when given orally (KISER et al. 1960). It was found that spiramycin was more effective than chlortetracycline or leucomycin. Erythromycin was the least effective. In later experiments WHITEHILL and KISER (1961) compared the effectiveness of oxytetracycline, chlortetracycline, dimethylchlortetracycline, and tetracycline against an experimental infection with *M. gallisepticum* in chicks and found chlortetracycline and dimethylchlortetracycline to be superior to the other two drugs. GROSS (1961) compared the effect of chlortetracycline, erythromycin, and two nitrofurans on an experimental "air sac disease." He found that the nitrofurans were effective in controlling the *E. coli* component of the infection but that chlortetracycline and erythromycin were not. They were effective in reducing the severity of lesions due to the pleuropneumonia-like organism (PPLO) (*M. gallisepticum*) component of the infection. Furaltadone had little effect on this component. GALE et al. (1967) reported on a series of experiments in which they compared tylosin and spiramycin with chlortetracycline in the feed against an infection with *M. gallisepticum* and/or *E. coli* in chicks. The *M. gallisepticum* infection alone was not highly lethal but reduced growth significantly. The *E. coli* infection was both lethal and retarded growth significantly among survivors. Tylosin and spiramycin were only slightly effective against the combined infections but chlortetracycline was highly effective. These authors also described experiments in turkey poults infected with two strains of *M. gallisepticum* and treated with subcutaneous injections of oxytetracycline, tetracycline, streptomycin, or tylosin. One strain, of turkey origin, was well controlled by the tetracyclines but neither streptomycin nor tylosin were effective. The other strain, of chicken origin, was well controlled by tylosin but less so by the tetracyclines.

Mycoplasma synoviae produces a subclinical upper respiratory infection which, under unknown conditions, may become systemic and result in an acute or chronic synovitis of chickens or turkeys. It involves primarily the synovial membranes of joints and tendon sheats, causing lameness – hence failure of the birds to eat properly – and resulting in poor growth and feed efficiency. Infected birds may be identified serologically but it is economically impractical to produce serologically negative flocks as is done with *M. gallisepticum*. Some broiler breeder flocks have been freed of *M. synoviae* by injecting the hatching eggs with tylosin or by heat treatment to prevent transmission of the organism through the egg. There is no satisfactory method of clearing the disease from turkey flocks (OLSON 1978).

SHELTON and OLSON (1959) found that chlortetracycline was more efficient than either oxytetracycline or tetracycline in controlling experimental infectious synovitis when given orally but that the effects of chlortetracycline and oxytetracycline were more nearly equal when they were administered intraperitoneally. OLSON and SAHU (1976) measured the efficacy of chlortetracycline at 55, 110, or 220 mg/kg feed against strains of *M. synoviae* isolated in the period 1954–1955 compared with the efficacy against strains isolated in 1963–1973. The 55-mg/kg level prevented mortality by all strains and reduced morbidity. The higher levels controlled mortality and morbidity, cleared the chicks of the organism, but did not entirely prevent lesions, especially in birds infected with strains isolated during the later period. Positive agglutination tests, reflecting the development of immunity, occurred almost entirely in birds on the two lower levels of antibiotic.

A study of the effect of a low-calcium diet on the control of *M. gallisepticum* infection by chlortetracycline was reported by HEISHMAN et al. (1962). The levels used in an attempt to clear the birds of the infectious agent were very high, 1,100 or 1,650 mg/kg feed, but the 0.85% calcium in the feed might have reduced the effectiveness of the antibiotic. The highest level of chlortetracycline was effective in shortening the time of infection, as was the lower level when fed for 5–6 weeks of the 10-week experimental period, but when fed for 3–4 weeks there was an increase in the number of isolations when the drug was withdrawn. The final weight of the medicated birds was higher than that of infected, nonmedicated birds in all cases. It has been shown (GALE and BAUGHN 1965) that the addition of 1.5% sodium sulfate to a broiler feed containing 1.3% calcium will increase chlortetracycline blood levels over the range from 27.5 to 440 mg/kg. This increase in antibiotic absorption could be significant in controlling disease as was shown in an experimental *M. gallisepticum* infection in chicks. Levels of 27.5–440 mg/kg chlortetracycline with 1.5% sodium sulfate increased weight gain over similar levels without sodium sulfate. Presumably the sodium sulfate acted by forming insoluble calcium sulfate in the chicks gut, thus allowing better absorption of the chlortetracycline.

The emergence of resistance to streptomycin, spiramycin, and chlortetracycline by *M. gallisepticum* in ovo was investigated by KISER et al. (1961). They found that resistance to streptomycin emerged rapidly, in about 5 passages, and that resistance to spiramycin emerged in about 10 passages but that resistance to chlortetracycline did not appear during 15 passages of *M. gallisepticum* in embryonated eggs.

2. Pasteurellosis

Pasteurella multocida is the etiological agent of avian pasteurellosis, also known as fowl cholera. Chickens, turkeys, and ducks are susceptible as are sparrows, robins, starlings, and crows. It was more prevalent in the 1940s than after the improvement of management practices and the more widespread use of antibiotics in the feed. The organism is usually transmitted by feed or water contaminated by mucus from the mouth or upper respiratory passages of infected birds. It may also be introduced into a flock by other farm animals, especially pigs or cats, or by infected crates or other equipment. It is not transmitted in ovo (HEDDLESTON and RHOADES 1978).

LITTLE (1948) was the first to show that chlortetracycline in the feed was effective in reducing mortality due to experimental *P. multocida* infection in chicks. DONAHUE and OLSON (1972) showed that *P. multocida* of turkey origin was sensitive in vitro to chlor- and oxytetracycline, erythromycin, novobiocin, and penicillin among the drugs permitted in feed. WALSER and DAVIS (1975) confirmed the work of DONAHUE and OLSON using field isolates of *P. multocida* from Georgia turkeys. OLSON (1977a) tested the effectiveness of chlortetracycline in the feed at 0.0055% and of Rofenaid at 0.01% in vaccinated and unvaccinated birds against *P. multocida* in turkeys. Both vaccination and medication were effective in reducing mortality. In another experiment turkeys were given *P. multocida* in the drinking water while they were on feed containing chlortetracycline at 55, 110, or 220 mg/kg. The inoculated medicated birds showed reduced mortality and improved weight gain compared with the noninoculated, nonmedicated birds (OLSON 1977b).

Transferable antibiotic resistance occurs rarely in *Pasteurella* but CURTIS and OLLERHEAD (1979) reported transferable tetracycline resistance in *P. multocida* isolated from an outbreak of fowl cholera in turkeys.

II. Ducks

1. Pasteurellosis

Pasteurellosis in ducks may be caused by *P. anatipestifer* as well as by *P. multocida*. This disease was diagnosed in semi-wild, pen-raised mallard ducks in South Carolina. A fatal *Pasteurella* meningitis was adequately controlled by chlortetracycline in the mash at 550 mg/kg for 7 days (ELEAZER et al. 1973). However, chlortetracycline at 0.044% in the diet was ineffective in controlling an experimental infection with *P. anatipestifer* in white Pekin ducklings. Novobiocin at 0.0386% or spectinomycin at 0.022% or a combination of lincomycin at 0.011% and spectinomycin at 0.022% in the feed were very effective (SANDHU and DEAN 1980).

III. Chickens

1. Escherichia coli Infections

Escherichia infections are usually associated with *M. gallisepticum* infections but they may occasionally occur alone as acute, fulminating septicemias in very young birds. Only a relatively small number of serotypes are highly pathogenic for chicks. Three serotypes used in an experimental infection to test the efficacy of drugs in feed were: O2a : K1 : H5, O78 : K80 : H9, and O10 : K? : H7. These three serotypes produced a high incidence of fatal infections when introduced into the thoracic air sacs of 2-week-old chicks. Furazolidone at 0.011% or 0.022% in the feed satisfactorily controlled these infections. The protection afforded by chlortetracycline at 550 mg/kg or oxytetracycline at 220 mg/kg was less satisfactory (HEBERT and CHANG 1969).

Another study involved experimental infection of 7-day-old chicks in the post-thoracic air sac with a culture of *E. coli* O2 : K1 : H5. Since this experiment was designed to test the effect of feeding low levels of chlortetracycline on subsequent treatment of an experimental infection with the same drug, the chicks were given chlortetracycline 55 mg/kg for 7 days, they were infected, and when the infection was established they were treated with chlortetracycline at 220 mg/kg, chloromycetin at 110 mg/kg, or ampicillin at 440 mg/kg. Previous treatment with low-level chlortetracycline did not reduce the effectiveness of subsequent treatment with the same or other antibiotics. Treatment with ampicillin at 440 mg/kg was more effective and with chloramphenicol at 110 mg/kg was less effective than treatment with chlortetracycline at 220 mg/kg (FAGERBERG et al. 1978).

IV. Cattle

1. Rumenitis-Liver Abscess Complex

This syndrome is frequently found in beef cattle in feedlots. It is a sequence of acute inflammation of the forestomachs, due to mechanical injury or, usually, excess lactic acid formed when cattle are shifted too quickly from a diet high in roughage to one high in grain. This inflammation is accompanied by penetration of the stomach wall by *Fusobacterium necrophorum*, which then establishes itself in the liver, causing abscesses. These abscesses may be chronic, in which case the animals grow more slowly and consume more feed per kilogram of gain. Considerable economic loss results from condemnation of livers, poor performance, or significant mortality. In acute cases there may be high mortality, as much as 50% of affected animals (JENSEN and MACKEY 1979c).

Chlortetracycline at 70 mg/head per day in the feed reduces the incidence of liver abscesses in feedlot cattle. FLINT and JENSEN (1958) attained reductions of 20%–90% in incidence of infections. FURR and CARPENTER (1967) and FURR et al. (1968a, b) and HARVEY et al. (1968) achieved similar results.

Overall a reduction of about 65% was achieved. Higher levels, 140 or 280 mg/head per day, yielded better results (AMERICAN CYANAMID TECHNICAL INFORMATION BULLETIN 25-3, 11/75). BROWN et al. (1975) also showed that chlortetracycline at 70 mg/head per day or tylosin at 75 mg/head per day would reduce the incidence of liver abscesses and improve the growth and feed efficiency of feedlot cattle.

2. Shipping Fever Pneumonia

Shipping fever pneumonia is an acute respiratory disease of young cattle. The etiology is complex and includes a myxovirus and *P. hemolytica* or *P. multocida*. Stress from shipping, vaccination, castration, dehorning, temperature extremes, and feed and water deprivation may precipitate the disease. Shipping fever is probably the most important disease of feedlot cattle in the United States. It reduces growth rate and feed efficiency and may cause the death of as many as 20% of affected animals. The most frequent victims are calves following weaning and young cattle shortly after they have been received in feedlots (JENSEN and MACKEY 1979b). Incidence of the disease may be reduced by feeding chlortetracycline or oxytetracycline at the rate of 350 mg/head per day for 28 days or 350 mg chlortetracycline and 350 mg sulfamethazine/head per day for 28 days (PERRY et al. 1971). PERRY (1980) cited seven studies in which daily gain was improved an average of 23% and feed efficiency was improved an average of 19% by feeding the same combination for 29 days. WOODS et al. (1973) compared the combination of chlortetracycline and sulfamethazine with an antiserum. The medicated ration and the antiserum, alone or in combination, were effective in preventing clinical disease but the calves given the medicated feed showed the best weight gains.

3. Foot Rot

Foot rot is an acute or chronic infection of the interdigital and coronary skin of cattle, caused by *Fusobacterium necrophorum,* usually with other bacterial species. It results in lameness, caused by swelling and necrosis of the tissues. This results in loss of appetite and therefore failure to grow at a normal rate. Feed efficiency is also impaired.

Chlortetracycline fed at 70 mg/head per day to cattle weighing up to 318 kg or 100 mg/head per day for cattle weighing more than 318 kg will greatly reduce or completely prevent foot rot. In one study (JOHNSON et al. 1957) there were 172 cases of foot rot in 681 untreated cattle and only 2 in 684 cattle treated with chlortetracycline.

4. Anaplasmosis

Anaplasmosis is an infection of the red blood cells of cattle by *Anaplasma marginale*. This organism is considered by JENSEN and MACKEY (1979a) to be a rickettsia but it has also been considered to be a protozoan. It is characterized by anemia which, especially in older animals, may be fatal. It is transmitted by ticks, by biting flies, or by use of contaminated hypodermic needles or surgical instruments. Young animals may show little evidence of infection but may become carriers.

The spread of infection within a herd may be prevented by feeding chlortetracycline at 1.1 mg/kg body weight per day during the fly and tick season (BROCK et al. 1957). The recommended level is 350 mg/head per day for cattle weighing less than 318 kg, 500 mg/head per day for cattle weighing 318–454 kg, and 1.1 mg/kg b.w. per day for those weighing 454–680 kg. The carrier state of anaplasmosis may be eliminated by feeding chlortetracycline at the rate of 12.1 mg/kg b.w. per day for 60 days (FRANKLIN et al. 1965, TWIEHAUS and ANTHONY 1963). RICHEY et al. (1977) succeeded in eliminating the carrier or latent infection by feeding chlortetracycline at 1.1 mg/kg b.w. per day for 120 days. SWEET and STAUBER (1978) achieved the same effect with 11 mg chlortetracycline/kg b.w. per day for 45 days.

5. Leptospirosis

Leptospira pomona is the usual cause of the disease in cattle. Leptospirosis does not appear to be much of a problem in cattle in the United States at this time. It may be spread in urine to cattle from swine or deer as well as within a herd by carrier cattle. The principal economic loss is due to abortions and decreased milk yields. The mortality rate is low.

Chlortetracycline has been shown to be quite effective in ovo against *L. pomona (*KISER et al. 1958). RINGEN and OKAZAKI (1958) showed that chlortetracycline at 1.1 mg/kg b.w. per day would prevent infection of calves with *L. pomona,* but would allow development of immunity; 0.22 mg/kg b.w. per day was ineffective.

V. Sheep

An early study (COLBY et al. 1950) suggested that chlortetracycline would be poorly tolerated by sheep. Later studies have failed to confirm this early finding, which was based on dosing by capsule rather than in the feed. Significant disease prevention properties for chlortetracycline in sheep have been reported.

1. Enterotoxemia

Enterotoxemia or "overeating disease" may cause significant losses in lambs in a feedlot. JOHNSON et al. (1956) showed that 55 mg chlortetracycline/kg feed fed for 21 days followed by 22 mg/kg for 27 days or 22 mg/kg throughout the feeding period prevented enterotoxemia in lambs in a feedlot. When the chlortetracycline was discontinued at the end of the first 21 days significant losses occurred.

2. Vibrionic Abortion

Campylobacter (Vibrio) fetus is an important cause of abortion in ewes. FRANK et al. (1958) showed that chlortetracycline at 80 mg/head per day would greatly reduce the incidence of abortion in artificially infected ewes. In a later study FRANK et al. (1959) confirmed their earlier results and showed that ewes given a suspension of *V. fetus*-infected tissue while receiving chlortetracycline in the feed would acquire immunity to a later infection with the same organism.

3. Pneumonia

A study by CREMPION et al. (1973) showed that chlortetracycline or a combination of chlortetracycline and sulfamethazine was effective in reducing mortality in lambs in a feedlot and later on range when given at the rate of 100 mg/head per day or 100 mg each drug/head per day. The lambs receiving medicated feed showed greater weight gains than those not so treated.

4. Ovine Coccidiosis

AJAYI and TODD (1977) fed a combination of chlortetracycline and sulfamethazine at levels of 100 or 500 mg/head per day of the combination to lambs experimentally infected with a mixed coccidial inoculum. A partial resistance to the coccidia developed in nonmedicated lambs and lambs given the lower dose of drug. The infection was suppressed to such an extent in the group given the higher dose that they failed to develop immunity and died after the drug was withdrawn.

VI. Swine

1. Swine Enzootic Pneumonia

Mycoplasma hyopneumoniae is the principal etiological agent of swine enzootic pneumonia. It is the opinion of SWITZER and ROSS (1975) that this may be the most important disease of swine in the world. The organism apparently effects only swine and is probably transmitted by aerosol from sow to pigs. The disease is most severe in young pigs 3–10 weeks of age. Mortality from the uncomplicated disease is usually low but morbidity within a herd may be high. The disease is much more severe if it is complicated by infection with *P. hemolytica* or *P. multocida*. It will also be potentiated by ascarid larvae migrating through the lungs or in animals infected with lungworms.

Chlortetracycline, at levels of 55–110 mg/kg feed, prevented the occurrence of lesions of swine enzootic pneumonia (SEP) in experimentally inoculated pigs. Tylosin and erythromycin failed to prevent lesion development (HUHN 1971 a). In another study HUHN (1971 b) showed that chlortetracycline at 400 mg/kg feed would not prevent infection of very young pigs but would suppress lesions of SEP. EGGERT et al. (1980) experimentally challenged young pigs that were being given feed with 55, 110, or 220 ppm chlortetracycline with *M. hyopneumoniae*. The 110- and 220-ppm levels maintained weight gains and feed efficiency at or above the rate of nonchallenged, nonmedicated controls but the percentage of pigs with negative complement fixation titers to *M. hyopneumoniae* was higher in the pigs on 110 ppm than in the nonchallenged controls. In five field trials chlortetracycline at 220 ppm in the feed was shown to be effective in controlling SEP.

2. Atrophic Rhinitis

Atrophic rhinitis, caused by *Bordetella bronchiseptica*, is very widespread in the United States and elsewhere. It is not fatal but may cause a serious retardation of growth and may predispose the animals to respiratory disease; hence it is of considerable economic consequence (SWITZER and FARRINGTON 1975).

In 1956 GOUGE et al. (1956) reported that the use of 55–220 g chlortetracycline/kg feed would improve the rate of weight gain and feed efficiency of pigs naturally infected with atrophic rhinitis. SWITZER (1963) found that pigs naturally infected with *Bordetella bronchiseptica* had reduced symptoms of atrophic rhinitis when given a mixture of chlortetracycline 110 mg, sulfamethazine 110 mg, and penicillin G (as procaine penicillin) 55 mg/kg feed. When chlortetracycline and sulfamethazine were tried separately it was found that sulfamethazine but not chlortetracycline would clear *B. bronchiseptica* from the nasal passages of the pigs. Performance data for these pigs were not obtained. WOODS et al. (1972) found that *B. bronchiseptica* was not isolated from pigs fed the combination of chlortetracycline, sulfamethazine, and penicillin. *Mycoplasma hyorhinis* was not found in the pigs receiving high levels of chlortetracycline but was found in all the other groups.

3. Cervical Abscesses

Cervical abscesses are usually caused by a *Streptococcus pyogenes* group E. These abscesses are rarely fatal but will cause a decrease in rate of weight gain and feed efficiency. The most readily observable loss is due to the condemnation of the heads of the pigs at slaughter. GOUGE et al. (1957) showed that chlortetracycline at 55 mg/kg feed would prevent an experimental infection with *S. pyogenes* group E. These experimental results were later confirmed by field experiments which showed that 55–110 g chlortetracycline/kg feed would greatly decrease or completely prevent the occurrence of cervical abscesses and improve the rate of weight gain and feed efficiency (GOUGE et al. 1958).

4. Leptospirosis

Leptospirosis in swine may be more prevalent than is usually thought because the disease is usually mild and of short duration. The problem is that infected animals frequently become carriers and shed leptospires in the urine. The organism infects the animal by way of breaks in the skin or through the mucous membranes of the conjunctiva. The disease in swine is usually caused by *Leptospira pomona* and may spread to swine from cattle, sheep, goats, and horses and from wildlife, e.g., deer, skunks, opossums, or rodents. The principal economic loss is caused by abortion of infected sows or pigs that are stillborn or die within a few days of birth. The organism may also be spread to humans (HANSON and FERGUSON 1975).

FERGUSON et al. (1956) showed that chlortetracycline at 440 mg/kg feed would prevent abortion due to leptospira in pregnant sows and prevent spread of the disease in a herd. Howarth (1956) was able to abolish the carrier state in an infected herd by use of 440 g chlortetracycline/kg feed for 14 days. Two hundred and twenty milligrams per kilogram will aid in preventing the spread of the disease within a herd.

D. Public Health Considerations

I. Epidemiology of Antibiotic Resistance

The wisdom of using tetracycline antibiotics in animal feeds has been questioned because of potential public health risks. Fundamental to this issue is an assessment of the possibility that the large pool of antibiotic-resistant bacteria in animals is an important source of antibiotic resistance in human clinical medicine. Practical considerations include whether or not government restrictions on feed antibiotics could help preserve antibiotic effectiveness in humans.

In the early 1960s, it was first appreciated that antibiotic resistance could be transferred from one bacterium to another (Watanabe 1963). This is accomplished by the passage of genetic material between bacterial cells.

Resistance plasmids or R-factors are small circular strands of DNA varying in size but often sufficiently large to carry genetic determinants specifying resistance to several antimicrobial agents. The plasmid DNA replicates in much the same manner as the host cells' chromosomal DNA and cell division yields plasmid-bearing daughter cells resistant to one or more antimicrobials. In the presence of inhibitory levels of tetracyclines, bacteria resistant to tetracyclines possess a selective advantage over antibiotic-sensitive bacteria. Because resistance to several antibiotics may be genetically controlled on a single plasmid, an antibiotic such as a tetracycline may select for resistance to several unrelated antimicrobial agents. The public health implications of this phenomenon were immediately apparent. Multiple antibiotic resistance may be achieved not by a very rare series of independent mutations in the same organism, but by the single transfer of genes specifying resistance to several antimicrobial agents. Without doubt, the frequent appearance of multiple resistance in human bacterial pathogens limits the practitioners' choice of drugs and often makes it necessary to conduct careful antibiotic sensitivity determinations before a rational course of treatment may be prescribed.

It was known quite early in the history of animal feed antibiotics that their use provided a selective pressure for antibiotic resistance in the animal's gut microflora. The immediate concern was that the improvements in growth promotion and feed efficiency would quickly be lost because of the development of such resistance. This proved not to be the case and systematic comparisons of tetracycline effects in livestock over a period of many years confirmed that improvements in growth and feed utilization were maintained (Bird 1980; Heth and Bird 1962; Teague et al. 1966; Begin 1971). During the same period, progress in genetics, nutrition, control of pathogenic protozoa, and advances in general husbandry provided similar improvements in the efficiency of meat production. As the use of feed antibiotics in livestock and poultry production became more widespread, the potential public health consequences of this practice began to be considered. It was appreciated that tetracyclines and other antimicrobials increased antibiotic resistance in the microflora of meat animals. The public health questions most often asked were, "Does this practice ultimately influence antibiotic resistance in bacteria isolated from humans?" and if it does, "Is there a reduced effectiveness of antibacterial therapy in humans because of this practice?" Complicating the answer to these questions was the undeniable influence of therapeutic uses in animals and humans on the development of antibiotic resistance in general. Nevertheless, it seemed important to try to determine whether livestock and poultry provided significant sources of antibiotic resistance which interfered with the treatment of bacterial infections in humans.

The possibility was considered that the food chain provided a source of resistant animal bacteria that could be inadvertently consumed by people eating meat. Evidence existed to show that meat products and eggs had frequently provided *Salmonella* sufficient to produce gastroenteritis in humans (CENTERS FOR DISEASE CONTROL 1981).

Since *Salmonella* is found with irregular frequency in humans and animals, it is not a part of the normal gut microflora. In contrast, *E. coli* is a commensal found consistently in the gut of mature animals and man although this organism usually represents less than 0.1% of the organisms in the large intestine (SAVAGE 1980). Since *E. coli* from livestock frequently carried transmissible plasmids with antibiotic resistance genes (R-factors), this easily isolated species was a logical subject for investigation in the effort to study the epidemiology of antibiotic resistance.

SMITH (1969) carried out a series of experiments in England which had clear relevance to the question of transfer of *E. coli* and R-factors from animals to man. He was able to isolate antibiotic-sensitive hemolytic *E. coli* from a human, prepare a nalidixic acid (NA)-resistant mutant of the strain, and establish the mutant as the dominant *E. coli* in the same human. Thus, an essentially native coliform strain could serve as a potential plasmid recipient in vivo and could be easily isolated on medium containing nalidixic acid. The human volunteer consumed 24-h broth cultures of plasmid-bearing *E. coli* isolated from a pig, ox, fowl, and human. The exposure varied from a single dose of 10^4 to daily doses of 10^9 colony forming units (cfu) for 7 days. SMITH demonstrated that when the largest numbers of animal *E. coli* were used, plasmid transfer to the resident NA-resistant *E. coli* could be demonstrated, but in extremely low numbers. Neither the plasmids which transferred to the resident strain in vivo nor the animal *E. coli* persisted for more than a few days. SMITH concluded that the amount of animal *E. coli* needed to demonstrate in vivo R-factor transfer in these experiments was far above the numbers that human beings would be expected to consume under natural conditions. He cautioned that although these were data collected from a few *E. coli* strains in a single individual, they did not indicate that animals are an important source of resistant *E. coli* for man.

Similar experiments have been conducted in which large numbers of animal *E. coli* have been deliberately consumed by volunteers and then monitored to determine whether they persist for an extended period in the human gut. COOKE et al. (1972) worked with three volunteers and twelve *E. coli* strains. Eight of the strains were of human origin and four were from animals. In twelve experiments with the animal *E. coli*, the organism in general persisted for short periods. The one exception was an experiment in which 10^{11} freeze-dried bovine *E. coli* were ingested in a capsule and the organism was isolated from the volunteer for 120 days. The remaining 11 experiments with animal *E. coli* resulted in shedding for an average of 6 days following dosages ranging from 10^5 to 10^{11}.

Generally, studies reporting accidental ingestion of animal *E. coli* by humans have confirmed that persistence is of short duration. LEVY et al. (1976) reported studies with 11 members of a farm family. Two *E. coli* strains isolated from chicks were used as recipients of a temperature-sensitive chloramphenicol-resistance plasmid. The chick *E. coli* bearing the new plasmid was introduced into the chicks by cloacal gavage. Subsequently, the plasmid-marked *E. coli* was isolated from a young family member 2 days after exposure and from one of the laboratory workers who had handled the animals. In the latter case the positive sample was taken a week after exposure to the chicks. Isolation in each case was on one occasion. Curiously, the plasmid isolated from the family member was no longer transferable nor did it bear specificity for tetracycline resistance, part of the original antibiogram.

LINTON et al. (1977) reported the results of studies in which five volunteers handled, cooked, and consumed 15 chickens obtained commercially. Extensive *E. coli* serotyping and plasmid identification studies strongly support the suggestion that on one of the 15 occasions, *E. coli* from a chicken carcass was inadvertently ingested. Two of the chick *E. coli* strains were excreted by the volunteer for a short period, with one of them persisting for 10 days.

Another approach in examining the potential transfer of plasmid-bearing bacteria between animals and humans has been to compare *E. coli* serotypes in humans and animals. BETTELHEIM et al. (1974) examined *E. coli* serotypes from 55 humans, 67 animals, and 48 samples of meat. They reported sharp differences in serotype distribution found in strains from man and animals. They concluded that "The results suggest either that animal strains of *E. coli* are not reaching the general human population outside hospital to any great extent, or, if they do so, are failing to implant in the bowel."

II. Salmonella

1. Poultry

a) Salmonellosis-Paratyphoid Infections

Paratyphoid infections of poultry are defined as infections with any of the motile salmonellae, i.e., infections with *Salmonella gallinarum*, which causes fowl typhoid, and *S. pullorum*, which causes pullorum disease, are excluded. These two species are quite host specific and are nonmotile. Paratyphoid infections of poultry are of considerable economic and public health concern. They occur worldwide and may be spread from poultry and poultry products to humans.

The disease manifestation in humans is usually an acute gastroenteritis but it may cause a serious septicemic disease, especially in the very young, the very old, or persons whith impaired immunity. The disease in young birds may be very severe, with high mortality. In older birds the infection may be asymptomatic but the birds may spread the infection to other birds, the environment, and other animals. Salmonellae are ubiquitous and infect both warm- and cold-blooded animals and insects.

Salmonella typhimurium, S. infantis, and *S. heidelberg* were the serotypes most frequently isolated from chickens; and *S. heidelberg, S. saint-paul,* and *S. anatum* were most frequently isolated from turkeys as reported to the Centers for Disease Control in 1978 (CDC 1981) of the United States Public Health Service.

In 1971 SOJKA et al. (1974) conducted a survey in England of salmonella cultures isolated from cattle (1,333), sheep (295), pigs (83), poultry (409), and other animals and miscellaneous sources (132), a total of 2,252 isolates of 43 serotypes. They found that the serotypes most frequently isolated from poultry were *S. typhimurium* and *S. montevideo*. Only 2.8% of the *S. typhimurium* cultures were resistant to chlortetracycline and only 0.8% of all other serotypes were resistant to that drug. Chlortetracycline and oxytetracycline were banned from use in England in feed of poultry and swine without a veterinary prescription in March of 1971. Their use in calves without a prescription had never been permitted. Since much of the *E. coli* isolated from animals at that time was resistant to the tetracyclines it would appear that salmonella may continue to be sensitive to tetracyclines even in the presence of high levels of resistant *E. coli* in animals.

GARSIDE et al. (1960) had demonstrated the emergence of resistance to chlortetracycline in *S. typhimurium* inoculated into chicks being given various levels of that drug. Although resistance was shown to emerge, mortality in the birds infected with resistant strains and treated with chlortetracycline was less than that in chicks infected with sensitive strains and treated with chlortetracycline, 16% and 23% respectively.

RANTALA (1974) showed that the presence in the feed of 20 or 100 ppm chlortetracycline enhanced the ability of *S. infantis* to colonize the ceca and small intestine of chicks. This colonization was not prevented by pretreating the chicks with a culture of intestinal bacteria but was prevented by 10 ppm nitrovin.

A series of experiments was carried out by JAROLMEN et al. (1976) on the effect of chlortetracycline in the feed on the salmonella reservoir in chicks inoculated with large numbers of *S. typhimurium* at 5 days of age. The number of salmonellae isolated from birds receiving 220 mg chlortetracycline/kg feed was very much smaller than that recovered from nonmedicated birds, in spite of the fact that there were large numbers of chlortetracycline-resistant salmonella in birds in the medicated group. This latter result could be expected since the birds were given medicated feed at 1 day of age and by 5 days of age, when they were inoculated orally with massive numbers of salmonella, the *E. coli* component of their intestinal flora was solidly resistant to tetracycline and capable of transferring this resistance to salmonella in vitro. Similar experiments were done by EVANGELISTI et al. (1975) and GIRARD et al. (1976) using oxytetracycline 220 mg/kg or a combination of 220 mg oxytetracycline and 220 mg neomycin/kg feed. An important difference was that the chicks used were 8 days old when given the medicated feed and probably had an established intestinal flora. The number of salmonellae isolated from the medicated group was much smaller and they were isolated for a much shorter time. Also only a few resistant salmonellae were isolated from the medicated birds and in no case did they become established in the chick's intestine.

MACKENZIE and BAINES (1974) infected 11-day-old birds with a culture of *S. typhimurium* resistant to chlor- and oxytetracycline. The birds were given chlor- or oxytetracycline in the drinking water at 110 mg/liter for 5 days starting 1 day after oral inoculation with 8×10^{10} viable cells of *S. typhimurium*. The birds shed salmonellae throughout the 7 days of the trial and mortality was 1 of 11 and 2 of 11 for the chlortetracycline- and oxytetracycline-treated groups respectively compared with 4 of 11 for infected nonmedicated birds.

The effect of antibiotic therapy on the fecal excretion of *S. typhimurium* by experimentally infected chicks was studied by SMITH and TUCKER (1975). They found that oxytetracycline at 500 mg/kg feed did not enhance shedding of *S. typhimurium*. Their birds were inoculated orally at 3 days of age and given medicated feed starting 3 days later. Oxytetracycline-resistant *S. typhimurium* was not isolated from this group. When the birds were given 100 mg oxytetracycline/kg feed fecal excretion of *S. typhimurium* was not affected but isolates with transferable resistance to ampicillin, spectinomycin, streptomycin, sulfonamides, and chloramphenicol, as well as tetracycline, were seen in the group on oxytetracycline. There were groups of birds on each of these antimicrobials in the experiment.

Two experiments on the effect of different levels of chlortetracycline, ranging from 33 to 440 mg/kg feed, on the shedding and emergence of resistance to *S. typhimurium* in experimentally inoculated turkey poults were done by NIVAS et al. (1976). They found that the antibiotic decreased shedding and that there was a dose response in this effect. There was a minimal emergence of transferable drug resistance to chlortetracycline and they believed that some change in phage type occurred in the organisms from medicated groups.

The effect of feeding low levels of chlortetracycline on subsequent therapy of an *S. typhimurium* infection in chicks was investigated by QUARLES et al. (1977). They found that chlortetracycline at either 55 or 220 mg/kg reduced mortality by about the same amount in control and pretreated chicks.

2. Cattle

Salmonellosis in cattle is less serious from a public health standpoint in the United States than it is in poultry or swine; nevertheless it does occur and beef is sometimes implicated in outbreaks of food poisoning though the beef itself may not be at fault. One incident was apparently caused by a contaminated liquid containing spices and flavorings injected into the beef before cooking and then cooking at a low temperature (KISER 1980). *S. typhimurium* and *S. dublin* are the serotypes most frequently isolated from cattle (CDC 1981) in the United States. SOJKA et al. (1974) reported that 3.4% of the*S. typhimurium* isolated from cattle in Great Britain was resistant to chlortetracycline and that only 0.7% of 832 cultures of *S. dublin* were resistant to that drug.

The influence of chlortetracycline with sulfamethazine in feed on the incidence, persistence, and antibiotic resistance of *S. typhimurium* in experimentally inoculated calves was studied by LAYTON et al. (1975). They gave

8- or 9-week-old calves 350 mg chlortetracycline or 350 mg chlortetracycline plus 350 mg sulfamethazine/head per day for 5 days before and 26 days after inoculating them orally with more than 10^9 cfu tetracycline-sensitive *S. typhimurium*. Four calves died during the study. The deaths were unrelated to treatment groups. The amount of salmonella shed by the nonmedicated calves was considerably greater than that shed by the medicated calves though the numbers of salmonella shed by all three groups dropped very rapidly. At the end of the experiment, 26 days after challenge, five calves were still positive for salmonella though the numbers were very low and there were no differences between groups. Chlortetracycline-resistant salmonella were isolated from nine calves during the experiment; and five were from the nonmedicated group. No more than two samples were positive from any one calf. Thus the resistant strain did not become established in the calves even though they were receiving chlortetracycline in the feed.

Two similar experiments were done with oxytetracycline in calves (EVANGELISTI et al. 1975; GIRARD et al. 1976). The data from these studies showed there was no increase, and probably there was a decrease, in the incidence and quantity of shedding of *S. typhimurium* in the medicated versus the nonmedicated groups. No tetracycline-resistant salmonella were isolated during either experiment.

3. Swine

Salmonellosis in swine occurs worldwide and is caused by many serotypes of salmonella. *Salmonella choleraesuis* var. *kunzendorf* and *S. typhisuis* are host adapted to swine though the latter is seldom reported in the United States. The disease affects pigs of all ages. It ranges in severity from a mild enterocolitis to a fulminating septicemia quickly terminating in death. The former is more frequent in older pigs. The septicemic form occurs almost exclusively in weanling pigs. In spite of its wide distribution and the fact that it can spread from and to other animals and humans, BARNES and SORENSEN (1975) expressed the opinion that salmonellosis in swine has decreased in the United States since the period 1940–1970. *S. choleraesuis* var. *kunzendorf*, *S. typhimurium*, *S. derby*, and *S. agona* were the four serotypes most frequently reported from swine in 1978 (CDC 1981).

SOJKA et al. (1974) surveyed salmonella from swine in Great Britain for resistance to antibiotics. There were 54 isolates of *S. choleraesuis*, 12 of *S. typhimurium*, and 17 of other serotypes. None of the *S. typhimurium* and only 1.5% of the other serotypes were resistant to chlortetracycline.

Several groups of workers in the United States did experiments which were designed to determine the effect of tetracyclines in the feed on shedding and emergence of resistance in salmonella in swine. *Salmonella typhimurium* is the serotype most frequently isolated from humans and the second most frequently isolated serotype in swine (CDC 1981). GUTZMANN et al. (1976) studied the effect of chlortetracycline 220 mg/kg or chlortetracycline 110 mg, sulfamethazine 110 mg, and penicillin 55 mg/kg feed on weanling swine experimentally infected orally with antibiotic-sensitive *S. typhimurium* and on the incidence and persistence of antibiotic resistance in the salmonella. The salmonella disappeared somewhat more rapidly from the treated groups than from the nontreated groups. Very few antibiotic-resistant salmonellae were isolated, although there were large numbers of antibiotic-resistant *E. coli* in the pig's intestines competent to transfer resistance to the salmonella. As many resistant salmonella were isolated from the nontreated as from the treated groups and antibiotic-resistant salmonella did not persist in any pig. Evangelisti et al. (1975) and Girard et al. (1976) did very similar experiments using oxytetracycline 165 mg/kg or a combination of oxytetracycline 165 mg/kg and neomycin sulfate 165 mg/kg, with very similar results.

In another experiment Williams et al. (1978) infected young pigs with a chlortetracycline-sensitive *S. typhimurium* and treated them with chlortetracycline at 110 mg/kg feed. None of these pigs died and the salmonella disappeared more rapidly from the medicated than from nonmedicated pigs. When a chlortetracycline-resistant strain of *S. typhimurium* was used to infect the pigs the results were quite different. The organism persisted in greater numbers for a longer time in the treated than in the untreated animals.

Wilcock and Ollander (1978) studied the effect of antibiotics in the feed on the duration and severity of clinical disease, growth rate, and salmonella shedding of pigs inoculated orally with an antibiotic-resistant strain of *S. typhimurium*. In the first experiment all pigs were given 110 mg oxytetracycline and 110 mg neomycin/kg feed continuously. One group was given an additional 440 mg oxytetracycline/kg during periods of diarrhea and another group was given nitrofurazone in the water during periods of diarrhea. During the first 60 days the group challenged with salmonella grew more slowly than controls. Among the infected pigs the nonmedicated group grew as well as the medicated groups and had somewhat less diarrhea. The strain of salmonella used was resistant to tetracyclines, streptomycin, and sulfonamides. The uninfected control group shed salmonella sporadically but the organism apparently was not the same serotype as that used to infect the pigs.

In the second experiment there was an uninfected group receiving control feed. The three groups of pigs challenged with salmonella included nonmedicated, sporadically medicated during periods of scouring, and continuously medicated. In general, after the first 30 days, the challenged group receiving no medication did as well as the medicated groups or the uninfected group. There were deaths in all groups except the continuously medicated group but they were apparently unrelated to the salmonella infection. The noninoculated group shed *S. anatum* throughout most of the trial. In general, the medication had little effect on the shedding of the salmonella, which, as in the first experiment, was resistant to tetracycline, streptomycin, and sulfonamides.

III. Tissue Residues

One part of the demonstration of safety of the use of an antibiotic in animal feed is the determination of its ability to be absorbed from the gastrointestinal tract, its distribution throughout the body tissues, and its excretion. The tetracyclines are well absorbed and widely distributed but they are rapidly excreted. In the United States, if a drug to be used in animal feed is absorbed the Food and Drug Administration is required to set a tolerance, i.e., an amount in tissue which is deemed safe for human consumption. This tolerance is based on extensive toxicological work including studies of possible carcinogenicity and teratogenicity. A method must be developed for analyzing tissues for the presence of drug and this method must be sensitive enough to detect the drug when it is present in an amount equal to or less than the tolerance. Sometimes the prevention or treatment of disease in animals requires a level of drug in the feed high enough to result in a level in the animal tissues that is above the tolerance. In that case the drug must be removed from the feed for a period sufficiently long for the drug to be excreted so that the tissue level is below the tolerance before the animal may be slaughtered for food. This withdrawal period varies in different countries. Recently German registration authorities have attempted to extend the withdrawal period for feed tetracyclines to result in no detectable residues in edible tissues. A common method for detecting residues in Germany is the *Hemmstofftest*. A portion of tissue, usually muscle, is placed on an agar plate which has been inoculated with a sensitive bacterial strain. After incubation, a zone of growth inhibition around the tissue is evidence for a positive test but not necessarily for a specific antibiotic. Authorities are primarily concerned about the selection of antibiotic-resistant bacteria in the intestine of humans consuming meat-containing residues. HIRSH et al. (1974) demonstrated that 1,000 mg oxytetracycline/day in four equal doses for 9 days favored the selection of tetracycline-resistant *E. coli* in humans. In contrast, 50 mg/day did not select the resistant organism. ROLLINS et al. (1974) demonstrated that 2 ppm tetracycline in the diets of dogs, guinea pigs, and rats failed to select antibiotic-resistant lactose-fermenting microflora. These studies suggest that tetracyclines in animal feeds are unlikely to result in residues in meat sufficient to select a population of antibiotic-resistant organisms in humans.

1. Chlortetracycline

a) Chickens and Turkeys

Two sets of experiments were carried out in chickens by GALE et al. (1968). The first set involved feeding chicks 220 mg chlortetracycline/kg feed containing 0.8% calcium plus an arsanilic acid derivative and/or coccidiostat and sodium sulfate from 1 day through 3 weeks of age. This is the highest level of chlortetracycline used in chicken feed.

The tissue levels at the time of withdrawal were below the established tolerance. The average values in parts per million (ppm) with the range in parenthesis were: muscle, 0.24 (0.08–0.43); liver, 0.53 (0.22–0.90); and kidney, 1.89 (1.08–2.50). At 3 days after withdrawal muscle was negative; liver, 0.04 (negative–0.05); and kidney, 0.27 (0.10–0.34). The limit of detectability of chlortetracycline in muscle or liver was 0.025 ppm and 0.04 ppm in kidney. The second set of experiments involved feeding 10-week-old broilers very high levels of chlortetracycline for 5 days in a feed containing only 0.4% calcium to enhance absorption of the drug. Antibiotic concentrations were determined in muscle, liver, kidney, and fat at 0, 1, 3, and 6 days after withdrawal. Levels of drug were 880, 1,320, 1,760, and 2,200 mg/kg feed. At the time of withdrawal of the medicated feed the average values for muscle were: 880 mg/kg, 0.38 ppm; 1,329 mg/kg, 0.54 ppm; 1,760 mg/

kg, 0.56 ppm; and 2,200 mg/kg, 0.63 ppm. Liver concentrations were higher: 0.90, 1.30, 1.27, and 1.55 ppm for 880, 1,360, 1,760, and 2,200 mg/kg, respectively. Residues in kidney were much higher: 6.44, 6.93, 10.4, and 11.8 ppm for 880, 1,360, 1,760, and 2,200 mg/kg, respectively. Very littel chlortetracycline had penetrated the fat; there was less than 0.2 ppm for any level in the feed. After 24 h withdrawal the level in muscle and kidney had decreased to 0.07 ppm or less for each of the concentrations in feed.

The most precipitous decrease was in kidney, where concentrations were less than 0.5 ppm even in the 2,000 mg/kg group. At 3 days withdrawal levels in muscle and liver were less than 0.1 ppm and in kidney average values were no higher than 0.31 ppm for any level in the feed. It is clear from these results that chlortetracycline is very rapidly excreted by chickens.

Katz et al. (1972a) developed a method for assay of chlortetracycline in chicken tissue that was slightly more sensitive and gave slightly higher values for residues of chlortetracycline in muscle than the standard Food and Drug Administration procedure. They fed levels of 55, 110, 165, and 220 mg chlortetracycline/kg feed and assayed tissues after 3, 6, 9, and 12 weeks of feeding. Blood levels were below 0.1 mg/g for all levels at all times. Levels in muscle were less than 0.1 mg/g for all feed levels at 3 and 9 weeks and all but the 220-mg/kg level at 12 weeks of feeding. The levels in muscle at 6 weeks were higher than at 3 or 9 weeks and higher at the 110-mg/kg level than for either the 165- or 220-mg/kg level. This result was not explained and did not occur in either liver or kidney tissue, though liver and kidney levels were higher in 6-week than in 3-, 9-, or 12-week samples. Conceivably the birds were eating more feed per kilogram body weight at that time though it would not be expected that they would be eating more feed per kilogram body weight at 6 than at 3 weeks of age. Liver assays showed no more than 0.2 μg/g tissue for any level in the feed at any time and kidney samples were less than 1.5 μg/g for any sample at any time. No residue was found in muscle, blood, or liver at 24 h withdrawal and kidney levels were less than 0.07 μg/g at 3 days withdrawal. Tissues from this experiment lost 30%–40% of their chlortetracycline content after being stored at −20 °C for 30 days followed by 7 days of storage at 7 °C. Boiling of tissues destroyed all of the antimicrobial activity due to almost complete conversion to isochlortetracycline. Sauteing of livers reduced the antimicrobial activity by 30%–70%. The same authors (Katz et al. 1972b) showed the presence of chlortetracycline residues in eggs from hens given 55, 110, 165, or 220 g chlortetracycline/kg feed for 30 days. Residues ranged from an average of 0.027 μg/g in 11% of the eggs from hens on 55 mg/kg to an average of 0.059 μg/g in 100% of eggs from hens on 220 mg/kg. Residues in eggs disappeared within 2 days after withdrawal of the 55-mg/kg level of the drug from the feed but 7 days were required for disappearance of the drug after withdrawal of the 220-mg/kg level. Cooking reduced the amount of chlortetracycline in eggs according to the method used. Soft boiling for 3 min and frying reduced the amount by 50%. Poaching reduced it by 70%.

Experiments in turkeys (Gale et al. 1968) suggest that they achieve somewhat higher levels in tissues than do chickens. In two experiments 440 mg/kg chlortetracycline/kg feed was fed to turkeys from 1 day to 3 or 4 weeks of age. The residues in muscle, liver, and kidney at the time of withdrawal were more than 1.0, about 2.0, and 5–12 ppm respectively. In a third experiment residues in muscle were less than 1.0 but in liver and kidney they were about the same as in the first two experiments. In all cases tissue residues at 1 day withdrawal were less than 1.0 ppm for muscle and liver and less than 4.0 ppm for kidney. The limit of detectability for chlortetracycline in muscle and liver was 0.025 ppm and 0.04 ppm. Turkeys given 440 mg chlortetracycline/kg feed acquire somewhat higher tissue levels than chickens on the same level, but at 1 day withdrawal their levels are also below established tolerances (SHOR et al. 1968).

b) Cattle

Feeder cattle are usually given 350 mg chlortetracycline/head per day for about 4 weeks followed by 70 mg/head per day to market weight. The tissue levels of chlortetracycline in cattle given 70 mg/head per day in feed are below the level of detectability in muscle and fat and barely detectable, if at all, in liver and kidney. The level of detectability is 0.025 ppm. When cattle weighing about 159 kg are given 350 mg/head per day chlortetracycline, i.e., about 2 mg/kg body weight, the levels in muscle and fat are not detectable or barely so. In liver and kidney they will be 0.25 ppm or less at the time of withdrawal and 0.1 ppm or less 2 days after withdrawal. Cattle may be given 5 mg/kg body weight per day (11 mg/kg) for 60 days to cure the carrier state of anaplasmosis. When cattle were thus treated the tissue levels at the time of withdrawal were: muscle, 0.22 ppm; liver, 1.0 ppm; kidney, 2.5 ppm; and fat, negative. At 3 days after withdrawal the levels were: muscle, 0.04 ppm; liver, 0.18 ppm; and kidney, 0.56 ppm. At 10 days withdrawal muscle, liver, and fat levels were negative and kidney levels were 0.05 ppm. The limit of detectability in these tissues was 0.025 ppm in muscle or fat and 0.04 ppm in liver or kidney (GALE et al. 1968).

From the above data it seems unlikely that meat from chickens, turkeys, swine, or cattle given approved levels of chlortetracycline in the feed would have tissue levels of the drug above established tolerances at the time of withdrawal. There are two other characteristics of chlortetracycline which make it unlikely that there would be any of the drug in meat as consumed. First, chlortetracycline in meat degrades on storage, even at refrigerator temperatures. When 2.0 ppm chlortetracycline was added to ground beef and stored at 10 °C the antibacterial activity was reduced by one-half in 2 days and below the level of detectability in 4 days. Rounds of beef were infused with chlortetracycline to a level of 5.0 ppm and held at 25 °C for 48 h and then at 1 °C. The antibacterial activity was reduced by one-half in 2 days. If the meat was refrigerated shortly after infusion the antibacterial activity was somewhat prolonged. Bacteria isolated from the treated meat were all sensitive to the antibiotic (WEISER et al. 1954).

Second, chlortetracycline is destroyed by cooking (BROQUIST and KOHLER 1953). It is converted to isochlortetracycline, which has a very low toxicity (SHIRK et al. 1957). A joint FAO/WHO Expert Committee on Food Additives set an Average Daily Intake (ADI) of 0–0.15 mg/kg per day chlortetracycline as being safe for humans. If a person who weighed 50 kg ate 0.5 kg meat containing 1.0 ppm chlortetracycline in 1 day, intake would be 0.01 mg/kg per day, well within the safe ADI (JOINT FAO/WHO EXPERT COMMITTEE 1969).

c) Swine

Feeder pigs averaging about 16 kg each were given feed containing 110 mg chlortetracycline/kg for 31 days. Pigs of this size will eat at a rate to give them about 8 mg drug/kg body weight per day. At the time of withdrawal the average level of chlortetracycline in muscle, liver, kidney, and fat was: 0.29 (0.23–0.34), 0.94 (0.60–1.80), 1.17 (0.85–1.45), and 0.06 (0.04–0.11) ppm. At 3 days withdrawal the level in muscle and fat was less than 0.025 ppm, and that in kidney and liver was 0.14 (0.11–0.16) and 0.12 (0.08–0.20) and at 5 days 0.10 (0.04–0.15) and 0.05 (0.05–0.05) ppm. The limit of detectability of chlortetracycline in tissues in the experiment was 0.025 ppm. A similar group of pigs was given feed containing 110 mg chlortetracycline/kg until they reached market weight (about 100 kg) 98 days later.

Older pigs eat less per kilogram body weight than young ones. The pigs in this experiment were eating enough to ingest about 5 mg chlortetracycline/kg body weight per day. Chlortetracycline levels in muscle, liver, and kidney were 0.04 (negative–0.06), 0.24 (0.14–0.20), and 0.26 (0.18–0.37) ppm; fat was negative. At 5 days withdrawal muscle and fat levels were negative, and liver and kidney contained 0.05 (negative–0.05) and 0.06 (0.04–0.07) ppm. The limit of detectability was 0.025 ppm in liver, kidney, or fat and 0.04 ppm in muscle (Gale et al. 1968). In this test another group of pigs, averaging about 15 kg in weight, were given feed containing 110 mg chlortetracycline, 110 mg sulfamethazine, and 55 mg penicillin G/kg as procaine penicillin for 14 weeks until they weighed about 100 kg. At the time of withdrawal the tissue levels of chlortetracycline in this group were slightly higher than in the group on chlortetracycline alone. Levels were 0.08 (0.07–0.09) ppm in muscle, 0.46 (0.30–0.54) ppm in liver, 0.51 (0.41–0.60) ppm in kidney, and negative in fat. At 5 days withdrawal there was no difference in tissue levels of the two groups (Messersmith et al. 1967).

From these experiments it seems likely that the tissue levels in swine on 110 mg chlortetracycline/kg feed would be below the tolerance, set by the FDA, at the time of withdrawal, i.e., less than 1.0 ppm in muscle, 2.0 ppm in liver, and 4.0 ppm in kidney.

2. Oxytetracycline

a) Chickens

An experiment was done in which chickens were fed 220 mg oxytetracycline/kg feed from 1 day to 8 weeks of age. The tissue levels at the time of withdrawal were: plasma 0.20 (0.11–0.29) ppm, muscle 0.3 (0.0–0.5) ppm, liver 1.2 (0.9–1.8) ppm, and kidney 5.6 (4.1–7.6) ppm. These values are very similar to those for tissues from chickens on the same level of chlortetracycline in feed except for the values for kidney, which are somewhat higher for oxytetracycline (Shor 1970).

Studies on oxytetracycline residues in tissues, organs, and eggs from chickens on 27.5, 55, 110, 165, or 220 mg oxytetracycline/kg feed for 3, 7, 9, or 11 weeks showed slightly higher levels of oxytetracycline in muscle than for chlortetracycline at the same level, but in only one instance, 220 mg/kg for 3 weeks, was the level higher than 0.2 mg/g. Blood, liver, and kidney levels were proportional to levels in muscle. Oxytetracycline disappeared rapidly from the tissues when the drug was withdrawn from the feed. No residues were found in any tissue after 24 h withdrawal. Oxytetracycline was destroyed by boiling. No measurable residues were found in eggs (KATZ et al. 1973).

b) Cattle

When heifers (weight not given) were fed 75 mg oxytetracycline/head per day for 21 days, muscle, fat, kidney, and liver levels were below the level of detectability, i.e., 0.25 ppm. Another experiment was done in which steers weighing about 386 kg each were given 0.5, 1.0, or 2.0 g oxytetracycline/head per day for 14 days. Muscle, kidney, and fat levels were negative at 1 day withdrawal in steers being fed 0.5 g/head per day but liver contained 0.11 (negative–0.32) ppm oxytetracycline. The group on 1.0 g/head per day had 1.47 (negative–4.40) ppm in liver. Muscle, kidney, and fat levels were negative at 1 day withdrawal. Muscle, liver, and fat were negative in the group on 2 g/head per day. Kidney had a residue of 0.22 (negative–0.40) ppm at 1 day withdrawal. All tissues in all groups were negative at 3 days withdrawal. The results of this test were anomalous since it would not be expected that there would be residues of the magnitude found in the livers of animals on 0.5 or 1.0 g/head per day but none in kidney. Also the residue in kidney in the group on 2.0 g/head per day was very small considering the levels in liver in the groups on the lower doses. The level of detectability in muscle, liver, and kidney was 0.25 ppm and 0.15 ppm in fat. In an experiment in heifers of 248 kg average weight the animals received: (a) 2 g oxytetracycline/head per day during days 109–118 of a 118-day feeding period; (b) 2.0 g/head per day for days 0–5, 75 mg/head per day for days 6–107, and 2.0 g/head per day for days 100–117; and (c) 75 mg/head per day for days 1–106 and 2.0 g/head per day for days 107–116. At 2 days withdrawal group (a) had residues of 0.55 and 0.18 ppm in muscle. Liver, kidney, and fat levels were negative. At 3 days withdrawal one animal had a residue of 0.34 ppm in kidney; all other tissue levels were negative. At 4 days withdrawal all tissues from group (c) were negative. The results for group (a) were anomalous since there should be no residue in muscle if liver and kidney were negative (Johnson 1970).

c) Swine

An experiment in which pigs weighing 84 kg were fed 110 mg oxytetracycline/kg feed for 14 days before slaughter showed no residues in muscle, liver, kidney, or fat at the time of withdrawal. The limit of detectability of oxytetracycline in this experiment was 0.25 ppm. In another experiment gilts (weight not mentioned) were given 220 mg oxytetracycline/kg feed for 21 days. At the time of withdrawal muscle and fat levels were negative, i.e., less than 0.25 ppm, and liver and kidney contained 0.37 and 0.71 ppm respectively. At 1 day withdrawal all tissue levels were below 0.25 ppm. In a third experiment pregnant gilts weighing about 104 kg each were given 550 mg oxytetracycline/kg feed for 21 days. At 1 day withdrawal muscle contained about 0.25 ppm and liver and kidney about 0.43 and 0.89 ppm respectively. The fat level was negative. At 3 days withdrawal all tissues were below 0.25 ppm except kidney. At 5 days after withdrawal all tissue levels were negative (KLINE 1970).

d) Fish

MCCRAKEN et al. (1976) investigated the absorption of oxytetracycline by fish given medicated feed and found a build-up in muscle over the first 3 days of feeding of 750 mg oxytetracycline/kg fish per day for 14 days. The excretion of the drug by the fish was strongly affected by the temperature of the water in which the fish were held. A temperature of 10 °C resulted in much more rapid excretion than a temperature of 5 °C.

E. Government Restrictions

I. Great Britain and Europe

Probably the first example of a national government's concern with the public health implications of feed antibiotics was the formation of the Netherthorpe Committee in Great Britain in 1960. This was a joint Agricultural and Medical Research Council Committee whose charge was to determine whether the practice of using antibiotics in animal feeds constituted a public or animal health hazard. A scientific subcommittee, chaired by Professor A. A. Miles, considered the question carefully while interviewing a large number of appropriate experts. After 16 months, a report was issued by the Scientific Subcommittee in which the continuing value of feed antibiotics was confirmed and the failure to identify evidence regarding adverse consequences was acknowledged. The Netherthorpe Committee issued its report in 1962, agreeing with the recommendations of its subcommittee. The report added that the public health questions should continue to be monitored carefully.

It was during the period between 1960 and 1965 that it became widely recognized that antibiotic resistance might be transmitted from cell to cell by plasmids. Adding to the level of concern was an outbreak of antibiotic-resistant *Salmonella typhimurium* phage-type 29 in calves in England (ANDERSON and LEWIS 1965). Cases of infection in humans were reported. The Enteric Reference Laboratory in London found in 1965 that 576 (23%) human salmonella isolates and 1,297 (73%) calf isolates were phage-type 29. The vast majority of these were antibiotic resistant (ANDERSON 1968). This situation was considered by ANDERSON to be the result of a combination of poor management and excessive use of antibiotics in animals. Calves had been deprived of colostrum, shipped at a very tender age by truck to a central point in England, and often treated with very large doses of antibiotics in an effort to control the apparent clinical disease. The resultant public response to media coverage of this outbreak resulted in meetings in April and June 1965 of the Scientific Subcommittee of the Netherthorpe Committee. After a thorough consideration of the phenomenon of transmissible antibiotic resistance and the salmonella outbreak in calves, it reconfirmed its earlier decision that no change in existing regulations was warranted. The full Netherthorpe Committee was convened in early 1966 and recommended that "an appropriate body with sufficiently wide terms of reference should consider the evidence about the use of antibiotics in both animal husbandry and veterinary medicine and its implications in the field of public health." The consequence of this recommendation was the establishment of a Joint Committee on the Use of Antibiotics in Animal Husbandry and Veterinary Medicine. This committee under the leadership of Professor Michael M. Swann was appointed in July 1968 by the Minister of Agriculture, Fisheries, and Food and the Minister of Health. The charge to the Committee was "to obtain information about the present and prospective uses of antibiotics in animal husbandry and veterinary medicine, with particular reference to the phenomenon of infective drug resistance, to consider the implications for animal husbandry and also for human and animal health, and to make recommendations."

The Swann Report was published in November 1969 and it acknowledged the usefulness of antibiotics in animal husbandry. However, the committee recommended that the permitted uses of antibacterials in animals be divided into two broad categories. Certain products were to continue to be used as feed additives for growth promotion and feed efficiency. Others, such as the tetracyclines, were to be used only by order of a veterinarian for control of animal disease. These recommendations were implemented in England in March 1971. During the years following these events in England, European Economic Community members and most nonmembers, which previously had allowed free sale of antibacterials for animals, instituted similar regulations, and most of Europe now requires a veterinary order before tetracyclines may be used in animals.

The effect of these controls on the overall use of tetracyclines in European livestock is difficult to assess. LINTON (1981) has suggested that in England there was an initial reduction in the use of "therapeutic" antibacterials following restrictions but that by 1977 the amount was equivalent to pre-Swann levels. There is no question that a considerable amount of chlortetracycline and oxytetracycline continues to be used throughout Europe.

Tetracycline resistance levels in animal coliforms in the years since restrictions were implemented have remained high. JACKSON (1981) reported the results of surveys to determine antibiotic resistance in animal *E. coli* in the United Kingdom during the years 1971–1977. A total of 94,827 isolates derived mainly from disease outbreaks in cattle, sheep, pigs, and poultry were examined for resistance to six antibiotics. Tetracycline resistance in these isolates in the years 1971 through 1977 was 50.0%, 44.8%, 42.1%, 40.8%, 39.4%, 40.3%, and 43.7%. Data on antibiotic resistance supplied by the Central Veterinary Laboratory were published in the *Veterinary Record,* June 7, 1980. These indicated that *E. coli* resistance to the tetracyclines showed a steady rise in frequency between 1975 and 1979. This was true of isolates from sheep, cattle, and pigs. Similar increases were reported for chloramphenicol, streptomycin, trimethoprim, neomycin, and ampicillin.

SMITH (1975) examined nonclinical random isolates from pigs at Chelmsford market in England. These are more likely to reflect the situation in healthy animals uncomplicated by recent disease therapy. He reported that in the 4 years following the implementation of the Swann restrictions, no appreciable reduction in resistance to tetracyclines could be detected. He further added "The failure of prohibition of the growth promotion use of tetracyclines to markedly reduce the amount of tetracycline resistant *E. coli* in the pig population stresses the fallacy of assuming that the ecological changes brought about largely by the persistent and widespread use of antibiotics can be reversed simply by reverting to a policy of withdrawal."

The question of the success or failure of the Swann restrictions has recently been the subject of serious debate in England. This was provoked in part by an epidemic of antibiotic-resistant *Salmonella typhimurium* in calves in the United Kingdom (THRELFALL et al. 1980). These authors stated that the current regulations had failed to prevent or control drug resistance in *S. typhimurium* phage-type 204 in bovines in Great Britain and that more stringent regulations might be appropriate. They charged that the responsibility lies with the veterinary profession and that the misuse of antibacterials in controlling the infection had promoted the establishment and maintenance of resistance in this strain. An editorial in the *British Medical Journal* on May 17, 1980, indicated that members of the medical profession must also be blamed for uncritical prescribing of antibiotics. In acknowledging the failure of the regulations based on the Swann Report, the editorial concluded: "Exactly why they failed, and when, may not be easy to discover; but clearly the present state of affairs is unsatisfactory and dangerous and more stringent regulations are needed."

RICHMOND (1980) sharply disagreed with the approach favored by those calling for still greater controls on antibiotics in animal agriculture. He emphasized that it was naive to expect antibiotic sensitivity to be restored by reducing antibiotic use. Resistant strains of bacteria had long since evolved to a point where persistence in the animal gut was inevitable, whether or not antibiotic pressure was continued. RICHMOND added, "...it now seems of nugatory advantage to attempt to control the situation by concentrating on antibiotic use." He concluded, "Is it not time that we concentrated on the old-fashioned but nevertheless well-tried methods for controlling communicable disease and really made them work?"

LINTON (1981) also disagreed with those calling for more stringent regulations, saying they were unlikely to have any effect unless pushed to unacceptable and impractical levels. He further expressed the opinion that Swann succeeded by being a failure. "The report focused attention on the growing problems of antibiotic resistance and, by its failure, has forced the opinion that the control of infections by multiply resistant pathogens must be pursued along conventional epidemiological lines and not solely by imposing more stringent restrictions on antibiotic use."

In October 1981, a symposium organized by the Association of Veterinarians in Industry was held at the Royal College of Physicians in London. The symposium was titled "Ten Years on from Swann" and was the result of "the need for a review of the concepts of the original Swann Report on the use of antibiotics in Agriculture." The editors of the proceedings concluded "The papers presented at the Symposium ... clearly demonstrated that many of these concepts have changed during the intervening years" (JOLLEY et al. 1981). The following year Lord SWANN (1982) presented a similar opinion concerning the outcome of his committee's 1969 recommendations, saying that they "had only got it very partly right" and "The time has come for a new committee of inquiry to have a fresh look, in the light of the present knowledge, at the best use of antibiotics."

II. United States

The Food and Drug Administration (FDA) controls the use of antibiotics in animal feeds in the United States. The Agency requires proof of safety and efficacy before registration is approved. If the FDA wishes to remove an approved drug from the market, it may do so quickly if "a clear and present danger" can be shown to exist. A less precipitous action may be taken by the FDA against approved drugs by requiring that the product sponsors satisfy questions with regard to safety or efficacy of the products. If after receiving such information, the Agency is not satisfied, a Notice of an Opportunity for a Hearing is published in the *Federal Register* in which the technical arguments supporting the FDA case are presented. The product sponsors or interested parties then are given a period of time, usually 2 or 3 months, to request on FDA hearing. The request must be accompanied by data, literature citations, statements from experts, and legal and scientific arguments showing why the proposed action by the FDA should not be taken.

This could be removal of the product from the market or imposition of new conditions or constraints on its use. For example, restricting product use to the order of a veterinarian would be such a constraint.

In April 1970, the Commissioner of the FDA, Dr. Charles C. Edwards, appointed a Task Force to study the controversy surrounding the use of animal feed antibiotics (KISER 1976). The Swann Report in England had been issued the previous year. The Task Force was made up of ten government scientists, four from universities, and one executive from the feed industry. A representative from the Canadian Food and Drug Directorate also participated. In addition to a study of the existing scientific literature, the Task Force members interviewed microbiologists, veterinarians, infectious disease experts, and officials of agricultural trade groups. Eight of the Antibiotic Task Force members traveled in England to confer with experts in the Ministry of Agriculture, Fisheries and Foods, the Department of Health and Social Security, the Association of the British Pharmaceutical Industry, the British Veterinary Association, the National Farmers Union, and the Swann Committee. Expert advice was also sought from Dr. E. S. Anderson and Dr. H. Williams Smith.

In January 1972, the Task Force Report was made public and shortly thereafter FDA Commissioner Edwards issued a Proposed Statement of Policy in the *Federal Register*. This charged that subtherapeutic antibiotics in animals could select for resistance in pathogenic and nonpathogenic bacteria and that such bacteria could be found on meat reaching the consumer. It further stated that antibiotic resistance was increasing in the bacteria of both animals and man and inferred that a potential for adverse effects to public health existed. The Proposed Statement of Policy provoked considerable public comment and protest from the agricultural community. These included meat producers, congressmen, researchers in animal sciences, and academicians from universities strong in agriculture. In April 1973, the final Statement of Policy issued with emphasis redirected to salmonella. Also of concern was the possible linkage of antibiotic resistance and genes coding for enterotoxin production on the same plasmid or on separate plasmids in the same organisms. The implication was that antibiotic use in animal feeds might serve to increase the prevalence of *E. coli* with the capacity to produce enteric disease in swine and cattle. The salmonella risk was said to center on the possibility that tetracyclines and penicillin might alter the animals' microflora in such a way as to promote establishment and shedding of salmonella. Such an event would be regarded as potentially increasing the risk, through the food chain, of salmonella disease in humans.

The FDA directed chlor- and oxytetracycline sponsors to conduct experiments in which salmonella shedding was monitored in target animals receiving antibiotic or control diets. The FDA further indicated specific conditions under which these tests should be conducted. For example, challenge levels of salmonella were to be extremely high in order to increase the chances of acquisition of R-plasmids from the indigenous animal flora. Antibiotic resistance was to be monitored throughout in salmonella and initially in *E. coli*. Product sponsors were also required to submit other information on the safety and efficacy of the tetracyclines.

All four of the United States sponsors of tetracyclines used in animal feeds submitted the required data in support of the safety of their products. Studies of salmonella shedding in pigs, calves, and chickens were to be submitted to the FDA by 20 April, 1974, and all other work by 20 April, 1975. The dozen or so industry-sponsored experiments all showed that the feed products did not promote salmonella establishment or increase the incidence of resistant salmonella and in several tests seemed to reduce it (EVANGELISTI et al. 1975; GIRARD et al. 1976; LAYTON et al. 1975; JAROLMEN et al. 1976; GUTZMANN et al. 1976).

During 1976, a subcommittee of the FDA's National Advisory Food and Drug Committee held a series of four meetings to consider the new data and the current status of the feed antibiotics controversy. The three members of the subcommittee and four expert advisors heard opinions and were presented data by industry and FDA scientists. The subcommittee, headed by Dr. J. Mosier of Kansas State University, was directed to make recommendations on the feed uses of tetracyclines, penicillin, and sulfaquinoxaline. Its final report to the full NAFD committee recommended no change for sulfaquinoxaline because of its utility as a coccidiostat, but that the uses of penicillin and tetracyclines in animal feeds should be restricted. The subcommittee report was discussed extensively at a meeting of the full Committee in January 1977 and it was decided, without opposition, to accept the recommendations on sulfaquinoxaline and penicillin but that restrictions on tetracyclines were not justified. This followed a discussion and conclusion that adequate substitutes for the prophylactic uses of tetracyclines were not available to the United States meat producer.

Several weeks after the NAFDC decision, the new FDA Commissioner, Dr. Donald Kennedy, decided not to accept the Committee recommendations and proceeded to take action to impose restrictions on penicillin and tetracycline feed additives. Notices of Opportunity for Hearings were published in the *Federal Register*. These were lengthy descriptions of the FDA position with extensive literature citations and analyses of pertinent published data, reports submitted to the FDA, and data from the FDA research laboratories at Beltsville, Maryland. Product sponsors responded by requesting hearings and presenting extensive expert opinion to support their requests. It was shortly thereafter that the FDA organized three regional meetings in Iowa, North Carolina, and Texas in order to measure the opinion of the agricultural community on the FDA's plan to restrict penicillin and tetracyclines to a veterinarian's order. Livestock producers, feed executives, animal scientists, veterinarians, and others had opportunities to speak at these meetings. The response was overwhelmingly opposed to the FDA proposal, with particular criticism directed toward the specific methods of control which the FDA had published. The primary point made was that the vast geographical areas in the United States and shortage of large animal veterinarians, particularly poultry experts, made the FDA proposal impractical. Producers were worried that attention to serious disease problems would be delayed by the difficulty of getting a veterinary order and obtaining the services of a feed mill to prepare promptly the appropriate medicated feed. The outcome of these meetings was that FDA withdrew its original proposal on the mechanism of antibiotic controls and admitted that more work was needed to overcome the difficulties.

Several prestigious groups in the United States have recently studied the controversy on animal feed additives. The Office of Technology Assessment in Washington, a government group which advises Congress on difficult technical issues, published a report on animal feed additives in July 1979. The Council for Agricultural Science and Technology (CAST) formed a committee made up of university scientists to study the issues. The original request for the study was submitted by an Alabama Congressman in January 1977 with the final report issuing in March 1981. The interim 4-year period was marked by acrimonious disagreement, charges of prejudice, attempts at reconciliation, and finally resignations from the committee by several microbial geneticists.

The National Academy of Sciences assembled a group of appropriate experts in 1979 to consider the subject of animal uses of penicillin and tetracyclines and possible effects on human health. This was in response to a Congressional mandate to FDA to determine the status of existing evidence and to weigh the value of epidemiological studies in helping to arrive at a regulatory decision. The March 1980 NAS report stated that the public health risks of feed antibiotics had been neither proven nor disproven. Committee members doubted whether a "comprehensive, all-encompassing study" could be carried out. Nevertheless, three epidemiological studies were suggested: (1) a comparison of antibiotic resistance in the intestinal flora of vegetarians and nonvegetarians; (2) antibiotic resistance studies of abattoir workers, their families, and neighborhood controls, a measure to see what effect high exposure to animal bacteria had on resistance in humans and their contacts; and (3) a study to see whether female workers in slaughterhouses had a higher than normal incidence of antibiotic-resistant urinary tract infections. The NAS also suggested a study in livestock to distinguish the effect of subtherapeutic and therapeutic uses in animals. The report stated, "The proportionate contributions to resistance made by subtherapeutic and therapeutic uses of antimicrobials in animals and in humans urgently need resolution."

The United States Congress took steps to limit the FDA's options in the Appropriations Bills of 1980, 1981, and 1982. The Agency was directed to use 1.5 million dollars to carry out epidemiological studies as recommended by the NAS. It further directed that the FDA should take no restrictive action until the studies had been completed or evidentiary hearings had been held. The FDA was left with the unenviable task of planning a research program that the NAS indicated would be technically difficult and possibly unproductive. Congressional members and their constituents from agricultural sections of the country were concerned that unjustified restrictions would make this important technology unavailable to animal agriculture. The economic effect of proposed restrictions at the consumer level was estimated to be between 1.0 billion and 3.5 billion dollars annually (CAST report of 1981). These figures were calculated by making certain assumptions concerning the extent of restrictions and the effectiveness and availability of substitutes. The FDA elected to fund epidemiological studies on the enteric pathogens *Campylobacter jejuni* and *Salmonella*. This work was carried out in Seattle, Washington, and Dubuque, Iowa, and was designed to examine the possibility that livestock, through the meat supply, were significant sources of infection in humans and that antibiotic resistance in these organisms was a consequence of antibiotic uses in meat animals. In 1984 studies of the sort suggested by the NAS were funded through the Animal Health Institute by several member companies. These included an examination of antibiotic resistance in the indigenous bacterial flora of vegetarians and nonvegetarians as well as a comparison of resistant urinary tract infections in female slaughterhouse workers and appropriately matched controls.

III. Far East

In June 1975, the Australian National Health and Medical Research Council established a Working Party on Antibiotics in Animal Husbandry. The charter of this group was "To consider the effects upon human medicine of the utilization of certain antibiotics in veterinary medicine and animal husbandry, and to make recommendations to Council through the Medicine Advisory Committee and the Public Health Advisory Committee." Care was taken to include members with veterinary and animal husbandry experience, in addition to microbiologists, physicians, and public health experts. The working party convened on four occasions in 1976 and early 1977. They excluded consideration of antibiotic residues in their deliberations and concentrated on the epidemiology of antibiotic resistance. A great deal of weight was given to the studies of this issue which had been carried out in other countries; these included the Swann Report from England, the report of a 1973 WHO meeting in Bremen, and the report of the Antibiotics in Animal Foods Subcommittee of the FDA's National Advisory Food and Drug Committee. A paucity of relevant information in Australia meant that the Swann, Bremen, and FDA reports were very influential in shaping the opinion of the working group. Particular consideration was given to veterinary uses of chloramphenicol and cloxacillin, two antibiotics considered to be of critical importance in the control of certain human diseases. Emphasis was also placed on the use of tetracyclines, penicillin, and sulfonamides in animal feeds. After these subjects were considered, the working group recommended that penicillins, tetracyclines, cephalosporins, sulfonamides, trimethoprim, aminoglycoside antibiotics, and chloramphenicol should be no longer permitted for use as growth promotants. They further recommended that tylosin and other macrolide antibiotics should be permitted for sale but that the situation be reviewed as new data become available. One concern was that macrolide resistance in gram-positive organisms would at some time in the future become clinically significant and that agricultural practices might contribute to that situation. The veterinary use of chloramphenicol was strongly discouraged by the working group since the antibiotic occupies a singular place in the defense against certain serious gram-negative infections in humans. This point had also been made in the Swann Report.

The National Health and Medical Research Council can advise Australian states regarding regulations and restrictions but the use of these products is defined by appropriate Acts in each state. Three states adopted restrictions recommended by the Council. These currently include Western Australia, South Australia, and Tasmania and involve about 35% of the total Australian market for the products affected by restrictive regulations.

Indonesian regulations involving agricultural uses of tetracyclines went into effect in May 1980. Products are now divided into two classes based on ten separate criteria. Class I products require a veterinary prescription for their use whereas class II products are free sale. The restrictions were influenced to a great extent by similar actions in other countries, primarily England and Australia. Most antibiotics are in class I and a veterinary prescription is required for their use. In practice, this has had little influence on the use of these products in poultry and pig production since necessary prescriptions are readily available, usually from veterinarians employed by the large producers.

References

Ajayi JA, Todd AC (1977) Relationship between two levels of Aureomycin-sulfamethazine supplementation and acquisition of resistance to ovine coccidiosis. Br Vet J 133:166–174

Anderson ES (1968) Transferable antibiotic resistance. Science April:71–76

Anderson ES, Lewis MJ (1965) Drug resistance and its transfer in *Salmonella typhimurium*. Nature 206:579–583

Barnes DM, Sorensen DK (1975) Salmonellosis. In: Dunne HW, Leman AD (eds) Diseases of swine. Iowa State University Press, Ames, pp 554–564

Bartley EE, Fountaine FC, Atkeson FW (1950) The effects of an APF concentrate containing Aureomycin on the growth and well-being of young dairy calves. J Anim Sci 9:646–647

Bartley EE, Fountaine FC, Atkeson FW, Fryer HC (1953) Antibiotics in dairy cattle nutrition: 1. The effect of an Aureomycin product (Aurofac) on the growth and well-being of young dairy calves. J Dairy Sci 36:103–111

Begin JJ (1971) The effect of antibiotic supplementation on growth and energy utilization of chicks. Poult Sci 50:1496–1500

Bettelheim KA, Bushrod FM, Chandler ME, Cooke EM, O'Farrell S, Shooter RA (1974) *Escherichia coli* serotype distribution in man and animals. J Hyg Camb 73:467–471

Bird HR (1968) Effectiveness of antibiotics in broiler feeds. World Poult Sci J 24:309–312

Bird HR (1980) Chick growth response to dietary antibiotics remains undiminished after 30 years. Feedstuffs 52 (Sept 29) 16, 24

Bird HR, Lillie RJ, Sizemore JR (1952) Environment and stimulation of chick growth by antibiotics. Poult Sci 31:907

Bolsen KK, Hatfield EE, Garrigus US, Lamb PE, Doane BB (1968) Effect of sources of supplement nitrogen and minerals, level of chlortetracycline and moisture content of corn on the performance of ruminants fed all-concentrate diets. J Anim Sci 27:1663–1668

Braude R, Wallace HD, Cunha TJ (1953) The value of antibiotics in the nutrition of swine: review. Antibiot Chemother 3:271–291

Brock WE, Pearson CC, Staley EE, Kliewer IO (1957) The prevention of anaplasmosis by feeding chlortetracycline. J Am Vet Med Assoc 130:445–446

Broquist HP, Kohler AR (1953) Studies of the antibiotic potency in meat of animals fed chlortetracycline. In: Welch H, Marti-Ibanez F (eds) Antibiotics annual 1953–1954. Medical Encyclopedia, New York, pp 409–415

Brown H, Bing RF, Grueter HP, Mc Askill JW, Cooley CO, Rathmacher RP (1975) Tylosin and chlortetracycline for the prevention of liver abscesses, improved weight gains and feed efficiency in feedlot cattle. J Anim Sci 40:207–213

Bunyan J, Jeffries L, Sayer JR, Gulliver AL, Coleman K (1977) Antimicrobial substances and chick growth promotion: the growth-promoting activities of antimicrobial substances, including fifty-two used either in therapy or as dietary additives. Br Poult Sci 18:283–294

Carpenter LE (1950 a) Effect of Aureomycin on the growth of weaned pigs. Arch Biochem 27:469–471

Carpenter LE (1950 b) Effect of an APF concentrate containing Aureomycin on gestating and lactating swine. J Anim Sci 9:651

Catron DV, Hoerlein AB, Bennett PC, Cuff PW, Homeyer PG (1950 a) Effect of vitamin B_{12}, APF and antibiotics on enteritis in swine. J Anim Sci 9:651

Catron DV, Speer VC, Maddock HM, Vohs RL (1950 b) Effect of different levels of Aureomycin with and without vitamin B_{12} on growing-fattening swine. J Anim Sci 9:652

Catron DV, Maddock HM, Speer VC, Vohs RL (1951) Effect of different levels of Aureomycin, with and without vitamin B_{12} on growing fattening swine. Antibiot Chemother 1:31–40

Centers for Disease Control (1981) Salmonella surveillance: annual summary 1978, issued January 1981. Centers for Disease Control, Atlanta

Clawson AJ, Alsmeyer WL (1973) Chemotherapeutics for pigs. J Anim Sci 37:918–926

Colby RW, Rau FA, Miller JC (1950) The effect of various antibiotics on fattening lambs. J Anim Sci 9:652

Cooke EM, Hettiaratchy IGT, Buck AC (1972) Fate of ingested *Escherichia coli* in normal persons. J Med Microbiol 5:361–369

Crempion C, Weir WC, Crenshaw G (1973) Medicated feed as a preventive for pneumonia in California range lambs. J Am Vet Med Assoc 162:112–116

Cuff PW, Maddock HM, Speer VC, Catron DV (1950) Rations for slow-growing (runt) pigs. J Anim Sci 9:653

Cunha TJ, Burnside JE, Buschman DM, Glasscock RS, Pearson AM, Shealy AL (1949) Effect of vitamin B_{12}, animal protein factor and soil for pig growth. Arch Biochem 23:324–326

Cunha TJ, Edwards HM, Meadows GB, Benson RH, Pearson AM, Glasscock RS (1950 a) APF, B_{12}, B_{13} and related factors for the pig. J Anim Sci 9:653

Cunha TJ, Meadows GB, Edwards HM, Sewell RF, Shawver CB, Pearson AM, Glasscock RS (1950 b) Effect of Aureomycin and other antibiotics on the pig. J Anim Sci 9:653

Curtis PE, Ollerhead GE (1979) Transferable oxytetracycline resistance in avian *Pasteurella multocida.* Vet Res 104:327 apr 7

Donahue JM, Olson LD (1972) The in vitro sensitivity of *Pasteurella multocida* of turkey origin to various chemotherapeutic agents. Avian Dis 16:506–511

Eggert RG, Maddock HM, Johnson DD (1980) Chlortetracycline for the prevention of mycoplasmal pneumonia in swine. J Anim Sci 51 (Suppl 2) (abstract:196)

Eleazer TH, Blalock HG, Harnell JS, Derieux WT (1973) *Pasteurella anatipestifer* as a cause of mortality in semiwild pen-raised mallard ducks in South Caroline. Avian Dis 17:855–857

Elliott RF, Johnson DD, Shor AL (1964) Effect of chlortetracycline, sulfamethazine and procaine penicillin on the performance of starting pigs. J Anim Sci 23:154–159

Evangelisti DG, English AR, Girard AE, Lynch JE, Solomons IA (1975) Influence of subtherapeutic levels of oxytetracycline on *Salmonella typhimurium* in swine, calves and chickens. Antimicrob Agents Chemother 8:664–672

Fagerberg DJ, Quarles CL, George BA, Fenton JM, Rollins LD, Williams LP, Hancock CB (1978) Effect of low level chlortetracycline feeding on subsequent therapy of *Escherichia coli* infection in chickens. J Anim Sci 46:1397–1412

Felsman RJ, Wise MB, Harvey RW, Barrick ER (1973) Effect of added dietary levels of copper and an antibiotic on performance and certain blood constituents of calves. J Anim Sci 36:157–160

Ferguson LC, Lococo S, Smith HR, Hamdy AH (1956) The control and treatment of swine leptospirosis during a naturally occurring outbreak. J Am Vet Med Assoc 129:263–265

Flint JC, Jensen R (1958) The effect of chlortetracycline, fed continuously during fattening, on the incidence of liver abscesses in beef cattle. Am J Vet Res 19:830–832

Frank FW, Scrivener LH, Bailey JW, Meinershagen WA (1958) Chlortetracycline as a preventive of vibrionic abortion in sheep. J Am Vet Med Assoc 132:24–26

Frank FW, Meinershagen WA, Scrivener HL, Bailey JW (1959) Antibiotics for the control of vibriosis in ewes. Am J Vet Res 20:973–976

Franklin TE, Huff JW, Grumbles LC (1965) Chlortetracycline for elimination of anaplasmosis in carrier cattle. J Am Vet Med Assoc 147:353–356

Furr RD, Carpenter JA Jr (1967) A comparison of antibiotics in high grain sorghum finishing rations. J Anim Sci 26:919

Furr RD, Hansen KR, Carpenter JA Jr, Sherrod LB (1968 a) Effect of different nitrogen sources and antibiotics on all-concentrate finishing rations. J Anim Sci 27:1110

Furr RD, Hansen KR, Carpenter JA Jr, Sherrod LB (1968 b) Mineral and chlortetracycline supplementation to all-concentrate NPN supplemented feedlot rations. J Anim Sci 27:1110

Gale GO, Baughn CO (1965) The effects of sodium sulfate in diets containing chlortetracycline hydrochloride on chicks infected with *Mycoplasma gallisepticum*. Poult Sci 44:342–344

Gale GO, Layton HW, Shor AL, Kemp GA (1967) Chemotherapy of experimental mycoplasma infections. Ann NY Acad Sci 143:239–255

Gale GO, Abbey A, Shor AL (1968) Disappearance of chlortetracycline residues from the edible tissues of animals fed rations containing the drug. 1 cattle and swine. In: Hobby GL (ed) Antimicrobial agents and chemotherapy. American Society for Microbiology, Ann Arbor, pp 749–756

Garside JS, Gordon RF, Tucker JF (1960) The emergence of resistant strains of *Salmonella typhimurium* in the tissues and alimentary tract of chickens following the feeding of antibiotics. Res Vet Sci 1:184–199

Girard AE, English AR, Evangelisti DA, Lynch JE, Solomons AJ (1976) Influence of subtherapeutic levels of a combination of neomycin and oxytetracycline on *Salmonella typhimurium* in swine, calves and chickens. Antimicrob Agents Chemother 10:89–95

Gouge HE, Bolton R, Alson MC (1956) The effect of feeding chlortetracycline to pigs with atrophic rhinitis. In: Antibiotic annual 1955–1956. Medical Encyclopedia, New York, pp 768–772

Gouge HE, Brown RG, Elliottt RF (1957) The control of laboratory-induced cervical jowl abscesses in swine by the continuous feeding of various levels of chlortetracycline. J Am Vet Med Assoc 131:324–326

Gouge HE, Elliott RF, Roekel OK Van (1958) Effect of chlortetracycline on incidence of cervical abscesses and weight gains of swine. J Anim Sci 17:34–41

Gross WB (1961) The effect of chlortetracycline, erythromycin and nitrofurans as treatments for experimental "air sac disease." Poult Sci 40:833–841

Gross WB, Johnson EP (1953) Effect of drugs on the agents causing infectious sinusitis and chronic respiratory disease (air sac infection) in chickens. Poult Sci 32:260–263

Gutzmann F, Layton H, Simkins K, Jarolmen H (1976) Influence of antibiotic supplemented feed on occurrence and persistence of *Salmonella typhimurium* in experimentally infected swine. Am J Vet Res 37:649–656

Hanson LE, Ferguson LC (1975) Leptospirosis. In: Dunne HW, Leman AD (eds) Diseases of swine, 4th edn. Iowa State University Press, Ames, pp 476–491

Harvey RW, Wise MM, Blumer TN, Barrick ER (1968) Influence of added roughage and chlortetracycline to all-concentrate rations for fattening steers. J Anim Sci 27:1438–1444

Hebert TJ, Chang TS (1969) The effect of furazolidone and other drugs on artificially induced *Escherichia coli* infection in chickens. Poult Sci 48:2063–2069

Heddleston KK, Rhoades KR (1978) Avian pasteurellosis. In: Hofstad MS (ed) Diseases of poultry, 7th edn. Iowa State University Press, Ames, pp 143–199

Heishman JO, Olsen NO, Cunningham CJ (1962) Control of chronic respiratory disease. IV. The effect of a low calcium diet and high concentrations of chlortetracycline on the isolation of mycoplasma from experimentally infected chicks. Avian Dis 6:165–170

Heth DA, Bird HR (1962) Growth response of chicks to antibiotics from 1950 to 1961. Poult Sci 41:755–760

Hirsh DC, Burton GC, Blendon DC (1974) The effect of tetracycline upon the establishment of *Escherichia coli* of bovine origin in the enteric tract of man. J Appl Bacteriol 37:327–333

Hogue DE, Warner RG, Loosli JK, Grippin JK (1957) Comparison of antibiotics for dairy calves on two levels of milk feeding. J Dairy Sci 40:1072–1078

Howarth JA (1956) Effect of Aureomycin and Polyotic in an outbreak of leptospirosis of swine. J Am Med Assoc 129:268–271

Huhn RG (1971 a) The action of certain antibiotics and ether on swine enzootic pneumonia. Can J Comp Med 35:1–4

Huhn RG (1971 b) Swine enzootic pneumonia: age susceptibility and treatment schemata. Can J Comp Med 35:77–81

Jackson G (1981) A survey of antibiotic resistance of *Escherichia coli* isolated from farm animals in Great Britain in 1971–1977. Vet Rec 108:325–328

Jarolmen H, Shirk RJ, Langworth BF (1976) Effect of chlortetracycline feeding on the *Salmonella typhimurium* reservoir in chickens. J Appl Bacteriol 40:153–161

Jensen R, Mackey DR (1979 a) Anaplasmosis. In: Jensen R, Mackey DR (eds) Diseases of feedlot cattle, 3rd edn. Lea and Febiger, Philadelphia, pp 41–45

Jensen R, Mackey DR (1979 b) Diseases caused by bacteria: shipping fever pneumonia. In: Jensen R, Mackey DR (eds) Diseases of feedlot cattle. Lea and Febiger, Philadelphia, pp 59–65

Jensen R, Mackey DR (1979 c) Diseases caused by bacteria: rumenitis-liver abscess complex. In: Jensen R, Mackey DR (eds) Diseases of feedlot cattle. Lea and Febiger, Philadelphia, pp 80–84

Jensen R, Mackey DR (1979 d) Diseases caused by bacteria: foot rot. In: Jensen R, Mackey DR (eds) Diseases of feedlot cattle. Lea and Febiger, Philadelphia, pp 91–95

Johnson WP (1970) Tissue residues in cattle fed antibiotics – a review. In: Proc of the Antibiotic presentations to the U.S. Food and Drug Administration Task Force on the use of antibiotics in animal feeds. Animal Health Institute, Washington DC, pp 176–187

Johnson WP, Elliott RF, Shor AL (1956) The effect of chlortetracycline on the incidence of enterotoxemia and weight gains in lambs maintained under commercial feedlot conditions. J Anim Sci 15:781–787

Johnson WP, Algeo J, Kleck J (1957) The effect of chlortetracycline supplementation on the incidence of foot rot and feedlot performance in cattle. Vet Med 52:375–378

Joint FAO/WHO Expert Committee on Food Additives (1969) Twelfth report specifications for the identity and purity of food additives and their toxicological evaluation: some antibiotics. World Health Organization, Tech Report Series No 430, Geneva, p 41

Jolly DW, Miller DJS, Ross DB, Simm PD (1981) Ten Years on from Swann. Royal College of Veterinary Surgeons, Wellcome Library, London

Jukes TH, Stokstad ELR, Taylor AR, Cunha TJ, Edwards HM, Meadows GB (1950) Growth promoting effect of Aureomycin on the pig. Arch Biochem 26:324–325

Jukes TM (1977) The history of the "antibiotic growth effect." Fed Proc 37:2514–2518

Katz SE, Fassbender CA, Dorfman D, Dowling JJ Jr (1972 a) Chlortetracycline residues in broiler tissues and organs. JAOA 55:134–138

Katz SE, Fassbender CA, Dowling JJ Jr (1972b) Chlortetracycline residues in eggs from hens on chlortetracycline-supplemented diets. JAOA 55:128–133

Katz SE, Fassbender CA, Dowling JJ Jr (1973) Oxytetracycline residues in tissues, organs and eggs of poultry fed supplemented rations. JAOA 56:77–81

Kiser JS (1961) Increasing the effectiveness of antibiotics as chemotherapeutic agents. Antibiot Chemother 11:261–266

Kiser JS (1976) A perspective on the use of antibiotics in animal feeds. J Anim Sci 42:1058–1072

Kiser JS (1980) Transmission of food borne diseases: implications of the subtherapeutic use of antimicrobials. In: The effects on human health of subtherapeutic use of antimicrobials in animal feed. National Academy of Sciences, Washington DC, p 227

Kiser JS, Clemente J, Popken F (1958) A comparison of the effectiveness of several antibiotics against an experimental infection with *Leptospira icterohemorrhagiae* or *L. pomona* in chick embryos. Antibiotics Annual 1957–1958:259–267

Kiser JS, Popken F, Clemente J (1960) Antibiotic control of an experimental *Mycoplasma gallisepticum* (PPLO) infection in chickens. Ann NY Acad Sci 79:593–607

Kiser JS, Popken F, Clemente J (1961) The development of resistance to spiramycin, streptomycin and chlortetracycline by *Mycoplasma gallisepticum* in chick embryos. Avian Dis 5:283–291

Kline RM (1970) Antibiotic residue studies in edible swine tissue. In: Proceedings of the antibiotic presentations to the U.S. Food and Drug Administration Task Force on the use of antibiotics in animal feed. Animal Health Institute, Washington DC, pp 290–308

Langlois BE, Cromwell GL, Hays VW (1978) Influence of chlortetracycline in swine feed on reproductive performance and on incidence and persistence of antibiotic resistant enteric bacteria. J Anim Sci 46:1369–1382

Lassiter CA (1955) Antibiotics as growth stimulants for dairy cattle: a review. J Dairy Sci 38:1102–1138

Lassiter CA, Brown LD, Duncan CW (1957) Effect of Aureomycin, erythromycin and hygromycin on the growth rate and well-being of young calves. J Dairy Sci 42:1712–1717

Layton HW, Langworth BF, Jarolmen H, Simkins KL (1975) Influence of chlortetracycline and chlortetracycline and sulfamethazine supplemented feed on the incidence, persistence and antibiotic susceptibility of *Salmonella typhimurium* in experimentally inoculated calves. Zentralbl Veterinarmed (B) 22:461–472

Levy SB, Fitzgerald GB, Macone AB (1976) Spread of antibiotic-resistant plasmids from chicken to chicken and from chicken to man. Nature 260:40–42

Libby DA, Schaible PJ (1955) Observations on growth responses to antibiotics and arsonic acids in poultry feeds. Science 121:733–734

Linton AH (1981) Has Swann failed? Vet Rec 108:328–331

Linton AH, Howe K, Bennett PM, Richmond MH, Whiteside EJ (1977) The colonization of the human gut by antibiotic resistant *Escherichia coli* from chickens. J Appl Bacteriol 43:465–469

Little PA (1948) Use of Aureomycin on some experimental infections in animals. Ann NY Acad Sci 51:246–253

Loosli JK, Wallace HD (1950) Influence of APF and Aureomycin on growth of dairy calves. Proc Soc Exp Biol Med 75:531–533

MacKenzie MM, Bains BS (1974) The effect of antibacterials on experimentally induced *Salmonella typhimurium* in chickens. Poult Sci 53:307–310

McCracken A, Fidgeon S, O'Brien JJ, Anderson D (1976) An investigation of antibiotic and drug residues in fish. J Appl Bacteriol 40:61–66

McGinnis J, Berg LR, Stern JR, Wilcox RA, Bearse GE (1950) The effect of Aureomycin and streptomycin on the growth of chicks and turkeys. Poult Sci 29:771

Messersmith RE, Johnson DD, Elliott RE, Drain JJ (1966) Value of chlortetracycline in breeding rations for sows. J Anim Sci 25:752–755

Messersmith RE, Sass B, Berger H, Gale GO (1967) Safety and tissue residue evaluations in swine fed rations containing chlortetracycline, sulfamethazine and penicillin. J Am Vet Med Assoc 151:719–724

Moore PR, Evanson A, Luckey TD, McCoy E, Elvehjen CA, Hart EB (1946) Use of sulfasuxidine, streptothricin, and streptomycin in nutritional studies with the chick. J Bio Chem 165:437–441

Morrill JL, Dayton AD, Mickelson R (1977) Cultured milk and antibiotics for young calves. J Dairy Sci 60:1105–1109

Nivas SC, York MD, Pomeroy BS (1976) Effect of different levels of chlortetracycline in the diet of turkey poults artificially infected with *Salmonella typhimurium*. Poult Sci 55:2176–2189

Olson LD (1977 a) Comparison of low-level Rofenaid, low-level chlortetracycline and vaccination with a commercial bacterin for preventing the pulmonary form of fowl cholera in turkeys. Avian Dis 21:160–166

Olson LD (1977 b) Evaluation of Aureomycin® for prevention of arthritic, pulmonary and cranial forms of fowl cholera in turkeys. Poult Sci 56:1102–1106

Olson NO (1978) Avian mycoplasmosis: *Mycoplasma synoviae* infection. In: Hofstad MS (ed) Diseases of poultry 7th edn. Iowa State University Press, Ames, pp 261–270

Olson NO, Sahu SP (1976) Efficacy of chlortetracycline against *Mycoplasma synoviae* isolated in two periods. Avian Dis 20:221–229

Perry TW (1980) Shipping fever. In: Perry TW (ed) Beef cattle feeding and nutrition. Academic, New York, pp 300–301

Perry TW, Beeson WM, Mohlor MT, Harrington RB (1971) Value of chlortetracycline and sulfamethazine for conditioning feeder cattle after transit. J Anim Sci 32:137–140

Quarles CL, Fagerberg DJ, Greathouse GA (1977) Effect of low level feeding of chlortetracycline on subsequent therapy of chicks infected with *Salmonella typhimurium*. Poult Sci 56:1674–1675

Rantala M (1974) Nitrovin and tetracycline: a comparison of their effects on salmonellosis in chicks. Br Poult Sci 15:299–303

Richey EJ, Brock WE, Kliewer TO, Jones EW (1977) Low levels of chlortetracycline for anaplasmosis. Am J Vet Res 38:171–172

Richmond MH (1980) Why has Swann failed? Br Med J 280:1615–1616

Ringen LM, Okazaki W (1958) The prophylactic effect of chlortetracycline given orally on bovine leptospirosis. J Am Vet Med Assoc 133:214–215

Rollins LD, Gaines SA, Pocurull DW, Mercer HD (1974) Animal models for determining the no effect level of an antimicrobial drug on drug resistance in the lactose fermenting enteric flora. Antimicrob Agents Chemother 7:661–665

Ruiz ME, Speer VC, Hays VW, Switzer WP (1968) Effect of feed intake and antibiotics on reproduction in gilts. J Anim Sci 27:1602–1606

Rusoff LL (1950) APF supplements for calves. J Anim Sci 9:666

Sandhu TS, Dean WF (1980) Effect of chemotherapeutic agents on *Pasteurella anatipestifer* infection in white Peking ducklings. Poult Sci 59:1027–1030

Savage DC (1980) Impact of antimicrobials on the microbial ecology of the gut. In: The effects in human health of subtherapeutic use of antimicrobials in animal feeds. National Academy of Sciences, Washington DC

Shelton DC, Olson NO (1959) Control of infectious synovitis: 7. Comparison of tetracycline antibiotics. Poult Sci 38:1309–1315

Shirk RJ, Whitehill AR, Hines LR (1957) A degradation product in cooked, chlortetracycline-treated poultry. In: Welch H, Marti-Ibanez F (eds) Antibiotics annual 1956–1957. World Encyclopedia, New York, pp 843–848

Shor AL (1970) Tissue residue levels in poultry products. In: Proceedings of the antibiotic presentations to the U.S. Food and Drug Administration Task Force on the use of antibiotics in animal feeds. Animal Health Institute, Washington DC, pp 95–115

Shor AL, Abbey A, Gale GO (1968) Disappearance of chlortetracycline residues from edible tissues: chickens and turkeys. In: Hobby GL (ed) Antimicrobial agents and chemotherapy 1967. American Society for Microbiology, Ann Arbor, pp 757–762

Sieburth JM, McNiell J, Stern JR, McGinnis J (1952) The effect of antibiotics and fecal preparations on growth of turkey poults. Poult Sci 31:625–627
Smith HW (1969) Transfer of antibiotic resistance from animal and human strains of *Escherichia coli* to resident *E. coli* in the alimentary tract of man. Lancet 1:1174–1176
Smith HW (1975) Persistence of tetracycline resistance in pig *E. coli*. Nature 258:628–630
Smith HW, Tucker JF (1975) The effect of antibiotic therapy on the fecal excretion of *Salmonella typhimurium* by experimentally infected chickens. J Hyg 75:275–292
Sojka WJ, Hudson EB, Slavin G (1974) A survey of drug resistance in *Salmonella* isolated from animals in England and Wales during 1971. Br Vet J 130:128–137
Speer VC, Vohs RL, Catron DV, Maddock HM, Culburtson CC (1950) Effect of Aureomycin and animal protein factor on healthy pigs. Arch Biochem 29:452
Stokstad ELR, Jukes TH (1950) Further observations on the animal protein factor. Proc Soc Exp Biol Med 73:523–528
Stokstad ELR, Jukes TH, Pierce J, Page AC Jr, Franklin AL (1949) The multiple nature of the animal protein factor. J Biol Chem 180:647–654
Swann MM (1982) Lord Swann calls for new committee on antibiotics. Vet Rec 111:287–288
Sweet VH, Stauber EH (1978) Anaplasmosis: a regional serological survey and oral antibiotic therapy in infected herds. J Am Vet Med Assoc 172:1310–1312
Switzer WP (1963) Elimination of *Bordetella bronchiseptica* from the nasal cavity of swine by sulfonamide therapy. Vet Med 58:571–574
Switzer WP, Farrington PO (1975) Infectious atrophic rhinitis. In: Dunne HW, Leman AD (eds) Diseases of swine, 4th ed. Iowa State University Press, Ames, pp 687–711
Switzer WP, Ross RF (1975) Mycoplasmal diseases: swine enzootic pneumonia. In: Dunne HW, Lemon AD (eds) Diseases of swine, 4th edn. Iowa State University Press, Ames, pp 749–764
Taylor JH, Gordon WS, Burell P (1954) The effect of supplementing the diet of thoroughbred foals with Aureomycin hydrochloride. Vet Rec 66:744–748
Teague HS, Grifo AP Jr, Rutledge EA (1966) Response of growing finishing swine to different levels and methods of feeding chlortetracycline. J Anim Sci 25:693–700
Terrill SW, Becker DE, Adams CR, Meade RJ (1952) Response of growing fattening pigs to bacitracin, Aureomycin and other supplements. J Anim Sci 11:84–91
Threlfall EJ, Ward LR, Ashley AS, Rowe B (1980) Plasmid-encoded trimethoprim resistance in multiresistant epidemic *Salmonella typhimurium* phage types 204 and 193 in Britain. Brit Med J 28:1210–1211
Twiehaus MJ, Anthony HD (1963) Feeding trials to control bovine-carrier anaplasmosis. Vet Med 58:596
Utley PR, Hollis DC, McCormick WC (1972) Feedlot performance of heifers fed melangesterol acetate and oxytetracycline separately and in combination. J Anim Sci 34:339–341
Wahlstrom RC, Libal GW (1975) Effects of dietary antimicrobials during early growth and on subsequent performance. J Anim Sci 40:655–659
Waibel PE, Abbott OJ, Baumann CA, Bird HR (1954) Disappearance of the growth response of chicks to dietary antibiotics in an "old" environment. Poult Sci 33:1141–1146
Waibel PE, Johnson EL, Hassing JW (1960) Comparison of various dietary antibiotics for turkey poults. Poult Sci 39:611–613
Walser MM, Davis RB (1975) In vitro characterization of field isolates of *Pasteurella multocida* from Georgia turkeys. Avian Dis 19:525–532
Watanabe T (1963) Infective heredity of multiple drug resistance in bacteria. Bacteriol Rev 27:87–115
Weiser HH, Kunkle LE, Deatherage FE (1954) The use of antibiotics in meat processing. Appl Microbiol 2:88–94
Whitehair CK, Heidebrecht AA, Ross OB (1951) Antibiotics for digestive disturbances in young pigs. Vet Med 46:81–83

Whitehill AR, Kiser JS (1961) The effectiveness of several tetracyclines in the control of an experimental PPLO (*Mycoplasma gallisepticum*) infection in chickens. Avian Dis 5:188–195
Whitehill AR, Oleson JJ, Hutchings BL (1950) Stimulatory effect of Aureomycin on the growth of young chicks. Proc Soc Exp Biol Med 74:11–13
White-Stevens R, Zeibel HG (1954) The effect of chlortetracycline (Aureomycin) on the growth efficiency of broilers in the presence of chronic respiratory disease. Poult Sci 33:1164–1174
Wilcock B, Ollander H (1978) Influence of oral antibiotic feeding on the duration and severity of clinical disease, growth performance and pattern of shedding in swine inoculated with *Salmonella typhimurium*. JAVMA 172:472–477
Williams RD, Rollins LD, Pocurell DW, Selwyn M, Mercer HD (1978) Effect of feeding chlortetracycline on the reservoir of *Salmonella typhimurium* in experimentally infected swine. Antimicrob Agents Chemother 14:710–719
Wong SC, James CG (1953) The susceptibility of the agents of chronic respiratory disease of chickens and infectious sinusitis of turkeys to various antibiotics. Poult Sci 32:589–593
Woods GT, Jensen AH, Gossling J, Rhoades HE, Nickelson WF (1972) The effect of medicated feed on the nasal microflora and weight gains of pigs. Can J Comp Med 36:49–54
Woods GT, Mansfield ME, Cmarick GF (1973) Effect of certain biologic and antibacterial agents on development of acute respiratory tract disease in weaned beef calves. J Am Vet Med Assoc 162:974–978
Yamamoto R (1978) Avian mycoplasmosis: *Mycoplasma melagridis* infection. In: Hofstad MS (ed) Diseases of poultry, 7th edn. Iowa State University Press, Ames, pp 250–260
Yoder HW Jr (1978) Avian mycoplasmosis: *Mycoplasma gallisepticum*. In: Hofstad MS (ed) Diseases of poultry, 7th edn. Iowa State University Press, Ames, pp 250–260

Subject Index

Handbook of Experimental Pharmacology

Continuation of "Handbuch der experimentellen Pharmakologie"

Springer-Verlag
Berlin
Heidelberg
New York
Tokyo

Volume 37
Angiotensin

Volume 38: Part 1
Antineoplastic and Immunosuppressive Agents I

Part 2
Antineoplastic and Immunosuppressive Agents II

Volume 39
Antihypertensive Agents

Volume 40
Organic Nitrates

Volume 41
Hypolipidemic Agents

Volume 42
Neuromuscular Junction

Volume 43
Anabolic-Androgenic Steroids

Volume 44
Heme and Hemoproteins

Volume 45: Part 1
Drug Addiction I

Part 2
Drug Addiction II

Volume 46
Fibrinolytics and Antififibronolytics

Volume 47
Kinetics of Drug Action

Volume 48
Arthropod Venoms

Volume 49
Ergot Alkaloids and Related Compounds

Volume 50: Part 1
Inflammation

Part 2
Anti-Inflammatory Drugs

Volume 51
Uric Acid

Volume 52
Snake Venoms

Volume 53
Pharmacology of Ganglionic Transmission

Volume 54: Part 1
Adrenergic Activators and Inhibitors I

Part 2
Adrenergic Activators and Inhibitors II

Volume 55
Psychotropic Agents

Part 1
Antipsychotics and Antidepressants

Part 2
Anxiolytics, Gerontopsychopharmacological Agents and Psychomotor Stimulants

Part 3
Alcohol and Psychotomimetics, Psychotropic Effects of Central Acting Drugs

Handbook of Experimental Pharmacology

Continuation of "Handbuch der experimentellen Pharmakologie"

Editorial Board
G. V. R. Born, A. Farah,
H. Herken, A. D. Welch

Springer-Verlag
Berlin
Heidelberg
New York
Tokyo

Volume 56, Part 1 + 2
Cardiac Glycosides

Volume 57
Tissue Growth Factors

Volume 58
Cyclic Nucleotides

Part 1: **Biochemistry**

Part 2: **Physiology and Pharmacology**

Volume 59
Mediators and Drugs in Gastrointestinal Motility

Part 1: **Morphological Basis and Neurophysiological Control**

Part 2: **Endogenous and Exogenous Agents**

Volume 60
Pyretics and Antipyretics

Volume 61
Chemotherapy of Viral Infections

Volume 62
Aminoglycoside Antibiotics

Volume 63
Allergic Reactions to Drugs

Volume 64
Inhibition of Folate Metabolism in Chemotherapy

Volume 65
Teratogenesis and Reproductive Toxicology

Volume 66
Part 1: **Glucagon I**

Part 2: **Glucagon II**

Volume 67
Part 1
Antibiotics Containing the Beta-Lactam Structure I

Part 2
Antibiotics Containing the Beta-Lactam Structure II

Volume 68, Part 1 + 2
Antimalarial Drugs

Volume 69
Pharmacology of the Eye

Volume 70
Part 1
Pharmacology of Intestinal Permeation I

Part 2
Pharmacology of Intestinal Permeation II

Volume 71
Interferons and Their Applications

Volume 72
Antitumor Drug Resistance

Volume 73
Radiocontrast Agents

Volume 74
Antieliptic Drugs

Volume 75
Toxicology of Inhaled Materials

Volume 76
Clinical Pharmocology of Antiangial Drugs

Volume 77
Chemotherapy of Gastrointestinal Helminths

MIX
Papier aus verantwortungsvollen Quellen
Paper from responsible sources
FSC® C105338

If you have any concerns about our products,
you can contact us on
ProductSafety@springernature.com

In case Publisher is established outside the EU,
the EU authorized representative is:
Springer Nature Customer Service Center GmbH
Europaplatz 3, 69115 Heidelberg, Germany

Printed by Libri Plureos GmbH
in Hamburg, Germany